KU-375-560

# Molecular Hematology

# Dedication

We would like to dedicate this book to our families, especially Val, Fraser and Peter, who provided constant encouragement and support throughout the project.

WH 120 PRO  £145

369 0299515

MONKLANDS HOSPITAL
LIBRARY
MONKSCOURT AVENUE
AIRDRIE ML60JS
☎ 01236712005

This book is due for return on or before the last date shown below.

# Molecular Hematology

## THIRD EDITION

Edited by

## Drew Provan MD FRCP FRCPath

Senior Lecturer
Centre for Haematology
Institute of Cell and Molecular Science
Barts and The London School of Medicine & Dentistry
The Royal London Hospital
London, UK

## John G. Gribben MD DSc FMedSci

Professor
Centre for Experimental Cancer Medicine
Institute of Cancer
Barts and The London School of Medicine & Dentistry
London, UK

**(W)WILEY-BLACKWELL**

A John Wiley & Sons, Ltd., Publication

MONKLANDS HOSPITAL
LIBRARY
MONKSCOURT AVENUE
AIRDRIE ML60 1S
☎ 01236712005

This edition first published 2010, © 2010, 2005, 2000 by Blackwell Publishing Ltd

Blackwell Publishing was acquired by John Wiley & Sons in February 2007. Blackwell's publishing program has been merged with Wiley's global Scientific, Technical and Medical business to form Wiley-Blackwell.

*Registered office:* John Wiley & Sons Ltd, The Atrium, Southern Gate, Chichester, West Sussex, PO19 8SQ, UK

*Editorial offices:* 9600 Garsington Road, Oxford, OX4 2DQ, UK

The Atrium, Southern Gate, Chichester, West Sussex, PO19 8SQ, UK

111 River Street, Hoboken, NJ 07030-5774, USA

For details of our global editorial offices, for customer services and for information about how to apply for permission to reuse the copyright material in this book please see our website at www.wiley.com/wiley-blackwell

The right of the author to be identified as the author of this work has been asserted in accordance with the Copyright, Designs and Patents Act 1988.

All rights reserved. No part of this publication may be reproduced, stored in a retrieval system, or transmitted, in any form or by any means, electronic, mechanical, photocopying, recording or otherwise, except as permitted by the UK Copyright, Designs and Patents Act 1988, without the prior permission of the publisher.

Wiley also publishes its books in a variety of electronic formats. Some content that appears in print may not be available in electronic books.

Designations used by companies to distinguish their products are often claimed as trademarks. All brand names and product names used in this book are trade names, service marks, trademarks or registered trademarks of their respective owners. The publisher is not associated with any product or vendor mentioned in this book. This publication is designed to provide accurate and authoritative information in regard to the subject matter covered. It is sold on the understanding that the publisher is not engaged in rendering professional services. If professional advice or other expert assistance is required, the services of a competent professional should be sought.

The contents of this work are intended to further general scientific research, understanding, and discussion only and are not intended and should not be relied upon as recommending or promoting a specific method, diagnosis, or treatment by physicians for any particular patient. The publisher and the author make no representations or warranties with respect to the accuracy or completeness of the contents of this work and specifically disclaim all warranties, including without limitation any implied warranties of fitness for a particular purpose. In view of ongoing research, equipment modifications, changes in governmental regulations, and the constant flow of information relating to the use of medicines, equipment, and devices, the reader is urged to review and evaluate the information provided in the package insert or instructions for each medicine, equipment, or device for, among other things, any changes in the instructions or indication of usage and for added warnings and precautions. Readers should consult with a specialist where appropriate. The fact that an organization or Website is referred to in this work as a citation and/or a potential source of further information does not mean that the author or the publisher endorses the information the organization or Website may provide or recommendations it may make. Further, readers should be aware that Internet Websites listed in this work may have changed or disappeared between when this work was written and when it is read. No warranty may be created or extended by any promotional statements for this work. Neither the publisher nor the author shall be liable for any damages arising herefrom.

*Library of Congress Cataloging-in-Publication Data*

Molecular hematology / edited by Drew Provan, John G. Gribben. – 3rd ed.
p. ; cm.
Includes bibliographical references and index.
ISBN 978-1-4051-8231-7 (hardcover : alk. paper)
1. Blood–Diseases–Molecular aspects. I. Provan, Andrew. II. Gribben, John.
[DNLM: 1. Hematologic Diseases. 2. Molecular Biology. WH 120 M7187 2010]
RC636.M576 2010
616.1′5–dc22
2009032167

A catalogue record for this book is available from the British Library.

Set in 10 on 12 pt Minion by Toppan Best-set Premedia Limited
Printed and bound in Singapore by Fabulous Printers Pte Ltd

1  2010

# Contents

*Color plates can be found facing pages 176 and 304*

# Contributors

**Nancy C Andrews MD, PhD**
Dean and Vice Chancellor for Academic Affairs, Professor of Pediatrics, Professor of Pharmacology and Cancer Biology, Duke University School of Medicine, Durham, NC, USA

**Eyal C Attar MD**
Instructor in Medicine, Harvard Medical School, Massachusetts General Hospital, Boston, MA, USA

**Luciano Baronciani PhD**
Research Assistant, Angelo Bianchi Bonomi Hemophilia and Thrombosis Center, University of Milan and IRCCS Maggiore Hospital, Mangiagalli and Regina Elena Foundation, Milan, Italy

**Anthony J Bench MA, PhD**
Senior Scientist, Haemato-Oncology Diagnostics Service, Department of Haematology, Addenbrooke's Hospital, part of Cambridge University Hospitals NHS Foundation Trust, Cambridge, UK

**P Leif Bergsagel MD**
Professor of Medicine, Division of Hematology-Oncology, Comprehensive Cancer Center, Mayo Clinic Arizona, Scottsdale, AZ, USA

**Dominique Bonnet PhD**
Group Leader, Haematopoietic Stem Cell Laboratory, Cancer Research UK London Research Institute, London, UK

**M Mansour Ceesay MB ChB, MSc, MRCP, FRCPath**
Clinical Research Fellow, Department of Haematological Medicine, King's College Hospital, London, UK

**Chetan E Chitnis MSc, MA, PhD**
Principal Investigator/Staff Research Scientist, Malaria Group, International Centre for Genetic Engineering and Biotechnology, Aruna Asaf Ali Marg, New Delhi, India

**Wee Joo Chng MB ChB, MRCP, FRCPath**
Associate Professor and Consultant, National University Cancer Institute, National University Health System, Singapore; Senior Principal Investigator, Cancer Science Institute, National University of Singapore, National University Hospital, Singapore

**Kenneth J Clemetson PhD, ScD, CChem, FRSC**
Emeritus Professor, University of Berne, Theodor Kocher Institute, Berne, Switzerland

**Jorge Cortes MD**
Internist and Professor, Deputy Chair, Department of Leukemia, University of Texas M.D. Anderson Cancer Center, Houston, TX, USA

**Björn Dahlbäck MD, PhD**
Professor of Blood Coagulation Research, Department of Laboratory Medicine, Section of Clinical Chemistry, Lund University, University Hospital, Malmö, Sweden

**Riccardo Dalla-Favera MD**
Director, Institute for Cancer Genetics and Herbert Irving Comprehensive Cancer Center, Columbia University, New York, NY, USA

**Francesco Dazzi MD, PhD**
Chair and Head, Stem Cell Biology, Department of Haematology, Imperial College London, London, UK

**Silvana Debernardi PhD**
Scientist, Cancer Research UK, Medical Oncology Unit, Barts and The London School of Medicine & Dentistry, London, UK

**William E Evans PharmD**
Director and Chief Executive Officer, St Jude Children's Research Hospital, Memphis, TN, USA

**Jude Fitzgibbon PhD**
Non-Clinical Senior Lecturer, Centre for Medical Oncology, Institute of Cancer, Barts and The London School of Medicine & Dentistry, London, UK

**Tomas Ganz PhD, MD**
Professor of Medicine and Pathology, Department of Medicine, David Geffen School of Medicine at UCLA, Los Angeles, CA, USA

**Paul LF Giangrande MD, FRCP, FRCPath, FRCPCH**
Consultant Haematologist, Oxford Haemophilia and Thrombosis Centre, Churchill Hospital, Oxford, UK

**D Gary Gilliland MD, PhD**
Professor of Medicine, Howard Hughes Medical Institute, Brigham and Women's Hospital; Dana-Farber Cancer Institute, Harvard Medical School, Boston, MA, USA

**Anthony R Green PhD, FRCP, FRCPath, FMedSci**
Professor of Haemato-oncology, Cambridge University Department of Haematology, Cambridge Institute for Medical Research; Addenbrooke's Hospital, part of Cambridge University Hospitals NHS Foundation Trust, Cambridge, UK

**John G Gribben MD, DSc, FMedSci**
Professor, Centre for Experimental Cancer Medicine, Institute of Cancer, Barts and The London School of Medicine & Dentistry, London, UK

**Andreas Hillarp PhD**
Associate Professor and Hospital Chemist, Department of Laboratory Medicine, Section of Clinical Chemistry, Lund University, University Hospital, Malmö, Sweden

**Wendy Ingram MB BS, MRCP, FRCPath**
Clinical Research Fellow, Department of Haematological Medicine, King's College Hospital, London, UK

**Leo Kager MD**
Associate Professor of Pediatrics, St Anna Children's Hospital, Vienna, Austria

**Hagop Kantarjian MD**
Professor of Medicine and Chairman, Department of Leukemia, University of Texas M.D. Anderson Cancer Center, Houston, TX, USA

**Anastasios Karadimitris PhD, MRCP, FRCPath**
Reader and Honorary Consultant Haematologist, Department of Haematology, Imperial College London, Hammersmith Hospital Campus, London, UK

**Ulf Klein PhD**
Assistant Professor in Pathology & Cell Biology, and Microbiology & Immunology, Herbert Irving Comprehensive Cancer Center, Columbia University, New York, NY, USA

**D Mark Layton MD**
Reader in Haematology, Division of Investigative Science, Imperial College London, London, UK

**Anthony G Letai MD, PhD**
Assistant Professor in Medicine, Harvard Medical School, Dana-Farber Cancer Institute, Boston, MA, USA

**Debra M Lillington PhD**
Head of Cytogenetics, ICRF Medical Oncology Laboratory, Barts and The London School of Medicine & Dentistry, London, UK

**Lucio Luzzatto MD**
Scientific Director, National Institute for Cancer Research, Istituto Scientifico Tumori, Genova, Italy

**Pier Mannuccio Mannucci MD**
Professor of Internal Medicine, Angelo Bianchi Bonomi Hemophilia and Thrombosis Center, University of Milan and IRCCS Maggiore Hospital, Mangiagalli and Regina Elena Foundation, Milan, Italy

**Jeffrey A Medin PhD**
Senior Scientist, Ontario Cancer Institute; Professor, Department of Medical Biophysics and the Institute of Medical Science, University of Toronto, University Health Network, Toronto, ON, Canada

**Graham Molineux PhD**
Executive Director, Hematology-Oncology Research, Amgen Inc., Thousand Oaks, CA, USA

**Paul Moss MD PhD**
Professor of Haematology and Head of School of Cancer Sciences, University of Birmingham, Birmingham, UK

**Ghulam J Mufti DM, FRCP, FRCPath**
Head, Department of Haematological Medicine, King's College Hospital and King's College London, London, UK

**Ronald L Nagel MD**
Irving D. Karpas Professor of Medicine, Head of Division of Hematology, Albert Einstein College of Medicine, New York, NY, USA

**Cristina Navarrete PhD**
National Head of Histocompatibility and Immunogenetics Services, NHS Blood and Transplant, London, UK; Reader in Immunology, Department of Immunology and Molecular Pathology, University College London, London, UK

**Adrian C Newland MA, FRCP, FRCPath**
Professor of Haematology, Department of Haematology, Barts and The London School of Medicine & Dentistry, London, UK

**Susan O'Brien MD**
Professor and Internist, Department of Leukemia, University of Texas M.D. Anderson Cancer Center, Houston, TX, USA

**Willem H Ouwehand MD, PhD**
NHSBT Consultant Haematologist; Lecturer in Haematology, Department of Haematology, University of Cambridge, Cambridge, UK

**Carolyn J Owen MD, MDres(UK), FRCPC**
Assistant Professor, Division of Hematology and Hematological Malignancies, University of Calgary, Foothills Medical Centre, Calgary, AB, Canada

**Drew Provan MD, FRCP, FRCPath**
Senior Lecturer, Centre for Haematology, Institute of Cell and Molecular Science, Barts and The London School of Medicine & Dentistry, The Royal London Hospital, London, UK

**Alfonso Quintás-Cardama MD**
Hematology/Oncology Fellow, Department of Leukemia, University of Texas M.D. Anderson Cancer Center, Houston, TX, USA

**David J Roberts DPhil, MRCP, FRCPath**
Professor of Haematology and Consultant Haematologist, National Health Service Blood and Transplant (Oxford), John Radcliffe Hospital, Oxford, UK

**David T Scadden MD**
Gerald and Darlene Jordan Professor, Harvard Medical School; Co-director, Harvard Stem Cell Institute; Director, Center for Regenerative Medicine, Massachusetts General Hospital, Boston, MA, USA

**John W Semple PhD**
Senior Staff Scientist, St Michael's Hospital; Professor of Pharmacology Medicine and Laboratory Medicine and Pathobiology, University of Toronto; Adjunct Scientist, Canadian Blood Services, Toronto, ON, Canada

**Jonathan S Stamler MD**
George Barth Geller Professor in Cardiovascular Research, Department of Medicine, Divisions of Cardiovascular and Pulmonary Medicine and Professor of Biochemistry, Duke University Medical Center, Durham, NC, USA

**Stephen J Szilvassy PhD**
Principal Scientist, Hematology-Oncology Research, Amgen Inc., Thousand Oaks, CA, USA

**David C Taussig MCRP, FRCPath, PhD**
Clinical Senior Lecturer, Department of Medical Oncology, Barts and The London School of Medicine & Dentistry, London, UK

**Marilyn J Telen MD**
Wellcome Professor of Medicine, and Chief, Division of Hematology, Duke University Medical Center, Durham, NC, USA

**George S Vassiliou MRCP, FRCPath**
Cancer Research UK Clinician Scientist and Honorary Consultant Haematologist, Wellcome Trust Sanger Institute, Cambridge, UK

**David Weatherall MD, FRCP, FRS**
Regius Professor of Medicine Emeritus, Weatherall Institute of Molecular Medicine, John Radcliffe Hospital, Oxford, UK

**Bryan D Young PhD, FMedSci**
Head of Cancer Genomics Group, Head of Medical Oncology Laboratory, Centre for Medical Oncology, Barts and The London School of Medicine & Dentistry, The Royal London Hospital, London, UK

# Foreword

In 1968, after a quest lasting 30 years, X-ray analysis of crystalline horse hemoglobin at last reached the stage when I could build a model of its atomic structure. The amino acid sequences of human globin are largely homologous to those of horse globin, which made me confident that their structures are the same. By then, the amino acid substitutions responsible for many abnormal human hemoglobins had been determined. The world authority on them was the late Hermann Lehmann, Professor of Clinical Biochemistry at the University of Cambridge, who worked in the hospital just across the road from our Laboratory of Molecular Biology. I asked him to come over to see if there was any correlation between the symptoms caused by the different amino acids substituted in the abnormal hemoglobin and their positions in the atomic model. The day we spent going through them proved one of the most exciting in our scientific lives. We found hemoglobin to be insensitive to replacements of most amino acid residues on its surface, with the notable exception of sickle cell hemoglobin. On the other hand, we found the molecule to be extremely sensitive to even quite small alterations of internal non-polar contacts, especially those near the hemes. Replacements at the contact between the α and β subunits affected respiratory function.

In sickle cell hemoglobin an external glutamate was replaced by a valine. We wrote: "*A non-polar instead at a polar residue at a surface position would suffice to make each molecule adhere to a complementary site at a neighbouring one, that site being created by the conformational change from oxy to deoxy haemoglobin.*" This was soon proved to be correct. We published our findings under the title: "The Molecular Pathology of Human Haemoglobin." Our paper marked a turning point because it was the first time that the symptoms of diseases could be interpreted in terms of changes in the atomic structure of the affected protein. In the years that followed, the structure of the contact between the valine of one molecule of sickle cell hemoglobin and that of the complementary site of its neighbor became known in some detail. At a meeting at Arden House near Washington in 1980, several colleagues and I decided to use this knowledge for the design of anti-sickling drugs, but after an effort

lasting 10 years, we realized that we were running up against a brick wall. Luckily, the work was not entirely wasted, because we found a series of compounds that lower the oxygen affinity of hemoglobin and we realized that this might be clinically useful. One of those compounds, designed by DJ Abraham at the University of Virginia in Richmond, is now entering phase 3 clinical trials. On the other hand, our failure to find a drug against sickle cell anemia, even when its cause was known in atomic detail, made me realize the extreme difficulty of finding drugs to correct a malfunction of a protein that is caused by a single amino acid substitution. Most thalassemias are due not to amino acid substitutions, but to either complete or partial failure to synthesize α- or β-globin chains. Weatherall's chapter shows that, at the genetic level, there may be literally hundreds of different genetic lesions responsible for that failure. Correction of such lesions is now the subject of intensive work in many laboratories.

Early in the next century, the human genome will be complete. It will reveal the amino acid sequences of all the 100 000 or so different proteins of which we are made. Many of these proteins are still unknown. To discover their functions, the next project now under discussion is a billion dollar effort to determine the structures of all the thousands of unknown proteins within 10 years. By then we shall know the identity of the proteins responsible for most of the several thousand different genetic diseases. Will this lead to effective treatment or will medical geneticists be in the same position as doctors were early in this century when the famous physician Sir William Osler confined their task to the establishment of diagnoses? Shall we know the cause of every genetic disease without a cure?

Our only hope lies in somatic gene therapy. The chapter on Molecular Therapeutics describes the many ingenious methods now under development. So far, none of these has produced lasting effects, apparently because the transferred genes are not integrated into the mammalian genome, but a large literature already grown up bears testimony to the great efforts now underway to overcome this problem. My much-loved teacher William Lawrence Bragg used to say *"If you go on hammering away at a problem, eventually it seems to get tired, lies down and lets you catch it."* Let us hope that somatic gene therapy will soon get tired.

M.F. Perutz
*Cambridge*

Perutz MF, Lehmann H. (1968) Molecular pathology of human haemoglobin. *Nature*, **219**, 902–909.

Perutz MF, Muirhead H, Cox JM, Goaman LCG. (1968) Three-dimensional Fourier synthesis of horse oxyhaemoglobin at 2.8 Å resolution: the atomic model. *Nature*, **219**, 131–139.

# Preface to the third edition

In the five years since the second edition of *Molecular Hematology*, the specialty continues to move forward apace, both in terms of the management of blood diseases and also in the basic science underpinning modern hematology. With each edition we have intentionally expanded the book, and this third edition sees six new chapters. For example, we now have a chapter dealing with the *History and Development of Molecular Biology*, written by Paul Moss, which will be of value to those less familiar with molecular biology. "Big pharma" is using pharmacogenomics in drug development and we felt that we should include a chapter by Leo Kager and William Evans, outlining exactly what *Pharmacogenomics* is, and how it is of value in drug discovery. One often-neglected area of non-malignant hematology is *Anemia of Chronic Disease*. At long last we have seen some good basic science in this area and a chapter dealing with this common anemia was much needed. Tomas Ganz is a recognized expert in this field and has written a chapter on this topic. Malaria and its interactions with the red cell is poorly appreciated but our understanding of the processes involved in malaria infection has improved hence the inclusion of a chapter on the *Molecular Pathology of Malaria* by David Roberts on this topic. Transplantation and stem cell biology has seen major advances and we have two new chapters dealing with these topics, namely the *Molecular Basis of Transplantation* by Francesco Dazzi and *Cancer Stem Cells* by David Taussig with Dominic Bonnet.

The original chapters remain, and have been thoroughly updated. Many of these have been taken over by new authors and have been completely rewritten.

We hope that by adding new topics to the book with each edition we have covered the most important topics in modern hematology. Doubtless there are subjects we have omitted and for this we apologize. We are, as always; open to suggestions from readers for topics we have not included. We will try to commission these for future editions.

Completing this book has been a lengthy but worthwhile task and we hope readers enjoy the final result. Perhaps if we can stimulate trainee hematologists they may be more tempted to become involved in the science of hematology and later contribute to the body of knowledge, as researchers.

## Acknowledgments

As ever, the team at Wiley-Blackwell have been incredibly patient with us and we are hugely indebted to Maria Khan, Associate Publishing Director, Medicine, Rebecca Huxley, Senior Production Editor, Jennifer Seward, Development Editor, and Alice Nelson, Project Manager. Let's hope the fourth edition does not try their patience quite as much.

Drew Provan (*a.b.provan@qmul.ac.uk*)
John Gribben (*j.gribben@qmul.ac.uk*)
February 2010

# Abbreviations

| | |
|---|---|
| **AAV** | adeno-associated virus |
| **ADA** | adenosine deaminase |
| **ADR** | adverse drug reaction |
| **AE1** | anion exchanger protein 1 |
| **AGM** | aorta–gonad–mesonephros (region) |
| **ALAS** | δ-aminolevulinate synthase |
| **ALCL** | anaplastic large cell lymphoma |
| **ALG** | antilymphocyte globulin |
| **ALK** | anaplastic lymphoma kinase |
| **ALL** | acute lymphoblastic leukemia |
| **AMA** | apical merozoite antigen |
| **AML** | acute myeloid leukemia (Chapters 2, 4, 8, 9, 12) |
| **AML** | acute myelogenous leukemia (Chapters 5, 6) |
| **AP** | accelerated phase (CML) |
| **APC** | activated protein C; antigen-presenting cell |
| **APL** | acute promyelocytic leukemia |
| **ASCT** | autologous stem cell transplantation |
| **AT** | antithrombin |
| **ATRA** | all-*trans*-retinoic acid |
| **B-CLL** | B-cell chronic lymphocytic leukemia |
| **BCR** | breakpoint cluster region |
| **BFU-E** | burst-forming units, erythroid |
| **BMF** | bone marrow failure |
| **BMPR** | bone morphogenetic protein receptor |
| **BMT** | bone marrow transplantation |
| **BP** | blast phase (CML) |
| **BSS** | Bernard–Soulier syndrome |
| **CAFC** | cobblestone area-forming cell |
| **CBF** | core-binding factor |
| **Cbl** | cobalamin |
| **CCR** | complete cytogenetic response |
| **CDA** | congenital dyserythropoietic anemia |
| **CDAE1** | N-terminal cytoplasmic domain of anion exchanger protein 1 |
| **CDKI** | cyclin-dependent kinase inhibitor |
| **CDR** | complementarity-determining region; common deleted region |
| **CEL** | chronic eosinophilic leukemia |
| **CFC** | colony-forming cell |
| **CFU** | colony-forming unit |
| **CFU-E** | colony-forming units – erythroid |
| **CFU-S** | colony-forming units – spleen |
| **CGH** | comparative genomic hybridization |
| **CH** | heavy-chain constant region |
| **CHOP** | cyclophosphamide, doxorubicin, vincristine, prednisone (regimen) |
| **CHR** | complete hematological response |
| **CIDR** | cysteine-rich interdomain region |
| **CLL** | chronic lymphocytic leukemia |
| **CLP** | common lymphoid progenitor |
| **CML** | chronic myeloid leukemia |
| **CMML** | chronic myelomonocytic leukemia |
| **CMR** | complete molecular response |
| **CNL** | chronic neutrophilic leukemia |
| **CNSHA** | chronic non-spherocytic hemolytic anemia |
| **CNV** | copy number variation |
| **CP** | chronic phase (CML) |
| **CR** | complete response |
| **CSC** | cancer stem cell |
| **CSF** | colony-stimulating factor |
| **CSP** | circumsporozoite protein |
| **CTLA** | cytotoxic T-lymphocyte antigen |
| **CVS** | chorionic villus sampling |
| **DBA** | Diamond–Blackfan anemia |
| **DC** | dyskeratosis congenita |
| **DLBL** | diffuse large B-cell lymphoma |
| **DLI** | donor lymphocyte infusion |
| **2,3-DPG** | 2,3-diphosphoglycerate |
| **EBA** | erythrocyte binding antigen |
| **EBMT** | European Group for Blood and Marrow Transplantation |
| **EBP** | erythrocyte-binding protein |
| **ECOG** | Eastern Cooperative Oncology Group |
| **EEC** | endogenous erythroid colony |
| **EFS** | event-free survival |
| **EGF** | epidermal growth factor |
| **EPO** | erythropoietin |
| **EPOR** | erythropoietin receptor |
| **ERT** | enzyme replacement therapy |

| | | | |
|---|---|---|---|
| **ESA** | erythropoiesis-stimulating agent | **IPI** | International Prognostic Index |
| **EST** | expressed sequence tag | **IPPS** | International Prognostic Scoring System |
| **ET** | essential thrombocythemia | **ISC** | irreversibly sickled cell |
| **FA** | Fanconi anemia | **ITD** | internal tandem duplication |
| **FAB** | French–American–British (classification of myelodysplastic syndromes) | **ITP** | idiopathic thrombocytopenic purpura |
| | | **IVIg** | intravenous immunoglobulin |
| **FACS** | fluorescence-activated cell sorter | **IVS** | intervening sequence |
| **FcR** | Fc receptor | **kb** | kilobase pair (1000 base pairs) |
| **FDA** | Food and Drug Administration | **KSS** | Kearns–Sayre syndrome |
| **FGFR** | fibroblast growth factor receptor | **KTLS** | c-kit$^{pos}$Thy-1.1$^{low}$Lin$^{neg}$Sca-1$^{pos}$ cellular phenotype |
| **FISH** | fluorescence in situ hybridization | | |
| **FPD** | familial platelet disorder | **LCR** | locus control region |
| **G6PD** | glucose 6-phosphate dehydrogenase | **LD** | linkage disequilibrium |
| **G-CSF** | granulocyte colony-stimulating factor | **LFA** | leukocyte function-associated antigen |
| **Ge** | Gerbich erythrocyte antigen | **LIF** | leukemia inhibitory factor |
| **GEP** | gene expression profiling | **LOH** | loss of heterozygosity |
| **GM-CSF** | granulocyte macrophage colony-stimulating factor | **LRR** | leucine-rich repeat |
| | | **LTC-IC** | long-term culture-initiating cell |
| **GP** | glycoprotein | **LTR** | long terminal repeat |
| **GPC, GPD** | glycophorin C, glycophorin D | **LV** | lentivirus |
| **GPI** | glycosylphosphatidylinositol | **MALT** | mucosa-associated lymphoid tissue |
| **GT** | Glanzmann thrombasthenia | **MCD** | mast cell diseases |
| **GVH** | graft-versus-host | **MCH** | mean corpuscular hemoglobin |
| **GVHD** | graft-versus-host disease | **MCHC** | mean corpuscular hemoglobin concentration |
| **GVL** | graft-versus-leukemia | | |
| **HCL** | hairy cell leukemia | **MCR** | major cytogenetic response |
| **HDAC** | histone deacetylase | **M-CSF** | macrophage colony-stimulating factor |
| **HDN** | hemolytic disease of the newborn | **MCV** | mean cell volume |
| **HES** | hypereosinophilic syndrome | **MDS** | myelodysplastic syndrome |
| **HGF** | hematopoietic growth factor | **M-FISH** | multiplex fluorescence in situ hybridization |
| **HLA** | human leukocyte antigen | **MGUS** | monoclonal gammopathy of undetermined significance |
| **HMCL** | human multiple myeloma cell line | | |
| **HNA** | human neutrophil antigens | **MHC** | major histocompatibility complex |
| **HPA** | human platelet antigen | **MIF** | macrophage inhibitory factor |
| **HPFH** | hereditary persistence of fetal hemoglobin | **MIP** | macrophage inflammatory protein |
| **HPP-CFC** | high proliferative potential colony-forming cell | **MLL** | mixed lineage leukemia |
| | | **MM** | multiple myeloma |
| **HRD** | hyperdiploid | **MMLV** | Moloney murine leukemia virus |
| **HSC** | hematopoietic stem cell | **MMR** | major molecular response |
| **HSCT** | hematopoietic stem cell transplantation | **MPB** | mobilized peripheral blood |
| **HSV** | herpes simplex virus | **MPD** | myeloproliferative disorder |
| **IAA** | idiopathic aplastic anemia | **MRD** | minimal residual disease |
| **IBMTR** | International Bone Marrow Transplant Registry | **MSP** | merozoite surface protein |
| | | **mtDNA** | mitochondrial DNA |
| **ICAM** | intercellular adhesion molecule | **MTX** | methotrexate |
| **ICL** | inter- and intra-strand DNA cross-links | **MTXPG** | methotrexate polyglutamate |
| **IFN** | interferon | **NAITP** | neonatal/fetal alloimmune thrombocytopenia |
| **Ig** | immunoglobulin | | |
| **IL** | interleukin | **NGF** | nerve growth factor |
| **IMF** | idiopathic myelofibrosis | **NHL** | non-Hodgkin lymphoma |
| **INR** | International Normalized Ratio | **NHRD** | non-hyperdiploid |
| **IOV** | inside-out vesicle (of red cell) | **NK** | natural killer (cell) |

| | |
|---|---|
| **NO** | nitric oxide |
| **NOD/SCID** | non-obese diabetic/severe combined immunodeficiency (mouse) |
| **NPM** | nucleophosmin |
| **OS** | overall survival |
| **PBSC** | peripheral blood stem cells |
| **PCL** | plasma cell leukemia |
| **PCR** | polymerase chain reaction |
| **PDGFR** | platelet-derived growth factor receptor |
| **PECAM** | platelet endothelial cell adhesion molecule |
| **PEG-MGDF** | pegylated megakaryocyte growth and development factor |
| **PETS** | paraffin-embedded tissue section |
| **PfEMP** | *Plasmodium falciparum* erythrocyte membrane protein |
| **PI3K** | phosphatidylinositol 3-kinase |
| **PKC** | protein kinase C |
| **PML** | promyelocytic leukemia (only as gene name in Ch. 4) |
| **PMPS** | Pearson marrow–pancreas syndrome |
| **PNH** | paroxysmal nocturnal hemoglobinuria |
| **PR** | partial response |
| **PT** | prothrombin |
| **PTD** | partial tandem duplication |
| **PUBS** | periumbilical blood sampling |
| **PV** | polycythemia vera |
| **RA** | refractory anemia |
| **RAEB** | refractory anemia with excess blasts |
| **RAEB-T** | refractory anemia with excess blasts in transformation |
| **RAR** | retinoic acid receptor |
| **RARS** | refractory anemia with ringed sideroblasts |
| **RBC** | red blood cell |
| **RCR** | replication-competent retrovirus |
| **RFLP** | restriction fragment length polymorphism |
| **RT-PCR** | reverse transcriptase polymerase chain reaction |
| **SA** | sideroblastic anemia |
| **SAGE** | serial analysis of gene expression |
| **SAO** | Southeast Asian ovalocytosis |
| **SBT** | sequencing-based typing |
| **SCF** | stem cell factor |
| **SCID** | severe combined immunodeficiency |
| **SDF** | stromal derived factor |

| | |
|---|---|
| **SDS-PAGE** | sodium dodecylsulfate–polyacrylamide gel electrophoresis |
| **SF** | steel factor |
| **SFK** | SRC family kinase |
| **SKY** | spectral karyotyping |
| **SLE** | systemic lupus erythematosus |
| **SMM** | smoldering myeloma |
| **SNO-Hb** | *S*-nitrosohemoglobin |
| **SNP** | single-nucleotide polymorphism |
| **SP** | side population |
| **SSOP** | sequence-specific oligonucleotide probing |
| **SSP** | sequence-specific priming |
| **STAT** | signal transducer and activation of transcription |
| **TAA** | tumor-associated antigen |
| **TBI** | total body irradiation |
| **TCR** | T-cell receptor |
| **TdT** | terminal deoxynucleotidyltransferase |
| **TF** | tissue factor |
| **TFPI** | tissue factor pathway inhibitor |
| **TFR** | transferrin receptor |
| **TGF** | transforming growth factor |
| **THF** | tetrahydrofolate |
| **TKD** | tyrosine kinase domain |
| **TKI** | tyrosine kinase inhibitor |
| **TNF** | tumor necrosis factor |
| **TNFR** | tumor necrosis factor receptor |
| **TPMT** | thiopurine *S*-methyltransferase |
| **TPO** | thrombopoietin |
| **TRALI** | transfusion-related acute lung injury |
| **TRAP** | thrombospondin-related adhesive protein |
| **UPD** | uniparental disomy |
| **V, D, J, C** | variable, diversity, joining and constant regions |
| **VCAM** | vascular cell adhesion molecule |
| **VH** | heavy-chain variable region |
| **VWD** | von Willebrand disease |
| **VWF** | von Willebrand factor |
| **vWF:RCo** | von Willebrand factor ristocetin cofactor activity |
| **WCP** | whole-chromosome painting probe |
| **WHO** | World Health Organization |
| **WPSS** | WHO classification-based prognostic scoring system |

# Chapter 1 Beginnings: the molecular pathology of hemoglobin

## David Weatherall

*Weatherall Institute of Molecular Medicine, John Radcliffe Hospital, Oxford, UK*

## Historical background

Linus Pauling first used the term "molecular disease" in 1949, after the discovery that the structure of sickle cell hemoglobin differed from that of normal hemoglobin. Indeed, it was this seminal observation that led to the concept of *molecular medicine*, the description of disease mechanisms at the level of cells and molecules. However, until the development of recombinant DNA technology in the mid-1970s, knowledge of events inside the cell nucleus, notably how genes function, could only be the subject of guesswork based on the structure and function of their protein products. However, as soon as it became possible to isolate human genes and to study their properties, the picture changed dramatically.

Progress over the last 30 years has been driven by technological advances in molecular biology. At first it was possible only to obtain indirect information about the structure and function of genes by DNA/DNA and DNA/RNA hybridization; that is, by probing the quantity or structure of RNA or DNA by annealing reactions with molecular probes. The next major advance was the ability to fractionate DNA into pieces of predictable size with bacterial restriction enzymes. This led to the invention of a technique that played a central role in the early development of human molecular genetics, called *Southern blotting* after the name of its developer, Edwin Southern. This method allowed the structure and organization of genes to be studied directly for the first time and led to the definition of a number of different forms of molecular pathology.

Once it was possible to fractionate DNA, it soon became feasible to insert the pieces into vectors able to divide within bacteria. The steady improvement in the properties of cloning vectors made it possible to generate libraries of human DNA growing in bacterial cultures. Ingenious approaches were developed to scan the libraries to detect genes of interest; once pinpointed, the appropriate bacterial colonies could be grown to generate larger quantities of DNA carrying a particular gene. Later it became possible to sequence these genes, persuade them to synthesize their products in microorganisms, cultured cells or even other species, and hence to define their key regulatory regions.

The early work in the field of human molecular genetics focused on diseases in which there was some knowledge of the genetic defect at the protein or biochemical level. However, once linkage maps of the human genome became available, following the identification of highly polymorphic regions of DNA, it was possible to search for any gene for a disease, even where the cause was completely unknown. This approach, first called *reverse genetics* and later rechristened *positional cloning*, led to the discovery of genes for many important diseases.

As methods for sequencing were improved and automated, thoughts turned to the next major goal in this field, which was to determine the complete sequence of the bases that constitute our genes and all that lies between them: the Human Genome Project. This remarkable endeavor was finally completed in 2006. The further understanding of the functions and regulation of our genes will require multidisciplinary research encompassing many different fields. The next stage in the Human Genome Project, called *genome annotation*, entails analyzing the raw DNA sequence in order to determine its biological significance. One of the main ventures in the era of functional genomics will be in what is termed *proteomics*, the large-scale analysis of the protein

*Molecular Hematology*, 3rd edition. Edited by Drew Provan and John Gribben.
© 2010 Blackwell Publishing.

products of genes. The ultimate goal will be to try to define the protein complement, or proteome, of cells and how the many different proteins interact with one another. To this end, large-scale facilities are being established for isolating and purifying the protein products of genes that have been expressed in bacteria. Their structure can then be studied by a variety of different techniques, notably X-ray crystallography and nuclear magnetic resonance spectroscopy. The crystallographic analysis of proteins is being greatly facilitated by the use of X-ray beams from a synchrotron radiation source.

In the last few years both the utility and extreme complexity of the fruits of the genome project have become apparent. The existence of thousands of single-nucleotide polymorphisms (SNPs) has made it possible to search for genes of biological or medical significance. The discovery of families of regulatory RNAs and proteins is starting to shed light on how the functions of the genome are controlled, and studies of acquired changes in its structure, *epigenetics*, promise to provide similar information. However, a full understanding of the interactions of these complex regulatory systems, presumably by major advances in systems biology, is still a long way in the future.

During this remarkable period of technical advance, considerable progress has been made toward an understanding of the pathology of disease at the molecular level. This has had a particular impact on hematology, leading to advances in the understanding of gene function and disease mechanisms in almost every aspect of the field.

The inherited disorders of hemoglobin – the thalassemias and structural hemoglobin variants, the commonest human monogenic diseases – were the first to be studied systematically at the molecular level and a great deal is known about their genotype–phenotype relationships. This field led the way to molecular hematology and, indeed, to the development of molecular medicine. Thus, even though the genetics of hemoglobin is complicated by the fact that different varieties are produced at particular stages of human development, the molecular pathology of the hemoglobinopathies provides an excellent model system for understanding any monogenic disease and the complex interactions between genotype and environment that underlie many multigenic disorders.

In this chapter I consider the structure, synthesis and genetic control of the human hemoglobins, describe the molecular pathology of the thalassemias, and discuss briefly how the complex interactions of their different genotypes produce a remarkably diverse family of clinical phenotypes; the structural hemoglobin variants are discussed in more detail in *Chapter 15*. Readers who wish to learn more about the methods of molecular genetics, particularly as applied to the study of hemoglobin disorders, are referred to the reviews cited at the end of this chapter.

## The structure, genetic control and synthesis of normal hemoglobin

### Structure and function

The varying oxygen requirements during embryonic, fetal and adult life are reflected in the synthesis of different structural hemoglobins at each stage of human development. However, they all have the same general tetrameric structure, consisting of two different pairs of globin chains, each attached to one heme molecule. Adult and fetal hemoglobins have $\alpha$ chains combined with $\beta$ chains (Hb A, $\alpha_2\beta_2$), $\delta$ chains (Hb $A_2$, $\alpha_2\delta_2$) and $\gamma$ chains (Hb F, $\alpha_2\gamma_2$). In embryos, $\alpha$-like chains called $\zeta$ chains combine with $\gamma$ chains to produce Hb Portland ($\zeta_2\gamma_2$), or with $\varepsilon$ chains to make Hb Gower 1 ($\zeta_2\varepsilon_2$), while $\alpha$ and $\varepsilon$ chains form Hb Gower 2 ($\alpha_2\varepsilon_2$). Fetal hemoglobin is heterogeneous; there are two varieties of $\gamma$ chain that differ only in their amino acid composition at position 136, which may be occupied by either glycine or alanine; $\gamma$ chains containing glycine at this position are called $^G\gamma$ chains, those with alanine $^A\gamma$ chains (Figure 1.1).

The synthesis of hemoglobin tetramers consisting of two unlike pairs of globin chains is absolutely essential for the effective function of hemoglobin as an oxygen carrier. The classical sigmoid shape of the oxygen dissociation curve, which reflects the allosteric properties of the hemoglobin molecule, ensures that, at high oxygen tensions in the lungs, oxygen is readily taken up and later released effectively at the lower tensions encountered in the tissues. The shape of the curve is quite different to that of myoglobin, a molecule that consists of a single globin chain with heme attached to it, which, like abnormal hemoglobins that consist of homotetramers of like chains, has a hyperbolic oxygen dissociation curve.

The transition from a hyperbolic to a sigmoid oxygen dissociation curve, which is absolutely critical for normal oxygen delivery, reflects cooperativity between the four heme molecules and their globin subunits. When one of them takes on oxygen, the affinity of the remaining three increases markedly; this happens because hemoglobin can exist in two configurations, deoxy(T) and oxy(R), where T and R represent the tight and relaxed states, respectively. The T configuration has a lower affinity than the R for ligands such as oxygen. At some point during the addition of oxygen to the hemes, the transition from the T to the R configuration occurs and the oxygen affinity of the partially liganded molecule increases dramatically. These allosteric changes result from interactions between the iron of the heme groups and various bonds within the hemoglobin tetramer, which lead to subtle spatial changes as oxygen is taken on or given up.

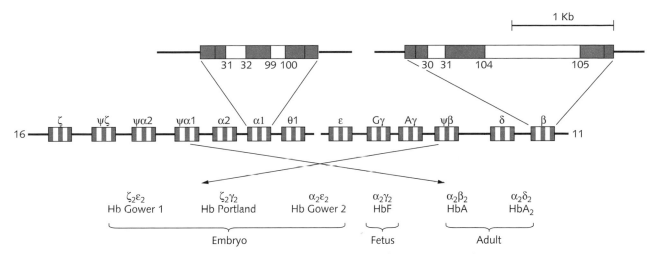

**Fig. 1.1 The genetic control of human hemoglobin production in embryonic, fetal and adult life**

The precise tetrameric structures of the different human hemoglobins, which reflect the primary amino acid sequences of their individual globin chains, are also vital for the various adaptive changes that are required to ensure adequate tissue oxygenation. The position of the oxygen dissociation curve can be modified in several ways. For example, oxygen affinity decreases with increasing $CO_2$ tension (the Bohr effect). This facilitates oxygen loading to the tissues, where a drop in pH due to $CO_2$ influx lowers oxygen affinity; the opposite effect occurs in the lungs. Oxygen affinity is also modified by the level of 2,3-diphosphoglycerate (2,3-DPG) in the red cell. Increasing concentrations shift the oxygen dissociation curve to the right (i.e., they reduce oxygen affinity), while diminishing concentrations have the opposite effect. 2,3-DPG fits into the gap between the two $\beta$ chains when it widens during deoxygenation, and interacts with several specific binding sites in the central cavity of the molecule. In the deoxy configuration the gap between the two $\beta$ chains narrows and the molecule cannot be accommodated. With increasing concentrations of 2,3-DPG, which are found in various hypoxic and anemic states, more hemoglobin molecules tend to be held in the deoxy configuration and the oxygen dissociation curve is therefore shifted to the right, with more effective release of oxygen.

Fetal red cells have greater oxygen affinity than adult red cells, although, interestingly, purified fetal hemoglobin has an oxygen dissociation curve similar to that of adult hemoglobin. These differences, which are adapted to the oxygen requirements of fetal life, reflect the relative inability of Hb F to interact with 2,3-DPG compared with Hb A. This is because the $\gamma$ chains of Hb F lack specific binding sites for 2,3-DPG.

In short, oxygen transport can be modified by a variety of adaptive features in the red cell that include interactions

between the different heme molecules, the effects of $CO_2$ and differential affinities for 2,3-DPG. These changes, together with more general mechanisms involving the cardiorespiratory system, provide the main basis for physiological adaptation to anemia.

## Genetic control of hemoglobin

The $\alpha$- and $\beta$-like globin chains are the products of two different gene families which are found on different chromosomes (Figure 1.1). The $\beta$-like globin genes form a linked cluster on chromosome 11, spread over approximately 60 kb (kilobase or 1000 nucleotide bases). The different genes that form this cluster are arranged in the order 5′–$\epsilon$–$^G\gamma$–$^A\gamma$–$\psi\beta$–$\delta$–$\beta$–3′. The $\alpha$-like genes also form a linked cluster, in this case on chromosome 16, in the order 5′–$\zeta$–$\psi\zeta$–$\psi\alpha$1–$\alpha$2–$\alpha$1–3′. The $\psi\beta$, $\psi\zeta$ and $\psi\alpha$ genes are pseudogenes; that is, they have strong sequence homology with the $\beta$, $\zeta$ and $\alpha$ genes but contain a number of differences that prevent them from directing the synthesis of any products. They may reflect remnants of genes that were functional at an earlier stage of human evolution.

The structure of the human globin genes is, in essence, similar to that of all mammalian genes. They consist of long strings of nucleotides that are divided into coding regions, or exons, and non-coding inserts called *intervening sequences* (IVS) or introns. The $\beta$-like globin genes contain two introns, one of 122–130 base pairs between codons 30 and 31 and one of 850–900 base pairs between codons 104 and 105 (the exon codons are numbered sequentially from the 5′ to the 3′ end of the gene, i.e., from left to right). Similar, though smaller, introns are found in the $\alpha$ and $\zeta$ globin genes. These introns and exons, together with short non-coding sequences at the 5′ and 3′ ends of the genes, represent

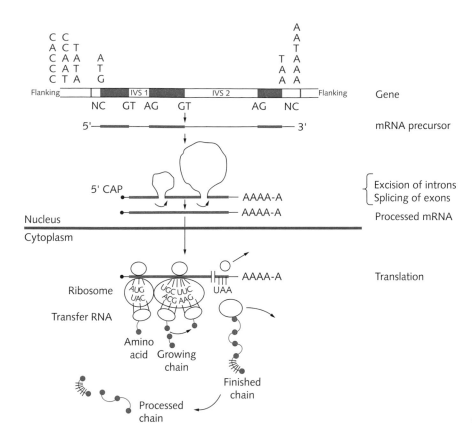

**Fig. 1.2 The mechanisms of globin gene transcription and translation**

the major functional regions of the particular genes. However, there are also extremely important regulatory sequences which subserve these functions that lie outside the genes themselves.

At the 5′ non-coding (flanking) regions of the globin genes, as in all mammalian genes, there are blocks of nucleotide homology. The first, the ATA box, is about 30 bases upstream (to the left) of the initiation codon; that is, the start word for the beginning of protein synthesis (*see below*). The second, the CCAAT box, is about 70 base pairs upstream from the 5′ end of the genes. About 80–100 bases further upstream there is the sequence GGGGTG, or CACCC, which may be inverted or duplicated. These three highly conserved DNA sequences, called *promoter elements*, are involved in the initiation of transcription of the individual genes. Finally, in the 3′ non-coding region of all the globin genes there is the sequence AATAAA, which is the signal for cleavage and polyA addition to RNA transcripts (*see section Gene action and globin synthesis*).

The globin gene clusters also contain several sequences that constitute regulatory elements, which interact to promote erythroid-specific gene expression and coordination of the changes in globin gene activity during development. These include the globin genes themselves and their promoter elements: enhancers (regulatory sequences that

increase gene expression despite being located at a considerable distance from the genes) and "master" regulatory sequences called, in the case of the β globin gene cluster, the *locus control region* (LCR), and, in the case of the α genes, HS40 (a nuclease-hypersensitive site in DNA 40 kb from the α globin genes). Each of these sequences has a modular structure made up of an array of short motifs that represent the binding sites for transcriptional activators or repressors.

## Gene action and globin synthesis

The flow of information between DNA and protein is summarized in Figure 1.2. When a globin gene is transcribed, messenger RNA (mRNA) is synthesized from one of its strands, a process which begins with the formation of a transcription complex consisting of a variety of regulatory proteins together with an enzyme called RNA polymerase (*see below*). The primary transcript is a large mRNA precursor which contains both intron and exon sequences. While in the nucleus, this molecule undergoes a variety of modifications. First, the introns are removed and the exons are spliced together. The intron/exon junctions always have the same sequence: GT at their 5′ end, and AG at their 3′ end. This appears to be essential for accurate splicing; if there is a mutation at these sites this process does not occur. Splicing reflects a complex series of intermediary stages and the interaction of a number of different nuclear proteins. After the exons are joined, the mRNAs are modified and stabilized; at their 5′ end a complex CAP structure is formed, while at their 3′ end a string of adenylic acid residues (polyA) is added. The mRNA processed in this way moves into the cytoplasm, where it acts as a template for globin chain production. Because of the rules of base pairing, i.e., cytosine always pairs with thymine, and guanine with adenine, the structure of the mRNA reflects a faithful copy of the DNA codons from which it is synthesized; the only difference is that, in RNA, uracil (U) replaces thymine (T).

Amino acids are transported to the mRNA template on carriers called transfer RNAs (tRNAs); there are specific tRNAs for each amino acid. Furthermore, because the genetic code is redundant (i.e., more than one codon can encode a particular amino acid), for some of the amino acids there are several different individual tRNAs. Their order in the globin chain is determined by the order of codons in the mRNA. The tRNAs contain three bases, which together constitute an anticodon; these anticodons are complementary to mRNA codons for particular amino acids. They carry amino acids to the template, where they find the appropriate positioning by codon–anticodon base-pairing. When the first tRNA is in position, an initiation complex is formed between several protein initiation factors together with the two subunits that constitute the ribosomes. A second tRNA moves in alongside and the two amino acids that they are carrying form a peptide bond between them; the globin chain is now two amino acid residues long. This process is continued along the mRNA from left to right, and the growing peptide chain is transferred from one incoming tRNA to the next; that is, the mRNA is translated from 5′ to 3′. During this time the tRNAs are held in appropriate steric configuration with the mRNA by the two ribosomal subunits. There are specific initiation (AUG) and termination (UAA, UAG and UGA) codons. When the ribosomes reach the termination codon, translation ceases, the completed globin chains are released, and the ribosomal subunits are recycled. Individual globin chains combine with heme, which has been synthesized through a separate pathway, and then interact with one like chain and two unlike chains to form a complete hemoglobin tetramer.

## Regulation of hemoglobin synthesis

The regulation of globin gene expression is mediated mainly at the transcriptional level, with some fine tuning during translation and post-translational modification of the gene products. DNA that is not involved in transcription is held tightly packaged in a compact, chemically modified form that is inaccessible to transcription factors and polymerases and which is heavily methylated. Activation of a particular gene is reflected by changes in the structure of the surrounding chromatin, which can be identified by enhanced sensitivity to nucleases. Erythroid lineage-specific nuclease-hypersensitive sites are found at several locations in the β globin gene cluster. Four are distributed over 20 kb upstream from the ε globin gene in the region of the β globin LCR (Figure 1.3). This vital regulatory region is able to establish a transcriptionally active domain spanning the entire β globin gene cluster. Several enhancer sequences have been identified in this cluster. A variety of regulatory proteins bind to the LCR, and to the promoter regions of the globin genes and to the enhancer sequences. It is thought that the LCR and other enhancer regions become opposed to the promoters to increase the rate of transcription of the genes to which they are related.

These regulatory regions contain sequence motifs for various ubiquitous and erythroid-restricted transcription factors. Binding sites for these factors have been identified in each of the globin gene promoters and at the hypersensitive-site regions of the various regulatory elements. A number of the factors which bind to these areas are found in all cell types. They include Sp1, Yy1 and Usf. In contrast, a number of transcription factors have been identified, including GATA-1, EKLF and NF-E2, which are restricted in their distribution to erythroid cells and, in some cases, megakaryocytes and mast cells. The overlapping of erythroid-specific and ubiquitous-factor binding sites in several cases suggests that competitive binding may play an important part in the regulation of erythroid-specific genes. Another binding factor, SSP, the stage selector protein, appears to interact specifically with ε and γ genes. Several elements involving the chromatin and histone acetylation required for access of these regulatory proteins have been identified.

The binding of hematopoietic-specific factors activates the LCR, which renders the entire β globin gene cluster transcriptionally active. These factors also bind to the enhancer and promoter sequences, which work in tandem to regulate the expression of the individual genes in the clusters. It is likely that some of the transcriptional factors are developmental stage-specific, and hence may be responsible for the differential expression of the embryonic, fetal and adult globin genes. The α globin gene cluster also contains an element, HS40, which has some structural features in common with the β LCR, although it is different in aspects of its structure. A number of enhancer-like sequences have also been identified, although it is becoming clear that there are fundamental differences in the pattern of regulation of the two globin gene clusters.

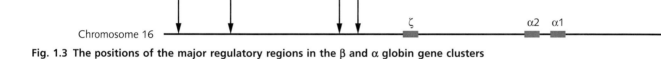

**Fig. 1.3 The positions of the major regulatory regions in the β and α globin gene clusters**
The arrows indicate the position of the erythroid lineage-specific nuclease-hypersensitive sites. HS, hypersensitive.

In addition to the different regulatory sequences outlined above, there are also sequences which may be involved specifically with "silencing" of genes, notably those for the embryonic hemoglobins, during development.

Some degree of regulation is also mediated by differences in the rates of initiation and translation of the different mRNAs, and at the post-transcriptional level by differential affinity for different protein subunits. However, this kind of post-transcriptional fine tuning probably plays a relatively small role in determining the overall output of the globin gene products.

### Regulation of developmental changes in globin gene expression

During development, the site of red cell production moves from the yolk sac to the fetal liver and spleen, and thence to bone marrow in the adult. Embryonic, fetal and adult hemoglobin synthesis is approximately related in time to these changes in the site of erythropoiesis, although it is quite clear that the various switches, between embryonic and fetal and between fetal and adult hemoglobin synthesis, are beautifully synchronized throughout these different sites. Fetal hemoglobin synthesis declines during the later months of gestation and Hb F is replaced by Hb A and Hb A$_2$ by the end of the first year of life.

Despite a great deal of research, very little is known about the regulation of these different switches from one globin gene to another during development. Work from a variety of different sources suggests that there may be specific regions in the α and β globin gene clusters that are responsive to the action of transcription factors, some of which may be developmental-stage-specific. However, proteins of this type have not yet been isolated, and nothing is known about their regulation and how it is mediated during development.

## The molecular pathology of hemoglobin

As is the case for most monogenic diseases, the inherited disorders of hemoglobin fall into two major classes. First, there are those that result from reduced output of one or other globin genes, the *thalassemias*. Second, there is a wide range of conditions that result from the production of *structurally abnormal globin chains*; the type of disease depends on how the particular alteration in protein structure interferes with its stability or function. Of course, no biological classification is entirely satisfactory and those which attempt to define the hemoglobin disorders are no exception. There are some structural hemoglobin variants which happen to be synthesized at a reduced rate and hence are associated with a clinical picture similar to thalassemia. And there are other classes of mutations which simply interfere with the normal transition from fetal to adult hemoglobin synthesis, a family of conditions given the general title *hereditary persistence of fetal hemoglobin*. Furthermore, because these diseases are all so common and occur together in particular populations, it is not uncommon for an individual to inherit a gene for one or other form of thalassemia and a structural hemoglobin variant. The heterogeneous group of conditions that results from these different mutations and interactions is summarized in Table 1.1.

Over recent years, determination of the molecular pathology of the two common forms of thalassemia, α and β, has provided a remarkable picture of the repertoire of mutations that can underlie human monogenic disease. In the sections that follow I describe, in outline, the different forms of molecular pathology that underlie these conditions.

**Table 1.1** The thalassemias and related disorders.

| α Thalassemia | γ Thalassemia |
|---|---|
| α⁰ | |
| α⁺ | δ Thalassemia |
|   Deletion (−α) | |
|   Non-deletion (αᵀ) | εγδβ Thalassemia |
| | |
| β Thalassemia | Hereditary persistence of |
| β⁰ | fetal hemoglobin |
| β⁺ | Deletion |
| Normal Hb A₂ |   (δβ)⁰ |
| "Silent" | Non-deletion |
| |   Linked to β globin genes |
| δβ Thalassemia |    ᴳγβ⁺ |
| (δβ)⁺ |    ᴬγβ⁺ |
| (δβ)⁰ |   Unlinked to β globin genes |
| (ᴬγδβ)⁰ | |

## The β thalassemias

There are two main classes of β thalassemia, β⁰ thalassemia, in which there is an absence of β globin chain production, and β⁺ thalassemia, in which there is variable reduction in the output of β globin chains. As shown in Figure 1.4, mutations of the β globin genes may cause a reduced output of gene product at the level of transcription or mRNA processing, translation, or through the stability of the globin gene product.

### Defective β globin gene transcription

There are a variety of mechanisms that interfere with normal transcription of the β globin genes. First, the genes may be either completely or partially deleted. Overall, deletions of the β globin genes are not commonly found in patients with β thalassemia, with one exception: a 619-bp deletion involving the 3′ end of the gene is found frequently in the Sind populations of India and Pakistan, where it constitutes about 30% of the β thalassemia alleles. Other deletions are extremely rare.

A much more common group of mutations, which results in a moderate decrease in the rate of transcription of the β globin genes, involves single nucleotide substitutions in or near the TATA box at about −30 nucleotides (nt) from the transcription start site, or in the proximal or distal promoter elements at −90 nt and −105 nt. These mutations result in decreased β globin mRNA production, ranging from 10 to 25% of the normal output. Thus, they are usually associated with the mild forms of β⁺ thalassemia. They are particularly common in African populations, an observation which explains the unusual mildness of β thalassemia in this racial

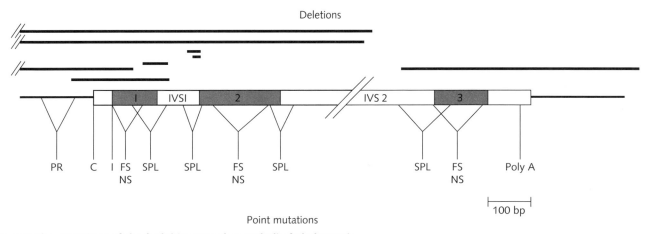

**Fig. 1.4 The mutations of the β globin gene that underlie β thalassemia**
The heavy black lines indicate the length of the deletions. The point mutations are designated as follows: PR, promoter; C, CAP site; I, initiation codon; FS, frameshift and nonsense mutations; SPL, splice mutations; Poly A, poly A addition site mutations.

group. One particular mutation, C→T at position −101 nt to the β globin gene, causes an extremely mild deficit of β globin mRNA. Indeed, this allele is so mild that it is completely silent in carriers and can only be identified by its interaction with more severe β thalassemia alleles in compound heterozygotes.

**Mutations that cause abnormal processing of mRNA**

As mentioned earlier, the boundaries between exons and introns are marked by the invariant dinucleotides GT at the donor (5′) site and AG at the acceptor (3′) site. Mutations that affect either of these sites completely abolish normal splicing and produce the phenotype of β⁰ thalassemia. The transcription of genes carrying these mutations appears to be normal, but there is complete inactivation of splicing at the altered junction.

Another family of mutations involves what are called *splice site consensus sequences*. Although only the GT dinucleotide is invariant at the donor splice site, there is conservation of adjacent nucleotides and a common, or consensus, sequence of these regions can be identified. Mutations within this sequence can reduce the efficiency of splicing to varying degrees because they lead to alternate splicing at the surrounding cryptic sites. For example, mutations of the nucleotide at position 5 of IVS-1 (the first intervening sequence), G→C or T, result in a marked reduction of β chain production and in the phenotype of severe β⁺ thalassemia. On the other hand, the substitution of C for T at position 6 in IVS-1 leads to only a mild reduction in the output of β chains.

Another mechanism that leads to abnormal splicing involves *cryptic splice sites*. These are regions of DNA which, if mutated, assume the function of a splice site at an inappropriate region of the mRNA precursor. For example, a variety of mutations activate a cryptic site which spans codons 24–27 of exon 1 of the β globin gene. This site contains a GT dinucleotide, and adjacent substitutions that alter it so that it more closely resembles the consensus donor splice site result in its activation, even though the normal splice site is intact. A mutation at codon 24 GGT→GGA, though it does not alter the amino acid which is normally found in this position in the β globin chain (glycine), allows some splicing to occur at this site instead of the exon–intron boundary. This results in the production of both normal and abnormally spliced β globin mRNA and hence in the clinical phenotype of severe β thalassemia. Interestingly, mutations at codons 19, 26 and 27 result in both reduced production of normal mRNA (due to abnormal splicing) and an amino acid substitution when the mRNA which is spliced normally is translated into protein. The abnormal hemoglobins produced are Hb Malay, Hb E and Hb Knossos, respectively. All

these variants are associated with a mild β⁺ thalassemia-like phenotype. These mutations illustrate how sequence changes in coding rather than intervening sequences influence RNA processing, and underline the importance of competition between potential splice site sequences in generating both normal and abnormal varieties of β globin mRNA.

Cryptic splice sites in introns may also carry mutations that activate them even though the normal splice sites remain intact. A common mutation of this kind in Mediterranean populations involves a base substitution at position 110 in IVS-1. This region contains a sequence similar to a 3′ acceptor site, though it lacks the invariant AG dinucleotide. The change of the G to A at position 110 creates this dinucleotide. The result is that about 90% of the RNA transcript splices to this particular site and only 10% to the normal site, again producing the phenotype of severe β⁺ thalassemia (Figure 1.5). Several other β thalassemia mutations have been described which generate new donor sites within IVS-2 of the β globin gene.

Another family of mutations that interferes with β globin gene processing involves the sequence AAUAAA in the 3′ untranslated regions, which is the signal for cleavage and polyadenylation of the β globin gene transcript. Somehow, these mutations destabilize the transcript. For example, a T→C substitution in this sequence leads to only one-tenth of the normal amount of β globin mRNA transcript and hence to the phenotype of a moderately severe β⁺ thalassemia. Another example of a mutation which probably leads to defective processing of function of β globin mRNA is the single-base substitution A→C in the CAP site. It is not yet understood how this mutation causes a reduced rate of transcription of the β globin gene.

There is another small subset of rare mutations that involve the 3′ untranslated region of the β globin gene and these are associated with relatively mild forms of β thalassemia. It is thought that these interfere in some way with transcription but the mechanism is unknown.

**Mutations that result in abnormal translation of β globin mRNA**

There are three main classes of mutations of this kind. Base substitutions that change an amino acid codon to a chain termination codon prevent the translation of β globin mRNA and result in the phenotype of β⁰ thalassemia. Several mutations of this kind have been described; the commonest, involving codon 17, occurs widely throughout Southeast Asia. Similarly, a codon 39 mutation is encountered frequently in the Mediterranean region.

The second class involves the insertion or deletion of one, two or four nucleotides in the coding region of the β globin gene. These disrupt the normal reading frame, cause a

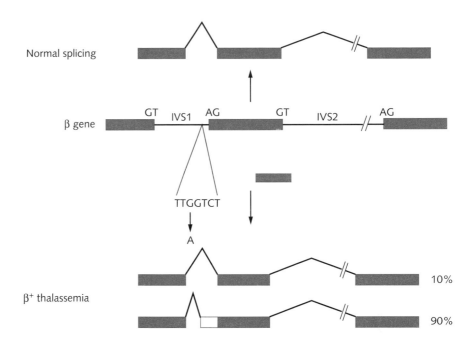

**Fig. 1.5 The generation of a new splice site in an intron as the mechanism for a form of β⁺ thalassemia**
*For details see text.*

frameshift, and hence interfere with the translation of β globin mRNA. The end result is the insertion of anomalous amino acids after the frameshift until a termination codon is reached in the new reading frame. This type of mutation always leads to the phenotype of $\beta^0$ thalassemia.

Finally, there are several mutations which involve the β globin gene initiation codon and which, presumably, reduce the efficiency of translation.

**Unstable β globin chain variants**

Some forms of β thalassemia result from the synthesis of highly unstable β globin chains that are incapable of forming hemoglobin tetramers, and which are rapidly degraded, leading to the phenotype of $\beta^0$ thalassemia. Indeed, in many of these conditions no abnormal globin chain product can be demonstrated by protein analysis and the molecular pathology has to be interpreted simply on the basis of a derived sequence of the variant β chain obtained by DNA analysis.

Recent studies have provided some interesting insights into how complex clinical phenotypes may result from the synthesis of unstable β globin products. For example, there is a spectrum of disorders that result from mutations in exon 3 which give rise to a moderately severe form of β thalassemia in heterozygotes. It has been found that nonsense or frameshift mutations in exons I and II are associated with the absence of mRNA from the cytoplasm of red cell precursors. This appears to be an adaptive mechanism, called *nonsense-mediated decay*, whereby abnormal mRNA of this type is not transported to the cytoplasm, where it would act as a

template for the production of truncated gene products. However, in the case of exon III mutations, apparently because this process requires the presence of an intact upstream exon, the abnormal mRNA is transported into the cytoplasm and hence can act as a template for the production of unstable β globin chains. The latter precipitate in the red cell precursors together with excess α chains to form large inclusion bodies, and hence there is enough globin chain imbalance in heterozygotes to produce a moderately severe degree of anemia.

**The α thalassemias**

The molecular pathology of the α thalassemias is more complicated than that of the β thalassemias, simply because there are two α globin genes per haploid genome. Thus, the normal α globin genotype can be written αα/αα. As in the case of β thalassemia, there are two major varieties of α thalassemia, $\alpha^+$ and $\alpha^0$ thalassemia. In $\alpha^+$ thalassemia one of the linked α globin genes is lost, either by deletion (−) or mutation (T); the heterozygous genotype can be written −α/αα or $\alpha^T\alpha/\alpha\alpha$. In $\alpha^0$ thalassemia the loss of both α globin genes nearly always results from a deletion; the heterozygous genotype is therefore written −−/αα. In populations where specific deletions are particularly common, Southeast Asia (SEA) or the Mediterranean region (MED), it is useful to add the appropriate superscript as follows: $-\!-^{SEA}/\alpha\alpha$ or $-\!-^{MED}/\alpha\alpha$. It follows that when we speak of an "α thalassemia gene" what we are really referring to is a haplotype; that is, the state and function of both of the linked α globin genes.

### α⁰ Thalassemia

Three main molecular pathologies, all involving deletions, have been found to underlie the α⁰ thalassemia phenotype. The majority of cases result from deletions that remove both α globin genes and a varying length of the α globin gene cluster (Figure 1.6). Occasionally, however, the α globin gene cluster is intact but is inactivated by a deletion which involves the major regulatory region HS40, 40 kb upstream from the α globin genes, or the α globin genes may be lost as part of a truncation of the tip of the short arm of chromosome 16.

As well as providing us with an understanding of the molecular basis for α⁰ thalassemia, detailed studies of these deletions have yielded more general information about the mechanisms that underlie this form of molecular pathology. For example, it has been found that the 5′ breakpoints of a number of deletions of the α globin gene cluster are located approximately the same distance apart and in the same order along the chromosome as their respective 3′ breakpoints; similar findings have been observed in deletions of the β globin gene cluster. These deletions seem to have resulted from illegitimate recombination events which have led to the deletion of an integral number of chromatin loops as they pass through their nuclear attachment points during chromosomal replication. Another long deletion has been characterized in which a new piece of DNA bridges the two breakpoints in the α globin gene cluster. The inserted sequence originates upstream from the α globin gene cluster, where normally it is found in an inverted orientation with respect to that found between the breakpoints of the deletion. Thus it appears to have been incorporated into the junction in a way that reflects its close proximity to the deletion breakpoint region during replication. Other deletions seem to be related to the family of Alu-repeats, simple repeat sequences that are widely dispersed throughout the genome; one deletion appears to have resulted from a simple homologous recombination between two repeats of this kind that are usually 62 kb apart.

A number of forms of α⁰ thalassemia result from terminal truncations of the short arm of chromosome 16 to a site about 50 kb distal to the α globin genes. The telomeric consensus sequence $TTAGGG_n$ has been added directly to the site of the break. Since these mutations are stably inherited, it appears that telomeric DNA alone is sufficient to stabilize the ends of broken chromosomes.

Quite recently, two other molecular mechanisms have been identified as the cause of α⁰ thalassemia which, though rare, may have important implications for an understanding of the molecular pathology of other genetic diseases. In one case, a deletion in the α globin gene cluster resulted in a widely expressed gene (*LUC7L*) becoming juxtaposed to a structurally normal α globin gene. Although the latter retained all its important regulatory elements, its expression was silenced. It was found in a transgenic mouse model that transcription of antisense RNA mediated the silencing of the α globin gene region, findings that provide a completely new mechanism for genetic disease. In another case of α⁰ thalassemia, in which no molecular defects could be detected in the α globin gene cluster, a gain-of-function regulatory polymorphism was found in the region between the α globin genes and their upstream regulatory elements. This alteration creates a new promoter-like element that interferes with the normal activation of all downstream α-like globin genes.

In short, detailed analysis of the molecular pathology of the α⁰ thalassemias has provided valuable evidence not only about how large deletions of gene clusters are caused, but also about some of the complex mechanisms that may underlie cases in which the α gene clusters remain intact but in which their function is completely suppressed.

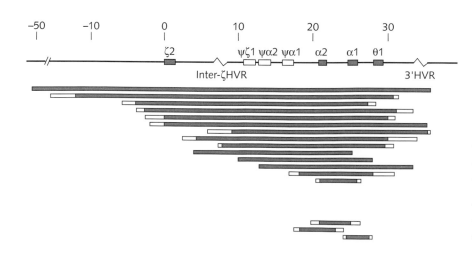

**Fig. 1.6 Some of the deletions that underlie α⁰ and α⁺ thalassemia**
The colored rectangles beneath the α globin gene cluster indicate the lengths of the deletions. The unshaded regions indicate uncertainty about the precise breakpoints. The three small deletions at the bottom of the figure represent the common α⁺ thalassemia deletions. HVR, highly variable regions.

### α⁺ Thalassemia

As mentioned earlier, the α⁺ thalassemias result from the inactivation of one of the duplicated α globin genes, either by deletion or point mutation.

*α⁺ Thalassemia due to gene deletions* There are two common forms of α⁺ thalassemia that are due to loss of one or other of the duplicated α globin genes, $-\alpha^{3.7}$ and $-\alpha^{4.2}$, where 3.7 and 4.2 indicate the size of the deletions. The way in which these deletions have been generated reflects the underlying structure of the α globin gene complex (Figure 1.7). Each α gene lies within a boundary of homology, approximately 4 kb long, probably generated by an ancient duplication event. The homologous regions, which are divided by small inserts, are designated X, Y and Z. The duplicated Z boxes are 3.7 kb apart and the X boxes are 4.2 kb apart. As the result of misalignment and reciprocal crossover between these segments at meiosis, a chromosome is produced with either a single ($-\alpha$) or triplicated ($\alpha\alpha\alpha$) α globin gene. As shown in Figure 1.7, if a crossover occurs between homologous Z boxes 3.7 kb of DNA are lost, an event which is described as a rightward deletion, $-\alpha^{3.7}$. A similar crossover between the two X boxes deletes 4.2 kb, the leftward deletion $-\alpha^{4.2}$. The corresponding triplicated α gene arrangements are called $\alpha\alpha\alpha^{\text{anti}3.7}$ and $\alpha\alpha\alpha^{\text{anti}4.2}$. A variety of different points of crossing over within the Z boxes give rise to different length deletions, still involving 3.7 kb.

*Non-deletion types of α⁺ thalassemia* These disorders result from single or oligonucleotide mutations of the particular α globin gene. Most of them involve the α2 gene but, since the output from this locus is two to three times greater than that from the α1 gene, this may simply reflect ascertainment bias due to the greater phenotypic effect and, possibly, a greater selective advantage.

Overall, these mutations interfere with α globin gene function in a similar way to those that affect the β globin genes. They affect the transcription, translation or post-translational stability of the gene product. Since the principles are the same as for β thalassemia, we do not need to describe them in detail with one exception, a mutation which has not been observed in the β globin gene cluster. It turns out that there is a family of mutations that involves the α2 globin gene termination codon, TAA. Each specifically changes this codon so that an amino acid is inserted instead of the chain terminating. This is followed by "read-through" of α globin mRNA, which is not normally translated until another in-phase termination codon is reached. The result is an elongated α chain with 31 additional residues at the C-terminal end. Five hemoglobin variants of this type have been identified. The commonest, Hb Constant Spring, occurs at a high frequency in many parts of Southeast Asia. It is not absolutely clear why the read-through of normally untranslated mRNAs leads to a reduced output from the α2 gene, although there is considerable evidence that it in some way destabilizes the mRNA.

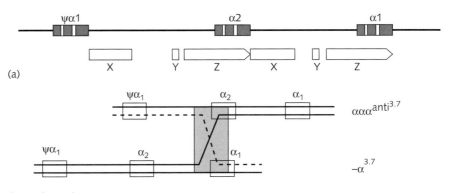

(b) Rightward crossover

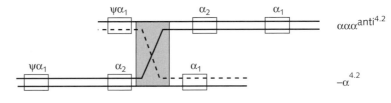

(c) Leftward crossover

**Fig. 1.7 Mechanisms of the generation of the common deletion forms of α⁺ thalassemia**
(a) The normal arrangement of the α globin genes, with the regions of homology X, Y and Z. (b) The crossover that generates the $-\alpha^{3.7}$ deletion. (c) The crossover that generates the $-\alpha^{4.2}$ deletion.

## α Thalassemia/mental retardation syndromes

There is a family of mild forms of α thalassemia which is quite different to that described in the previous section and which is associated with varying degrees of mental retardation. Recent studies indicate that there are two quite different varieties of this condition, one encoded on chromosome 16 (ATR-16) and the other on the X chromosome (ATR-X).

The ATR-16 syndrome is characterized by relatively mild mental handicap with a variable constellation of facial and skeletal dysmorphisms. These individuals have long deletions involving the α globin gene cluster, but removing at least 1–2 Mb. This condition can arise in several ways, including unbalanced translocation involving chromosome 16, truncation of the tip of chromosome 16, and the loss of the α globin gene cluster and parts of its flanking regions by other mechanisms.

The ATR-X syndrome results from mutations in a gene on the X chromosome, Xq13.1–q21.1. The product of this gene is one of a family of proteins involved in chromatin-mediated transcriptional regulation. It is expressed ubiquitously during development and at interphase it is found entirely within the nucleus in association with pericentromeric heterochromatin. In metaphase, it is similarly found close to the centromeres of many chromosomes but, in addition, occurs at the stalks of acrocentric chromosomes, where the sequences for ribosomal RNA are located. These locations provide important clues to the potential role of this protein in the establishment and/or maintenance of methylation of the genome. Although it is clear that *ATR-X* is involved in α globin transcription, it also must be an important player in early fetal development, particularly of the urogenital system and brain. Many different mutations of this gene have been discovered in association with the widespread morphological and developmental abnormalities which characterize the ATR-X syndrome.

## α Thalassemia and the myelodysplastic syndrome

Since the first description of Hb H (*see later section*) in the red cells of a patient with leukemia, many examples of this association have been reported. The condition usually is reflected in a mild form of Hb H disease, with typical Hb H inclusions in a proportion of the red cells and varying amounts of Hb H demonstrable by hemoglobin electrophoresis. The hematological findings are usually those of one or other form of the myelodysplastic syndrome. The condition occurs predominantly in males in older age groups. Very recently it has been found that some patients with this condition have mutations involving *ATR-X*. The relationship of these mutations to the associated myelodysplasia remains to be determined.

## Rarer forms of thalassemia and related disorders

There are a variety of other conditions that involve the β globin gene cluster which, although less common than the β thalassemias, provide some important information about mechanisms of molecular pathology and therefore should be mentioned briefly.

### The δβ thalassemias

Like the β thalassemias, the δβ thalassemias, which result from defective δ and β chain synthesis, are subdivided into the $(\delta\beta)^+$ and $(\delta\beta)^0$ forms.

The $(\delta\beta)^+$ thalassemias result from unequal crossover between the δ and β globin gene loci at meiosis with the production of δβ fusion genes. The resulting δβ fusion chain products combine with α chains to form a family of hemoglobin variants called the hemoglobin Lepores, after the family name of the first patient of this kind to be discovered. Because the synthesis of these variants is directed by genes with the 5′ sequences of the δ globin genes, which have defective promoters, they are synthesized at a reduced rate and result in the phenotype of a moderately severe form of δβ thalassemia.

The $(\delta\beta)^0$ thalassemias nearly all result from long deletions involving the β globin gene complex. Sometimes they involve the $^A\gamma$ globin chains and hence the only active locus remaining is the $^G\gamma$ locus. In other cases the $^G\gamma$ and $^A\gamma$ loci are left intact and the deletion simply removes the δ and β globin genes; in these cases both the $^G\gamma$ and the $^A\gamma$ globin gene remains functional. For some reason, these long deletions allow persistent synthesis of the γ globin genes at a relatively high level during adult life, which helps to compensate for the absence of β and δ globin chain production. They are classified according to the kind of fetal hemoglobin that is produced, and hence into two varieties, $^G\gamma(^A\gamma\delta\beta)^0$ and $^G\gamma^A\gamma(\delta\beta)^0$ thalassemia; in line with other forms of thalassemia, they are best described by what is not produced: $(^A\gamma\delta\beta)^0$ and $(\delta\beta)^0$ thalassemia, respectively. Homozygotes produce only fetal hemoglobin, while heterozygotes have a thalassemic blood picture together with about 5–15% Hb F.

### Hereditary persistence of fetal hemoglobin

Genetically determined persistent fetal hemoglobin synthesis in adult life is of no clinical importance except that its genetic determinants can interact with the β thalassemias or structural hemoglobin variants; the resulting high level of Hb F production often ameliorates these conditions. The different forms of hereditary persistence of fetal hemoglobin (HPFH) result from either long deletions involving the δβ globin gene cluster, similar to those that cause (δβ)$^0$ thalassemia, or from point mutations that involve the promoters of the $^G$γ or $^A$γ globin gene. In the former case there is no β globin chain synthesis and therefore these conditions are classified as (δβ)$^0$ HPFH. In cases in which there are promoter mutations involving the γ globin genes, there is increased γ globin chain production in adult life associated with some β and δ chain synthesis in *cis* (i.e., directed by the same chromosome) to the HPFH mutations. Thus, depending on whether the point mutations involve the promoter of the $^G$γ or $^A$γ globin gene, these conditions are called $^G$γ β$^+$ HPFH and $^A$γ β$^+$ HPFH, respectively.

There is another family of HPFH-like disorders in which the genetic determinant is not encoded in the β chain cluster. In one case the determinant encodes on chromosome 6, although its nature has not yet been determined.

It should be pointed out that all these conditions are very heterogeneous and that many different deletions or point mutations have been discovered that produce the rather similar phenotypes of (δβ)$^0$ or $^G$γ or $^A$γ β$^+$ HPFH.

## Genotype–phenotype relationships in the thalassemias

It is now necessary briefly to relate the remarkably diverse molecular pathology described in the previous sections to the phenotypes observed in patients with these diseases. It is not possible to describe all these complex issues here. Rather we shall focus on those aspects that illustrate the more general principles of how abnormal gene action is reflected in a particular clinical picture. Perhaps the most important question that we will address is why patients with apparently identical genetic lesions have widely differing disorders, a problem that still bedevils the whole field of medical genetics, even in the molecular era.

### The β thalassemias

As we have seen, the basic defect that results from the 200 or more different mutations that underlie these conditions is reduced β globin chain production. Synthesis of the α globin chain proceeds normally and hence there is imbalanced globin chain output with an excess of α chains (Figure 1.8). Unpaired α chains precipitate in both red cell precursors and their progeny with the production of inclusion bodies. These interfere with normal red cell maturation and

survival in a variety of complex ways. Their attachment to the red cell membrane causes alterations in its structure, and their degradation products, notably heme, hemin (oxidized heme) and iron, result in oxidative damage to the red cell contents and membrane. These interactions result in intramedullary destruction of red cell precursors and in shortened survival of such cells as they reach the peripheral blood. The end result is an anemia of varying severity. This, in turn, causes tissue hypoxia and the production of relatively large amounts of erythropoietin; this leads to a massive expansion of the ineffective bone marrow, resulting in bone deformity, a hypermetabolic state with wasting and malaise, and bone fragility.

A large proportion of hemoglobin in the blood of β thalassemics is of the fetal variety. Normal individuals produce about 1% of Hb F, unevenly distributed among their red cells. In the bone marrow of β thalassemics, any red cell precursors that synthesize γ chains come under strong selection because they combine with α chains to produce fetal hemoglobin and therefore the degree of globin chain imbalance is reduced. Furthermore, the likelihood of γ chain production seems to be increased in a highly stimulated erythroid bone marrow. It seems likely that these two factors combine to increase the relative output of Hb F in this disorder. However, it has a higher oxygen affinity than Hb A and hence patients with β thalassemia are not able to adapt to low hemoglobin levels as well as those who have adult hemoglobin.

The greatly expanded, ineffective erythron leads to an increased rate of iron absorption; this, combined with iron received by blood transfusion, leads to progressive iron loading of the tissues, with subsequent liver, cardiac and endocrine damage.

The constant bombardment of the spleen with abnormal red cells leads to its hypertrophy. Hence there is progressive splenomegaly with an increased plasma volume and trapping of part of the circulating red cell mass in the spleen. This leads to worsening of the anemia. All these pathophysiological mechanisms, except for iron loading, can be reversed by regular blood transfusion which, in effect, shuts off the ineffective bone marrow and its consequences.

Thus it is possible to relate nearly all the important features of the severe forms of β thalassemia to the primary defect in globin gene action. However, can we also explain their remarkable clinical diversity?

#### Phenotypic diversity

Although the bulk of patients who are homozygous for β thalassemia mutations or compound heterozygotes for two different mutations have a severe transfusion-dependent

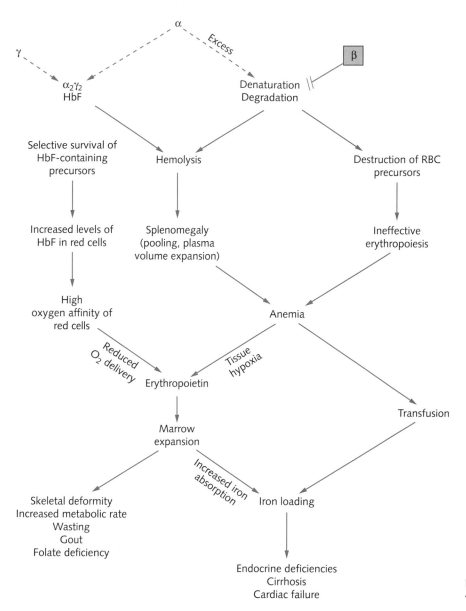

**Fig. 1.8 The pathophysiology of β thalassemia**

phenotype, there are many exceptions. Some patients of this type have a milder course, requiring few or even no transfusions, a condition called β thalassemia intermedia. A particularly important example of this condition is illustrated by the clinical findings in those who inherit β thalassemia from one parent and Hb E from the other, a disorder called Hb E/β thalassemia. Because the mutation that produces Hb E also opens up an alternative splice site in the first exon of the β globin gene, it is synthesized at a reduced rate and therefore behaves like a mild form of β thalassemia. It is the commonest hemoglobin variant globally and Hb E/β thalassemia is the commonest form of severe thalassemia in many Asian countries. It has an extraordinarily variable phenotype, ranging from a condition indistinguishable from β

thalassemia major to one of such mildness that patients grow and develop quite normally and never require transfusion.

Over recent years a great deal has been learnt about some of the mechanisms involved in this remarkable phenotypic variability. In short, it reflects both the action of modifying genes and variability in adaptation to anemia and, almost certainly, the effects of the environment. Given the complexity of these interactions, it is helpful to divide the genetic modifiers of the β thalassemia phenotype into primary, secondary and tertiary classes (Table 1.2).

The primary modifiers are the different β thalassemia alleles that can interact together. For example, compound heterozygotes for a severe $β^0$ thalassemia mutation and a milder one may have an intermediate form of β thalassemia

**Table 1.2** Mechanisms for the phenotypic diversity of the β thalassemias.

**Genetic modifiers**
Primary: alleles of varying severity
Secondary: modifiers of globin chain imbalance
  α Thalassemia
  Increased α globin genes: ααα or αααα
  Genes involved in unusually high Hb F response
Tertiary: modifiers of complications
  Iron absorption, bone disease, jaundice, infection

**Adaptation to anemia***
Variation in oxygen affinity ($P_{50}$) of hemoglobin
Variation in erythropoietin response to anemia

**Environmental**
Nutrition
Infection
Others

*There may be genetic variation in the adaptive mechanisms.

of varying severity depending on the degree of reduction in β globin synthesis under the action of the milder allele. This is undoubtedly one mechanism for the varying severity of Hb E/β thalassemia; it simply reflects the variable action of the β thalassemia mutation that is inherited together with Hb E. However, this explanation is not relevant in cases in which patients with identical β thalassemia mutations have widely disparate phenotypes.

The secondary modifiers are those which directly affect the degree of globin chain imbalance. Patients with β thalassemia who also inherit one or other form of α thalassemia tend to have a milder phenotype because of the reduction in the excess of α globin genes caused by the coexistent α thalassemia allele. Similarly, patients with severe forms of thalassemia who inherit more α genes than normal because their parents have triplicated or quadruplicated α gene arrangements tend to have more severe phenotypes. Other patients with severe thalassemia alleles appear to run a milder course because of a genetically determined ability to produce more γ globin chains and hence fetal hemoglobin, a mechanism that also results in a reduced degree of globin chain imbalance. It is now clear that several gene loci are involved in this mechanism; the best characterized is a polymorphism in the promoter region of the $^{G}$γ globin gene that appears to increase the output from this locus under conditions of hemopoietic stress. However, there are clearly other genes involved in increasing the output of Hb F. Recent genome-wide linkage studies have shown clear evidence that there are determinants on chromosomes 6 and 8 and a par-

ticularly strong association has been found with *BCL11A*, a transcription factor known to be involved in hematopoiesis. The exact mechanism for the associated increase in Hb F in β thalassemia and in sickle cell anemia remains to be determined.

The tertiary modifiers are those that have no effect on hemoglobin synthesis but which modify the many different complications of the β thalassemias, including osteoporosis, iron absorption, jaundice, and susceptibility to infection.

Although neglected until recently, it is also becoming apparent that variation in adaptation to anemia and the environment may also play a role in phenotypic modification of the β thalassemias. For example, patients with Hb E/β thalassemia have relatively low levels of Hb F and hence their oxygen dissociation curves are more right-shifted than patients with other forms of β thalassemia intermedia with significantly higher levels of Hb F. Very recent studies also suggest that the erythropoietin response to severe anemia for a given hemoglobin level varies considerably with age; patients during the first years of life have significantly higher responses to the same hemoglobin level than those who are older. This observation may go some way to explaining the variation in phenotype at different ages that has been observed in children with Hb E/β thalassemia. Finally, it is clear that further studies are required to dissociate the effects on the phenotype of genetic modifiers and environmental factors.

Thus the phenotypic variability of the β thalassemias reflects several layers of complex interactions involving genetic modifiers together with variation in adaptation and, almost certainly, the environment. These complex interactions are summarized in Table 1.2.

## The α thalassemias

The pathophysiology of the α thalassemias differs from that of the β thalassemias mainly because of the properties of the excess globin chains that are produced as a result of defective α chain synthesis. While the excess α chains produced in β thalassemia are unstable and precipitate, this is not the case in the α thalassemias, in which excess γ chains or β chains are able to form the soluble homotetramers $γ_4$ (Hb Bart's) and $β_4$ (Hb H) (Figure 1.9). Although these variants, particularly Hb H, are unstable and precipitate in older red cell populations, they remain soluble sufficiently long for the red cells to mature and develop relatively normally. Hence there is far less ineffective erythropoiesis in the α thalassemias and the main cause of the anemia is hemolysis associated with the precipitation of Hb H in older red cells. In addition, of course, there is a reduction in normal hemoglobin synthesis, which results in hypochromic, microcytic erythrocytes. Another important factor in the pathophysiology of the α

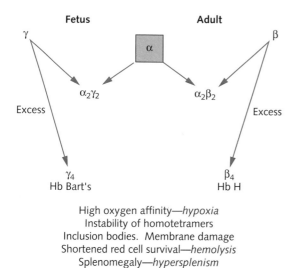

**Fig. 1.9 The pathophysiology of α thalassemia**

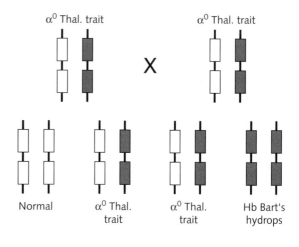

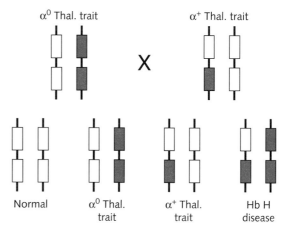

**Fig. 1.10 The genetics of the common forms of α thalassemia**
The open boxes represent normal α genes and the green boxes deleted α genes. The mating shown at the top shows how two α⁰ thalassemia heterozygotes can produce a baby with the Hb Bart's hydrops syndrome. In the mating at the bottom, between individuals with α⁰ and α⁺ thalassemia, one in four of the offspring will have Hb H disease.

thalassemias is the fact that Hb Bart's and Hb H are useless oxygen carriers, having an oxygen dissociation curve similar to that of myoglobin. Hence the circulating hemoglobin level may give a false impression of the oxygen-delivering capacity of the blood and patients may be symptomatic at relatively high hemoglobin levels.

The different clinical phenotypes of the α thalassemias are an elegant example of the effects of gene dosage (Figure 1.10). The heterozygous state for $\alpha^+$ thalassemia is associated with minimal hematological changes. That for $\alpha^0$ thalassemia (the loss of two α globin genes) is characterized by moderate hypochromia and microcytosis, similar to that of the β thalassemia trait. It does not matter whether the α genes are lost on the same chromosome or on opposite pairs of homologous chromosomes. Hence the homozygous state for $\alpha^+$ thalassemia, $-\alpha/-\alpha$, has a similar phenotype to the heterozygous state for $\alpha^0$ thalassemia ($--/\alpha\alpha$).

The loss of three α globin genes, which usually results from the compound heterozygous states for $\alpha^0$ and $\alpha^+$ thalassemia, is associated with a moderately severe anemia with the production of varying levels of Hb H. This condition, hemoglobin H disease, is characterized by varying anemia and splenomegaly with a marked shortening of red cell survival.

Finally, the homozygous state for $\alpha^0$ thalassemia ($--/--$) is characterized by death *in utero* or just after birth, with the clinical picture of hydrops fetalis. These babies produce no α chains and their hemoglobin consists mainly of Hb Bart's with variable persistence of embryonic hemoglobin. This is reflected in gross intrauterine hypoxia; although these babies may have hemoglobin values as high as 8–9 g/dL, most of it is unable to release its oxygen. This is reflected in the hydropic changes, a massive outpouring of nucleated red

cells, and hepatosplenomegaly with persistent hematopoiesis in the liver and spleen.

## Structural hemoglobin variants

The structural hemoglobin variants are described in detail in *Chapter 15*. Here, their molecular pathology and genotype–phenotype relationships are briefly outlined.

### Molecular pathology

The molecular pathology of the structural hemoglobin variants is much less complex than that of the thalassemias. The majority result from missense mutations – base substitutions that produce a codon change which encodes a different amino acid in the affected globin chain. Rarely, these variants result from more subtle alterations in the structure of the α/β globin chains. For example, shortened chains may result from internal deletions of their particular genes, while elongated chains result from either duplications within genes or frameshift mutations which allow the chain termination codon to be read through and in which additional amino acids are added to the C-terminal end. The majority of the 700 or more structural hemoglobin variants are of no clinical significance but a few, because they interfere with the stability or functions of the hemoglobin molecule, are associated with a clinical phenotype of varying severity.

## Genotype–phenotype relationships

### The sickling disorders

The sickling disorders represent the homozygous state for the sickle cell gene, sickle cell anemia, and the compound heterozygous state for the sickle cell gene and various structural hemoglobin variants, or β thalassemia. The chronic hemolysis and episodes of vascular occlusion and red cell sequestration that characterize sickle cell anemia can all be related to the replacement of the normal β6 glutamic acid by valine in Hb S. This causes a hydrophobic interaction with another hemoglobin molecule, triggering aggregation into large polymers. It is this change that causes the sickling distortion of the red blood cell and hence a marked decrease in its deformability. The resulting rigidity of the red cells is responsible for the vaso-occlusive changes that lead to many of the most serious aspects of all the sickling disorders.

The different conformations of sickle cells (banana-shaped or resembling a holly leaf) reflect different orientations of bundles of fibers along the long axis of the cell, the three-dimensional structure of which is constituted by a rope-like polymer composed of 14 strands. The rate and extent of polymer formation depend on the degree of oxygenation, the cellular hemoglobin concentration, and the presence or absence of Hb F. The latter inhibits polymerization and hence tends to ameliorate sickling. Polymerization of Hb S causes damage to the red cell membrane, the result of which is an irreversibly sickled cell. Probably the most important mechanism is cellular dehydration resulting from abnormalities of potassium/chloride cotransport and $Ca^{2+}$-activated potassium efflux. This is sufficient to trigger the $Ca^{2+}$-dependent (Gardos) potassium channel, providing a mechanism for the loss of potassium and water and leading to cellular dehydration.

However, the vascular pathology of the sickling disorders is not entirely related to the rigidity of sickled red cells. There is now a wealth of evidence that abnormal interactions between sickled cells and the vascular endothelium play a major role in the pathophysiology of the sickling disorders. Recently it has been demonstrated that nitric oxide may also play a role in some of the vascular complications of this disease. It has been found that nitric oxide reacts much more rapidly with free hemoglobin than with hemoglobin in erythrocytes and therefore it is possible that such decompartmentalization of hemoglobin into plasma, as occurs in sickle cell disease and other hemolytic anemias, diverts nitric oxide from its homeostatic vascular function.

### Unstable hemoglobin variants

There is a variety of different mechanisms underlying hemoglobin stability resulting from amino acid substitutions in different parts of the molecule. The first is typified by amino acid substitutions in the vicinity of the heme pocket, all of which lead to a decrease in stability of the binding of heme to globin. A second group of unstable variants results from amino acids that simply disrupt the secondary structure of the globin chains. About 75% of globin is in the form of α helix, in which proline cannot participate except as part of one of the initial three residues. At least 11 unstable hemoglobin variants have been described that result from the substitution of proline for leucine, five that are caused by the substitution of alanine by proline, and three in which proline is substituted for histidine. Another group of variants that causes disruption of the normal configuration of the hemoglobin molecule involves internal substitutions that somehow interfere with its stabilization by hydrophobic interactions. Finally, there are two groups of unstable hemoglobins that result from gross structural abnormalities of the globin subunits; many are due to deletions involving regions at or near interhelical corners. A few of the elongated globin chain variants are also unstable.

### Abnormal oxygen transport

There is a family of hemoglobin variants associated with high oxygen affinity and hereditary polycythemia. Most result from amino acid substitutions that affect the equilibrium between the R and T states (*see section Structure and function*). Thus, many of them result from amino acid substitutions at the $α_1$–$β_2$ interface, the C-terminal end of the β chain, and at the 2,3-DPG binding sites.

### Congenital cyanosis due to hemoglobin variants

There is a family of structural hemoglobin variants that is designated Hb M, to indicate congenital methemoglobinemia, and is further defined by their place of discovery. The iron atom of heme is normally linked to the imidazole group of the proximal histidine residue of the $\alpha$ and $\beta$ chains. There is another histidine residue on the opposite side, near the sixth coordination position of the heme iron; this, the so-called distal histidine residue, is the normal site of binding of oxygen. Several M hemoglobins result from the substitution of a tyrosine for either the proximal or distal histidine residue in the $\alpha$ or $\beta$ chain.

## Postscript

In this short account of the molecular pathology of hemoglobin we have considered how mutations at or close to the $\alpha$ or $\beta$ globin genes result in a diverse family of clinical disorders due to the defective synthesis of hemoglobin or its abnormal structure. Work in this field over the last 30 years has given us a fairly good idea of the repertoire of different mutations that underlie single-gene disorders and how these are expressed as discrete clinical phenotypes. Perhaps more importantly, however, the globin field has taught us how the interaction of a limited number of genes can produce a remarkably diverse series of clinical pictures, and something of the basis for how monogenic diseases due to the same mutation may vary widely in their clinical expression.

## Further reading

Bank A. (2006) Regulation of human fetal hemoglobin: new players, new complexities. *Blood*, **107**, 435–443.

Gibbons RJ, Wada T. (2004) ATRX and X-linked (alpha)-thalassemia mental retardation syndrome. In: Epstein CJ, Erickson RP, Wynshaw-Boris A (eds). *Inborn Errors of Development*. Oxford: Oxford University Press, pp. 747–757.

Higgs DR. (2004) Ham-Wasserman lecture: gene regulation in hematopoiesis: new lessons from thalassemia. *Hematology. American Society of Hematology Education Program*, 1–13.

Steinberg MH, Forget BG, Higgs DR, Weatherall DJ. (2008) *Disorders of Hemoglobin*, 2nd edn. Cambridge: Cambridge University Press.

Weatherall DJ. (2001) Phenotype–genotype relations in monogenic disease: lessons from the thalassaemias. *Nature Reviews. Genetics*, **2**, 245–255.

Weatherall DJ. (2004) Thalassaemia: the long road from bedside to genome. *Nature Reviews. Genetics*, **5**, 625–631.

Weatherall DJ, Clegg JB. (2001) *The Thalassaemia Syndromes*. Oxford: Blackwell.

# Chapter 2 Molecular cytogenetics and array-based genomic analysis

**Debra M Lillington[1], Silvana Debernardi[2] & Bryan D Young[3]**

[1] ICRF Medical Oncology Laboratory, Barts and The London School of Medicine & Dentistry, London, UK
[2] Cancer Research UK, Medical Oncology Unit, Barts and The London School of Medicine & Dentistry, London, UK
[3] Cancer Genomics Group, Medical Oncology Laboratory, Barts and The London School of Medicine & Dentistry, The Royal London Hospital, London, UK

## Introduction

The use of cytogenetics and molecular cytogenetic analysis in hematology has both increased and improved over the last decade. Fluorescence *in situ* hybridization (FISH) has been incorporated into most diagnostic laboratories to complement chromosome analysis and further improve its accuracy. In the era of risk-adapted and mutation-directed therapy, accurate assessment of genetic status is of paramount importance. In many current studies, patients are stratified on the basis of their cytogenetic or molecular rearrangements, since numerous disease- or subtype-specific abnormalities have independent prognostic outcomes. Such is the specificity of certain chromosomal rearrangements that molecular cytogenetic information can provide an unequivocal diagnosis of the type of malignancy. In national treatment trials for acute myeloid leukemia (AML) and acute lymphoblastic leukemia (ALL), cytogenetic information is vital to treatment stratification, and in other diseases, such as chronic lymphoblastic leukemia and myeloma, the impact of chromosomal abnormalities is now recognized.

Chromosomal analysis of metaphase cells provides a global assessment of karyotype and still plays a major role in modern tumor cytogenetics. FISH is used as a rapid sensitive test to complement G-band analysis, allowing the detection of cryptic or subtle changes. In addition, FISH can be used to screen non-dividing cell populations, such as bone marrow smears, tumor imprints and paraffin-embedded tissue sections (PETS). A vast array of FISH probes is currently available, aimed at detecting fusion genes, numerical abnormalities, chromosomal imbalance, chromosomal rearrangement and complex events. FISH has been further developed to allow the global detection of tumor-associated gain and loss using tumor DNA as a FISH probe against normal metaphase chromosomes. This technique is known as comparative genomic hybridization (CGH).

The recent introduction of high-resolution array-based techniques promises to further revolutionize the analysis of chromosomal aberrations in cancer. Oligonucleotide-based arrays can provide high-resolution analysis of copy number alterations. A variation of this approach is the single-nucleotide polymorphism (SNP) genotype array, which can provide both copy number and allelotype information. Gene expression profiling also offers exciting prospects in hematology and, coupled with the molecular cytogenetic and cytogenetic information, accurate diagnostic genetic analysis looks set to revolutionize patient management.

## FISH on metaphase chromosomes

The production of metaphase chromosomes from malignant cells plays a fundamental role in genetic analysis, allowing both G-banded chromosome analysis and subsequent FISH analysis. The chromosome offers a more versatile target than interphase cells since many types of FISH probes can be applied. In leukemia and lymphoma, gene fusions are relatively frequent and well characterized at the molecular level. These novel disease-associated fusion events arise through chromosomal translocations, inversions or insertions and are usually visible by routine karyotype analysis, although subtle abnormalities do exist and some of the recurrent rearrangements can be cryptic. FISH probes mapping to the unique sequences involved in these fusions are readily available and detect their respective abnormalities by one of two

*Molecular Hematology*, 3rd edition. Edited by Drew Provan and John Gribben.
© 2010 Blackwell Publishing.

methods. In the first strategy, probes mapping to the two genes involved are labeled in two distinct colors; as an example, the *BCR–ABL* (breakpoint cluster region–Abelson) fusion associated with the t(9;22)(q34;q11.2) is illustrated in Plate 2.1. *BCR* is represented by the green fluorescence and *ABL* by the red signal. The t(9;22) translocation results in both *BCR–ABL* and *ABL–BCR* fusions, and since the probe extends beyond the breakpoint for both genes, two fusion signals (red and green juxtaposed) are generated (dual fusion probes), one on the der(9), the other on the der(22). A normal 9 and a normal 22 (single red and green signal) will also exist. To further complicate the analysis, however, deviations from this pattern may exist since some patients carry deletions around the breakpoint and some harbor cryptic insertions of part of one gene, thereby generating only one of the fusion sequences (Plate 2.2). An alternative approach is to use four fluorescent probes to enhance the sensitivity and specificity to simultaneously detect translocations and deletions around the breakpoint, which may confer independent prognostic value. Plate 2.3 shows a cryptic insertion of part of the *RARA* gene (chromosome 17) into the *PML* locus (chromosome 15) in a patient with acute promyelocytic leukemia. The t(15;17)(q21;q11) translocation is the hallmark of acute promyelocytic leukemia and is cytogenetically visible in 90% of patients.

The second common type of FISH strategy is the "break apart" probe, specifically designed to detect abnormalities affecting one specific gene which rearranges with multiple partner loci, such as *MLL* (11q23). Over 60 different *MLL* gene translocations have been cytogenetically reported, and the FISH probe used most often for diagnosis consists of a probe mapping above the breakpoint labeled with one color and a second probe mapping below the breakpoint in another color. Translocations involving *MLL* therefore result in the separation of one set of probes (Plate 2.4) and the displaced *MLL* signal will map to the partner chromosome. Single-color probes extending across the breakpoints can also be used, resulting in a split signal.

Unique sequence probes can also be used to screen for copy number changes, particularly in cases with evidence of additional genetic material, by karyotyping such as double minute chromosomes, homogeneously staining regions or additional pieces of chromosomes. Double minute chromosomes and homogeneously staining regions are manifestations of gene amplification and in certain malignant diseases, particularly solid tumors, are well-recognized mechanisms for oncogene activation. FISH probes mapping to the genes commonly associated with amplification can very quickly confirm the presence of multiple copies of genes; an example is N-*myc* in neuroblastoma. Plate 2.5 shows a bone marrow aspirate infiltrated by neuroblastoma and multiple copies of N-*myc*. Alpha satellite probes are often used to determine chromosome number. Hyperdiploidy is a frequent phenomenon in ALL and is associated with a common pattern of gain, namely chromosomes 4, 6, 10, 14, 17, 18, 21 and X. Using a selected cocktail of alpha satellite probes mapping to these chromosomes, hyperdiploidy can be detected in both metaphase and interphase cells (Plate 2.6). Metaphase cells derived from leukemic blasts of patients with ALL can often have poor morphology and be difficult to fully characterize. In such situations FISH can be of particular value since it may help elucidate chromosomal gains and losses.

Whole-chromosome painting probes (WCPs), consisting of pools of DNA sequences mapping along the full length of a particular chromosome and labeled with a fluorochrome, can be used individually or in combination to characterize abnormalities whose origin is uncertain by G-banding. In simple karyotypes, requiring confirmation of a suspected rearrangement, two-color chromosome painting might be the most useful option (Plate 2.7). In more complex karyotypes, such as those associated with therapy-related leukemia, a mixture of WCPs mapping to all 24 human chromosomes (24-color karyotyping) is probably the most informative. Multiplex (M)-FISH/spectral karyotyping (SKY) is not used routinely for diagnostic purposes but has revealed cryptic rearrangements in several studies. M-FISH/ SKY uses a combinatorial labeling approach such that each individual chromosome paint is labeled with a unique combination of not more than five fluorochromes. The 24 differentially labeled paints are then applied in a single hybridization assay and visualization is achieved using one of two strategies. M-FISH uses a series of optical filters to collect the images from the different fluorochromes, which are then merged into a composite image; a pseudocolor is then assigned to each chromosome on the basis of its fluorochrome combination (Plate 2.8). SKY uses an interferometer with Fourier transformation to determine the spectral characteristics of each pixel in the image, and assigns a pseudocolor.

## FISH on nuclei

The non-dividing cell population can be examined using FISH probes to yield both diagnostic and prognostic molecular cytogenetic information. Interphase cells from the sample sent for cytogenetic analysis (peripheral blood, bone marrow, lymph node, etc.), tumor touch imprints, PETS and bone marrow smears can be used as the target for FISH. In these instances screening for a specific chromosomal abnormality is performed, thereby allowing detection or exclusion of a single event per FISH assay. Techniques that involve the use of whole or chromosome-specific probes cannot readily be applied to interphase cells. PETS are sometimes the only tumor sample available for analysis since the paraffin treatment preserves the morphology of the tumor, thereby enabling histological diagnosis. However, if histology is equivocal, FISH for a tumor-associated chromosomal abnormality can be extremely valuable for diagnostic purposes. FISH on PETS does have inherent technical problems not found with FISH on other sample types; for example, probe accessibility is reduced, the thickness of the section means that the resulting FISH signals may not all be visible in the same focal plane, and the cells may be very tightly packed, making analysis more difficult. Interphase cells can be used to assess the copy number of unique sequences/ alpha satellites or to look for chimeric fusion genes. Plate 2.9 illustrates two PETS screened for the presence of the *EWS/ FLI1* rearrangement associated with Ewing's sarcoma/primitive neuroectodermal tumor.

## Comparative genomic hybridization and SNP array analysis

CGH provides a global assessment of copy number changes, revealing regions of the chromosome that are either gained or lost in the tumor sample. A key feature of this technique is that dividing tumor cells are not required. DNA is extracted from the tumor, labeled (usually) with a green fluorochrome and compared with DNA from a normal reference labeled with a red fluorochrome. Labeled test and reference DNA are combined and hybridized to normal chromosomes and the resulting ratio of the two signals along the length of the chromosomes reflects the differences in copy number between the tumor and reference DNA samples (Plate 2.10). Regions of gain in the tumor DNA are represented by an increased green/red ratio whereas deletions are indicated by a reduced ratio. CGH requires 50% abnormal cells to be present within the tumor sample for reliable detection of genomic imbalance and will not easily detect regions involving less than 10 Mb of DNA unless it involves high-level amplification. Nevertheless, CGH is particularly applicable to the analysis of solid tumors since DNA can be readily extracted from them and the karyotype frequently involves loss or gain of whole or partial chromosomes.

The use of genomic DNA arrays as the hybridization target allows much higher resolution for the detection of copy number changes. Currently the highest resolution is provided by commercial oligonucleotide arrays. Array CGH has the potential to provide a highly sensitive and unbiased global assessment of gene copy number. Additionally such arrays can detect small focal deletions which are well below the level of detection of conventional cytogenetics. Oligonucleotide arrays have been developed that are directed against known SNPs. Several million SNPs have been defined

in the human genome and the highest resolution arrays encode approximately 900 000 SNPs. Such arrays can be used to provide high-resolution genotype and copy number information for the entire genome of the cancer cell. They have been particularly useful in the detection of loss of heterozygosity (LOH) in leukemias. The application of SNP arrays to a series of AML samples has uncovered large-scale

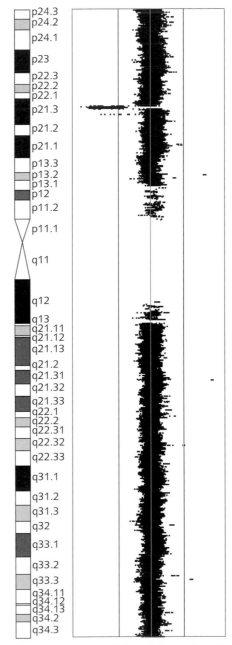

**Fig. 2.1** High-resolution SNP analysis (SNP6) reveals a microdeletion of the *CDKN2A* locus on chromosome 9p in an acute lymphoblastic leukemia.

regions of LOH that were not associated with copy number changes. These regions are the consequence of mitotic recombination and have been termed *acquired uniparental disomy*. It has been further shown that these events appear to render the cell homozygous for a pre-existing mutation in genes such *FLT3*, *WT1*, *CEBPA* and *RUNX1*.

The application of SNP arrays to a series of ALL samples has detected a high frequency of small focal deletions in certain genes. This appears to be much more frequent than in a similar series of AML samples and may be characteristic of ALL. An example of such a deletion affecting the *CDKN2A* gene on chromosome 9p is illustrated in Figure 2.1.

## Gene expression profiling

The introduction of microarrays for gene expression profiling now offers a new approach to molecular cytogenetics. Measurement of the expression of all the genes in a range of tissues or cell types allows the determination of the transcriptional status of the cell, identifying which genes are active and which are silent. Microarrays for expression profiling consist of systematic arrays of cDNA or oligonucleotides of known sequence that are spotted or synthesized at discrete loci on a glass or silicon surface. They allow the simultaneous analysis of a large number of genes at high resolution following the hybridization of labeled cDNA or cRNA derived from the samples to be examined. Microarray output is represented by a large number of individual data points that must be analyzed by a data-mining program in order to correlate the data, and to group them together in a meaningful manner. In recent years, the use of DNA microarrays has been largely devoted to the genetic profiling of tumor subtypes, with the aims of defining new classes with prognostic and diagnostic relevance and of increasing our knowledge of the mechanisms underlying the biology of these diseases. The pathological diagnosis and classification of human neoplasia is based on well-defined morphological, cytochemical, immunophenotypic and clinical criteria. For leukemia and lymphoma, the relevance of cytogenetics as one of the most valuable prognostic determinants at diagnosis has come from analysis of the leukemia karyotype. This has identified non-random somatically acquired translocations, inversions and deletions, which are often associated with specific morphological subtypes. However, leukemias with apparently normal karyotypes do exist and constitute the largest single subgroup (up to 40% of cases). Thus, the application of microarray analysis may improve the classification of leukemias and offer clues to the underlying etiology. A molecular classification would have the potential to define new subgroups with more prognostic and therapeutic significance, linking the expression profile to the outcome.

It could offer many advantages over conventional classification methods, including the possibility of deducing chromosomal data from non-dividing cells.

Three basic steps for efficient and effective data analysis are necessary: data normalization, data filtering, and pattern identification. To compare expression values directly, it is necessary to apply some sort of normalization strategy to the data, either between paired samples or across a set of experiments. To "normalize" in the context of DNA microarrays means to standardize the data so as to be able to differentiate between real (biological) variations in gene expression levels and variations due to the measurement process. Gene expression data can then be subjected to a variation filter, which excludes uninformative genes (i.e., genes showing minimal variation across the samples) and genes expressed below or above a user-defined threshold. This step facilitates the search for partners and groups in the data that can be used to assign biological meaning to the expression profiles, leading to the production of straightforward lists of increasing or decreasing genes or of more complex associations with the help of sophisticated clustering and visualization programs. Hierarchical clustering is used traditionally in phylogenetic analysis for the classification of organisms into trees; in the microarray context it is applied to genes and samples. Organisms sharing properties tend to be clustered together. The length of a branch containing two organisms can be considered a measure of how different the organisms are. It is possible to classify genes in a similar manner, gathering those whose expression patterns are similar into clusters in the tree. Such mock-phylogenetic trees are often referred to as dendrograms. Genes can also be grouped on the basis of their expression patterns using *k-means clustering*. The goal is to produce groups of genes with a high degree of similarity within each group and a low degree of similarity between groups. The self-organizing map is a clustering technique similar to k-means clustering, but in addition illustrates the relationship between groups by arranging them in a two-dimensional map. Self-organizing maps are useful for visualizing the number of distinct expression patterns in the data. A complex dataset can also be reduced to a few specified dimensions by applying multidimensional scaling, so that the relationships between groups can be more effectively visualized.

The first classification of cancer on the basis of gene expression showed that it was possible to distinguish between myeloid and lymphoid acute leukemias by the use of arrays with approximately 6800 human genes. Since then, the coverage of gene expression arrays has been expanded to include most known genes and more recently to include the exons of known genes. This approach has been applied successfully to the classification of hematological malignancies and a large variety of solid tumors. Acute lymphoid leukemias with rearrangements of the *MLL* gene were shown to have expression patterns that could allow them to be distinguished from ALLs and AMLs without the *MLL* translocations. Further microarray analysis of AML cases with a favorable outcome – AML M2 with t(8;21), AML M3 or M3v with t(15;17) and AML M4eo with inv(16) – has shown a specific pattern of predictor genes associated with the three subclasses. In a subsequent microarray study, AML samples were specifically chosen to represent the spectrum of known karyotypes common in AML and included examples with AML-FAB phenotypes from M1 to M5. Hierarchical clustering sorted the profiles into separate groups, each representing one of the major cytogenetic classes in AML [i.e., t(8;21), t(15;17), inv(16), 11q23] and a normal karyotype, as shown in Plate 2.11. Statistical analysis identified genes whose expression was strongly correlated with these chromosomal classes. Importantly in this study, the AMLs with a normal karyotype were characterized by distinctive upregulation of certain members of the class I homeobox A and B gene families, implying a common underlying genetic lesion. These data reveal novel diagnostic and therapeutic targets and demonstrate the potential of microarray-based dissection of AML. The cluster analysis presented here illustrates the potential of expression profiling to distinguish the major subclasses. An important conclusion of expression profiling studies is that the major cytogenetic events in AML have associated expression signatures. This could form the basis of customized DNA arrays designed to classify leukemia.

# Further reading

## FISH on metaphase chromosomes and nuclei

Bayani JM, Squire JA. (2002) Applications of SKY in cancer cytogenetics. *Cancer Investigation*, **20**, 373–386.

Dave BJ, Nelson M, Pickering DL et al. (2002) Cytogenetic characterization of diffuse large cell lymphoma using multi-color fluorescence in situ hybridization. *Cancer Genetics and Cytogenetics*, **132**, 125–132.

Dierlamm J, Stul M, Vranckx H et al. (1998) FISH identifies inv(16)(p13q22) masked by translocations in three cases of acute myeloid leukemia. *Genes, Chromosomes and Cancer*, **22**, 87–94.

Fischer K, Scholl C, Salat J et al. (1996) Design and validation of DNA probe sets for a comprehensive interphase cytogenetic analysis of acute myeloid leukemia. *Blood*, **88**, 3962–3971.

Grimwade D, Gorman P, Duprez E et al. (1997) Characterization of cryptic rearrangements and variant translocations in acute promyelocytic leukemia. *Blood*, **90**, 4876–4885.

Hagemeijer A, de Klein A, Wijsman J et al. (1998) Development of an interphase fluorescent in situ hybridization (FISH) test to detect t(8;21) in AML patients. *Leukemia*, **12**, 96–101.

Jabber Al-Obaidi MS, Martineau M, Bennett CF et al. (2002) ETV6/AML1 fusion by FISH in adult acute lymphoblastic leukemia. *Leukemia*, **16**, 669–74.

Johnson PW, Leek J, Swinbank K et al. (1997) The use of fluorescent in situ hybridization for detection of the t(2;5)(p23;q35) translocation in anaplastic large-cell lymphoma. *Annals of Oncology*, **8** (Suppl 2), 65–69.

Kasprzyk A, Secker-Walker LM. (1997) Increased sensitivity of minimal residual disease detection by interphase FISH in acute lymphoblastic leukemia with hyperdiploidy. *Leukemia*, **11**, 429–435.

Kearney L, Bower M, Gibbons B et al. (1992) Chromosome 11q23 translocations in both infant and adult acute leukemias are detected by in situ hybridisation with a yeast artificial chromosome. *Blood*, **80**, 1659–1665.

Ketterling RP, Wyatt WA, VanWier SA et al. (2002) Primary myelodysplastic syndrome with normal cytogenetics: utility of "FISH panel testing" and M-FISH. *Leukemia Research*, **26**, 235–240.

Lu XY, Harris CP, Cooley L et al. (2002) The utility of spectral karyotyping in the cytogenetic analysis of newly diagnosed pediatric acute lymphoblastic leukemia. *Leukemia*, **16**, 2222–2227.

Mancini M, Nanni M, Cedrone M et al. (1995) Combined cytogenetic, FISH and molecular analysis in acute promyelocytic leukaemia at diagnosis and in complete remission. *British Journal of Haematology*, **91**, 878–884.

Mathew P, Sanger WG, Weisenburger DD et al. (1997) Detection of the t(2;5)(p23;q35) and NPM–ALK fusion in non-Hodgkin's lymphoma by two-color fluorescence in situ hybridization. *Blood*, **89**, 1678–1685.

Monteil M, Callanan M, Dascalescu C et al. (1996) Molecular diagnosis of t(11;14) in mantle cell lymphoma using two-colour interphase fluorescence in situ hybridization. *British Journal of Haematology*, **93**, 656–660.

Mrozek K, Heinonen K, Theil KS et al. (2002) Spectral karyotyping in patients with acute myeloid leukemia and a complex karyotype shows hidden aberrations, including recurrent overrepresentation of 21q, 11q, and 22q. *Genes, Chromosomes and Cancer*, **34**, 137–153.

Nanjangud G, Rao PH, Hegde A et al. (2002) Spectral karyotyping identifies new rearrangements, translocations, and clinical associations in diffuse large B-cell lymphoma. *Blood*, **99**, 2554–2561.

Paternoster SF, Brockman SR, McClure RF et al. (2002) A new method to extract nuclei from paraffin-embedded tissue to study lymphomas using interphase fluorescence in situ hybridization. *American Journal of Pathology*, **160**, 1967–1972.

Schrock E, du Manoir S, Veldman T et al. (1996) Multicolor spectral karyotyping of human chromosomes. *Science*, **273**, 494–497.

Siebert R, Matthiesen P, Harder S et al. (1998) Application of interphase fluorescence in situ hybridization for the detection of the Burkitt translocation t(8;14)(q24;q32) in B-cell lymphomas. *Blood*, **91**, 984–990.

Sinclair PB, Green AR, Grace C et al. (1997) Improved sensitivity of BCR–ABL detection: a triple-probe three-color fluorescence in situ hybridization system. *Blood*, **90**, 1395–1402.

Speicher MR, Gwyn Ballard S, Ward DC. (1996) Karyotyping human chromosomes by combinatorial multi-fluor FISH. *Nature Genetics*, **12**, 368–375.

Suijkerbuijk RF, Matthopoulos D, Kearney L *et al.* (1992) Fluorescent in situ identification of human marker chromosomes using flow sorting and Alu element-mediated PCR. *Genomics*, **13**, 355–362.

Takashima T, Itoh M, Ueda Y *et al.* (1997) Detection of 14q32.33 translocation and t(11;14) in interphase nuclei of chronic B-cell leukemia/lymphomas by in situ hybridization. *International Journal of Cancer*, **72**, 31–38.

Telenius H, Pelmear AH, Tunnacliffe A *et al.* (1992) Cytogenetic analysis by chromosome painting using DOP-PCR amplified flow-sorted chromosomes. *Genes, Chromosomes and Cancer*, **4**, 257–263.

Ueda Y, Nishida K, Miki T *et al.* (1997) Interphase detection of BCL6/IgH fusion gene in non-Hodgkin lymphoma by fluorescence in situ hybridization. *Cancer Genetics and Cytogenetics*, **99**, 102–107.

Van Limbergen H, Poppe B, Michaux L *et al.* (2002) Identification of cytogenetic subclasses and recurring chromosomal aberrations in AML and MDS with complex karyotypes using M-FISH. *Genes, Chromosomes and Cancer*, **33**, 60–72.

Veldman T, Vignon C, Schrock E *et al.* (1997) Hidden chromosome abnormalities in haematological malignancies detected by multicolour spectral karyotyping. *Nature Genetics*, **15**, 406–410.

von Bergh A, Emanuel B, van Zelderen-Bhola S *et al.* (2000) A DNA probe combination for improved detection of MLL/11q23 breakpoints by double-color interphase-FISH in acute leukemias. *Genes, Chromosomes and Cancer*, **28**, 14–22.

## CGH and SNP array analysis

Avet-Loiseau H, Andree-Ashley LE, Moore D *et al.* (1997) Molecular cytogenetic abnormalities in multiple myeloma and plasma cell leukemia measured using comparative genomic hybridization. *Genes, Chromosomes and Cancer*, **19**, 124–133.

Avet-Loiseau H, Vigier M, Moreau A *et al.* (1997) Comparative genomic hybridization detects genomic abnormalities in 80% of follicular lymphomas. *British Journal of Haematology*, **97**, 119–122.

Barth TFE, Dohner H, Werner CA *et al.* (1998) Characteristic pattern of chromosomal gains and losses in primary large B-cell lymphomas of the gastrointestinal tract. *Blood*, **91**, 4321–4330.

Bentz M, Plesch A, Stilgenbauer S *et al.* (1998) Minimal sizes of deletions detected by comparative genomic hybridization. *Genes, Chromosomes and Cancer*, **21**, 172–175.

Cai WW, Mao JH, Chow CW *et al.* (2002) Genome-wide detection of chromosomal imbalances in tumors using BAC microarrays. *Nature Biotechnology*, **20**, 393–396.

Carter NP, Fiegler H, Piper J. (2002) Comparative analysis of comparative genomic hybridization microarray technologies: report of a workshop sponsored by the Wellcome Trust. *Cytometry*, **49**, 43–48.

Cigudosa JC, Rao PH, Calasanz MJ *et al.* (1998) Characterization of nonrandom chromosomal gains and losses in multiple myeloma by comparative genomic hybridization. *Blood*, **91**, 3007–3010.

El-Rifai W, Elonen E, Larramendy M *et al.* (1997) Chromosomal breakpoints and changes in DNA copy number in refractory acute myeloid leukemia. *Leukemia*, **11**, 958–963.

Fitzgibbon J, Iqbal S, Davies A *et al.* (2007) Genome-wide detection of recurring sites of uniparental disomy in follicular and transformed follicular lymphoma. *Leukemia*, **21**, 1514–1520.

Forozan F, Karhu R, Kononen J *et al.* (1997) Genome screening by comparative genomic hybridization. *Trends in Genetics*, **13**, 405–409.

Gupta M, Raghavan M, Gale RE *et al.* (2008) Novel regions of acquired uniparental disomy discovered in acute myeloid leukemia. *Genes Chromosomes and Cancer*, **47**, 729–739.

Haas O, Henn T, Romanakis K *et al.* (1998) Comparative genomic hybridization as part of a new diagnostic strategy in childhood hyperdiploid acute lymphoblastic leukemia. *Leukemia*, **12**, 474–481.

Houldsworth J, Mathew S, Rao PH *et al.* (1996) REL proto-oncogene is frequently amplified in extranodal diffuse large cell lymphoma. *Blood*, **87**, 25–29.

Joos S, Otano-Joos MI, Ziegler S *et al.* (1996) Primary mediastinal (thymic) B-cell lymphoma is characterized by gains of chromosomal material including 9p and amplification of the REL gene. *Blood*, **87**, 1571–1578.

Kallioniemi A, Kallioniemi OP, Sudar D *et al.* (1992) Comparative genomic hybridization for molecular cytogenetic analysis of solid tumors. *Science*, **258**, 818–821.

Karhu R, Knuutila S, Kallioniemi OP *et al.* (1997) Frequent loss of the 11q14–24 region in chronic lymphocytic leukemia: a study by comparative genomic hybridization. Tampere CLL Group. *Genes, Chromosomes and Cancer*, **19**, 286–290.

Karhu R, Siitonen S, Tanner M *et al.* (1997) Genetic aberrations in pediatric acute lymphoblastic leukemia by comparative genomic hybridization. *Cancer Genetics and Cytogenetics*, **95**, 123–129.

Monni O, Oinonen R, Elonen E *et al.* (1998) Gain of 3q and deletion of 11q22 are frequent aberrations in mantle cell lymphoma. *Genes, Chromosomes and Cancer*, **21**, 298–307.

Paszek-Vigier M, Talmant P, Mechinaud F *et al.* (1997) Comparative genomic hybridization is a powerful tool, complementary to cytogenetics, to identify chromosomal abnormalities in childhood acute lymphoblastic leukaemia. *British Journal of Haematology*, **99**, 589–596.

Paulsson K, Cazier JB, Macdougall F *et al.* (2008) Microdeletions are a general feature of adult and adolescent acute lymphoblastic leukemia: unexpected similarities with pediatric disease. *Proceedings of the National Academy of Sciences of the United States of America*, **105**, 6708–6713.

Raghavan M, Lillington DM, Skoulakis S *et al.* (2005) Genome-wide single nucleotide polymorphism analysis reveals frequent partial uniparental disomy due to somatic recombination in acute myeloid leukemias. *Cancer Research*, **65**, 375–378.

Rao PH, Houldsworth J, Dyomina K *et al.* (1998) Chromosomal and gene amplification in diffuse large B-cell lymphoma. *Blood*, **92**, 234–240.

Solinas-Toldo S, Lampel S, Stilgenbauer S *et al.* (1997) Matrix-based comparative genomic hybridization: biochips to screen for genomic imbalances. *Genes, Chromosomes and Cancer*, **20**, 399–407.

Wessendorf S, Schwaenen C, Kohlhammer H *et al.* (2003) Hidden gene amplifications in aggressive B-cell non-Hodgkin lymphomas detected by microarray-based comparative genomic hybridization. *Oncogene*, **22**, 1425–1429.

## Expression profiling

Armstrong SA, Staunton JE, Silverman LB *et al.* (2002) MLL translocations specify a distinct gene expression profile that distinguishes a unique leukemia. *Nature Genetics*, **30**, 41–47.

Debernardi S, Lillington DM, Chaplin T *et al.* (2003) Genome-wide analysis of acute myeloid leukemia with normal karyotype reveal a unique pattern of homeobox gene expression distinct from those with translocation-mediated fusion events. *Genes, Chromosomes and Cancer*, **37**, 149–158.

Golub TR. (2001) Genomic approaches to the pathogenesis of hematologic malignancy. *Current Opinion in Hematology*, **8**, 252–261.

Golub TR. (2001) Genome-wide views of cancer. *New England Journal of Medicine*, **344**, 601–602.

Golub TR, Slonim DK, Tamayo P *et al.* (1999) Molecular classification of cancer: class discovery and class prediction by gene expression monitoring. *Science*, **286**, 531–537.

Schoch C, Kohlmann A, Schnittger S *et al.* (2002) Acute myeloid leukemias with reciprocal rearrangements can be distinguished by specific gene expression profiles. *Proceedings of the National Academy of Sciences of the United States of America*, **99**, 10008–10013.

Shipp MA, Ross KN, Tamayo P *et al.* (2002) Diffuse large B-cell lymphoma outcome prediction by gene-expression profiling and supervised machine learning. *Nature Medicine*, **8**, 68–74.

Tamayo P, Slonim D, Mesirov J *et al.* (1999) Interpreting patterns of gene expression with self-organizing maps: methods and application to hematopoietic differentiation. *Proceedings of the National Academy of Sciences of the United States of America*, **96**, 2907–2912.

Yeang CH, Ramaswamy S, Tamayo P *et al.* (2001) Molecular classification of multiple tumor types. *Bioinformatics*, **17**, S316–S322.

Yeoh EJ, Ross ME, Shurtleff SA *et al.* (2002) Classification, subtype discovery, and prediction of outcome in pediatric acute lymphoblastic leukemia by gene expression profiling. *Cancer Cell*, **1**, 133–143.

# Chapter 3 Stem cells

## Eyal C Attar[1] & David T Scadden[2]

[1] Harvard Medical School, Massachusetts General Hospital, Boston, MA, USA
[2] Harvard Medical School; Harvard Stem Cell Institute; and Center for Regenerative Medicine, Massachusetts General Hospital, Boston, MA, USA

## Introduction

The generation of sufficient numbers of blood cells to maintain homeostasis requires sustained production of mature cells. This process, called *hematopoiesis*, yields approximately $10^{10}$ blood cells daily, with capability for dramatic increases in the number and subsets of cells in response to physiological stress. Hematopoiesis is therefore a highly dynamic process dependent upon numerous modulating factors. Its prodigious production capability derives from the sustained presence of a cell type which is generally quiescent, but the descendants of which proliferate vigorously. This cell is the hematopoietic stem cell (HSC).

## Stem cell definitions and distinctions

Stem cells derive their name from their ability to produce daughter cells of different types. Stem cells are defined by a combination of the traits of self-maintenance and the ability to produce multiple, varied offspring. Putting this in more biological terms, stem cells have the unique and defining characteristics of *self-renewal* and of *differentiation into multiple cell types*. Thus, with each cell division there is an inherent asymmetry in stem cells that is generally not found with other cell types.

While their name implies that stem cells have specific intrinsic characteristics, there are multiple different types of stem cells, each defined by their production ability. *Totipotent* stem cells are capable of generating any type of cell in the body, including those of the extra-embryonic tissues, such as the placental tissues (Figure 3.1). *Pluripotent* stem cells may give rise to any type of cell found in the body except those of the extra-embryonic membranes. They can produce ectoderm, mesoderm or endoderm cells. Recently, it has also become possible to create pluripotent cell by "reprogramming" mature cells. Pluripotent stem cells include embryonic stem cells, isolated from the inner cell mass of the blastocyst, embryonic germ cells, isolated from embryonic gonad precursors, and embryonic carcinoma cells, isolated from teratocarcinomas. Pluripotent stem cells may be maintained indefinitely in culture under specialized conditions that prevent differentiation. In particular, embryonic stem cells have been used to generate "knockout" mice, animals harboring targeted gene disruptions via homologous recombination that permit the *in vivo* study of individual gene function. Lastly, *multipotent* stem cells, such as the HSCs of the bone marrow, are capable of giving rise to multiple mature cell types, but only those of a particular tissue, such as blood. Multipotent stem cells are found in adults, perhaps in all tissue, and function to replace dead or damaged tissue. Such stem cells are commonly referred to as "adult" stem cells.

## Hematopoietic stem cell concepts and their origin

### The cellular compartment model

The short-lived nature of most blood cells was first deduced in the 1960s using thymidine labeling of reinfused blood. These studies demonstrated that the maintenance of normal numbers of blood cells in the adult requires a process with the capacity to briskly generate large numbers of mature cells

*Molecular Hematology*, 3rd edition. Edited by Drew Provan and John Gribben.
© 2010 Blackwell Publishing.

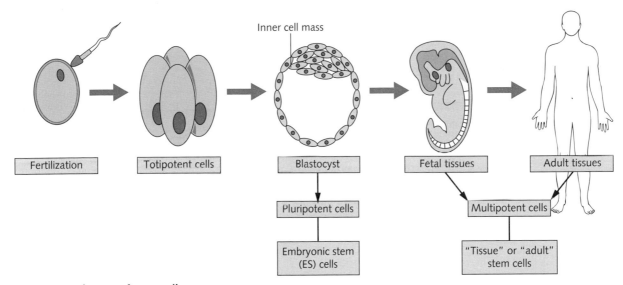

**Fig. 3.1 Sources and types of stem cells**
Adapted with gratitude from the National Institutes of Health Stem Cell Information website.

along multiple blood lineages. The early history of HSC research was largely shaped by cellular biology and animal transplantation experiments. It was advanced by experiments in the early 1960s demonstrating that injection of marrow cells could generate large hematopoietic colonies in the spleen of irradiated mice. Such colonies were the clonal progeny of single initiating cells, termed *colony-forming units, spleen* (CFU-S), and contained hematopoietic populations of multiple lineages. CFU-S were further transplantable, demonstrating the self-renewing nature of CFU-S. HSCs are a minor component of marrow cells, able both to generate large numbers of progeny differentiated along multiple lines and to renew themselves.

The field was further advanced by the use of *in vitro* cell culture techniques; in particular, solid-state cultures of marrow and spleen cells furthered understanding of the colony-forming capacity of individual hematopoietic cells. The original technique demonstrated clonal colonies of granulocytes and/or macrophages, termed *in vitro colony-forming cells* (CFCs), which are now considered lineage-committed progenitor cells. These cells could be separated from whole marrow cells and from CFU-S, were more numerous than CFU-S, and could be detected in splenic colonies as the progeny of CFU-S. These observations gave rise to the concept of the *three-compartment model of hematopoiesis*, the compartments being stem cells, progenitor cells, and dividing mature cells in increasing numbers; each compartment consists of the amplified progeny of cells in the preceding compartment.

Subsequent analyses have added further complexity to the compartment model of hematopoiesis. The term CFU-S

describes at least two groups of precursor cells. One group, arising from committed progenitors with little capacity for self-renewal, gives rise to colonies that peak in size by day 8, while a second, arising from a more primitive cell that is capable of self-renewal, yields colonies that peak in size at day 12. To further highlight the complexity of the hematopoietic hierarchy, a rarer population of hematopoietic cells provides longer-term repopulation of an irradiated host than CFU-S. These long-term repopulating cells have the capacity for sustained self-renewal and were considered the true adult stem cells. The presence of stromal cells in the cultures is important for the long-term culture of CFU-S and repopulating cells. Cells capable of long-term survival in culture on stroma were termed *long-term culture-initiating cells* (LTC-ICs) and *cobblestone area-forming cells* (CAFCs). These multipotential cell types were considered more primitive than lineage-committed progenitor cells but more mature than long-term repopulating cells.

Thus, a more complex version of the compartmental model has emerged. This provides a model with two populations of stem cells, the most immature group consisting of long-term repopulating cells and a more mature group of short-term repopulating cells. An intermediate group consisting of preprogenitor cells (blast colony-forming cells) follows, leading to a larger population of lineage-committed progenitor cells. This large group of committed progenitors is stratified on the basis of the number of progeny they are able to generate. The immediate progeny of progenitor cells, cluster-forming cells, have less proliferative capacity. Subsequent progenitors (CFCs) have the capacity to give rise to colonies of clonal origin in semisolid media containing

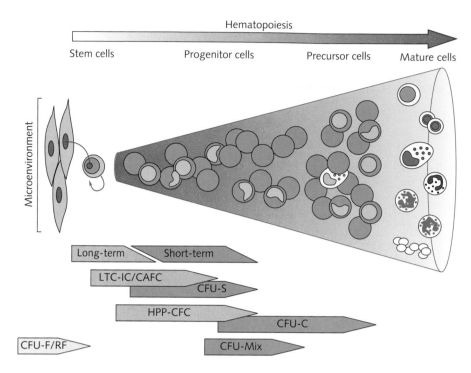

Long-term — Short-term

LTC-IC/CAFC

CFU-S

HPP-CFC

CFU-C

CFU-F/RF

CFU-Mix

**Fig. 3.2 Schematic view of hematopoiesis**
See text for definition of abbreviations. Modified from Figure 12.1 in *Hematology: Basic Principles and Practice*, 3rd edn (ed. R. Hoffman), 2000, with permission from Elsevier.

fully mature cells, permitting their analysis. A more mature set of precursor cells constitutes the bulk of bone marrow cells and has unique, identifiable features by light microscopy. Rapid division of precursor cells culminates in the production of mature cells. Although hematopoiesis proceeds according to this orderly scheme (Figure 3.2), special consideration must be given to the development of T and B lymphocytes. These cells are generated in the thymus and bone marrow, respectively, by a similar hierarchical process. Mature T and B lymphocytes enter peripheral lymphoid organs, where they encounter relevant antigens, leading to the production of new cells from reactivated mature cells. This process amplifies the *de novo* bone marrow formation of T and B lymphocytes. In addition, some members of this type of cell, memory T or B lymphocytes, are capable of sustained self-renewal. Their inability to produce multiple different types of daughter cells distinguishes them from stem cells.

In summary, the compartment model has given rise to terms that are generally applied to cells of hematopoietic origin. *Stem cells* are those that are multipotent and self-renewing. *Progenitor cells* have limited ability to self-renew and are likely to be unipotential or of very limited multipotential. *Precursor cells* are restricted to a single lineage, such as neutrophil precursors, and are the immediate precursors of the *mature cells* found in the blood. The mature cells are generally short-lived and preprogrammed to be highly responsive to cytokines, while the stem cells are long-lived, cytokine-resistant and generally quiescent.

## Models of lineage commitment

Several theories have emerged to describe the manner by which HSCs undergo lineage commitment and differentiate. Some studies support a *deterministic theory* whereby the stem cell compartment encompasses a series of closely related cells maturing in a stepwise process. Other studies suggest that hematopoiesis is a random, *stochastic* process. The stochastic theory is based on *in vitro* observations that multilineage colonies develop variable combinations of lineages and that such lineage choices occur independently of external influences.

Similar controversy exists regarding the role of cytokines in cell lineage determination. An *instructive* model suggests that cytokine signaling forces the commitment of primitive cells along a particular lineage. Ectopic expression of the granulocyte macrophage colony-stimulating factor (GM-CSF) receptor in a common lymphoid progenitor (CLP) population was capable of converting the cells from a lymphoid to a myeloid lineage. The influence of the GM-CSF receptor was sufficiently dominant to change the entire differentiation program of cells, but only the CLP stage of development. A *permissive* model postulates that decisions about cell fate occur independently of extracellular signals. This model suggests that cytokines serve only to allow certain lineages to survive and proliferate. Evidence supporting this model is provided by the ectopic expression of growth receptors in progenitor cells. Expression of the erythropoietin receptor in a macrophage progenitor results in macrophage colony formation, whereas expression of the macrophage colony-stimulating factor (M-CSF) receptor in an erythroid progenitor results in erythroid rather than macrophage colony formation. Replacing the thrombopoietin receptor (c-mpl) with a chimeric receptor consisting of the extracellular domain of c-mpl with the cytoplasmic domain of the granulocyte colony-stimulating factor (G-CSF) receptor results in normal platelet counts in homozygous "knock-in" mice. Therefore, the instructive and permissive models may both be correct, but at different stages of hematopoietic differentiation. Cells at earlier points in the differentiation cascade may be more plastic and susceptible to fate-altering stimuli, while more committed cells may be irreversibly determined, with only proliferation, cell death or the rate of differentiation susceptible to influence by external signals.

## Stem cell plasticity and transdifferentiation

*Plasticity* refers to the concept that HSC development is not limited to hematopoietic cells but may also include cells of other tissue types. Studies have suggested that bone marrow-derived cells may develop into other cell types such as neural cells. The possibility that HSCs have undergone *transdifferentiation* serves as one explanation for these phenomena. However, it has been shown that hematopoietic cells may fuse with somatic cells and this is more likely. The possibility that cells may convert from one cell type to another by reprogramming has now been well shown. However, such events are observed after genetic manipulation and it is not clear that this occurs in the body.

## Molecular regulation of hematopoiesis

The molecular nature of stem cell regulatory pathways has been determined using a variety of genetic approaches, including genetic loss-of-function and gain-of-function studies. These have provided several important concepts regarding the molecular control of hematopoiesis. First, some genes have binary functions and are either on or off in various biological states, while other genes function in a continuum and have different effects at different levels. Secondly, while perturbations in single genes may have dramatic cellular effects, cell cycle and lineage effects result from the combinatorial interplay of multiple genes and require coordinated expression of genes with both stimulatory and inhibitory functions. Finally, signal integration often depends on the assembly of large signaling complexes and the spatial proximity of molecules to facilitate interaction is therefore important.

## Cell-intrinsic regulators of hematopoiesis

### Cell cycle control

The quiescent nature of HSCs is supported by their low level of staining with DNA and RNA nucleic acid dyes, which is consistent with low metabolic activity. These studies have indicated a heterogeneity among stem cells with a subgroup that is deeply quiescent. Various studies have sought to determine the cell-intrinsic regulators of hematopoiesis involved in HSC cycle control.

Single-cell reverse transcriptase polymerase chain reaction (RT-PCR) has been used to profile pertinent transcription factors and other molecules in HSCs induced to differentiate along various lineages by the application of cytokines. This technique has demonstrated the presence of elevated levels of cyclin-dependent kinase inhibitors (CDKIs), suggesting that CDKIs present in HSCs function to exert a dominant inhibitory tone on HSC cell cycling. The bone marrow of some mouse strains deficient in CDKI $p21^{cip1/waf1}$ or $p18^{INK4a}$ have increased HSC cell cycling, suggesting that these CDKIs function as a dominant negative regulators of HSC proliferation. Other CDKIs, such as $p27^{kip}$, may serve as negative regulators of hematopoietic progenitor cells.

### Self-renewal, commitment, and lineage determination

Experimental results involving transcription factors have demonstrated cell-intrinsic roles in both global and lineage-specific hematopoietic development. Loss-of-function studies involving the transcription factors c-Myb, AML1 (CBF2), SCL (tal-1), LMO2 (Rbtn2), GATA-2 and TEL/ETV6 have demonstrated global effects on all hematopoietic lineages. Stem cells in animals deficient in these molecules fail to establish definitive hematopoiesis. To test the role of these genes in established hematopoiesis, a method of altering gene expression in the adult animal is required. A molecular technique to address this involves generating conditional knockouts. In these systems, transgenic animals are generated by swapping the wild-type gene of interest with a gene flanked at both ends with lox-p sites, target sites for Cre-recombinase. Such animals can then be mated with transgenic animals expressing the Cre-recombinase driven by different gene promotors. The Cre-recombinase can then be used to specifically excise the gene of interest in a global-, tissue- or developmental-specific manner, depending on the promoter driving the expression of the *Cre* gene. This approach is technically somewhat limited by the absence of stem cell-specific promoters thus far. However, this approach has aided the identification of critical roles for genes such as Notch-1, which are required for T-cell lineage induction, as

Notch-1-deficient mice die during embryogenesis because of a requirement for the protein in other tissues. An interferon-inducible promoter (Mx-Cre) can also be used to turn on Cre-recombinase at specific times by injecting animals with nucleotides, a means of inducing endogenous interferon. This approach has been useful in defining a very different role for SCL in maintaining hematopoiesis in the adult than in establishing it in the developing fetus. This gene product is absolutely required for establishing HSCs. Unexpectedly, there is not a requirement for SCL once the stem cell pool is present in the adult. Rather, SCL is required only for erythroid and megakaryocytic homeostasis. Therefore, transcription factor regulation of the stem cell compartment is highly dependent on the stage of development of the organism. Lineage-specific effects of transcription factors may also be stage-dependent.

Loss-of-function studies have also proved useful in identifying lineage-specific transcription factors. Mice genetically deficient in the transcription factor Ikaros lack T and B lymphocytes and natural killer cells, but maintain erythropoiesis and myelopoiesis. Mice lacking the ets-family transcription factor PU.1 demonstrate embryonic lethality. However, mutant embryos produce normal numbers of megakaryocytes and erythroid progenitors but have impaired erythroblast maturation and defective generation of progenitors for B and T lymphocytes, monocytes and granulocytes. While the outcome of such genetic lesions can be assessed, it remains unclear whether such lesions result in failure to establish a commitment program or the execution of an established program.

Gain-of-function studies have been used similarly to assess the roles of various global and lineage-specific transcription factors. Enforced expression of the *HoxB4* homeobox gene in HSCs confers heightened capacity for *in vivo* stem cell function. Similarly, ectopic expression of *HoxB4* in embryonic stem cells combined with *in vitro* culture on stroma induces a switch to the definitive hematopoiesis phenotype that is transplantable into adult recipients. Mice deficient in the Pax-5 transcription factor suffer from severe impairment of the B-lymphoid lineage. This phenotype may be rescued by reintroduction of wild-type Pax-5.

In alternative model systems, lineage reprogramming may be achieved by ectopic expression of transcription factors. Introduction of the erythrocytic lineage transcription factor GATA-1 reprograms avian myeloblast cells down eosinophilic and thromboblastic lineages. Introduction of the dominant negative retinoic acid receptor-alpha (RARα) into murine stem cells permits the establishment of permanent cell lines that grow in response to stem cell factor (SCF) and maintain the ability to differentiate along myeloid, erythroid and B-lineage lines. The points in the hematopoietic cascade at which specific transcription factors play a role are illustrated in Figure 3.3.

## Cell-extrinsic regulators

Ultimately, hematopoietic stem and progenitor cell decisions are regulated by the coordinated action of transcription factors as modified by extracellular signals. Extracellular signals in the form of hematopoietic growth factors are mediated via cell surface hematopoietic growth factor receptors. Hematopoietic growth factors exert specific effects when acting alone and may have different effects when combined with other cytokines. There are at least six receptor superfamilies, and most growth factors are members of the type I cytokine receptor family. The effects of various cytokines during myelopoiesis are illustrated in Figure 3.4.

### Type I cytokine receptors

Type I receptors do not possess intrinsic kinase activity but lead to phosphorylation of cellular substrates by serving as docking sites for adapter molecules with kinase activity. Examples of receptors in this family include leukemia inhibitory factor (LIF), interleukin (IL)-1, IL-2, IL-3, IL-4, IL-5, IL-6, IL-7, IL-9, IL-13, IL-18, GM-CSF, G-CSF, erythropoietin, prolactin, growth hormone, ciliary neurotrophic factor and c-mpl. These receptors share several features, including enhanced binding and/or signal transduction when expressed as heterodimers or homodimers, four cysteine residues and fibronectin type III domains in the extracellular domain, WSXWS ligand-binding sequence in the extracellular cytokine receptor domains, and lack of a known catalytic domain in the cytoplasmic portion. Another shared feature of receptors in this family is the ability to transduce signals that prevent programmed cell death (apoptosis).

Several exceptions to this family with intrinsic kinase activity are the hematopoietic growth factor receptors platelet-derived growth factor receptor (PDGFR), flt-3 receptor and c-fms, which are the ligands for steel factor (SF), Flt-ligand (FL) and M-CSF, respectively (Table 3.1).

### Type II cytokine receptors

This class includes the receptors for tissue factor, IL-10 and interferon (IFN)-γ. This family contains a type III fibronectin domain in the extracellular domain, like the type I family.

### Protein serine–threonine kinase receptors

This family includes the 30 members of the transforming growth factor (TGF)-β superfamily, which bind to their

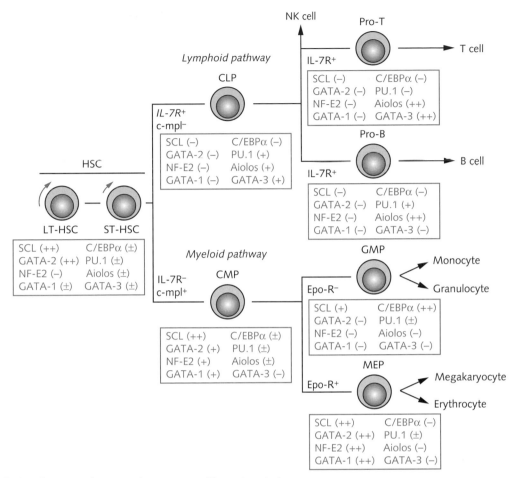

**Fig. 3.3 Transcription factors active at various stages of hematopoiesis**
CLP, common lymphoid progenitor; CMP, common myeloid progenitor; GMP, granulocyte monocyte progenitor; MEP, megakaryocyte erythrocyte progenitor; NK, natural killer. Redrawn from Akashi K, Traver D, Miyamoto T, Weissman IL. (2000) A clonogenic common myeloid progenitor that gives rise to all myeloid lineages. *Nature*, 404, 193–197, with permission.

receptors as homodimers. Members of this family include the three TGF-β receptors: type I (TbRI, 53 kDa), type II (TbRII, 75 kDa) and type III (TbRIII, 200 kDa). Members of this family have a profound inhibitory effect on the growth and differentiation of hematopoietic cells and on auxiliary hematopoietic cells. Binding of TFG-β requires TbRII. After binding, signal transduction occurs via activation of serine–threonine kinase cytoplasmic domains of the receptor chains, which results in the phosphorylation of Smad molecules on serines. Phosphorylated Smad complexes translocate to the nucleus, where they induce or repress gene transcription. TGF-β is the best-characterized negative regulator of hematopoiesis. It inhibits mitosis by inducing cell cycle inhibitors such as p21$^{cip1/waf1}$, p27$^{kip1}$ and p16$^{INK4a}$, inhibiting the cyclin-dependent kinases Cdk4 and Cdk6, and inducing phosphorylation of the retinoblastoma protein.

The TGF-β receptor family and its downstream mediators act as braking factors for a number of cell types and are frequently inactivated by somatic mutation in a number of cancers.

### Chemokine receptors

This family comprises seven transmembrane-spanning G-protein-coupled receptors that influence both cell cycle and cellular movement, or chemotaxis. These receptors are divided into three families, α or CXC, β or CC, and γ or C, on the basis of variability in cysteine residues. The best characterized is CXCR4, which mediates homing and engraftment of HSCs in bone marrow and is critical to hematopoietic development. IL-8 and macrophage inflammatory protein (MIP)-1α act as inhibitors of progenitor cell proliferation.

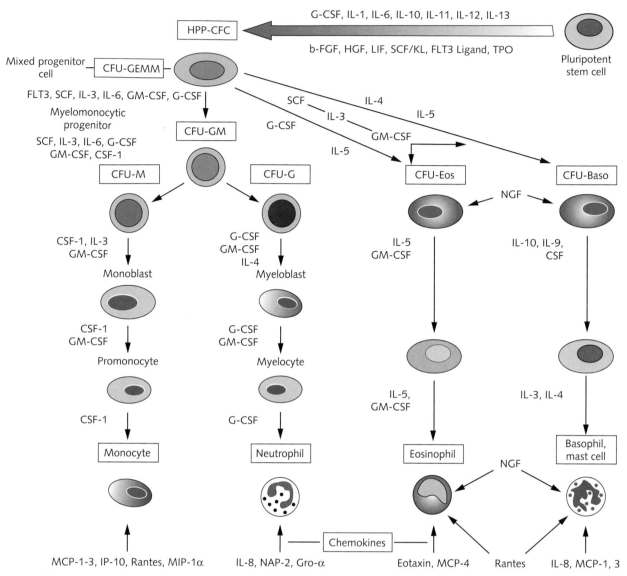

**Fig. 3.4 Cytokines active at various stages of hematopoiesis**
See text for definition of abbreviations. Modified from Figure 16.3 in *Hematology: Basic Principles and Practice,* 3rd edn (ed. R. Hoffman), 2000, with permission from Elsevier.

Members of this receptor family have also been implicated in cancer metastasis and the entry of HIV-1 into cells.

### Tumor necrosis factor receptor family

Members of the tumor necrosis factor (TNFR) family have varied effects, some having the ability to induce programmed cell death and others stimulating mesenchymal cells to secrete hematopoietic growth factors. These receptors contain Cys-rich extracellular domains and 80-amino acid cytoplasmic "death domains," which are required for transducing the apoptotic signal and inducing

NF-κB activation. Members of this family include TNFR1, TNFR2, fas, CD40, nerve growth factor (NGF) receptor, CD27, CD30 and OX40, each with at least one distinct biological effect.

## Components of the hematopoietic microenvironmental niche

While soluble factors influence stem cell fate, these factors are seen by the cell in the context of the cell–cell contact among heterologous cell types and cell–matrix contact that comprise the three-dimensional setting of the bone marrow.

**Table 3.1** Factors affecting hematopoietic control.

| Growth factor | Growth factor receptor | Produced by | Bioactivity | Deficient states |
|---|---|---|---|---|
| **Erythropoiesis** | | | | |
| EPO (erythropoietin) | EPO-R | Adult kidney Liver during development | Stimulates clonal growth of CFU-E and BFU-E subsets Suppresses erythroid progenitor cell apoptosis Induces bone marrow release of reticulocytes Induces erythroid globin synthesis | Anemia |
| SF (steel factor), kit ligand, mast cell growth factor | c-kit (CD117) | Fibroblasts Endothelial cells Bone marrow stroma | Promotes proliferation and differentiation of pre-CFC cells Acts synergistically with IL-3, GM-CSF and TPO to support growth of CFU-GEMM, BFU-E, and CFU-Mk Expansion of committed progenitor cells *in vivo* Stimulates mast cell hyperplasia, degranulation, and IgE-dependent mediator release | Anemia Mast cell deficiency |
| IGF-1 (insulin-like growth factor, somatomedin C) | IGF-1R | Liver | Induces DNA synthesis and has anti-apoptotic effects in erythroid progenitors Simulates erythroid colony growth in the absence of EPO at high doses | Growth retardation, neurological defects, homozygous deficiency lethal |
| **Granulopoiesis** | | | | |
| G-CSF (granulocyte colony-stimulating factor) | G-CSFR | Monocytes, macrophages, endothelial cells, fibroblasts | Stimulates growth of progenitors committed to neutrophil differentiation Activates neutrophil phagocytosis Stimulates quiescent HPCs to enter $G_1$/S Stimulates mobilization of HSCs and HPCs from bone marrow to periphery | Neutropenia, failure to develop neutrophilic leukocytosis in response to infection |
| GM-CSF (granulocyte macrophage colony-stimulating factor) | GM-CSFR | Mast cells, T lymphocytes, endothelial cells, fibroblasts, thymic epithelial cells | Stimulates multilineage hematopoietic progenitor cells Stimulates BFU-E and granulocyte, macrophage, and eosinophil colony growth | Susceptibility to infections caused by obligate intracellular organisms |
| M-CSF (macrophage colony-stimulating factor) | c-fms | Monocytes, macrophages, fibroblasts, epithelial cells, vascular endothelium, osteoblasts | Induces monocyte/macrophage growth and differentiation and activation | Macrophage and osteoclast deficiency, hematopoietic failure |
| Thrombopoietin | c-mpl | Bone marrow stroma, spleen, renal tubule, liver, muscle, brain | Stimulates *in vitro* growth of CFU-Mk, megakaryocytes and platelets Stimulates clonal growth of individual CD34$^+$CD38$^-$ cells Synergizes with SF, IL-3 and FL Primes response to platelet activators ADP, epinephrine and thrombin but no effect on aggregation | Thrombocytopenia |
| IL-5 | IL-5R | T lymphocytes | Stimulates eosinophil production and activation Activates cytotoxic T cells Induces immunoglobulin secretion | Inability to mount eosinophilic response |
| IL-11 | IL-11R | Fibroblasts, bone marrow stroma | Acts synergistically with IL-3 or SF to stimulate the clonal growth of erythroid (BFU-E and CFU-E) and primitive megakaryocytic (BFU-Mk) progenitors Shortens duration of $G_0$ of HPCs Quickens hematopoietic recovery after chemotherapy and radiation | No hematological defect |

**Table 3.1** *Continued*

| Growth factor | Growth factor receptor | Produced by | Bioactivity | Deficient states |
|---|---|---|---|---|
| **Lymphopoiesis** | | | | |
| IL-7 | IL-7R | Bone marrow stroma, spleen, thymus | Induces clonal growth of pre-B cells<br>Induces growth of pre-T cells | B- and T-cell lymphopenia |
| IL-2 | IL-2R | T lymphocytes | Induces proliferation and activation of T cells, B cells and NK cells | Fatal immunoproliferative disorder, loss of self-tolerance |
| IL-15 | IL-15R | Monocytes, macrophages, epithelial cells, skeletal muscle cells, bone marrow and thymic stroma | Induces proliferation and activation of T cells, B cells and NK cells | |
| IL-4 | IL-4R | T lymphocytes | Induces proliferation of activated B cells<br>Inhibits IL-2-stimulated proliferation of B cells<br>Induces T-cell proliferation | Defective T helper cell responses |
| IL-10 | | | Inhibits monocyte/macrophage-dependent synthesis of Th1- and Th2-derived cytokines | |
| **Early-acting factors** | | | | |
| IL-3 | IL-3R | T lymphocytes, mast cells | Stimulates multilineage colony growth and growth of primitive cell lines with multilineage potential<br>Stimulates BFU-E proliferation | No hematopoietic defect in steady state, deficient delayed-type hypersensitivity |
| FLT3-ligand (FL) | FLT-3R, flk2 | Most tissues, including spleen, lung, stromal cells, peripheral blood mononuclear cells | Weak colony-stimulating activity alone but synergizes with IL-3, GM-CSF, SF, IL-11, IL-6, G-CSF, IL-7, and others<br>Augments retroviral transduction of HSCs when added to cytokine cocktails<br>Mobilizes HSCs to periphery weakly alone but adds greatly to G-CSF | Reduction in pro-B cells, pre-B cells, B-cell colony-forming potential, reduced repopulating capacity of stem cells |
| IL-9 (T-cell growth factor) | IL-9R | T lymphocytes | Stimulates growth of BFU-E when combined with EPO<br>Stimulates clonal growth of fetal CFU-Mix and CFU-GM | |
| IL-6 | IL-6R | Macrophages, endothelial cells, fibroblasts, T lymphocytes | Synergistic with IL-3 for CFU-GEMM colony growth<br>Synergistic with IL-4 in inducing T-cell proliferation and colony growth<br>Synergistic with M-CSF in macrophage colony growth<br>Synergistic with GM-CSF in granulocyte colony growth<br>Co-induces differentiation of B cells | Reduced HSC and progenitor cell survival, reduced T-cell numbers, reduced proliferation and maturation of erythroid and myeloid cells |

BFU-E, burst-forming unit, erythroid; CFU-mix, colony-forming unit, mix; CFU-Mk, colony-forming unit, megakaryocyte; CFU-GM, colony-forming unit, granulocyte/macrophage; CFU-GEMM, colony-forming unit, granulocyte, erythroid, monocyte, megakaryocyte.

What actually constitutes the critical microenvironment for hematopoiesis is surprisingly poorly defined. The ability of primitive cells to mature *in vitro* in complex stromal cultures suggests that at least some elements of the regulatory milieu of the bone marrow can be recapitulated *ex vivo*. Studies based solely on *ex vivo* systems are suspect, however, as no fully satisfactory re-creation of stem cell expansion or self-renewal has been defined. Recognizing this limitation, it has been determined that mesodermal cells of multiple types are needed to enable hematopoietic support. These include adipocytes, fibroblastic cells and endothelium. Recently, *in vivo* studies have indicated that osteoblast lineage cells may perform a key regulatory role in stem cell self-renewal, and the activation of such cells can affect the number of stem cells. For example, expression of angiopoietin-1 by osteoblastic cells has been shown to modulate cell cycling.

## Trafficking of primitive hematopoietic cells

The migratory behavior characteristic of primitive hematopoietic cells is an area of intense research because of its relationship to bone marrow transplantation. Trafficking of HSCs can be divided into the components of homing, retention and engraftment. *Homing* describes the tendency of cells to arrive at a particular environment, while *retention* is their ability to remain in such an environment after arrival. Lastly, *engraftment* reflects the ability of cells to divide and form functional progeny in a given microenvironment. Much has been learned about trafficking from the ontogeny of mouse and human HSCs.

### Hematopoietic ontogeny

In both humans and mice, hematopoiesis occurs sequentially in distinct anatomical locations during development. These shifts in location are accompanied by changes in the functional status of the stem cells and reflect the changing needs of the developing organism. These are relevant for adult hematopoiesis since they offer insight into how the blood production process can be located in different places with distinct regulation.

There are essentially five sites of blood cell formation recognized in mammalian development, and these are best defined in the mouse. At about embryonic day 7.5 (E7.5), blood and endothelial progenitors emerge in the extra-embryonic yolk sac blood islands. The yolk sac supports the generation of primitive hematopoietic cells, which are primarily composed of nucleated erythrocytes. More sustained or definitive hematopoiesis may derive from the yolk sac, but this remains controversial. However, the aorta–gonad–mesonephros (AGM) region has been clearly identified as the first site of definitive hematopoiesis in both the mouse (E8.5) and the human. It is not clear if the yolk sac seeds the AGM region or if the hematopoietic cells arise there *de novo*. The placenta also appears to be a site of *de novo* HSC generation. By E10 in the mouse the fetal liver assumes the primary role of cell production. By E14 in the mouse and the second trimester of human gestation, the bone marrow becomes populated with HSCs and it takes over blood cell production, along with the spleen and thymus. The spleen remains a more active hematopoietic organ in the mouse than in the human.

The transition in the location of hematopoiesis is roughly associated with changes in HSC function. Primitive hematopoiesis and definitive hematopoiesis in the AGM region is dominated by the production of red blood cells and stem cells. As the organism and its vascular supply become more, platelet increases and, by late gestation, a full spectrum of innate and adaptive immune system cells are part of the production repertoire. Stem cell proliferation decreases and eventually reaches a state of relative quiescence shortly after gestation.

### Homing and engraftment of HSCs following infusion

Despite the use of HSC transplantation for over three decades, the exact mechanisms whereby bone marrow cells home to the bone marrow are not fully understood. Other than lectins, no adhesion receptors have been identified that are exclusively present on HSCs. Furthermore, no adhesion ligands, other than hemonectin, have been identified that are exclusively present in the bone marrow microenvironment.

When first infused, HSCs lodge in the microvasculature of the lung and liver; they then colonize the bone marrow, first passing through marrow sinusoids, migrating through the extracellular space of the bone marrow, and ultimately settle in the stem cell niches. Passage through endothelial barriers at first requires tethering, through endothelium-expressed addressins that bind hematopoietic cell selectins, and this is followed by firm attachment mediated by integrins.

Selectins are receptors expressed on hematopoietic cells (L- and P-selectins) and endothelium (E- and P-selectins). They have long extracellular domains containing an amino-terminal $Ca^{2+}$-binding domain, an epidermal growth factor domain, and a series of consensus repeats similar to those present in complement regulatory molecules. Ligands for selectins are sialylated fucosylglucoconjugates present on endothelium, termed *addressins*. L-selectin is present on $CD34^+$ hematopoietic progenitors while L-selectin and P-selectin are present on more mature myeloid and lymphoid cells. Tethering by selectins allows integrin-mediated adhesion to the endothelium. Integrins, a family of glycoproteins composed of α and β chains responsible for cell–extracellular matrix and cell–cell adhesion, provide not only firm attachment but also allow migration of hematopoietic cells through the endothelium and bone marrow extracellular space. The functional state of integrins is only loosely tied to their expression level and depends on ligand affinity modulation regulated by the β subunit in response to cytokines and other stimuli.

The process of migration depends on the establishment of adhesion at the leading edge of the cell and simultaneous release at the trailing edge. The rate of migration depends on dynamic changes in the strength of the cell–ligand interactions, which is dictated by the number of receptors and their affinity state and the strength of the adhesion receptor–cytoskeleton interactions. Cell–ligand interaction strength may also be modulated by cytokines. Thus, successful engraftment relies not only on the presence of several different adhesion receptors but also on their functional state and ability to facilitate both migration and adhesion.

## Egress of HSCs from bone marrow under physiological conditions

The majority of primitive HSCs are resident within the bone marrow space under steady-state physiological conditions. However, a population of CD34[+] cells capable of forming CFCs and LTC-ICs and capable of long-term repopulation may be found circulating in the peripheral blood and these may increase after physiological stressors such as exercise, stress and infection. Recent studies have suggested that a relatively large number of bone marrow-derived stem cells circulates during the course of a day and that these cells periodically transit back into an engraftable niche to establish hematopoiesis. Defining the processes involved is important in guiding new approaches to peripheral blood stem cell mobilization for transplantation.

Examining mice in which specific adhesion molecules have been deleted has revealed several key molecular determinants of stem cell localization in the bone marrow. Among these, the chemokine receptor CXCR4 has perhaps the most striking phenotype. In the absence of this receptor, stem cells fail to traffic from the fetal liver to the bone marrow. Partly because of these studies, others have defined that CXCR4 is relevant for the engraftment of transplanted stem cells and that the modulation of CXCR4 signaling can affect adult stem cell localization in the bone marrow versus peripheral blood. As described, the integrin and selectin families are also important molecular participants in stem cell location. For example, HSCs from animals that are heterozygous-deficient for β1 integrin cannot compete with wild-type cells

for the colonization of hematopoietic organs. Pre-incubation of HSCs with α4 integrin antibodies prior to transplantation results in decreased bone marrow and increased peripheral recovery of cells, while the continued presence of α4 antibodies prevents engraftment. Evidence for selectin involvement has been demonstrated in animals deficient for single selectins or combinations of selectins. Endothelial P-selectin mediates leukocyte rolling in the absence of inflammation, while L-, P- and E-selectins contribute to leukocyte rolling in the setting of inflammation. L-selectin is important in lymphocyte homing. Transplantation studies performed in animals deficient in P- and E-selectins demonstrate severely decreased engraftment due to impaired homing, an effect that is further compromised by blocking vascular cell adhesion molecule (VCAM)-1.

Mature hematopoietic cells are thought to migrate from the marrow to the blood by similar mechanisms, though these are not well defined. One purported mechanism is a shift in expression from molecules thought to interact with stromal proteins to those that interact with endothelium. For example, myeloid progenitors express functional α4β1 and α5β1 integrins that act to ensure that these progenitors are retained in the bone marrow through interactions with VCAM and fibronectin. Mature neutrophils, in contrast, express β2 integrins that permit interaction with ligands, such as intercellular adhesion molecule, expressed by endothelial cells. Mature neutrophils also express β1 integrins that permit interaction with collagen and laminin present in basal membranes, perhaps regulating a progressive shift in cell affinities for specific microenvironmental determinants that ultimately results in cell egress into the blood. Mobilization of murine HSCs induced by cyclophosphamide or G-CSF is accompanied by changes in integrin expression levels and functional changes in homing, thus linking cellular localization with adhesion molecule receptor expression.

## Manipulating hematopoietic stem cells for clinical use

### Mobilization of HSCs

Mobilization of HSCs in response to chemotherapy or cytokines was first documented in the 1970s and 1980s. This process may be induced by a variety of molecules, including cytokines such as G-CSF, GM-CSF, IL-7, IL-3, IL-12, SCF and flt-3 ligand; and chemokines such as IL-8, MIP-1α, Gro-β and SDF-1. The one that is most often used clinically is G-CSF, which may be combined with chemotherapeutic agents for added benefit. This mobilizing capability has resulted in a dramatic change in the manner by which HSCs are harvested for transplantation. Up to 25% of candidates for autologous transplantation are unable to mobilize sufficient cells to enable the procedure to be safely performed. The study of mobilization and its counterpart, engraftment, has implications of great significance for patient care. The ability of G-CSF to mobilize bone marrow HSCs has several apparent mechanisms. The first is reported to be the activation of neutrophils, causing the release of neutrophil elastases capable of cleaving CXCR4 on HSCs, thus reducing HSC–bone marrow interaction. Other receptors that undergo cleavage are VCAM-1 and c-kit. A second mechanism of G-CSF-induced mobilization is via CD26, an extracellular dipeptidase present on primitive HSCs that is able to cleave SDF-1 to an inactive form. Other proposed options for improving mobilization include coadministration of G-CSF and kit ligand, antibodies directed against VLA-4, and infusion of IL-8. The inhibition of the CXCR4 receptor by a small molecule has been shown to effectively mobilize HSCs into the blood of patients, including those with poor G-CSF-induced mobilization. This compound may be added to the available drugs for clinical HSC harvesting.

## Isolating stem cells for manipulation

### Characteristics of HSCs used for isolation

*Physical* Early attempts to isolate HSCs were based on cell size and density. In order to clarify whether the heterogeneity of CFU-S was due to differences in the input cells used, velocity sedimentation was performed to separate cells by size, demonstrating that smaller cells were more likely to produce secondary CFU-S than larger cells. HSCs are similar in size to mature lymphocytes and, when flow cytometry is performed, overlap the lymphocyte region on plots of forward and side scatter.

*Using cell-cycle-active drugs* Because HSCs are largely in a quiescent portion of the cell cycle ($G_0$ or $G_1$), investigators have used cell-cycle-active drugs to deplete bone marrow populations of cycling cells and thereby enrich for primitive HSCs. Treatment of mice with nitrogen mustard resulted in a 30-fold enrichment in CFU-S. HSCs may be isolated by *in vitro* treatment with 5-fluorouracil, and this remains the most commonly used agent. In addition, HSC populations may be further enriched by first stimulating cells to enter the cell cycle with the early-acting cytokines c-kit ligand and IL-3 before forcing them to metabolic death. This strategy is useful for human cells but not murine cells, probably because of different cycling characteristics. It should be noted that these techniques might result in a decrease in the quality of HSCs obtained.

*Markers of primitive HSCs* A variety of strategies have been used to identify potential HSC markers. CFU-S in rat bone marrow, fetal liver and neonatal spleen express Thy-1 antigen at high levels, and this was the first important HSC marker discovered. Pluripotent stem cells could be enriched from the bone marrow 150-fold on the basis of combination of size and Thy-1 expression. Negative selection of cells using soybean agglutination resulted in enrichment in the colony-forming unit culture assay (CFU-C). In addition, a fluorescence-activated cell sorter (FACS)-based negative selection strategy that involves labeling hematopoietic cells with a cocktail of antibodies directed against mature hematopoietic cell antigens has been developed. These lineage-directed antibodies include B220 (directed against mature B lymphocytes), CD8 (directed against T cells), Mac-1 (directed against macrophages), and Gr-1 (directed against granulocytes). When this negative selection protocol ($Lin^{neg}$) was combined with a positive selection protocol to enrich for cells that expressed low levels of Thy-1 ($Thy-1^{low}$), 200-fold enrichment of day-10 CFU-S could be achieved.

Using a magnetic bead selection strategy to enrich for Thy-1-expressing cells followed by a FACS-based strategy to deplete cells expressing lineage markers, murine cells were isolated that were found to express a newly defined stem cell antigen, Sca-1. These $Lin^{neg}Thy-1^{low}Sca-1^{pos}$ cells represented 1 in 1000 bone marrow cells and had heightened stem cell activity compared with whole bone marrow in the CFU-S assay. This highly selected cell population produced day-13 CFU-S at 1 colony per 10 cells and day-8 CFU-S at 1 per 100 cells. Also, these cells were 1000–2000-fold enriched in their ability to rescue irradiated animals and could give rise to all blood cell lineages. Self-renewal capability was demonstrated by the ability of these cells to rescue lethally irradiated animals upon secondary transplantation. Interestingly, the $Sca-1^{neg}$ population had similar CFU-S activity but could not produce T cells or confer radioprotection.

More recently, the receptor for SCF, c-kit, was demonstrated to be present on HSCs. Populations expressing this phenotype ($c-kit^{pos}Thy-1.1^{low}Lin^{neg}Sca-1^{pos}$), also known as KTLS, are 2000-fold enriched in HSC activity compared with unfractionated bone marrow. Thus, KTLS has come to be regarded by many as a profile that represents, but is not specific for, HSCs in the mouse. The presence of CD10 and absence of CD48 on KLS cells has also been shown to greatly enrich for HSCs. Equivalent markers are not as well defined in the human, though it is apparent that cells expressing kit ligand without lineage markers (including the CD38 antigen) are enriched in stem cells. The antigen CD34 has long been regarded as a marker for a stem cell population, but it is now clear that the vast majority of CD34$^+$ cells are progenitors, and stem cells may or may not express CD34. CD133 is a marker more recently shown to be expressed on primitive human hematopoietic cells. A summary of proposed HSC markers for the mouse and human is presented in Table 3.2.

*Supravital stains* Since HSCs are inherently quiescent, spend most of their time in inactive portions of the cell cycle and are resistant to toxins, exclusion of dyes has been used as a method of isolation. The DNA dye Hoechst 33342 was first used to separate quiescent cells from the bone marrow. Cells with low-intensity staining were enriched for high proliferative potential (HPP)-CFC and day-12 CFU-S. The red and blue emissions from this dye have been recently used to define a small subset of bone marrow cells known as the side population (SP). SP cells have extremely low fluorescence emission in these channels, resulting from efflux of Hoechst 33342 by multidrug resistance pumps that are highly expressed on HSCs. SP cells constitute approximately 0.1% of the bone marrow and are highly enriched in reconstitution potential.

The mitochondrial dye rhodamine-123 (Rh-123) has also been used to subdivide primitive stem cells. Mitochondria in quiescent cells bind low levels of Rh-123 and FACS can be used to separate Rh-123$^{low}$ cells. These cells were enriched for day-13 CFU-S and multilineage reconstituting potential.

The combination of supravital stains with fluorescent antibodies against cell surface markers provides the ability to enrich for highly primitive HSCs such that fewer than 10 cells are required to reconstitute hematopoiesis.

### Methods of isolation of HSCs

*FACS* While the flow cytometer may be used for analysis of cells, the apparatus may also physically sort cells of desired fluorescence or fluorescence pattern, size and granularity characteristics. Using a magnetic field, these cells may be diverted to a collection tube during analysis and later analyzed using techniques of molecular and cellular biology. Sorting is both expensive and labor-intensive as it requires costly machines, a high degree of expertise, and time to sort samples consisting of single-cell suspensions. Many FACS machines are now available with high-speed sorting. This was once a technique available to only a few laboratories, but many centers are developing "core" laboratories to provide cell analysis and sorting services for investigators. FACS may be used to isolate HSCs using both positive and negative selection strategies with fluorescence-labeled antibodies directed against primitive hematopoietic cell antigens, as described above.

*Magnetic bead columns* Large-volume isolation of HSC subsets has been facilitated by the use of magnetic bead columns. Using this system, cells are incubated with antibodies directed against primitive hematopoietic cells. These antibodies are typically coupled to a hapten. A second-step incubation is then performed using a magnetic microbead conjugated to a hapten that is able to bind the first-step hapten. The effect is to label HSCs with a magnetic bead. Cells are then passed through a column mounted adjacent to a magnet. Labeled cells are retained within the column and unbound cells can be washed through. Then, the column is removed from the magnet and the desired cells may be eluted.

Alternatively, negative selection may be performed by capturing only the cells that pass through the column. For example, a sample may be depleted of mature cells by labeling with antibodies directed against mature blood cell antigens (Lin$^{pos}$). Cells can then be passed over a column in which the mature cells adhere and immature cells pass through and may be isolated.

Systems of these types permit rapid isolation of large numbers of primitive cells of relatively high purity.

### *Ex vivo* expansion

Given the possible clinical applications of HSCs for such uses as bone marrow transplantation, there is increasing interest in strategies that both result in an increase in the quantity of HSCs and the ability to manipulate HSCs *ex vivo*. Thus, *ex vivo* expansion of HSCs represents a highly prioritized goal of clinically oriented HSC research.

The first benefit of expanding HSCs is to provide sufficient cells for transplantation when insufficient numbers exist. For example, cord blood represents a rich source of primitive CD34$^+$ cells that are less immunocompetent and are therefore transplantable across partial HLA disparity barriers. However, the absolute quantity of HSCs within a single cord blood is low and transplantation is followed by periods of aplasia. *Ex vivo* expansion would thereby facilitate

**Table 3.2** Proposed surface markers of primitive hematopoietic stem cells.

| Mouse | Human |
|---|---|
| CD34$^{low/-}$ | CD34$^+$ |
| Sca-1$^+$ | CD59$^+$ |
| Thy1$^{+/low}$ | Thy1$^+$ |
| CD38$^+$ | CD38$^{low/-}$ |
| C-kit$^+$ | C-kit$^{-/low}$ |
| lin$^-$ | lin$^-$ |
| CD150$^+$ | |
| CD48$^-$ | |

cord blood transplantation. Similarly, selective expansion of HSC subsets would permit the extension of tumor-free cells from patients with limited quantities of normal bone marrow due to bone marrow-infiltrating diseases, such as leukemia, for the purpose of autologous transplantation.

The second benefit of *ex vivo* manipulation is that HSCs have a relative growth advantage over other cell types, such as tumor cells. Therefore, *ex vivo* growth provides a purging effect. Furthermore, specific tumor cell purging may be achieved via the application of certain cytokines (IL-2, IFN-γ), antitumor agents such as 5-fluorouracil or cyclophosphamide, tumor-specific antibodies combined with complement-mediated lysis, and oncogene-specific tyrosine kinase inhibitors, in addition to other targeted therapies, such as antisense oligonucleotides, prior to use of the graft.

The third benefit is the support of gene transfer into HSCs for the purpose of gene therapy. A variety of gene-transfer mechanisms, including retroviral infection, are conveyed during mitosis. Thus, the *ex vivo* stimulation of cells using cytokines results in heightened transfer of exogenous genes to HSCs.

Strategies to expand HSCs *ex vivo* have used cytokine cocktails such as IL-11, flt3-ligand and SF, stimulation with the purified WNT-3a glycoprotein, neutralizing antibodies of TGF-β alone or in combination with inhibition of CDKI p27, inhibition of the CDKI p21, and stimulation with Notch ligands. Others have reported that angiopoietin-like factor 2 can be a potent HSC expansion stimulus in combination with other cytokines. While these efforts have resulted in encouraging laboratory results, none to date has translated into accepted clinical practice. Testing regarding these methods continues with intensity and relies heavily on specific functional analyses.

## Functional analysis of HSCs

Functional assays for HSCs do not actually measure the activity of HSCs but instead assess more differentiated progeny, such as progenitor and precursor cells. Whereas *in vitro* assays measure mature populations, *in vivo* assays detect the activity of primitive cells capable of homing and engrafting in the proper microenvironment to produce functional hematopoietic progeny.

In vitro *assays* The CFU-C measures hematopoietic progenitor function and is performed by plating cells in semisolid media containing methylcellulose and one or more cytokines. After 5–14 days, colonies comprising mature cell populations committed to either myeloid or lymphoid lineages may be observed. While most colonies obtained using this assay are composed of cells of a single lineage, less frequently multipotent progenitors can yield colonies containing multiple lineages. Another type of primitive cell, known as the HPP-CFC, which possesses a high degree of proliferative and multilineage potential, may be detected in this culture system. Formation of HPP-CFC colonies, characterized by size greater than 0.5 mm and multilineage composition, requires the use of multiple cytokines in order to proliferate.

The LTC-IC assay correlates more closely to HSCs. Here, hematopoietic cells are plated on top of stromal cell lines or irradiated primary bone marrow stroma. Primitive HSCs are able to initiate growth and to generate progeny *in vitro* for up to 12 weeks. Progenitor cells and mature myeloid cells are removed weekly to prevent overgrowth. Ultimately, HSCs, characterized by high proliferative and self-renewal capabilities, are able to sustain long-term culture and may be enumerated at the conclusion of the assay.

The CAFC assay represents a type of LTC-IC that similarly measures the ability of cells to initiate growth and generate progeny *in vitro* for up to 12 weeks. However, the readout is slightly different. Hematopoietic cells are plated at limiting dilution on top of a monolayer consisting of irradiated bone marrow stroma or a stromal cell line. The growth of colonies consisting of at least five small non-refractile cells reminiscent of cobblestones, found underneath the stromal layer, are counted. Such cultures are maintained using weekly half-media changes until up to 5 weeks after seeding. In this assay, more primitive cells appear later, and day-35 CAFCs represent a close correlate of a cell with *in vivo* long-term multilineage repopulating potential. LTC-ICs may be enumerated after day 35 by completely removing the CAFC medium, overlaying methylcellulose and counting the number of colonies produced after 8–10 days.

In vivo *assays* The CFU-S assay, first developed by Till and McCulloch in 1961, is described earlier in this chapter (*see section Hematopoietic stem cell concepts and their origin*). Bone marrow or spleen cells are transplanted to irradiated recipients and animals are killed after 8 or 12 days for analysis of spleen colonies, termed CFU-S$_8$ and CFU-S$_{12}$, respectively. Cells that give rise to CFU-S$_8$ are predominantly unipotential and produce erythroid colonies. CFU-S$_{12}$ colonies consist of several types of myeloid cells, including erythrocytes, megakaryocytes, macrophages and granulocytes. Cells giving rise to CFU-S$_{12}$ represent a more primitive population of multipotent cells than those that result in CFU-S$_8$.

The long-term repopulation assay is a more accurate measure of HSC activity. Whole collections of hematopoietic cells or fractionated subpopulations are transplanted to lethally irradiated syngeneic mice, typically by tail vein injection. Recipients are screened for ongoing hematopoiesis 8–10 weeks after transplantation. By this time, hematopoi-

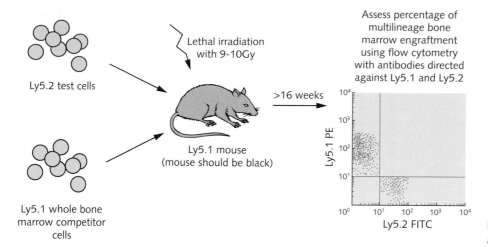

**Fig. 3.5 Competitive repopulation assay**

esis is firmly established and donor-derived blood is produced by transplanted HSCs. This assay requires that cells fulfill the two central features of HSCs: multilineage reconstitution, consistent with multipotentiality, and indefinite hematopoiesis, indicative of self-renewal.

Tracking of transplanted cells was originally conducted using radiation-induced chromosomal abnormalities or by retrovirally marking donor cells. However, a major advance in the ability to track transplanted cells has been the development of congenic mice with minor allelic differences in the leukocyte common antigen Ly5, which is expressed on all nucleated blood cells. The C57/BL6 ("black-6") strain contains the Ly5.2 antigen, while the BL6/SJL strain contains a separate allele, Ly5.1. However, these syngeneic strains may be transplanted interchangeably. Both antibodies are available with distinct fluorescent labels. FACS analysis using these antibodies permits measurement of donor-derived reconstitution of the nucleated blood lineages. However, erythrocytes and platelets do not express the Ly5 antigen and cannot be tracked using this technique. Instead, investigators use congenic strains with allelic variants of hemoglobin and glucose phosphate isomerase to track erythroid and platelet engraftment, respectively.

A modification of this assay permits quantitation of HSCs within the graft. Here, HSCs are quantified by transplanting limiting-dilution numbers of bone marrow into lethally irradiated recipients. Each recipient also receives $1 \times 10^5$ cells of the host's marrow to ensure survival during the period of pancytopenia immediately after irradiation. At 10–12 weeks, host peripheral blood is assessed to determine whether donor-derived reconstitution has occurred. Donor cells must constitute at least 1% of the peripheral blood to contend that at least one HSC was present in the donor population. Also, both lymphoid and myeloid lineages must demonstrate at least 1% donor derivations. The percentage of reconstituted animals in each group may be plotted against the number of input cells to determine a limiting-dilution estimate of the frequency of HSCs within the donor population. This assay is termed a *competitive repopulation assay*, as transplanted HSCs compete with the host's HSCs that survive irradiation-induced death, in addition to host cells transplanted with the graft. The HSCs detected are termed *competitive repopulation units*. The competitive repopulation assay using congenic mouse strains is depicted in Figure 3.5.

## Summary

Investigation of HSCs has been facilitated by the development of *in vitro* and *in vivo* assays of hematopoietic cell function followed by the identification of molecular cell surface markers that permit the isolation of purified subsets of cells with defined characteristics. Studies in this field have contributed greatly to the understanding of both general stem cell biology and hematopoiesis. Further investigation of cell-intrinsic and cell-extrinsic regulators of hematopoiesis will enable rational manipulation of HSCs and thereby extend the current uses of stem cells in clinical practice.

## Further reading

### Identification of stem cells and colony assays

Bradley TR, Metcalf D. (1966) The growth of mouse bone marrow cells in vitro. *Australian Journal of Experimental Biology and Medical Science*, **44**, 287–299.

Curry JL, Trentin JJ. (1967) Hemopoietic spleen colony studies. I. Growth and differentiation. *Developmental Biology*, **15**, 395–413.

Ichikawa Y, Pluznik DH, Sachs L. (1966) In vitro control of the development of macrophage and granulocyte colonies. *Proceedings of the National Academy of Sciences of the United States of America*, **56**, 488–495.

Metcalf D. (1984) *The Hematopoietic Colony Stimulating Factors.* Amsterdam: Elsevier.

Till J, McCulloch E. (1961) A direct measurement of the radiation sensitivity of normal mouse bone marrow cells. *Radiation Research*, **14**, 213–222.

## Lineage commitment

Morrison SJ, Hemmati HD, Wandycz AM *et al.* (1995) The purification and characterization of fetal liver hematopoietic stem cells. *Proceedings of the National Academy of Sciences of the United States of America*, **92**, 10302–10306.

Nakahata T, Ogawa M. (1982) Clonal origin of murine hemopoietic colonies with apparent restriction to granulocyte-macrophage-megakaryocyte (GMM) differentiation. *Journal of Cellular Physiology*, **111**, 239–246.

## Stem cell plasticity

Brazelton TR, Rossi FM, Keshet GI *et al.* (2000) From marrow to brain: expression of neuronal phenotypes in adult mice. *Science*, **290**, 1775–1779.

Camargo FD, Green R, Capetenaki Y *et al.* (2003) Single hematopoietic stem cells generate skeletal muscle through myeloid intermediates. *Nature Medicine*, **9**, 1520–1527.

Ferrari G, Cusella-De Angelis G, Coletta M *et al.* (1998) Muscle regeneration by bone marrow-derived myogenic progenitors. *Science*, **279**, 1528–1530.

Gussoni E, Soneoka Y, Strickland CD *et al.* (1999) Dystrophin expression in the mdx mouse restored by stem cell transplantation. *Nature*, **401**, 390–394.

Lagasse E, Connors H, Al-Dhalimy M *et al.* (2000) Purified hematopoietic stem cells can differentiate into hepatocytes in vivo. *Nature Medicine*, **6**, 1229–1234.

Mezey E, Chandross KJ, Harta G *et al.* (2000) Turning blood into brain: cells bearing neuronal antigens generated in vivo from bone marrow. *Science*, **290**, 1779–1782.

Orlic D, Kajstura J, Chimenti S *et al.* (2001) Bone marrow cells regenerate infarcted myocardium. *Nature*, **410**, 701–705.

Wagers AJ, Sherwood RI, Christensen JL *et al.* (2002) Little evidence for developmental plasticity of adult hematopoietic stem cells. *Science*, **297**, 2256–2259.

Wang X, Willenbring H, Akkari Y *et al.* (2003) Cell fusion is the principal source of bone-marrow-derived hepatocytes. *Nature*, **422**, 897–901.

## Molecular regulators of hematopoiesis

Cheng T, Rodrigues N, Dombkowski D *et al.* (2000) Stem cell repopulation efficiency but not pool size is governed by p27(kip1). *Nature Medicine*, **6**, 1235–1240.

Cheng T, Rodrigues N, Shen H *et al.* (2000) Hematopoietic stem cell quiescence maintained by p21cip1/waf1. *Science*, **287**, 1804–1808.

Kuhn R, Schwenk F, Aguet M *et al.* (1995) Inducible gene targeting in mice. *Science*, **269**, 1427–1429.

Orkin SH. (1996) Development of the hematopoietic system. *Current Opinion in Genetics and Development*, **6**, 597–602.

Reya T, Duncan AW, Ailles L *et al.* (2003) A role for Wnt signalling in self-renewal of haematopoietic stem cells. *Nature*, **423**, 409–414.

Shivdasani RA, Orkin SH. (1996) The transcriptional control of hematopoiesis. *Blood*, **87**, 4025–4039.

Shivdasani RA, Mayer EL, Orkin SH. (1995) Absence of blood formation in mice lacking the T-cell leukaemia oncoprotein tal-1/SCL. *Nature*, **373**, 432–434.

## Homing and engraftment

Cashman JD, Lapidot T, Wang JC *et al.* (1997) Kinetic evidence of the regeneration of multilineage hematopoiesis from primitive cells in normal human bone marrow transplanted into immunodeficient mice. *Blood*, **89**, 4307–4316.

Peled A, Petit I, Kollet O *et al.* (1999) Dependence of human stem cell engraftment and repopulation of NOD/SCID mice on CXCR4. *Science*, **283**, 845–848.

Wright DE, Wagers AJ, Gulati AP *et al.* (2001) Physiological migration of hematopoietic stem and progenitor cells. *Science*, **294**, 1933–1936.

## Isolation of stem cells

Baum CM, Weissman IL, Tsukamoto AS *et al.* (1992) Isolation of a candidate human hematopoietic stem-cell population. *Proceedings of the National Academy of Sciences of the United States of America*, **89**, 2804–2808.

Goodell MA, Brose K, Paradis G *et al.* (1996) Isolation and functional properties of murine hematopoietic stem cells that are replicating in vivo. *Journal of Experimental Medicine*, **183**, 1797–1806.

Spangrude GJ, Heimfeld S, Weissman IL. (1988) Purification and characterization of mouse hematopoietic stem cells. *Science*, **241**, 58–62.

# Chapter 4 The genetics of acute myeloid leukemias

## Carolyn J Owen[1] & Jude Fitzgibbon[2]

[1] Division of Hematology and Hematological Malignancies, University of Calgary, Foothills Medical Centre, Calgary, Canada
[2] Centre for Medical Oncology, Institute of Cancer, Barts and The London School of Medicine & Dentistry, London, UK

## Introduction

Acute myeloid leukemia (AML) is a heterogeneous disease with respect to clinical features and acquired genetic aberrations. AML patients are generally divided into three broad risk groups based on cytogenetic abnormalities, favorable, intermediate and adverse, with each having different cure rates. After age, these abnormalities are the most important predictors of outcome in AML. Unfortunately, even the favorable risk group has a high risk of relapse after conventional chemotherapy and the overall outcomes in AML are poor, with most patients succumbing to their disease. Outcomes are particularly poor for older adults (>60 years) who form the majority of AML cases.

Since the publication of the World Health Organization (WHO) classification of AML in 2001, significant progress has been made through the discovery of recurrent genetic aberrations that are not detectable by conventional cytogenetics. These "molecular markers" include mutations in specific genes as well as altered gene expression and/or methylation status of genes. Several of these new molecular markers have prognostic implications and can aid in the risk stratification of patients. The importance of these new molecular markers is manifest in the 2008 update of the WHO classification. In the 2001 classification, about 25% of newly diagnosed patients would be classified in the category of "AML with recurrent genetic abnormalities" while 70–75% will now be included in the same category in the 2008 update, which encompasses the newly defined molecular

aberrations. These recent insights have led to recommendations for complex risk-adapted strategies, aiming to improve treatment outcomes and minimize toxicity. Although these new insights are set to revolutionize treatment approaches in AML, none has yet had an effect on the routine management of AML as it stands today.

This chapter reviews the prognostically important recurrent genetic aberrations observed in AML. As most currently available data on the impact of genetic abnormalities in AML are derived from large trials enrolling younger patients (<60 years), the implications for older adults remain unclear.

## AML with recurrent cytogenetic abnormalities

Cytogenetic abnormalities in AML have long been known to have prognostic relevance. Several recurrent translocations are associated with a favorable prognosis when treated with appropriate therapeutic agents, while particular numeric chromosomal abnormalities, such as monosomies of chromosomes 5 and/or 7, are associated with a poor prognosis. Advances in molecular genetic research have enabled a better understanding of the mechanisms by which these translocations cause leukemia. Importantly, these studies have demonstrated that the pathogenesis of AML is one of a sequential acquisition of genetic aberrations, with a single aberration being insufficient alone to cause overt leukemia.

### Core-binding factor leukemias

The core-binding factor (CBF) is a key regulator of hematopoiesis and the most frequent target of chromosomal translocations associated with leukemia. This transcription factor is composed of two subunits, the α subunit encoded by

*Molecular Hematology*, 3rd edition. Edited by Drew Provan and John Gribben.
© 2010 Blackwell Publishing.

*RUNX1* (also called *AML1*) and the β subunit encoded by *CBFB*. Homozygous loss of function of either RUNX1 or CBFB in genetically engineered mice results in a complete lack of definitive hematopoiesis, indicating that both components of CBF are necessary for normal hematopoietic development. CBF AML is a relatively frequent subtype of adult AML, classified in the favorable risk category. Between 7 and 12% of *de novo* AML patients present with t(8;21) in which the *RUNX1* gene is fused to *RUNX1T1* (*ETO*), while another 10–12% of patients present with inv(16)/t(16;16) in which *CBFB* is fused to *MYH11*. The CBF partner gene in each case has constitutive activity leading to persistent expression of the RUNX1–RUNX1T1 (AML-ETO) or CBFβ–MYH11 fusion protein, causing recruitment of co-repressor complex and underexpression of genes regulated by the CBF complex.

Recent data from *in vitro* studies and transgenic animal models suggest a dominant-negative role for these fusion genes. RUNX1–RUNX1T1 acts as a dominant-negative inhibitor of the wild-type CBF with the fusion transcript retaining RUNX1's DNA binding and heterodimerization domains but lacking the C-terminal transcription activation domain. The mechanism of dominant-negative activity is less clear for CBFβ–MYH11 but both prevent transactivation of CBF targets. Despite this understanding, the precise mechanism by which these fusion proteins exert their leukemogenic effect remains to be elucidated. However, it is clear that the translocations alone are not sufficient to result in overt leukemia. For example, conditional alleles of RUNX1–RUNX1T1 expressed in adult hematopoietic progenitors are not sufficient to cause AML but result instead in a myeloproliferative phenotype. In these mouse models, it is necessary to treat animals with chemical mutagens to induce overt AML.

## Acute promyelocytic leukemia

As with the CBF genes, there are also multiple chromosomal translocations that involve the retinoic acid receptor *RARα* locus on chromosome 17. The subgrouping of patients with *RARα* translocations is particularly important because of the distinctly better prognosis that these individuals exhibit compared with other subtypes of AML. In t(15;17), the *RARα* gene fuses with a nuclear regulatory factor called the promyelocytic leukemia gene (*PML*), giving rise to the PML–RARα gene fusion product. Several less-frequent variant translocations with *RARα* also occur involving the *PLZF*, *NPM1*, *NuMA*, *STAT5B* or *PRKAR1A* genes. Each of these is associated with an acute promyelocytic leukemia (APL) characterized by a block in differentiation at the promyelocyte stage of hematopoietic development. The t(15;17) is the most frequent translocation causing APL and has been extensively studied. *PML–RARα* expression is associated with a block in differentiation due to aberrant recruitment of the nuclear co-repressor complex, similar to observations in the context of the RUNX1–RUNX1T1 and CBFβ–MYH11 fusions.

APL has a particular sensitivity to all-*trans*-retinoic acid (ATRA), a ligand for RARα, which has proven to be very effective therapy for this subtype of AML, when given in combination with induction chemotherapy containing anthracyclines with or without cytosine arabinoside. The efficacy of ATRA in the treatment of APL is related to the ability of ATRA to bind to the fusion protein, with resultant dissociation of the nuclear co-repressor complex. Promyelocytes are then able to engage normal hematopoietic differentiation programs that ultimately result in apoptotic cell death. However, many of the variant *RARα* translocations are not sensitive to ATRA, suggesting they have different functional effects to the *PML–RARα* translocation.

Similar to the CBF leukemias, expression of *PML–RARα* is not sufficient to induce AML. There are several lines of evidence supporting this assertion, including transgenic murine models of *PML–RARα*-induced AML. In this model, although the fusion gene is present in the germline and is expressed during embryonic and adult development, the animals do not develop AML until 3–6 months after birth, and even then with a modest penetrance of only 15–30%, and often with acquisition of secondary cytogenetic abnormalities.

## Mixed lineage leukemia gene rearrangements (11q23)

Abnormalities of 11q23 (containing the mixed lineage leukemia, *MLL*, gene) are found in 5–6% of AMLs. These abnormalities can occur at any age but are particularly common in children and after treatment with DNA topoisomerase II inhibitors. The *MLL* gene is the most promiscuous of genes involved in translocations in AML and has been reported fused with more than 30 partner genes. These translocations lead to fusion genes containing the N-terminus of *MLL* fused in-frame to the partner gene, most of which have subsequently been noted to have roles in normal hematopoiesis. Molecular studies have also shown that *MLL* is frequently rearranged by cryptic translocations that are not detectable by conventional cytogenetics.

The *MLL* gene is a transcription factor important for embryonic development and regulation of hematopoietic differentiation. Similar to *RUNX1* and *CBFB*, homozygous disruption of *MLL* in mice is lethal to the embryos because of disordered hematopoiesis. MLL is thought to function as both a transcriptional activator and a transcriptional repressor, using different domains within the protein. Importantly, the repression domain is more N-terminal to the activation domain such that oncogenic MLL fusion proteins are thought to retain their repression, while losing their transcriptional activation capability.

The prognostic impact of *MLL* translocations appears to be variable and may be determined by the partner gene. However, in general, 11q23 abnormalities confer an intermediate to poor prognosis.

## Numeric chromosomal abnormalities

In addition to translocations, numeric chromosomal abnormalities are noted on karyotyping of many AML cases. These numeric aberrations are non-random, with particular chromosomes being more likely to exhibit losses or gains. Acquired trisomy of chromosome 8 or 21 is frequently seen and is associated with an intermediate prognosis. More importantly, partial or complete loss of chromosome 5 and/ or 7 confers a very poor prognosis. Abnormalities of chromosome 7, usually in the form of monosomy or partial deletion of the long arm, constitute the second most frequent numeric chromosomal abnormality in *de novo* AML, after trisomy 8.

Many investigators have attempted to narrow the region of interest on chromosomes 5 and 7 in order to determine the deleted genes that result in leukemia; however, no single culprit gene has been conclusively identified. Two potential gene targets, *CTNNA1* and *EGR1*, have been reported on chromosome 5 but these require confirmation. However, recent investigations in myelodysplastic syndromes (MDS) involving deletion of the long arm of chromosome 5 (5q–) were successful. A novel investigational technique using RNA interference identified loss of the ribosomal subunit-encoding gene *RPS14* as the causative gene defect in the 5q– syndrome. The region of loss on chromosome 5 in AML is more centromeric to that in MDS with 5q–; however, many patients lose both regions, suggesting that deletion of *RPS14* may be a necessary "second hit" in some cases of AML.

Monosomy 7 is also interesting because it is the most commonly acquired abnormality in children with syndromes that predispose to AML, such as Fanconi anemia and other bone marrow failure syndromes. This suggests that monosomy 7 is a secondary genetic aberration and likely requires the presence of other mutations to cause AML.

## Molecular genetic aberrations not detectable by conventional cytogenetics

New molecular tests have rapidly advanced the field of AML genetics in the last several years and have revealed numerous novel leukemogenic mutations that can act in concert to cause AML. Analysis of the catalog of mutations that have been cloned in human acute leukemias has suggested that disease alleles can be broadly divided into two categories: those that confer a proliferative and/or survival advantage on hematopoietic progenitors and those that impair hematopoietic differentiation. This forms the basis of the theory of the multistep development of leukemia in which one mutation alone is not sufficient to transform a normal cell into a leukemic blast.

A summary of the recently discovered mutations in AML is presented below, focusing on gene mutations associated with a prognostic impact in patients with AML (Figures 4.1 and 4.2).

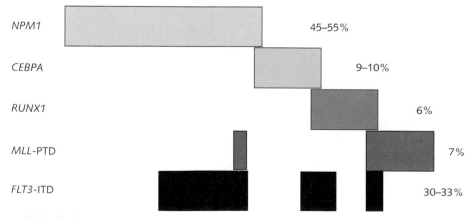

**Fig. 4.1 Frequencies and distributions of *NPM1*, *CEBPA*, *RUNX1*, *MLL*-PTD and *FLT3*-ITD mutations in normal-karyotype AML**

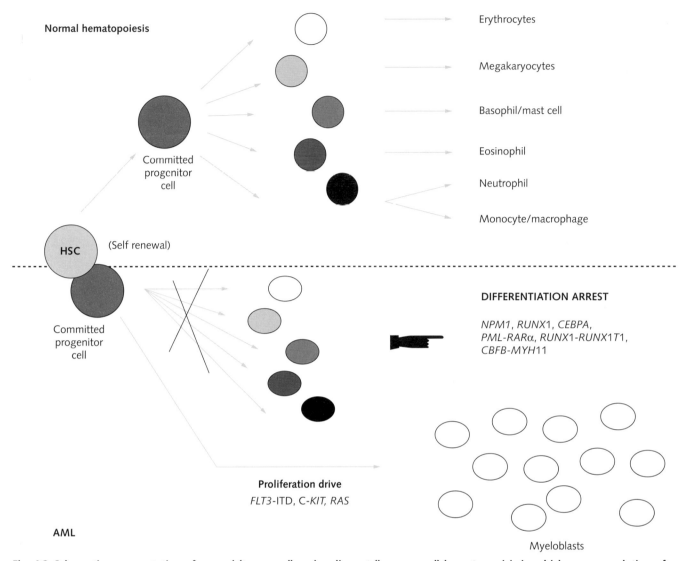

**Fig. 4.2** Schematic representation of normal (top panel) and malignant (lower panel) hematopoeisis in which an accumulation of gene mutations in the hematopoietic stem cell (HSC) or the committed progenitor cell leads to loss of normal differentiation, in concert with mutations conferring a proliferative advantage to the undifferentiated myeloblasts

## Mutations that confer a proliferative and/or survival advantage

### FLT3

*FLT3* (FMS-like tyrosine kinase 3) encodes a membrane-bound receptor tyrosine kinase with important roles in hematopoietic stem/progenitor cell survival, differentiation and proliferation. *FLT3* is constitutively activated by acquired mutation in approximately 30–35% of cases of AML. In 20–25% of cases, internal tandem duplications (ITDs) are noted in the juxtamembrane domain, ranging in size from 3 to 400 nucleotides, with the resultant transcripts always being in-frame and adding to the length of the protein. *FLT3* is normally expressed in myeloid and lymphoid progenitor cells and expression is lost as hematopoietic cells differentiate. In comparison, ITDs of *FLT3* result in constitutive activation of the tyrosine kinase. This results in subsequent activation of downstream signaling targets, including the phosphatidylinositol 3-kinase (PI3K)/AKT, Ras/MAPK and JAK2/STAT pathways. Mutations in *FLT3* also occur in the activation loop of the tyrosine kinase domain (TKD) in about 5–10% of AML cases. These also result in constitutive kinase activation but there is increasing evidence that the downstream signaling events are different in the setting of TKD versus ITD, such that their clinical implications are not equivalent.

AML with *FLT3*-ITD constitutes an important subset of AML cases that has a poor prognosis in most studies of children and adults. The clinical implications of TKD mutations remain controversial and larger studies are required to define if these also confer a poor prognosis. The frequency of *FLT3* mutations varies considerably in different cytogenetic subgroups of AML, with a particularly high frequency of 30–35% in normal-karyotype and t(15;17) AML cases. The poor prognosis of *FLT3*-ITD in normal-karyotype AML is conferred via increased relapse rates with subsequent reduced event-free survival (EFS) and overall survival (OS). The complete remission rate is not affected but several studies have shown that the duration of complete remission is significantly reduced in these patients. The significance of *FLT3*-ITD in t(15;17) cases is unclear but it does not appear to be an independent prognostic factor in APL patients.

The dosage of *FLT3*-ITD is another important complication. Most *FLT3*-ITDs are found in the heterozygous state but some cases are noted to have homozygous *FLT3*-ITD with complete loss of the wild-type allele. The homozygous *FLT3* mutation is thought to arise as a consequence of mitotic recombination resulting in segmental uniparental disomy. Prognosis appears to be worse for these patients and for other patients with high expression ratios of the mutated to wild-type *FLT3*. The presence of uniparental disomy in AML has been linked to homozygous mutations in several genes, which are known mutational targets in AML. This suggests that the mutation (such as *FLT3*-ITD) precedes mitotic recombination, which then acts as a "second hit" responsible for removal of the remaining wild-type allele. A similar mechanism was recently demonstrated for the *JAK2* gene in myeloproliferative disorders. Finally, the size of the duplicated segment may also affect EFS, with a suggestion that longer ITDs result in worsened outcomes.

The relatively high frequency of *FLT3*-ITD initially stimulated interest for its use as a marker of minimal residual disease (MRD). However, studies have shown that the mutational status of *FLT3* may change between diagnosis and relapse, with about 9% of patients losing their *FLT3*-ITD status. The length of the *FLT3*-ITD has also been noted to vary between diagnosis and relapse. This discordance between diagnosis and relapse suggests that *FLT3* mutations are not sufficient for the development of overt AML but may be secondary events in leukemogenesis. This is further demonstrated by murine bone marrow transplantation and "knock-in" models in which *FLT3*-ITD induces a myeloproliferative disease, but does not cause AML. The *FLT3*-ITD phenotype is similar to that reported in the murine bone marrow transplantation assay for other constitutively activated tyrosine kinases associated with myeloproliferative phenotypes in humans, including BCR-ABL, TEL-PDGFβR, TEL-ABL and TEL-JAK2. Taken together, these data indicate that constitutive activation of tyrosine kinases is sufficient to induce a myeloproliferative phenotype, but not AML.

### c-KIT

The c-*KIT* gene encodes c-KIT, a member of the type III receptor tyrosine kinase family, the same family as *FLT3*. c-KIT's ligand, stem cell factor (SCF), promotes c-KIT dimerization and phosphorylation, activating downstream signaling pathways important for proliferation, differentiation and migration of hematopoietic stem cells. Gain-of-function mutations in c-*KIT* occur at various sites within the tyrosine kinase causing constitutive kinase activation. The overall frequency of c-KIT mutations in AML is 5–10%. However, a much higher frequency of 12–45% is observed in the CBF leukemias. Interestingly, c-*KIT* mutations are not seen in APL. Thus, a significant functional redundancy is noted between c-*KIT* and *FLT3* mutations, with c-*KIT* mutations arising in CBF leukemias in which *FLT3* aberrations are absent and *FLT3* mutations arising in APL in which c-*KIT* mutations are absent. Occurrence of c-*KIT* and *FLT3* mutations within the same patient are also very rare. Like *FLT3*-ITD in normal-karyotype AML, certain c-*KIT* mutations confer a higher risk of relapse in CBF leukemias. Conflicting evidence has been reported on the impact of c-*KIT* mutations on survival in these cases, such that confirmatory studies are necessary to be confident of their adverse impact on survival.

## Mutations that affect hematopoietic differentiation

### NPM1

Nucleophosmin (*NPM1*) mutations were first reported in 2005 by Falini and colleagues as the most frequent genetic alteration in patients with normal-karyotype AML. NPM1 is a nucleolar phosphoprotein that continuously shuttles between the nucleus and the cytoplasm but with predominant nucleolar localization. NPM1 acts as a molecular chaperone in the nucleolus and is also involved in cell cycle progression and regulation of the alternate reading frame (ARF)/TP53 tumor-suppressor pathway. Mutations in *NPM1* occur in exon 12, with more than 95% consisting of a 4-bp insertion at position 960. This 4-bp insertion results in a frameshift within the C-terminal region of the NPM1 protein, resulting in loss of nucleolar localization and gain of a nuclear export signal. The mutant NPM1 protein (called

NPM1c+) therefore acquires aberrant cytoplasmic localization, which is readily detected by immunohistochemistry. This cytoplasmic localization is thought to be necessary for the leukemogenic activity of NPM1c+, although details of the exact mechanism are not yet known.

*NPM1* mutations occur predominantly in the normal-karyotype AML subgroup, with about 50% of this group affected. Mutations are very rarely observed in the favorable or adverse risk groups. These mutations are significantly associated with aberrations in *FLT3* (both ITD and TKD), with 60% of patients with *NPM1* mutations also carrying a *FLT3*-ITD. The prognostic relevance of *NPM1* mutations has been clarified in several large studies, with clear evidence that patients with NPM1c+/wild-type FLT3 have an improved prognosis over other normal-karyotype AML patients. These individuals have an EFS and OS with conventional chemotherapy which is similar to those with CBF leukemias. In most studies, the favorable outcome predicted by *NPM1* mutations is restricted to patients who lack the *FLT3*-ITD. Interestingly, initial studies suggest that *NPM1* mutations are very stable between diagnosis and relapse and thus are likely to constitute a primary event in leukemogenesis. Subsequent acquisition of *FLT3* or other secondary mutations is thought to be necessary to trigger overt AML development. The stability of *NPM1* mutations and their high frequency has stimulated interest in the use of this molecular marker as a target for MRD monitoring, which will hopefully be useful for the management of individual patients in the coming years.

### RUNX1

*RUNX1* is commonly dysregulated in AML, by translocations in t(8;21) CBF leukemia and by point mutations in intermediate-risk patients. Although point mutations occur in only 6–10% of *de novo* AMLs, they are much more frequent in specific subgroups, arising in about 20% of FAB M0 (undifferentiated) AML and about 25% of AML associated with myelodysplasia (MDS), including refractory anemia with excess blasts, AML with multilineage dysplasia and AML following MDS. These point mutations are yet more frequent in therapy-related MDS/AML and in radiation-associated MDS/AML (tested in survivors of the atomic bomb in Hiroshima).

Further evidence of RUNX1's involvement in the pathogenesis of AML has come from the analysis of pedigrees with an inherited predisposition to MDS/AML. Familial platelet disorder with propensity to develop myeloid malignancy (FPD/AML syndrome) is an autosomal dominant disorder caused by germline mutations in the *RUNX1* gene. Individuals with FPD/AML have a variable risk of developing overt MDS/AML (20–60% in different pedigrees) and a large range in age of presentation of MDS/AML (age 6–75 years). This latency suggests that secondary mutations are necessary to trigger MDS/AML and that a heterozygous *RUNX1* mutation is insufficient alone.

Secondary mutations are also required for overt leukemia development in *RUNX1*-mutated *de novo* MDS/AML. AML M0 cases frequently demonstrate biallelic *RUNX1* mutations and MDS cases demonstrate additional karyotypic abnormalities. *RUNX1* mutations are also frequently associated with acquired trisomy 21 in non-M0 MDS/AML, with two of the three *RUNX1* alleles carrying the mutation. Finally, *RUNX1* mutations are also strongly associated with trisomy 13. As *FLT3* resides on chromosome 13, trisomy 13 leads to increased expression of *FLT3* acting as the necessary secondary mutation.

### CEBPA

C/EBPα is a transcription factor that regulates genes involved in myeloid differentiation, particularly by inducing granulocytic development of bipotential myeloid progenitors. The protein consists of N-terminal transactivating domains, a DNA-binding domain and a C-terminal leucine-zipper region (bZIP), necessary for dimerization. The gene contains two translational start sites, yielding a 42-kDa and a smaller 30-kDa isoform. Somatic *CEBPA* mutations are noted in about 9% of AML cases and 70% of these mutations are detected in patients with normal-karyotype AML. The morphological features of the disease are distinctive, with a predominance of M1 and M2 subtypes. Mutations are usually N-terminal and out-of-frame and abolish the production of the full-length 42-kDa protein with upregulation of the truncated 30-kDa isoform. The 30-kDa C/EBPα isoform lacks the first transactivating domain but retains the bZIP region required for dimerization and is thus able to dimerize with the wild-type 42-kDa protein, and is thought to inhibit its function in a dominant-negative manner. *CEBPA* mutations in normal-karyotype AML patients are noted to confer a favorable prognosis, similar to the outcomes for patients with CBF leukemia, although most recent studies suggest that such favorable outcomes are associated with biallelic inactivation of the gene.

Similar to *RUNX1*, *CEBPA* mutations have been observed in very rare pedigrees with familial AML. The reported pedigrees were all noted to exhibit germline mutations in the N-terminal region of *CEBPA*. The nature and timing of *CEBPA* mutations in familial AML provides further insight into the sequence of molecular events in the development of leukemia. This insight comes particularly from second mutations targeting the remaining wild-type allele, which are commonly observed in familial and sporadic *CEBPA*-associated AML. Second mutations are usually C-terminal and are in-frame insertions or deletions, which result in interference with dimerization and subsequent loss of C/EBPα function. These appear necessary to cause overt leukemia in familial *CEBPA*-associated AML. Interestingly, one individual with a germline N-terminal *CEBPA* mutation was noted to relapse several years after his original diagnosis, but with a distinctive somatic C-terminal mutation different from that observed in his original AML. This implies that, rather than a true relapse, this individual developed two discrete secondary events and two unrelated episodes of AML. As with FPD/AML, the age of presentation of disease is extremely variable in familial *CEBPA*-associated AML, ranging from 4 to 39 years. However, the disease appears to have near-complete penetrance, suggesting that *CEBPA* mutations are primary leukemogenic events.

More recently, a series of patients with presumed sporadic *CEBPA*-mutated AML were investigated and 10% had evidence of a germline *CEBPA* mutation, suggesting that inherited *CEBPA* mutations account for 1% of all AMLs, a much higher frequency than previously appreciated.

### WT1

Mutations in Wilms tumor 1 (*WT1*) gene are observed in 10% of normal-karyotype AMLs. The precise role of *WT1* in normal and malignant hematopoiesis remains controversial but it has been implicated in the regulation of cell survival, proliferation and differentiation. Mutation in *WT1* has recently been observed to act as an independent negative prognostic indicator in AML by reducing the likelihood of achieving a complete remission and/or increasing relapse rates. *WT1* is also highly expressed in the majority of AMLs such that it can be used as a marker for MRD monitoring. Mutations are noted in heterozygous and homozygous states and show some association with *FLT3*-ITD, though larger studies are required to confirm this. Germline mutations in *WT1* are associated with the development of Wilms tumor and other nephrologic syndromes but not with the development of AML, again suggesting that isolated *WT1* mutations are insufficient to cause AML.

### MLL

As with *RUNX1*, the *MLL* gene was first noted to be aberrantly regulated in AML through translocations. Subsequently, *MLL* partial tandem duplications (PTDs) were reported in about 8% of normal-karyotype AML patients. These mutations are restricted to AML patients with normal karyotype or with trisomy 11. *MLL*-PTD was the first gene mutation shown to negatively affect prognosis in normal-karyotype AML patients, with most large studies confirming these initial findings. *MLL*-PTDs are interesting

because the presence of a heterozygous *MLL*-PTD has been associated with silencing of the wild-type allele in AML blasts. The mechanism for this silencing appears to involve epigenetic modifications (DNA methylation and histone modifications) rather than direct mutational effects. This suggests that epigenetic events may be sufficient to serve as secondary events in leukemogenesis. This mechanistic understanding is also important in identifying a new avenue for molecularly targeted therapy in AML through the use of hypomethylating agents and histone deacetylase inhibitors.

## Genes altered by overexpression

Several studies have suggested that overexpression of particular genes is also associated with poor outcomes in AML. The first of these, *BAALC* (brain and acute leukemia, cytoplasmic gene), has been demonstrated to be an independent adverse prognostic indicator in AML. High *BAALC* expression predicts worsened survival and resistance to induction chemotherapy. The mechanism of action for *BAALC* overexpression and its effects are not known. Similar results have been suggested for overexpression of *ERG* (ETS-related gene) and *MN1* (meningioma 1 gene), which have also been reported as new molecular markers conferring poor prognosis. Further studies are necessary to confirm these findings.

## AML therapies targeted by genetics

Traditional cytotoxic chemotherapy is effective in a minority of patients with AML. The majority of younger patients initially respond to treatment by achieving a complete remission, but most relapse and subsequently die of their disease. Current advances in molecular technologies in AML have provided numerous new targets for directed therapies in AML. The best example of targeted therapy in AML is the use of ATRA in APL in which ATRA overcomes the *PML–RARα*-induced differentiation block, leading to maturation of the malignant myeloblasts and promyelocytes.

Most recent work in targeted therapies for AML has been directed toward exploiting aberrantly regulated signal transduction pathways, including those constitutively activated by *FLT3*, c-KIT and *RAS* mutations. This approach of targeting constitutively activated kinases with selective small-molecule inhibitors has been validated by Druker and colleagues by demonstration of the efficacy of the ABL kinase inhibitor imatinib in *BCR-ABL*-positive chronic myelogenous leukemia. While signal transduction inhibitors appear promising in AML, no agent has yet demonstrated obvious clinical benefit when used as monotherapy.

*FLT3* mutations, being among the most common mutations in AML, are an attractive target for therapeutic intervention. Several FLT3-selective inhibitors are in use in clinical trials in humans. These include lestaurtinib (CEP-701), midostaurin (PKC412), tandutinib (MLN518), sunitinib (SU11248, Sutent) and sorafenib (BAY 043-9006, Nexavar). None of these agents are specific for FLT3 but all have FLT3-inhibitory activity *in vitro* and some also show activity against wild-type FLT3 AML samples, suggesting that the drugs may also work in part by FLT3-independent mechanisms. Many have cross-reactivity against other tyrosine kinases that are known to be dysregulated in AML. For example, MLN518 is also a potent inhibitor of KIT and platelet-derived growth factor receptor (PDGFR); CEP-701 also inhibits transforming tyrosine kinase protein (TRKA); PKC412 inhibits KIT, PDGFR and protein kinase C; and sunitinib also inhibits KIT and PDGFR.

Results of several phase I studies of FLT3 inhibitors have demonstrated rapid clearance of peripheral blood blasts but less substantial reductions in bone marrow blasts. Complete remissions have only rarely been seen with any of these agents as monotherapy. Clinical responses were noted to be brief and usually measured in weeks. For this reason, the test for FLT3 inhibitors will be with their efficacy when combined with traditional chemotherapy or other targeted agents. *In vitro* data have shown additive or synergistic interactions between FLT3 inhibitors and chemotherapy and several trials are underway to see if this approach may improve outcomes for AML patients. A few small studies have been reported with some encouraging results but larger ongoing trials are required to determine whether FLT3 inhibitors will provide benefit to AML patients.

Several other small-molecule inhibitors are also being investigated in AML. The growth-stimulating ras/raf/MAPK pathway is frequently constitutively activated in AML by *RAS* mutations or by other events. (Despite being frequent in AML, *RAS* mutations have not been discussed in this chapter because they have not demonstrated prognostic impact in AML.) RAS activation is dependent on the post-translational addition of a prenyl group by farnesyltransferase. Small molecules targeting RAS itself have proven difficult to produce; thus current attempts have focused on inhibition of RAS prenylation. Several small-molecule inhibitors of farnesyltransferase have been developed including two that have moved to human studies, tipifarnib (R115777, Zarnestra) and lonafarnib (SCH66336, Sarasar). Early tipifarnib studies were encouraging but, similar to FLT3 inhibitors, the responses were brief. Early results from a large Phase III trial of monotherapy with tipifarnib versus best supportive care in elderly patients over age 70 years suggest no benefit to the drug. Additionally, results from a large Phase I/II trial of tipifarnib plus cytotoxic chemotherapy in younger patients with AML and MDS are less encour-

aging. Confirmation of these results and other trials are awaited.

The newest line of investigation in signal transduction inhibition is via the PI3K pathway and its downstream effectors AKT and mTOR. Constitutive activation of this pathway is also frequently noted in AML, prompting investigation of several AKT and mTOR inhibitors. Most data are available for mTOR inhibitors, including sirolimus (rapamycin, Rapamune), temsirolimus (CCI-779, Torisel) and everolimus (RAD-001, Certican). Sirolimus and temsirolimus are already available as marketed agents for use as immunosuppressants. Several years of clinical experience with these agents as immunosuppressants has provided safety data that has enabled more rapid investigation in AML. Early *in vitro* studies have again been encouraging and trials in humans have begun and are eagerly awaited.

## Summary

Recurrent cytogenetic abnormalities are frequent in AML and many new molecular aberrations have also been discovered that are undetectable by conventional karyotyping. Studies suggest that at least two, and probably many more, mutations are required for the development of AML. Genotypic analysis of known leukemia oncogenes indicates that there are at least two broad complementation groups of mutations. One class of mutations, exemplified by *FLT3*-ITD or c-*KIT* mutations, confers a proliferative and/or survival advantage on hematopoietic progenitors. The second group of mutations, resulting in loss of function of hematopoietic transcription factors, result in a block in differentiation in hematopoietic development. It is thought that coexpression of a mutation that confers a proliferative and/or survival advantage and a mutation than impairs hematopoietic differentiation results in AML.

Many of these newly discovered genetic aberrations have prognostic implications and may be used to help risk-stratify patients for therapy. Currently, AML patients who are at high risk of relapse are recommended for allogeneic stem cell transplantation, a treatment with a relatively high morbidity and mortality. The decision of whether to proceed to transplantation is a difficult one for both the patient and the physician. As new molecular markers are detected which help us better risk-stratify individual patients, these treatment decisions will become clearer. New molecular discoveries are also helping to direct research toward novel targeted therapies. In the future, it may be possible to use combinations of molecularly targeted therapies, in selected clinical contexts, to improve outcomes and/or to reduce toxicity.

The future of molecular genetics in AML appears bright, with the rapid development of sensitive high-throughput investigational techniques leading to further discoveries of novel gene mutations such as the recent detection of mutations in the *TET2* (ten eleven translocation 2) and *ASXL1* (additional sex comb like 1) genes. Studies of aberrant gene expression and altered methylation may also provide new avenues for targeted therapies. Given the dismal prognosis for most patients with AML, these recent discoveries have brought new excitement to the field of leukemia research and have identified new avenues for the treatment of patients.

## Acknowledgments

Drs Owen and Fitzgibbon are supported by grants from Cancer Research UK and the Medical Research Council in the UK and the Sangara Family Fund through the Department of Leukemia/BMT of British Columbia in Canada.

## Further reading

### Acute myeloid leukemia

Mrozek K, Marcucci G, Paschka P *et al.* (2007) Clinical relevance of mutations and gene-expression changes in adult acute myeloid leukemia with normal cytogenetics: are we ready for a prognostically prioritized molecular classification? *Blood*, **109**, 431–448.

Renneville A, Roumier C, Biggio V *et al.* (2008) Cooperating gene mutations in acute myeloid leukemia: a review of the literature. *Leukemia*, **22**, 915–931.

Schlenk RF, Dohner K, Krauter J *et al.* (2008) Mutations and treatment outcome in cytogenetically normal acute myeloid leukemia. *New England Journal of Medicine*, **358**, 1909–1918.

### Molecular genetics of leukemia

Bullinger L, Valk PJ. (2005) Gene expression profiling in acute myeloid leukemia. *Journal of Clinical Oncology*, **23**, 6296–6305.

Huntly BJP, Gilliland DG. (2005) Leukemia stem cells and the evolution of cancer-stem-cell research. *Nature Reviews. Cancer*, **5**, 311–321.

Raghavan M, Lillington DM, Skoulakis S *et al.* (2005) Genome-wide single nucleotide polymorphism analysis reveals frequent partial uniparental disomy due to somatic recombination in acute myeloid leukemias. *Cancer Research*, **65**, 375–378.

Speck NA, Gilliland DG. (2002) Core-binding factors in haematopoiesis and leukemia. *Nature Reviews. Cancer*, **2**, 502–513.

### FLT3 in leukemia

Gale RE, Green C, Allen C *et al.* (2008) The impact of FLT3 internal tandem duplication mutant level, number, size, and interaction with NPM1 mutations in a large cohort of young adult patients with acute myeloid leukemia. *Blood*, **111**, 2776–2784.

Thiede C, Steudel C, Mohr B *et al.* (2002) Analysis of FLT3-activating mutations in 979 patients with acute myelogenous leukemia: association with FAB subtypes and identification of subgroups with poor prognosis. *Blood*, **99**, 4326–4335.

### NPM1 in leukemia

Falini B, Mecucci C, Tiacci E *et al.* (2005) Cytoplasmic nucleophosmin in acute myelogenous leukemia with normal karyotype. *New England Journal of Medicine*, **352**, 254–266.

Schnittger S, Schoch C, Kern W *et al.* (2005) Nucleophosmin gene mutations are predictors of favorable prognosis in acute myelogenous leukemia with a normal karyotype. *Blood*, **106**, 3733–3739.

### Further molecular markers in AML

Osato M. (2004) Point mutations in the RUNX1/AML1 gene: another actor in RUNX leukemia. *Oncogene*, **23**, 4284–4296.

### Familial AML

Michaud J, Wu F, Osato M *et al.* (2002) In vitro analyses of known and novel RUNX1/AML1 mutations in dominant familial platelet disorder with predisposition to acute myelogenous leukemia: implications for mechanisms of pathogenesis. *Blood*, **99**, 1364–1372.

Owen C, Barnett M, Fitzgibbon J. (2008) Familial myelodysplasia and acute myeloid leukemia: a review. *British Journal of Haematology*, **140**, 123–132.

Song W-J, Sullivan MG, Legare RD *et al.* (1999) Haploinsufficiency of CBFA2 (AML1) causes familial thrombocytopenia with propensity to develop acute myelogenous leukemia (FPD/AML). *Nature Genetics*, **23**, 166–175.

### Targeted therapy

Perl A, Carroll M. (2007) Exploiting signal transduction pathways in acute myelogenous leukemia. *Current Treatment Options in Oncology*, **8**, 265–276.

# Chapter 5 Secondary myelodysplasia/acute myelogenous leukemia: assessment of risk

## D Gary Gilliland[1] & John G Gribben[2]

[1] Howard Hughes Medical Institute, Brigham and Women's Hospital; Dana-Farber Cancer Institute, Harvard Medical School, Boston, MA, USA
[2] Centre for Experimental Cancer Medicine, Institute of Cancer, Barts and The London School of Medicine & Dentistry, London, UK

## Introduction

A major complication of chemotherapy and radiotherapy for the treatment of cancer is the subsequent development of therapy-related myelodysplastic syndromes and secondary acute myelogenous leukemia (t-MDS/AML). Although devastating in their impact, t-MDS/AML allow the opportunity to study the development of malignancy since many such patients have serial blood and bone marrow samples available from the time of initial therapy to their subsequent diagnosis with leukemia. There is abundant evidence that t-MDS/AML are clonal disorders that are the consequence of acquired somatic mutations and confer a proliferative and/or survival advantage on hematopoietic progenitors. No single mutation or gene rearrangement appears to be sufficient for the development of tMDS/AML. Indeed, the identification of a single gene rearrangement or point mutation may not necessarily be predictive of its subsequent development. Methods for assessing risk are based on the presence of clonal abnormalities in hematopoietic cells, including standard cytogenetics, interphase fluorescence *in situ* hybridization (FISH), analysis for loss of heterozygosity (LOH), polymerase chain reaction (PCR) for point mutations, and X-inactivation-based clonality assays. Each of these approaches has strengths and weaknesses, and they are discussed in more detail below.

The actuarial risk of developing therapy-related leukemia (t-MDS/AML) varies with the therapy used to treat the cancer. Although some agents are associated with particu-

larly increased risk, in general the more intensive the therapy, the higher the risk. The risk of the development of t-MDS/AML after high-dose chemoradiotherapy and autologous stem cell transplantation (ASCT) for lymphoma is substantial, ranging from 3% to as many as 24% of patients. In our own series of patients with non-Hodgkin lymphoma who have undergone high-dose therapy and ASCT at the Dana-Farber Cancer Institute, development of t-MDS/AML has emerged as the second most common cause of death, after relapse of disease, in these patients. On review of these cases, it became clear that strict criteria were required to make the diagnosis of secondary MDS. A number of patients have relative pancytopenia after ASCT and many patients have dysplastic features and cytogenetic abnormalities, but only 30% of these patients develop secondary MDS. The criteria that we use to define t-MDS are shown in Table 5.1. On the basis of these criteria, some patients initially reported to have developed t-MDS in the original report from this center have now been excluded, and it is of note that none of these patients has progressed to t-MDS or AML. The median time from high-dose therapy to the development of t-MDS was 47 months, with a range of 12–129 months after ASCT. The actuarial risk of development of t-MDS in these patients is shown in Figure 5.1. The prognosis of these patients remains dismal and they have a median survival after diagnosis of less than 1 year.

## Risk factors for t-MDS/AML after autologous stem cell transplantation

Because t-MDS/AML is frequently a fatal complication, there is a need to better understand the risk factors and to identify individuals at risk prior to ASCT. There are three

*Molecular Hematology*, 3rd edition. Edited by Drew Provan and John Gribben.
© 2010 Blackwell Publishing.

**Table 5.1** Criteria used to define t-MDS after ASCT at Dana-Farber Cancer Institute.

- Significant marrow dysplasia in at least two cell lineages
- Peripheral cytopenia without alternative explanation
- Blast counts in marrow defined by FAB classification

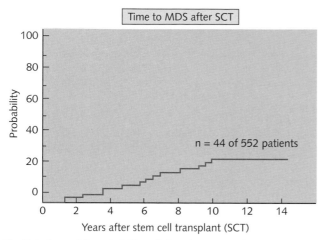

**Fig. 5.1 Actuarial probability of development of t-MDS/AML after ASCT**

contributors to the risk of t-MDS/AML in this context that have been identified: pretransplant therapy, the method of stem cell mobilization, and the transplant conditioning regimens.

The data implicating pretransplant therapy as a risk factor include the demonstration that patients who do not undergo ASCT have a risk of developing t-MDS/AML, although there is a relatively longer latency of development of t-MDS/AML in patients who have undergone ASCT. In patients who have undergone ASCT, there is increased risk with increased cumulative exposure to alkylating agents and with prior external beam irradiation. Specific cytogenetic abnormalities and clonal hematopoiesis have been identified at the time of stem cell harvest in patients who subsequently develop t-MDS/AML.

The method of stem cell collection may influence the risk of developing t-MDS/AML. For example, patients undergoing ASCT using peripheral blood stem cells (PBSC) have a higher risk of developing t-MDS/AML than those receiving bone marrow stem cells. There may be several explanations for this observation, including the possibility that previously only those patients who had inadequate marrow harvests had PBSC collected. It has also been reported that patients primed by receiving etoposide as part of their mobilization regimen had a higher risk of developing t-MDS/AML; this

included patients with 11q23 and 21q22 chromosomal abnormalities.

The use of total body irradiation (TBI) in the conditioning regimen is associated with an increased risk of t-MDS/AML after ASCT, although a randomized trial to determine the contribution of TBI to the risk of t-MDS/AML has not been done. Only one study has compared patients who did and did not receive TBI at a single institution, and this did not demonstrate increased incidence in patients who received a TBI-containing regimen.

## Therapy-related AML is a clonal disorder

There is abundant evidence that t-MDS and AML are clonal disorders. Multiple cytogenetic abnormalities, including deletions (5q, 7q, 20q), numerical abnormalities (trisomy 8, deletion 7), translocations [11q23, t(3;21), t(15;17)] and clonal point mutations of *RAS*, *FLT3* and *AML1*, have been identified in t-MDS/AML. Population-based analysis of clonality using X-inactivation assays in females has convincingly demonstrated that t-MDS/AML is a clonal disease. Thus, t-MDS/AML is a clonal disease that is the consequence of an acquired somatic mutation that confers a proliferative and/or survival advantage on hematopoietic progenitors.

## More than one mutation is necessary to cause AML

It is plausible to determine risk through the analysis of molecular markers of disease. However, no single mutation or gene rearrangement appears to be sufficient for the development of therapy-related AML.

Several lines of evidence support the requirement for second mutations in leukemias associated with mutations of core-binding factor (*CBF*), including analysis of the heritable FPD/AML syndrome (familial platelet disorder with propensity to develop AML), the *TEL/AML1* leukemias in syngeneic twins, and murine models of *AML1/ETO* and *CBFβ/MYH11* leukemias. In addition, point mutations that cause loss of function of AML1 have been identified in both inherited and sporadic leukemias. *CBF* is a heterodimeric transcription factor comprising *AML1* (also known as *RUNX1*) and *CBFβ* subunits. It is a common target of gene rearrangements as a consequence of chromosomal translocations, giving rise to the *AML1/ETO*, *CBFβ/MYH11* and *TEL/AML1* fusions. FPD/AML syndrome is an autosomal dominant trait characterized by a qualitative and quantitative platelet defect, progressive pancytopenia and dysplasia with age, and progression to AML associated with acquisition of secondary mutations. FPD/AML is caused by loss-of-function mutations in the *AML1* gene, demonstrating that mutations in the *AML1* component of *CBF* are not sufficient to cause leukemia, but require second mutations during the lifetime of affected individuals to cause leukemia. *TEL/AML1* leukemias have been studied in syngeneic twins, each of whom harbored the same clone of cells containing the TEL/AML1 gene rearrangement at the time of birth, presumably as a result of intrauterine transmission of a *TEL/AML1*-positive clone. However, despite the syngeneic host background and the carriage of an identical *TEL/AML1* clone, the twins developed leukemia at widely different ages, indicating the need for additional mutations to cause leukemia.

Murine models of leukemia also provide convincing evidence for "multiple-hit" pathogenesis of disease. Expression of either AML1/ETO or CBFβ/MYH11 fusion proteins alone in hematopoietic cells is not sufficient to cause leukemia, and chemical-induced mutagenesis must be added to generate a leukemia phenotype. Similar data emerge for *PML/RARα*-mediated leukemias in transgenic murine models. *PML/RARα* is expressed in promyelocytes in the germline of transgenic animals under the control of the cathepsin G promoter. However, despite germline expression, animals require 4–6 months to develop leukemia and have karyotypically evident second mutations. Similarly, in *MLL/AF9* "knock-in" mice there is a long latency required for the development of leukemia, and MLL/CBP leukemias in a murine bone marrow transplant model require long latencies, indicative of the need for second mutations.

Furthermore, leukemogenic fusions have been detected using sensitive PCR-based assays in normal individuals. Examples include *IgH/BCL2*, *BCR/ABL*, *MLL* tandem duplication and the *TEL/AML1* fusion. The frequency of these rearrangements is much higher in the general population than the risk of developing the respective leukemias. These data indicate that carriage of even a known leukemogenic fusion gene does not provide useful information about the likelihood of progression to leukemia. Indeed, there are currently no data demonstrating that PCR-detectable fusions are a risk factor for the eventual development of leukemia. Collectively, these data indicate that the identification of a single gene rearrangement or point mutation may not necessarily be predictive of the development of therapy-related AML in the post-ASCT setting.

## Methods for assessing the risk of therapy-related leukemia

Methods for assessing risk are based on the presence of clonal abnormalities in hematopoietic cells. These methods

---

**Table 5.2** Methods for assessing the risk of t-MDS/AML before and after ASCT.

- Standard cytogenetics
- Interphase FISH
- Loss of heterozygosity
- PCR for point mutations
- X-inactivation-based clonality

---

are shown in Table 5.2 and include standard cytogenetics, interphase FISH, analysis for LOH, PCR for point mutations, and X-inactivation-based clonality assays. Each of these approaches has strengths and weaknesses in this context.

*Standard cytogenetics* analyzes a limited number of cells that must be capable of mitosis and therefore lacks sensitivity and specificity. Most patients who develop t-MDS/AML after ASCT may have normal cytogenetics at the time of stem cell harvest, whereas some patients who have characteristic cytogenetic abnormalities will not develop t-MDS/AML.

*Interphase FISH* (Figure 5.2) circumvents some of the frailties of conventional cytogenetics. For example, abnormal clones (5q–, –7, +8, –11) were detectable in pre-ASCT specimens from 9 of 12 patients who developed t-MDS/AML. An advantage of interphase FISH is that hundreds of non-mitotic cells can be analyzed. However, the technique is locus-specific and requires prior selection of markers for analysis, such as 5q–, 7q– and +8. In addition, interphase FISH is not sensitive below the level of approximately 5–10% of cells. However, the identification of clonal abnormalities in a high percentage of cells may indicate a proliferative advantage for these cells, and may be more predictive of the development of t-MDS/AML. The specificity of interphase FISH is also unknown, since we do not know how many patients who do not develop t-MDS/AML have interphase FISH abnormalities at the time of stem cell harvest. The test has been validated only in retrospective studies, and it is time- and labor-intensive as a screening test.

*LOH analysis* is based on the loss of one allele at a particular locus, usually by PCR analysis. This strategy can be used to identify LOH and to define the excursion of large deletions (Figures 5.3 and 5.4). It is a population-based assay and requires prior selection of loci to be analyzed. It lacks sensitivity and is probably unable to detect fewer than 20% of cells with LOH at a given locus. However, it is more likely to be specific, in that a positive test indicates clonal expansion of cells with LOH. It is amenable to high-throughput strategies, but has not yet been validated as a predictor of post-ASCT t-MDS/AML in prospective studies, although such studies are underway.

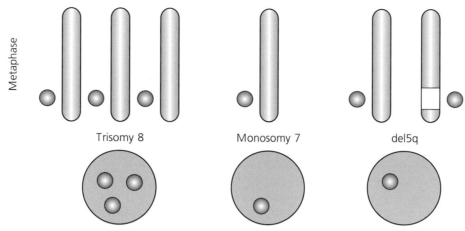

**Fig. 5.2 Applications of interphase FISH to detect trisomy, monosomy or chromosomal deletions**

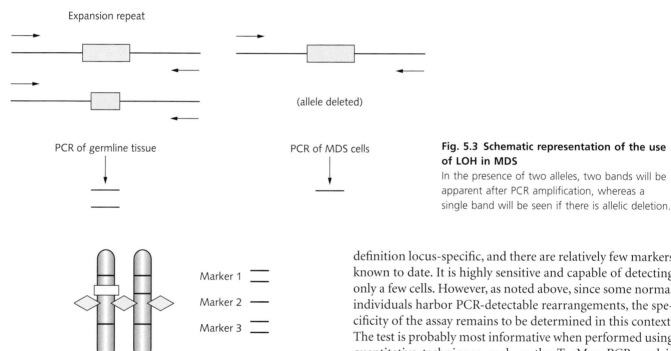

**Fig. 5.3 Schematic representation of the use of LOH in MDS**

In the presence of two alleles, two bands will be apparent after PCR amplification, whereas a single band will be seen if there is allelic deletion.

**Fig. 5.4 Schematic representation of the use of LOH to map deletions**

*PCR for point mutations or chromosomal translocations* is emerging as a potentially useful predictor of t-MDS/AML as we learn more about the molecular genetics of the disease. Markers that may be useful include mutations in *RAS*, *FLT3*, *AML1* and *MLL*. In addition, PCR can be used to identify fusion transcripts, including *AML1/EVI1*, *PML/RARα* and 11q23 gene rearrangements. The PCR approach is also by definition locus-specific, and there are relatively few markers known to date. It is highly sensitive and capable of detecting only a few cells. However, as noted above, since some normal individuals harbor PCR-detectable rearrangements, the specificity of the assay remains to be determined in this context. The test is probably most informative when performed using quantitative techniques, such as the TaqMan PCR, and is amenable to high-throughput analysis, but has not yet been validated as a predictor of t-MDS/AML.

*X-inactivation-based clonality assays* require no locus-specific information, or indeed any information about the nature of the mutation that causes t-MDS/AML (Figure 5.5). It detects only clonal populations of cells that have a proliferative advantage over normal polyclonal cells. It uses DNA, is PCR-based and is readily amenable to high-throughput analysis, but is only applicable to female patients. There are several potential pitfalls of this test, including false-positive results due to germline or acquired skewing of the pattern of X-inactivation. This problem can be overcome in part by the appropriate use of related tissue controls. However, the

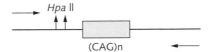

- Variable length CAG expansion repeat distinguishes the maternal from paternal X in >90% of females
- Variably methylated *Hpa* II sites distinguish active from inactive X chromosomes

(a)

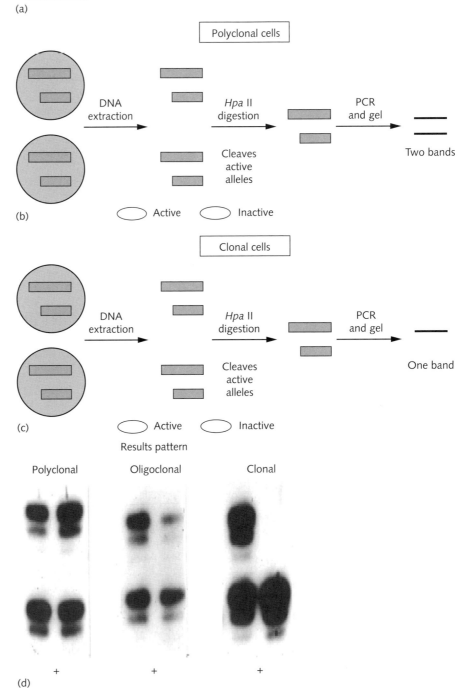

**Fig. 5.5 Human androgen receptor assay (HUMARA)**

(a) Schema of the assay, which uses the variable-length CAG repeat pattern to distinguish the maternal and paternal X chromosomes. (b) Two bands will be seen after PCR amplification in polyclonal cells where there is random inactivation. (c) A single band will be seen in a clonal population. (d) Results from patients studied, showing polyclonal, oligoclonal and clonal populations.

test may be difficult to interpret in cases with severe skewing of the X-inactivation pattern. This technique has been validated in retrospective studies and prospective studies are ongoing.

## Approaches for minimizing the risk of t-MDS/AML

It may be appropriate to minimize, where possible, agents that are particularly associated with the greatest risk, including alkylating agents, external beam irradiation and topoisomerase inhibitors. This can be accomplished in part by the identification of high-risk individuals who are likely to require ASCT as part of their therapy. Recent innovations in the application both of standard prognostic indicators and of global expression arrays may help in the identification of such patients, and efforts to assess risk using molecular markers should be further explored and validated. It seems advisable to avoid TBI as part of the conditioning regimen, although it may be best to directly determine the risk–benefit ratio of using TBI in a randomized trial. If standard cytogenetics are abnormal, allogeneic rather than autologous stem cell transplantation may be indicated. Selected FISH loci, such as 5q, 7q, +8, 20q and −11, should be explored prospectively as predictors of outcome, as should X-inactivation-based clonality assays. Effort should be devoted to pilot retrospective studies to evaluate the role and validity of genome-wide LOH screens, quantitative PCR for specific mutations and gene rearrangements, and the assessment of global expression patterns to identify signatures predictive of t-MDS/AML.

## Further reading

Castilla LH, Garrett L, Adya N et al. (1999) The fusion gene Cbfβ blocks myeloid differentiation and predisposes mice to acute myelomonocytic leukemia. *Nature Genetics*, **23**, 144–146.

Ford AM, Bennett CA, Price CM et al. (1998) Fetal origins of the TEL-AML1 fusion gene in identical twins with leukemia. *Proceedings of the National Academy of Sciences of the United States of America*, **95**, 4584–4588.

Friedberg JW, Neuberg D, Stone RM et al. (1999) Outcome in patients with myelodysplastic syndrome after autologous bone marrow transplantation for non-Hodgkin's lymphoma. *Journal of Clinical Oncology*, **17**, 3128–3135.

Mach-Pascual S, Legare RD, Lu D et al. (1998) Predictive value of clonality assays in patients with non-Hodgkin's lymphoma undergoing autologous bone marrow transplant: a single institution study. *Blood*, **91**, 4496–4503.

Pedersen-Bjergaard J, Andersen MK, Christiansen DH. (2000) Therapy-related acute myeloid leukemia and myelodysplasia after high-dose chemotherapy and autologous stem cell transplantation. *Blood*, **95**, 3273–3279.

Zimonjic DB, Pollock JL, Westervelt P et al. (2000) Acquired, nonrandom chromosomal abnormalities associated with the development of acute promyelocytic leukemia in transgenic mice. *Proceedings of the National Academy of Sciences of the United States of America*, **97**, 13306–13311.

# Chapter 6 Detection of minimal residual disease in hematological malignancies

## John G Gribben

*Centre for Experimental Cancer Medicine, Institute of Cancer, Barts and The London School of Medicine & Dentistry, London, UK*

## Introduction

Despite advances in the treatment of human hematological malignancies, a significant proportion of patients relapse, usually with the same malignant clone found at diagnosis. Detection of residual leukemia or lymphoma cells in marrow, blood or lymph nodes has relied on light microscopy and immunophenotyping. However, these techniques are not sensitive for the detection of small numbers of malignant cells. Other, more sensitive, methods are now available to assess whether early detection of residual tumor might allow intervention and prevent relapse of disease. Multiparameter flow cytometric analysis and molecular techniques, using polymerase chain reaction (PCR), offer highly sensitive detection of residual disease, and these techniques have been applied to a wide variety of diseases.

Many studies have now been carried out in a variety of disorders, and whilst it is true for many hematological cancers that persistence of residual detectable disease predicts which patients will do less well, this does not hold true for all diseases studied. It appears that patients with some malignancies may harbor residual tumor cells for many years without ever showing any evidence of clinical relapse. This is discussed in detail later in this chapter.

This chapter outlines the methods available, with particular emphasis on PCR amplification, and their clinical application to a variety of hematological malignancies, including lymphomas and leukemias. The molecular basis of leukemia and lymphoma is discussed in detail in Chapters 4 and 10.

## What is minimal residual disease?

Minimal residual disease (MRD) describes the *lowest level of disease detectable using available methods*. Previously, light microscopy, cytogenetic analysis and flow cytometry were standard techniques used for the detection of residual malignant cells in the blood and marrow of patients after treatment. However, the sensitivities of these methods do not allow identification of low levels of disease, nor do they allow accurate quantitation of malignant cell numbers. Since these residual malignant cells may be the source of ultimate relapse, there has been great interest in developing molecular techniques for the detection of residual tumor. For many years Southern blot hybridization was the gold standard for the detection of DNA sequence alterations at specific genetic loci, but it has now been superseded by PCR amplification of DNA sequences. Because of the power of PCR technology, we are now able to detect one residual malignant cell in a background of up to 1 million normal cells. Molecular targets for PCR-based approaches include chromosomal translocations and antigen receptor (immunoglobulin and T-cell receptor) gene rearrangements.

### Methods available for the detection of residual disease

Several methods have been used to determine the presence of residual neoplastic cells in blood, bone marrow or other tissue following therapy (Figure 6.1). The ideal assay system for the detection of small numbers of malignant cells in a marrow or blood sample should fulfill the following criteria: be applicable in most cases of the disease under investigation; be specific for the neoplastic cell type; be sensitive; and

*Molecular Hematology*, 3rd edition. Edited by Drew Provan and John Gribben.
© 2010 Blackwell Publishing.

| Technique | | Features | Sensitivity |
|---|---|---|---|
| Morphology | 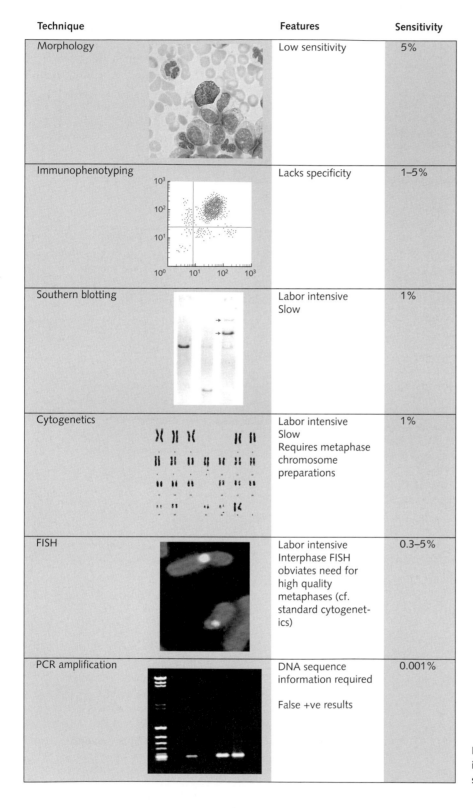 | Low sensitivity | 5% |
| Immunophenotyping | | Lacks specificity | 1–5% |
| Southern blotting | | Labor intensive Slow | 1% |
| Cytogenetics | | Labor intensive Slow Requires metaphase chromosome preparations | 1% |
| FISH | | Labor intensive Interphase FISH obviates need for high quality metaphases (cf. standard cytogenetics) | 0.3–5% |
| PCR amplification | | DNA sequence information required False +ve results | 0.001% |

**Fig. 6.1 Methods of detection of marrow infiltration in non-Hodgkin lymphoma showing the sensitivity of each**

be quantitative for prognostic purposes. Such methods include:
- morphology;
- cell culture assays;
- karyotypic analysis;
- fluorescence *in situ* hybridization (FISH) techniques;
- flow cytometry and immunophenotypic analyses;
- molecular analyses, including Southern blotting and PCR.

## Morphology

In acute leukemia, remission is the term used to describe a bone marrow containing fewer than 5% blast (i.e., leukemic) cells using conventional light microscopy, but this may still represent a considerable tumor burden since, at diagnosis, the leukemic cell number may be $10^{12}$ and, following therapy, the neoplastic cell number may drop only by 2 logs to $10^{10}$ even in the presence of fewer than 5% marrow blasts. Standard morphology alone is not a sensitive method for determining low levels of disease and is a poor indicator to attempt to predict impending relapse (Table 6.1).

## Cell culture assays

These involve growing T-cell-depleted marrow in culture after the patient has undergone treatment, followed by subsequent morphological, immunophenotypic and karyotypic analyses on the colonies produced. Due to the variability of culture techniques between and within laboratories, this method has proved unreliable and insensitive for detecting persisting blasts. In addition, culture techniques do not provide any estimate of cell number and hence provide little information about tumor cell burden.

## Karyotypic analysis

Detection of non-random chromosomal translocations is of great value in the diagnosis of leukemias and lymphomas. Chromosomal abnormalities are present in at least 70% of

**Table 6.1** Sensitivity of methods for MRD detection.

| | |
|---|---|
| Standard morphology | 1–5% |
| Cytogenetics | 5% |
| Fluorescence *in situ* hybridization | 0.3–5% |
| Immunophenotyping | $10^{-4}$ |
| Translocations | |
| PCR | $10^{-6}$ |
| Gene rearrangements | |
| Southern blotting | 1–5% |
| PCR | $10^{-4}$ to $10^{-6}$ |

patients with acute lymphoblastic leukemia (ALL) and 50% of patients with chronic lymphocytic leukemia (CLL). However, karyotypic analysis is of limited value following therapy, with a sensitivity of around 5%, making it little better than standard morphological analysis. In addition, cytogenetics relies on obtaining adequate numbers of suitable metaphases for analysis, which is difficult in some malignancies.

## Fluorescence *in situ* hybridization

FISH can detect smaller chromosomal abnormalities than standard karyotyping and allows analysis of interphase nuclei (cf. metaphase preparations in standard karyotyping). The method involves the binding of a nucleic acid probe to a specific chromosomal region. Preparations are counterstained with fluorescent dye, allowing the chromosomal region of interest to be detected. The technique is useful in the diagnosis of trisomies and monosomies and has been particularly useful in identifying deletions that have prognostic significance in CLL. The sensitivity of the technique is around 1%, making it considerably more useful than standard karyotyping for follow-up marrows in patients with leukemias or lymphomas, but is still of limited value for MRD detection.

## Flow cytometry and immunophenotyping

Immunophenotypic analysis using single monoclonal antibodies to cell membrane or cytoplasmic proteins lacks absolute specificity for leukemia or lymphoma cells and is therefore of limited value. Combining monoclonal antibodies allows the more specific detection of residual disease and quantitation is possible, although the tumor cell burden may be underestimated. The technique is further hampered by the lack of true "specific–specific" surface determinants and tumor-associated antigens are normal differentiation antigens present on developing hematopoietic progenitor cells. Using combinations of monoclonal antibodies and multicolor flow cytometric analysis, the sensitivity of this technique can be greatly enhanced. Except in the most expert hands, this technique is generally limited to a sensitivity of around $10^{-4}$ (i.e., 1 malignant cell in 10 000 normal cells).

## Molecular techniques: Southern blot hybridization

Initially described by its inventor, Professor Ed Southern, in the 1970s, Southern blotting involves the digestion of chromosomal DNA using bacterial restriction enzymes, with size separation of the DNA fragments using electric current and gel electrophoresis before transferring these to a nylon support membrane. A labeled probe for the gene of interest

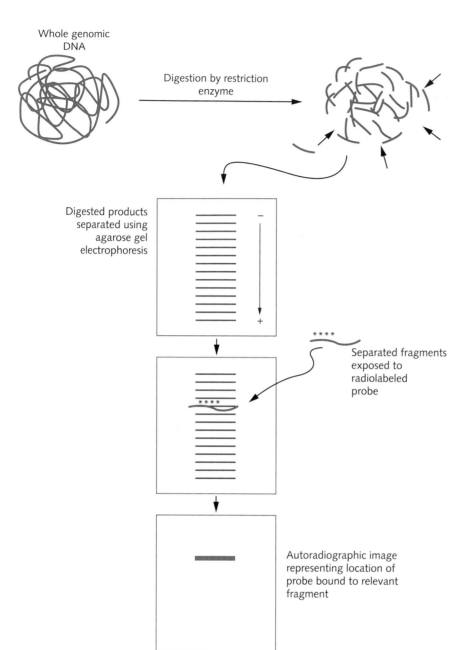

Whole genomic
DNA

Digestion by restriction
enzyme

Digested products
separated using
agarose gel
electrophoresis

\*\*\*\*

Separated fragments
exposed to
radiolabeled
probe

Autoradiographic image
representing location of
probe bound to relevant
fragment

**Fig. 6.2 Principle of Southern blotting**
Genomic DNA is digested using a restriction
enzyme, after which the fragments are
separated on the basis of size using agarose
gel electrophoresis, and are finally transferred
to a nylon membrane. Radiolabeled probe for
the gene of interest is hybridized to the DNA
on the membrane and, after removal of the
non-specifically hybridized probe, the location
and size of the fragment are determined using
autoradiography.

is applied, which binds to its complementary sequence on the membrane and visualization of the gene is by autoradiography (Figure 6.2).

Southern blotting is useful for the initial diagnosis of leukemia and lymphoma using probes specific for translocations or gene rearrangements. With Southern blotting, a non-germline or rearranged gene pattern may be seen in DNA from a population of cells where more than 1% of the total population is made up by a clone of malignant lymphoid cells. In other words, Southern blotting will detect a rearranged gene provided the cells containing the rearranged

gene exceed 1 in 100 normal cells. The disadvantage of Southern blotting is that the technique is not sufficiently sensitive for the detection of small numbers of malignant cells persisting after therapy and giving rise to disease relapse. For this reason, Southern blotting has been replaced by PCR for the detection of MRD.

**PCR amplification of DNA**

As described above, Southern blotting is a useful technique for assessing whether there is a clone of abnormal cells in blood, marrow or other tissue but is not useful if these cells are present in only very small amounts. In this case, techniques that involve amplification of specific DNA sequences are required. PCR has filled the void in this respect and has found a place in diagnostic laboratories investigating oncogenes, hematological malignancies, single-gene disorders and infectious diseases. Part of the attraction of a PCR-based approach is its extreme simplicity and the speed with which results are obtained.

## What is PCR amplification?

In the PCR reaction, two short oligonucleotide DNA primers are synthesized that are complementary to the DNA sequence on either side of the translocation or gene of interest. The region between the primers is filled in using a heat-stable bacterial DNA polymerase (*Taq*) from the hot-spring bacte-

rium *Thermus aquaticus*. After a single round of amplification has been performed, the whole process is repeated (Figure 6.3). This takes place 30 times (i.e., through 30 cycles of amplification) and leads to a million-fold increase in the amount of specific sequence. When the 30 cycles are complete, a sample of the PCR is electrophoresed on agarose or polyacrylamide gel. Information about the presence or absence of the region or mutation of interest is obtained by assessing the sizes and numbers of different PCR products obtained after 30 cycles of amplification.

The specificity of PCR can be further increased by the use of nested PCR, which involves reamplification of a small amount of the amplified product (obtained using outside, external, primers) using internal oligonucleotide primers.

PCR has the advantage that very little tissue sample is required for analysis and the technique can be applied to a variety of different sample types, for example fresh, unfixed, cryopreserved and formalin-fixed paraffin-embedded tissue

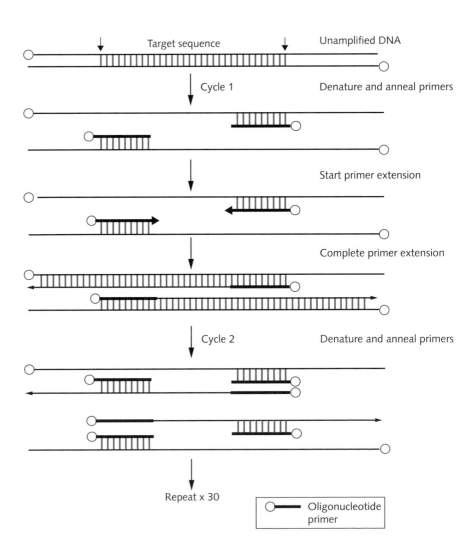

**Fig. 6.3 Simplified PCR schema**
Double-stranded DNA is denatured to allow binding of specific oligonucleotides on either side of the region of interest. *Taq* DNA polymerase extends the oligonucleotides before the double-stranded molecules are denatured and the process is repeated.

as well as hematoxylin and eosin-stained and formalin-fixed tissue.

PCR may be used to detect the presence of chromosomal translocations. The most commonly investigated rearrangements include the t(9;22) translocation in chronic myeloid leukemia (CML), t(15;17) in acute promyelocytic leukemia (APL), t(1;19) in a subset of pre-B-cell ALL, t(14;18) found in 85% of follicular and 15% of diffuse large cell lymphomas, and several others. Alternatively, in the lymphoid malignancies, if the tumor being investigated does not carry a translocation marker, PCR may be used to amplify rearranged antigen receptor [immunoglobulin or T-cell receptor (TCR)] genes.

## Molecular targets

### Chromosomal translocations

Translocations, which involve the transfer of DNA between chromosomes, are found in many of the hematological malignancies. Other chromosomal abnormalities include chromosomal deletions and inversions. Table 6.2 shows some of the translocations described in myeloid and lymphoid malignancies. As a result of chromosomal translocation, a gene from one chromosome ends up adjacent to a gene on the chromosome to which the DNA has been translocated, and this may have important consequences for the cell (and the patient). If a potentially cancerous gene (proto-oncogene), which is generally not transcriptionally active, abuts onto a gene that is being actively transcribed, this may result in upregulation of expression of that proto-oncogene. This is exactly the situation in many translocations described to date. In some cases, such as the translocation between chromosomes 14 and 18 found in many cases of follicular lymphoma, the *BCL-2* gene is moved to chromosome 14 and comes under the transcriptional control of the immunoglobulin heavy chain (IgH) gene, which is transcribed actively. The increase in BCL-2 protein prevents apoptosis (programmed cell death) and this may explain, in part, the underlying pathogenesis of some lymphomas.

The first non-random chromosome translocation described was the Philadelphia chromosome, in which reciprocal translocation of DNA between chromosomes 9 and 22 takes place. In t(9;22), the distal ends of chromosomes 9 and 22 are exchanged in a so-called reciprocal translocation; that is, there is no overall net loss or gain of genetic material. The C-*ABL* proto-oncogene from chromosome 9 becomes joined to *BCR* (breakpoint cluster region) on chromosome 22, resulting in a chimeric fusion protein that has tyrosine

**Table 6.2** PCR-amplifiable chromosomal translocations and gene rearrangements in human hematological disorders.

| Disease | Translocation | Genes involved |
|---|---|---|
| **Acute myeloid leukemia** | | |
| M2 | t(8;21) | ETO/AML1 |
| M2 or M4 | t(6;9) | DEK/CAN |
| M3 | t(15;17) | PML/RARα |
| M4 | inv(16) | CBFβ/MYH11 |
| **Acute lymphoblastic leukemia** | | |
| B-lineage | t(9;22) | BCR/ABL |
| | t(1;19) | E2A/PBX1 |
| | t(17;19) | HLF/E2A |
| | t(12;21) | TEL/AML1 |
| | t(4;11) | AF4/MLL |
| | t(8;14) | MYC/IgH |
| T-lineage | TAL interstitial deletion | TAL |
| | t(1;14) | TAL1/TCRδ |
| | t(10;14) | HOX11/TCRα |
| | t(11;14) | 11p13/TCRδ |
| **Lymphomas** | | |
| Follicular and diffuse NHL | t(14;18) | BCL-2/IgH |
| Mantle cell lymphoma | t(11;14) | BCL-1/IgH |
| Burkitt lymphoma | t(8;14) | MYC/IgH |
| Anaplastic lymphoma | t(2;5) | ALK/NPM |
| **Gene rearrangements** | | |
| Immunoglobulin heavy chain | B-cell lymphoma/leukemia | |
| T-cell receptors | T-cell lymphoma/leukemia | |

NHL, non-Hodgkin lymphoma.

kinase properties, and through some unknown mechanism leads to the typical CML phenotype (*discussed in detail in Chapter 7*).

### Detecting the presence of translocations
(Table 6.3)

#### Some translocations are disease-specific

Follicular lymphoma is characterized by t(14;18), which is found in almost 90% of cases. However, this translocation is found in other types of non-Hodgkin lymphoma (NHL), so that t(14;18) is not, in itself, diagnostic of one particular malignancy. APL is characterized by a reciprocal translocation between chromosomes 15 and 17. This is found in the

**Table 6.3** Detecting the presence of translocations.

**Standard cytogenetics**
If the translocation alters the appearance of banded chromosomes using standard cytogenetic analysis

**Fluorescence *in situ* hybridization**
Using metaphase or interphase techniques

**Polymerase chain reaction**
Requires the DNA on either side of the breakpoint to be sequenced to allow oligonucleotide primers to be constructed

majority of cases but, unlike t(14;18), t(15;17) is not found in any other neoplasm or in health and so serves as a diagnostic marker for this disease (although its absence does not exclude the diagnosis). Although t(9;22) is characteristic of CML, it is important to detect this in cases in which blastic transformation has occurred. In addition, t(9;22) occurs in a subset of patients with ALL and in these cases is associated with a particularly poor prognosis. It is therefore important to identify these patients at diagnosis since their prognosis and treatment differ from those for other cases of ALL.

More recently a number of chromosomal translocations that were thought to be leukemia- or lymphoma-specific have been found in the blood of normal individuals when assessed by PCR amplification, including t(14;18), t(8;14), t(2;5), t(9;22), t(4;11), t(15;17) and t(12;21). The implication of this finding is that these rearrangements are not themselves sufficient for malignant transformation of cells, in keeping with the "multiple-hit" hypothesis for tumor development.

**Translocations may be used for detecting residual disease**

Translocations serve as useful diagnostic disease markers at presentation for a variety of leukemias and lymphomas. For the detection of MRD, standard cytogenetic analysis for the detection of translocations is not sufficiently sensitive for follow-up but other techniques can be applied, including FISH and PCR. FISH techniques are constantly being improved (*see Chapter 2*) and may be of value for MRD detection. However, more sensitive MRD detection is possible using PCR in cases where the translocations are well characterized and DNA on either side of the breakpoints has been sequenced. MRD using the chromosomal translocations t(14;18) and t(9;22) and other translocations are described later.

## Antigen receptor gene rearrangements: immunoglobulin and TCR genes as molecular markers

Many hematopoietic malignancies have no detectable translocation suitable for PCR amplification, and in these cases an alternative strategy is required. In the lymphoid malignancies there is rearrangement of the antigen receptor at the immunoglobulin H (IgH) or TCR genes. The Ig and TCR molecules belong to a group of related proteins termed the immunoglobulin superfamily. Other members include CD8, the neural cell adhesion molecule (N-CAM) and the major histocompatibility complex (MHC). The Ig and TCR molecules have many similarities and have been shown to share common amino acid motifs. It is estimated that the immune system requires in excess of $10^{10}$ specific antibodies to respond to antigenic determinants encountered in the environment. If each Ig molecule were encoded separately in the germline, most of our genome would consist simply of Ig genes. Elegant work by Tonegawa demonstrated that Ig and TCR genes exist in the germline state as non-contiguous DNA segments that are rearranged during lymphocyte development (Table 6.4). Gene rearrangement involves recombination of germline gene segments that results in a permanently altered non-germline configuration (Figure 6.4). The process of Ig and TCR gene assembly ensures almost limitless variation of Ig and TCR molecules using only a limited amount of chromosomal DNA. Other features that ensure Ig and TCR variability include imprecise joining of individual V, D and J segments, duplication and inversion of segments, and somatic mutation (in Ig genes) of V, D and J.

### The immunoglobulin heavy chain locus

During normal lymphoid development, both B and T lymphocytes undergo rearrangement of their antigen receptor genes (i.e., Ig genes in B cells and TCR genes in T cells), and their clonal progeny bear this identical antigen receptor rearrangement. B-cell neoplasms, including NHL, ALL, myeloma and CLL, undergo irreversible somatic rearrangement of the IgH locus, providing a useful marker of clonality and the stage of differentiation in these tumors. Until recently, the lineage of Hodgkin lymphoma cells was unclear. PCR amplification of Ig genes has demonstrated that the vast majority of cases of Hodgkin disease are of B-cell lineage.

The human IGH locus at 14q32.33 spans 1250 kb. Unlike the light chain (IgL) locus, IgH contains diversity segments in addition to V, J and C segments. It consists of 123–129 IGHV genes, depending on the haplotypes, 27 IGHD

**Table 6.4** Immunoglobulin and T-cell receptor diversity is achieved through rearrangement of separate germline segments.

| | Diversity of immunoglobulin and TCR genes | | | | | | |
| --- | --- | --- | --- | --- | --- | --- | --- |
| | Immunoglobulin | | | T-cell receptor | | | |
| | H | κ | λ | α | β | γ | δ |
| V segments | 250 | 100 | 100 | 60 | 80 | 8 | 6 |
| D segments | 15 | 0 | 0 | 0 | 2 | 0 | 3 |
| J segments | 6 | 5 | 4 | 50 | 13 | 5 | 3 |
| VDJ recombination | 104 | 500 | 400 | 3000 | 2000 | 40 | 18 |
| N regions | 2 | 0 | 0 | 1 | 2 | 1 | 4 |
| N region additions | V–D, D–J | None | None | V–J | V–D, D–J | V–J | V–D1, D1–D2, D1–J |
| V domains | $10^{10}$ | $10^4$ | $10^4$ | $10^6$ | $10^9$ | $10^4$ | $10^{13}$ |
| V domain pairs | | $10^{14}$ | | | $10^{15}$ | | $10^{17}$ |

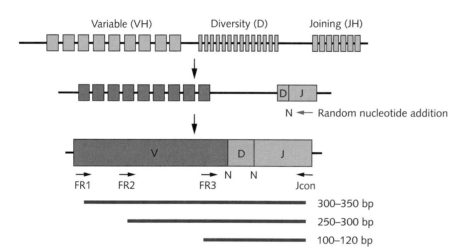

**Fig. 6.4 VDJ rearrangement**
Rearrangement of non-contiguous germline V-, D- and J-region segments generates a complete V–D–J complex, which serves as a useful marker of malignancy. FR1, FR2 and FR3 refer to framework regions 1, 2 and 3, respectively; N, random N nucleotides; Jcon, JH consensus primer. The sizes of the various PCR products are shown (FR1 + Jcon generates a fragment of 300–350 bp, and so on).

segments belonging to seven subgroups, nine IGHJ segments, and 11 IGHC genes; 82–88 IGHV genes belong to seven subgroups, whereas 41 pseudogenes, representing ancestral gene remnants (denoted by ψ), which are too divergent to be assigned to subgroups, have been assigned to four clans. Seven non-mapped IGHV genes have been described as insertion/deletion polymorphisms but have not yet been precisely located. The VH elements fall into seven families (VH1, VH2, VH3, VH4a, VH4b, VH5 and VH6). Unlike the TCR and IgL loci, the IgH locus contains multiple heavy-chain constant region (CH) segments (Figure 6.5), some 11 in total, including two pseudogenes (Cμ, Cδ, Cγ3, Cγ1, Cψε, Cα1, Cψγ, Cγ2, Cγ4, Cε and Cα2). Each C segment contains multiple exons corresponding to the functional domains in the heavy-chain protein (CH1, CH2, CH3, etc.). The multiple C elements correspond to the different classes of heavy chain encountered during class switching. Cμ generates IgM, Cα generates IgA, and so on. This mecha-

nism ensures that although the heavy chains are of varying class, they will all bear identical V–D–J sequences.

## Third complementarity-determining region

The third complementarity-determining region (CDR3) region of the IgH gene is generated early in B-cell development and is the result of rearrangement of germline sequences on chromosome 14. One diversity segment is joined to a joining region (D→J). The resulting D–J segment then joins one variable-region sequence (V→DJ), producing a V–D–J complex (Figure 6.4). The enzyme terminal deoxynucleotidyltransferase (TdT) inserts random nucleotides at two sites: the V–D and D–J junctions. At the same time random deoxynucleotides are removed by exonucleases. Antibody diversity is further increased by somatic mutation, a process that is not found in TCR genes. The final V–N–D–N–J sequence (CDR3) is unique to that cell, and if the cell multiplies to form a clone

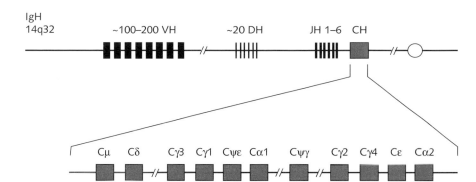

**Fig. 6.5 Genetic map of region 14q32**
The CH segments are shown toward the 3′
end of the region.

this region will act as a unique marker for that malignant clone. The V(D)J product corresponds to part of the variable region of the antibody molecule.

## TCR genes undergo a similar process of rearranging their germline segments to produce complete TCR genes

### Junctional region diversity

Imprecise recombination involving V(D)J region DNA enhances the number of possible different antibody molecule polypeptides due to loss or gain of additional nucleotides during the recombination event. The resulting V(D)J product may be functional (i.e., generates antibody molecules) or, if the reading frame is lost, non-functional. Whether functional or not, the CDR3 remains a unique marker for the malignant clone.

### TdT inserts N region nucleotides into the CDR3

N region nucleotide insertion is seen at the boundary of V, D or J coding segments and is template-independent. These N regions contain 1–12 nucleotides and are more often guanine or cytosine than adenine or thymidine, reflecting the role played by the enzyme TdT in this process.

### Combinatorial association

The TCR molecules are dimeric proteins, usually α plus β (TCR α:β), although 5% of circulating T cells bear the γ:δ TCR. The random combination of subunits in the TCR dimers further enhances the generation of diversity. The recombination events on one chromosome leading to the production of a functional molecule, such as TCR α:β, result in the inhibition of recombination at that locus on the other chromosome. This so-called allelic exclusion ensures that any given lymphocyte will express only one type of receptor molecule.

### Somatic hypermutation

This describes the random introduction of mutations within the V, D and J segments and is well documented in Ig genes but does not contribute to diversity in the TCR genes. Rearranged V-region sequences in B cells have been analyzed and found to differ from those of the germline V sequences from which they were generated. Most of these mutated V regions are found in the secondary immune response on rechallenge of B cells with antigen. During this process the antibody of the primary response (IgM) is switched to IgG or IgA. The somatic mutation rate has been estimated to be as high as $10^{-3}$ per base pair per cell generation, and the process occurs predominantly in variable regions of the molecule. The presence of somatic mutation can be useful in determining the stage of lineage in B-cell malignancies. In CLL it has been shown that cells either do or do not have mutated Ig genes. This has important prognostic significance since those patients who have undergone somatic hypermutation have a better prognosis than those who have no mutations.

## The clinical utility of the CDR3 DNA sequence

The description of V–D–J recombination may appear arcane, with no obvious relevance in clinical terms, but it is the formation of this unique recombination product that generates a powerful specific–specific marker that we can use for the detection of malignant clones and MRD. The DNA sequence within the V–D–J is determined by sequencing, following which the individual V, D and J segments are delineated. This allows accurate identification of the N region nucleotides (which are generated randomly by the enzyme TdT) that form the basis of the unique clone-specific (patient-specific) probe (Figure 6.6).

There are two sites available for design of the customized probe: the DNA of the V–N–D sequence and that of the D–N–J sequence. Does it matter which one we use to make

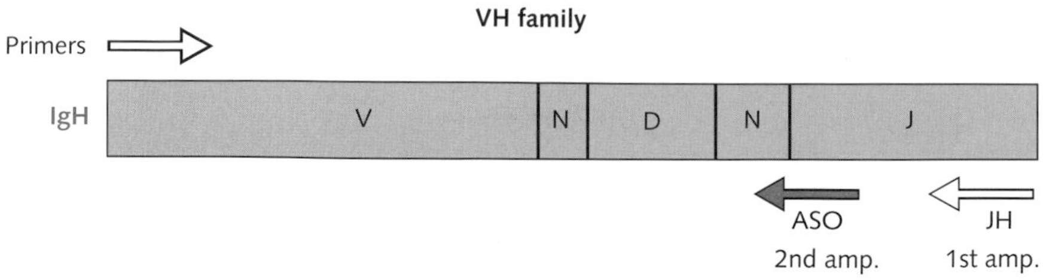

VH family

Primers

IgH

| V | N | D | N | J |

ASO
2nd amp.

JH
1st amp.

**Fig. 6.6 Semi-nested PCR of IgH region in patient with B-cell tumor**
V- and J-region primers are used to generate the initial PCR product. Using DNA sequence information, an allele-specific oligonucleotide (ASO) primer unique to that patient is constructed and used with the V primer to amplify an aliquot of the first-round PCR product.

the probes? The V–N–D sequence generally has a larger N region with more random nucleotides inserted, but the D–N–J site appears preferable for use as a clone-specific probe since there is less base deletion of the 3′ end of the framework region 3 (FR3) than of the 5′ end of the J region. In addition, the D–J segments appear to be inherently more stable than V–D segments. Finally, where there is V→V switching, as happens in some diseases such as ALL, the D–J segment remains unchanged and the probe will still detect the clone even if the V regions alter. The consensus view at present is that the D–N–J is probably the best DNA sequence to use to make probes for MRD detection.

## Quantitation of neoplastic cells using PCR

Until fairly recently, PCR amplification simply confirmed the presence (+) or absence (−) of tumor DNA sequences with little scope for quantifying the tumor bulk, particularly when using DNA as the PCR template. A band on agarose gel may represent the DNA from one cell, or many millions of cells. Clearly, this is of clinical importance if the information obtained is to be of value in determining the need for further chemotherapy, which is the main rationale for attempting to detect MRD in the first place.

In the early years of PCR detection of MRD the starting template was usually DNA, but more recently PCR amplification of reverse-transcribed mRNA (termed "complementary DNA" or cDNA) has been used. This refinement in PCR amplification has evolved where analysis of translocations such as t(9;22) or t(15;17) is impossible using a DNA template, simply because of the enormous size of the target being amplified. In these translocations the primer binding sites are so far apart on the DNA template that amplification is virtually impossible. However, the mRNA transcribed from these translocations undergoes considerable modification, with excision of introns making the mRNA counterpart of the translocation much smaller than the DNA.

Quantitation using competitive PCR templates has been possible for RNA-based PCR, and so we are able to quanti-

tate the tumor cell burden in those diseases where RNA is the nucleic acid used for the PCR assays. Diseases in which reverse transcriptase PCR (RT-PCR) is possible, with quantitation of the tumor burden, include CML [with t(9;22)], APL [t(15;17)] and acute myelogenous leukemia (AML)-M2 [t(8;21)].

DNA templates are more difficult to quantitate, although competitive PCR templates may be of value here also. Recent technologies such as the TaqMan real-time PCR machine may allow true quantitation using DNA as starting material. This system uses an internal oligonucleotide probe with added reporter and quenching activities (Figure 6.7). After primer and probe annealing, the reporter dye is cleaved off by the 5′–3′ nuclease activity of *Taq* DNA polymerase during primer extension (Figure 6.8). This cleavage of the probe separates the reporter from quencher dye, greatly increasing the reporter dye signal. The sequence detector is able to detect the fluorescent signal during thermal cycling. The advantages of this system are the elimination of post-PCR processing and the ability to examine the entire PCR process, not simply the end point of amplification. Moreover, since the probe is designed to be sequence-specific, non-specific amplification products are not detected.

## Use of PCR for detection of MRD in non-Hodgkin lymphoma

The standard technique used for the diagnosis of NHL is light microscopy of stained sections of lymph node or other tissue. This allows accurate classification of lymphoma subtype. In terms of detecting MRD, this technique has the limitation of detecting lymphoma cells only when they constitute approximately 5% or more of all cells (i.e., 1 malignant cell in 20 normal cells). Application of flow cytometric analysis for the detection of NHL has been hampered by the lack of lymphoma-specific monoclonal antibodies since all the cell surface antigens identified to date on the surface of lymphoma cells are also present on normal B cells or B-cell precursor cells (Table 6.5).

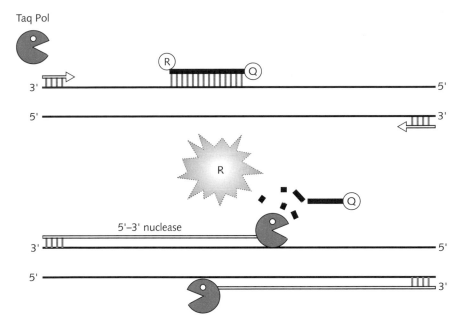

**Fig. 6.7 Real-time PCR amplification**
See text for details.

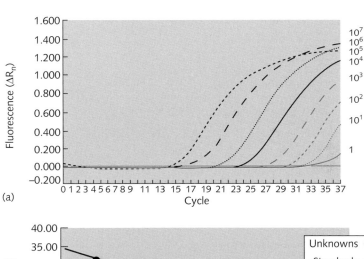

(a)

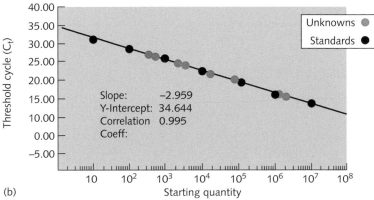

(b)

**Fig. 6.8 Standard curves generated for accurate quantitation of leukemic cell burden**

Quantitation by real-time PCR requires generation of a standard curve. A known amount of template DNA is diluted into genomic DNA and amplified by PCR. The threshold cycle is the cycle number at which reported fluorescence is first detected above background and is proportional to the amount of starting template DNA. The threshold cycle number is then plotted against the known amounts and a standard curve can be generated. The threshold cycle of the unknown samples can then be quantified by reading off the standard curve.

## Chromosomal translocations

As shown in Table 6.2, a number of chromosomal translocations and gene rearrangements associated with NHL have been identified; the breakpoints have been sequenced and are applicable for PCR amplification.

### t(14;18)

The most widely studied non-random chromosomal translocations in NHL is t(14;18), occurring in 85% of patients with follicular lymphoma and 30% of patients with diffuse large cell lymphoma. In t(14;18) the *BCL-2* proto-oncogene on chromosome 18 is juxtaposed with the IgH locus on chromosome 14 (Figure 6.9). The breakpoints have been cloned and sequenced, and have been shown to cluster at two main regions 3′ to the *BCL-2* coding region: the major

breakpoint region (MBR) within the 3′ untranslated region of the *BCL-2* gene, and the minor breakpoint cluster region (m-BCR) located 20 kb downstream. Juxtaposition of the transcriptionally active IgH with the *BCL-2* gene results in upregulation of the *BCL-2* gene product and subsequent resistance to programmed cell death by apoptosis.

The clustering of the breakpoints at these two main regions at the *BCL-2* gene and the availability of consensus regions of the IgH joining (J) regions make this an ideal candidate for PCR amplification to detect lymphoma cells containing the t(14;18) translocation. A major advantage in the detection of lymphoma cells bearing the *BCL-2*/IgH translocation is that DNA rather than RNA can be used to detect the translocation. In addition, since there is variation at the site of the breakpoint at the *BCL-2* gene, the PCR products for individual patients differ in size and have unique sequences. The size of the PCR product can be assessed by gel electrophoresis and used as confirmation that the expected size fragment is amplified from a specific patient.

### Other translocations in non-Hodgkin lymphoma

The t(11;14)(q13;q32) is associated with a number of B-cell malignancies, particularly mantle cell lymphomas. In this translocation the proto-oncogene *BCL-1* (also called *PRAD-1*) on chromosome 11 is juxtaposed to the IgH chain locus on chromosome 14.

One-third of anaplastic lymphomas express the chromosomal translocation t(2;5)(p23;q35), which involves a novel protein tyrosine kinase and nucleophosmin, resulting in a p80 fusion protein. This translocation is detected by RT-PCR

---

**Table 6.5** Clinical utility of PCR-based studies in patients with leukemia and lymphoma.

- Detection of bone marrow infiltration as part of staging procedure
- Detection of circulating lymphoma cells in peripheral blood
- Detection of minimal residual disease following therapy
- Assessing contribution of reinfused lymphoma cells to relapse in patients undergoing autologous bone marrow transplantation
- Assessing ability of purging techniques to eradicate residual malignant cells in marrow

---

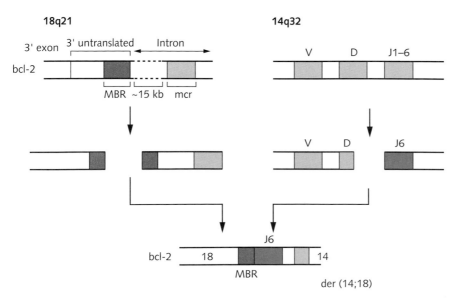

**Fig. 6.9 t(14;18) translocation**
In t(14;18) the *BCL-2* locus on chromosome 18 is juxtaposed to the IgH locus on chromosome 14. The breakpoints on chromosome 18 cluster at two main regions: the major breakpoint region (MBR) in the 5′ untranslated region of the *BCL-2* gene, and the minor cluster region (mcr) downstream in the intron. The chimeric gene product provides a unique tumor marker that can be PCR-amplified using primers upstream of the MBR or mcr region with consensus primers within the J region of the IgH gene.

where the mRNA sequence is converted into cDNA before PCR amplification.

## Use of molecular techniques for detection of MRD in lymphoma

Detection of MRD has clearly illustrated that patients in clinical complete remission often harbor malignant cells in low numbers. The clinical significance of the detection of such MRD is still being evaluated and remains unclear. The results of these studies will likely have great impact on the clinical management of patients as we understand more about the contribution of minimal disease to subsequent relapse. The prognostic significance of the achievement of molecular complete remission remains elusive, and few studies to date have demonstrated the importance of eradicating MRD in the patient to achieve cure. The majority of studies have been performed using as a target the t(14;18) in follicular lymphoma, but more recent studies have examined other translocations as well as Ig or TCR rearrangements and have been reporting similar results. These studies have suggested that the goal of therapy should be to eradicate the malignant clone and achieve molecular complete remission.

### PCR detection of bone marrow infiltration as a staging procedure

Lymphomas generally originate in lymphoid tissue, but as the disease progresses there may be spread to other sites, such as bone marrow and blood. At initial presentation all patients undergo staging investigations to determine the extent of disease as a means of planning treatment. A number of studies have examined the use of PCR detection of t(14;18) as a staging procedure to detect lymphoma cells in the bone marrow and peripheral blood at the time of initial presentation. However, PCR analysis cannot replace morphological assessment of bone marrow since not all patients have translocations detectable by PCR, and these techniques are essentially complementary. These PCR studies have all detected lymphoma cells in the bone marrow in a number of patients who had no overt evidence of marrow infiltration by morphology. Of great interest are those studies that have evaluated the clinical utility of MRD detection in those patients presenting with localized disease. Although patient numbers are small, a significant number can be found who would be upstaged from early-stage to advanced-stage disease by the results of PCR analysis. Whether PCR detection of minimal marrow infiltration will eventually lead to modifications in therapy in those patients currently treated with localized radiotherapy remains to be determined.

### PCR detection of MRD following chemotherapy

In follicular lymphoma, long-term analysis of patients after completion of conventional chemotherapy has shown that conventional-dose chemotherapy does not eradicate PCR-detectable disease, but this may not be associated with poor outcome. One study has shown no association between the presence or absence of PCR-detectable lymphoma cells and clinical outcome. Moreover, this confirms the previous observation that some patients can indeed remain in long-term continuous complete remission despite the presence of PCR-detectable lymphoma cells, strongly suggesting that the detection of residual lymphoma cells has no prognostic significance. Thus cells containing t(14;18) might not always represent residual lymphoma cells, but simply cells without the additional necessary cellular changes required for malignant transformation. However, an alternative explanation is that conventional chemotherapy might not cure any patients with advanced stage follicular lymphoma and that all patients with persistent lymphoma cells are destined to relapse. The long-term remission status of these small numbers of patients might therefore represent merely the very long duration of their disease course.

These studies suggest that conventional-dose chemotherapy did not result in molecular remission. More novel treatment approaches, including more aggressive induction therapy and combinations of monoclonal antibody therapy with chemotherapy and the use of stem cell transplantation, have all been reported to be capable of eradicating PCR-detectable disease, achieving so-called molecular complete remission. In all these circumstances, eradication of PCR-detectable disease has been shown to be associated with improved outcome in follicular lymphoma, strongly suggesting that eradication of MRD may be required for cure. With longer follow-up this question should be answered.

### Detection of circulating lymphoma cells in peripheral blood

Blood is less frequently involved than marrow at presentation, but becomes more frequent as disease progresses. Studies at the time of initial presentation have suggested a high level of concordance between the detection of lymphoma cells in the peripheral blood and bone marrow when assessed by PCR. However, other studies have found that the bone marrow is more likely than peripheral blood to contain infiltrating lymphoma cells in previously untreated patients. The presence of residual lymphoma in the bone marrow but not in the peripheral blood argues strongly that the marrow is indeed infiltrated with lymphoma in these patients and does not simply represent contamination from the peripheral blood. The findings of peripheral blood contamination with NHL when assessed by PCR are likely to have profound implications since there is now increasing interest in the use of peripheral blood stem cells, rather than bone marrow, as a source of hematopoietic progenitors. A number of studies have demonstrated that peripheral blood stem cell collections may also be contaminated with lymphoma cells when assessed by PCR techniques. In addition, much work is being performed to monitor the effects of chemotherapy and the growth factors that are used to mobilize hematopoietic progenitor cells, to ensure that these agents do not also mobilize lymphoma cells.

### Contribution of reinfused lymphoma cells to relapse after autologous stem cell transplantation

In low-grade NHL there has been increasing interest in the use of high-dose therapy as salvage therapy for patients who have failed conventional-dose chemotherapy regimens. The resulting ablation of a patient's marrow after high-dose therapy can be rescued by infusion of allogeneic or autologous stem cells. Autologous stem cell transplantation (ASCT) has several potential advantages over allogeneic stem cell transplantation for marrow rescue: there is no need for a histocompatible donor and there is no risk of graft-versus-host disease. ASCT can therefore be performed more safely, and in older patients, and has become a major treatment option for an increasing number of patients with hematological malignancies.

The major obstacle to the use of ASCT is that the infusion of occult tumor cells harbored within the stem cell collection may result in more rapid relapse of disease. To minimize the effects of the infusion of significant numbers of malignant cells, stem cells are collected when the patient either is in complete remission or has no evidence of lymphoma in the blood. In addition, a variety of methods have been developed to purge malignant cells from the stem cell collection in an attempt to eliminate any contaminating malignant cells and leave intact the hematopoietic stem cells that are necessary for engraftment. The development of purging techniques has led to a number of studies of ASCT in patients with either a previous history of bone marrow infiltration or even overt marrow infiltration at the time of bone marrow harvest. Because of their specificity, monoclonal antibodies are ideal agents for the selective elimination of malignant cells. Clinical studies have demonstrated that immunological purging can deplete malignant cells *in vitro* without significantly impairing hematological engraftment.

### Assessing purging efficacy by PCR

PCR has been used to assess the effectiveness of immunological purging in models using lymphoma cell lines and has shown itself to be a highly sensitive and efficient method for determining the efficacy of purging residual lymphoma cells. The efficacy of purging varies between the cell lines studied, making it likely that there would also be variability between patient samples.

PCR amplifications of the t(14;18), t(11;14) and IgH rearrangements have all been used to detect residual lymphoma cells in the bone marrow before and after purging in patients undergoing autologous bone marrow transplantation (BMT) to assess whether the efficiency of purging had any impact on disease-free survival. In one study, 114 patients with B-cell NHL and the *BCL-2* translocation were studied. Residual lymphoma cells were detected by PCR analysis in the harvested autologous bone marrow of all patients. Following three cycles of immunological purging using anti-B-cell monoclonal antibodies and complement-mediated lysis, PCR amplification detected residual lymphoma cells in 50% of these patients. The incidence of relapse was significantly increased in the patients who had residual detectable lymphoma cells compared with those in whom no lymphoma cells were detectable after purging.

### Detection of residual lymphoma cells in the marrow after transplantation is associated with increased incidence of subsequent relapse

Since PCR analysis detected residual lymphoma cells after conventional-dose chemotherapy in the majority of patients studied, it is not surprising that it has not been possible to determine any prognostic significance for the persistence of PCR-detectable lymphoma cells. At the Dana-Farber Cancer Institute, PCR analysis was performed on serial bone marrow samples obtained after ASCT to assess whether high-dose therapy might be capable of depleting PCR-detectable lymphoma cells. The persistence or reappearance of residual detectable lymphoma cells had a great adverse influence on the disease-free survival of patients in this study after high-dose therapy. In contrast to previous findings that all patients had bone marrow infiltration following conventional-dose therapy, no PCR-detectable lymphoma cells could be found in the most recent bone marrow sample obtained from more than 50% of patients following high-dose chemoradiotherapy and ASCT. A number of studies have now demonstrated that persistent detection of MRD by PCR following ASCT in patients with lymphoma identifies those patients who require additional treatment for cure, and also suggest that our therapeutic goal should be to eradicate all PCR-detectable lymphoma cells. In addition, quantitative PCR analysis has further shown that a rising tumor burden is a particularly poor prognostic feature.

## Use of PCR for detection of MRD in acute leukemias

### Acute lymphoblastic leukemia

The treatment of childhood ALL has been one of the great success stories of modern chemotherapy and cure rates approaching 80% have been achieved in recently reported series. ALL cells usually rearrange either the IgH or TCR genes or both, and these provide markers that can be used to assess the clinical significance of MRD detection in a disease with such a high likelihood of cure. It is now clear that early eradication of MRD is a powerful prognostic marker in childhood ALL. Most studies have suggested that modern aggressive induction regimens are often associated with rapid elimination of PCR-detectable disease and many studies are ongoing where treatment is intensified in children with higher levels of residual disease early in their treatment. Most studies have also demonstrated that a quantitative increase in tumor burden is almost invariably associated with impending relapse. The impact of MRD on outcome has been studied less extensively in adult ALL, but most studies have also suggested that failure to eradicate MRD has important prognostic significance and should influence future clinical management.

### t(12;21)

The *TEL/AML-1* gene rearrangement results from the cryptic reciprocal translocation t(12;21). This is the most common gene rearrangement found in childhood ALL and accounts for 25% of pre-B-cell ALL in children, but is rarely found in adult ALL. Most data are suggestive that the presence of this rearrangement is associated with a good prognosis. However, qualitative and quantitative PCR analysis studies have suggested that the persistence of residual leukemia cells or a slower rate of eradication of the leukemic cells is associated with poor prognosis.

### Acute promyelocytic leukemia

APL is associated with a balanced translocation between chromosomes 15 and 17, resulting in t(15;17)(q22;q21) and leading to rearrangement of the *RARα* gene (also termed *RARA*) on chromosome 17 and *PML* on chromosome 15 (Figure 6.10). With rearrangement of DNA, the chromosomal translocation produces two novel fusion genes involving *PML* and *RARα*, namely *PML/RARα* and *RARα/PML*. It is believed that *PML/RARα* is responsible for the development of aberrant hematopoiesis. There are two isoforms of the *PML/RARα* fusion gene: long and short. Patients who possess the short isoform have a poorer clinical outcome than those in whom the long isoform is found, but the exact mechanism involved is unclear at present.

The resultant fusion protein (PML/RARα) contains functional domains in both PML and RARα, and binds all-*trans* retinoic acid (ATRA), to which the leukemic cells in APL are exquisitely sensitive. In fact ATRA, which induces differentiation of the leukemic cells, may alone achieve remission in 80% of *de novo* cases of APL. Two classes of retinoic acid receptor mediate the effects of retinoids: RAR and RXR, both of which are members of a superfamily of related ligand-inducible transcriptional regulatory factors. RAR (α, β and γ) is activated by ATRA and 9-*cis*-retinoic acid. RXR (α, β and γ) is activated by 9-*cis*-retinoic acid only.

Patients with APL and t(15;17) who achieve remission are now regarded as good-risk patients, with a 60% chance of achieving long-term remission. The presence of the fusion gene may be inferred from cytogenetic analysis (i.e., the presence of typical translocation) or, more recently, by an RT-PCR method. In this, the *PML/RARα* mRNA is reverse-transcribed into cDNA, which is then used for PCR detection of the abnormal transcript. The RT-PCR assay has been used to quantitate residual leukemic cells in patients with APL undergoing chemotherapy.

Trial data suggest that persistence of t(15;17) determined by the PCR approach predicts outcome: those patients who fail to become PCR-negative or who become PCR-positive following a period of PCR negativity subsequently suffer overt clinical relapse. Quantitative PCR monitoring of *PML/RARα* can identify patients at high risk of relapse, suggesting that clinically practical monitoring at more frequent intervals may improve predictive accuracy for relapse or continuing complete remission in many patients with persistent, fluctuating MRD levels.

### Acute myelogenous leukemia

MRD monitoring in all AML treatment phases using real-time quantitative PCR for fusion transcripts (*CBFB/MYH11*; *RUNX1/RUNX1T1* fusion transcripts of *MLL* gene) and for the Wilms tumor (*WT1*) gene has demonstrated clinical utility in predicting relapse.

### t(8;21)

The non-random chromosomal translocation t(8;21) occurs in up to 10% of *de novo* AML cases. It is more common in AML with features of maturation. This gene fuses the *AML* gene on 21q22 with the *ETO* gene on 8q22. The breakpoints in this translocation invariably occur within defined regions

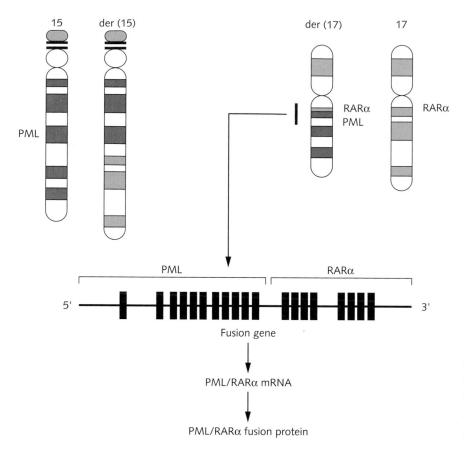

**Fig. 6.10 t(15;17)(q22;q21) translocation**
A balanced translocation involving the *RAR*α gene (at 17q21) and the *PML* gene (15q22) found in AML M3 (APL) in >90% of cases. The chimeric PML/RARα protein plays a role in the differentiation block characteristic of APL.

in the *AML* and *ETO* genes, resulting in a fairly uniform fusion product. Early studies of this translocation suggested that there was persistence of this transcript in almost all cases studied, even in patients in long-term remission. This suggests that the *AML1/ETO* translocation may be necessary, but in itself insufficient, for leukemic transformation. PCR analysis suggests that a quantitative increase in the fusion transcript is predictive of subsequent relapse.

## Use of PCR for detection of MRD in chronic leukemias

### Chronic myeloid leukemia

#### Detection of t(9;22) by PCR amplification

The translocation t(9;22), termed the Philadelphia chromosome, was described in 1960 by Nowell and Hungerford, and represented the first non-random chromosomal abnormality shown to be associated with a specific neoplasm, namely CML (although it is found in other disorders). The t(9;22) is formed by the fusion of the *BCR* gene on chromosome 22 with the *ABL* proto-oncogene on chromosome 9 and occurs

in the vast majority of patients with CML and in up to 20% of adult patients with ALL. The CML cells transcribe an 8.5-kb chimeric mRNA that is translated into a 210-kDa protein (p210) with tyrosine kinase activity. The breakpoints at the *ABL* gene can occur at any point up to 200 kb upstream in the intron and therefore cannot easily be amplified by PCR using genomic DNA as described earlier in this chapter. In contrast, the chimeric mRNA will usually be of two possible types: *BCR* between exons 13 and 14 is fused 5' of exon 2 of *ABL*, generating the b2a2 product; an alternative product, b3a2, is generated when the breakpoint is located between exons 14 and 15 of *BCR*. It is therefore possible to amplify the chimeric mRNA by first reverse-transcribing to cDNA. Using this technique, it is possible to detect one leukemic cell in up to $10^6$ normal cells (*see Chapter 7*).

#### MRD monitoring in tyrosine kinase inhibitor therapy in CML

Imatinib induces complete cytogenetic response in most patients with CML, but MRD remains detectable by RT-PCR in many cases. These cells retain full leukemogenic potential since disease recurrence occurs after discontinuation of imatinib, an indication that the residual *BCR/ABL*-positive cells retain full leukemogenic potential. Whereas most patients who fail to respond or relapse after initial response harbor mutations in the kinase domain of BCR/ABL that impair drug binding, the mechanisms responsible for persistence of MRD in responding patients are not well understood. Continuous monitoring using quantitative assessment of MRD during continuous drug therapy allows assessment of initial response, can predict relapse, even in cases achieving complete cytogenetic remission, and is an independent prognostic factor for progression-free survival.

## Detection of MRD after bone marrow transplantation in CML

Before the widespread use of tyrosine kinase inhibitors in CML, allogeneic BMT was treatment of choice for suitable patients. However, 20% of patients transplanted in the chronic phase and more than 50% of patients transplanted in the accelerated phase or blast crisis relapse. Considerable effort has been made to establish whether persistence of MRD after allogeneic BMT is predictive of relapse. Early studies yielded conflicting results about the clinical implications of persistence of PCR-detectable disease. However, a recent large study from Seattle, including analysis of data from 346 patients, showed a clear association between the relapse and persistence of PCR-detectable disease. Detection of MRD early after BMT does not necessarily suggest a poor prognosis, and a PCR-positive sample 3 months after BMT was not informative for the clinical outcome. In contrast, a PCR-positive bone marrow or peripheral blood sample at or after 6 months post-BMT was closely associated with subsequent relapse. Statistical analysis of the data revealed that the PCR assay for the *BCR/ABL* fusion transcript 6–12 months after BMT is an independent predictor of subsequent relapse. In contrast, no clear prediction of clinical outcome could be made in patients who tested PCR-positive more than 3 years after BMT. This study and others have clearly demonstrated that most patients are PCR-positive 3 months after BMT, indicating that BMT preparative regimens alone do not eradicate CML cells effectively. Nevertheless, since this treatment leads to cure in more than 50% of patients, other mechanisms (e.g., immunological mechanisms) must be responsible for tumor eradication.

## Chronic lymphocytic leukemia

This is the commonest leukemia in adults and predominantly affects the elderly. A full description of CLL and its molecular abnormalities is provided in *Chapter 10*. Most are B-cell neoplasms (95%) which demonstrate a variety of cytogenetic abnormalities that are of value for molecular diagnosis and residual disease detection. Karyotypic abnor-

malities include trisomy 12 and deletions or translocations of chromosomes 11 and 13. Since these tumors are of B-cell origin, rearranged IgH genes may be used to confirm clonality and to detect residual tumor following chemotherapy and, in younger poor-risk patients, BMT. Most studies in CLL have suggested that eradication of MRD predicts for improved outcome. The variety of MRD techniques and the lack of standardization have made it difficult to interpret and compare different clinical trials. Two techniques are widely used to assess MRD in CLL: PCR detection of IGVH rearrangements and multiparameter flow cytometric analysis. An international standardized approach has been adopted for flow cytometric analysis of MRD in CLL and compared with real-time quantitative PCR. Assessment of 50 CLL-specific monoclonal antibody combinations identified three (CD5/CD19 with CD20/CD38, CD81/CD22 and CD79b/CD43) that had low interlaboratory variation and low false-positive results. There was close correlation between four-color flow cytometry and PCR when levels of disease were above 0.01%. Allele-specific oligonucleotide PCR appears to be approximately 1 log more sensitive than four-color flow cytometric assessment, which has the advantage of being more applicable and does not require sequencing of the IGVH rearrangement.

BMT is generally precluded in most patients with CLL due to the advanced age of the patients affected. However, recent studies of younger patients with aggressive disease who have undergone either autologous or reduced intensity conditioning allogeneic BMT have shown that PCR-detectable disease is often present at, or shortly after, transplantation, but this does not predict relapse. In the largest single-center study, the methods used for the analysis involved PCR amplification of the IgH locus with sequencing of the CDR3 products, before constructing patient-specific oligonucleotide probes, which were then used to probe the PCR products from marrow or blood samples taken after transplantation. Data suggest that patients who remain PCR-positive in the months following transplantation or who become PCR-positive, having been PCR-negative initially, tend to relapse. Those who remain PCR-negative or become negative remain in clinical and morphological remission (Figure 6.11). Obviously, with an indolent, slow-growing disease like CLL, we must wait some years before the data can be interpreted fully, since it may be that ultimately all patients will relapse.

## Problems with PCR analysis for detection of MRD

The major concern with PCR-based disease detection will always be the fear of false-positive results because of the

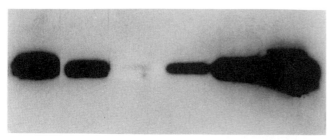

**Fig. 6.11 Detection of relapse of CLL in a patient undergoing autologous bone marrow transplantation using PCR**
In the samples before (pre) and after (post) purging of the patient's marrow, PCR positivity is clearly seen. Six months after autologous bone marrow transplantation no PCR-detectable signal is seen. However, 15, 27 and 32 months after the transplant, PCR positivity is easily detected. These findings were confirmed clinically and using standard morphological examination of the patient's bone marrow.

ability of the technique to amplify even minute amounts of contaminating DNA. Unlike cell culture assays, it is not possible to determine whether cells detected by PCR are clonogenic (i.e., capable of division and causing relapse). Cells bearing a translocation may be committed progenitors incapable of further proliferation, or might have been sufficiently damaged by previous exposure to chemotherapy or radiotherapy to be already dead but still detectable by PCR analysis. A potential problem with the use of PCR of the *BCL-2/IgH* translocation is that this translocation may not be specific for lymphoma cells. Cells bearing the translocation have been detected in hyperplastic lymphoid tissue in healthy individuals with no evidence of lymphoma, and more recently have been shown to occur rarely in normal B cells.

## Conclusions

Methodologies have been developed for the sensitive detection of MRD in lymphoma and leukemia that are applicable to many patients. The question that now remains to be answered is the clinical utility of these techniques and development of standardized approaches that lead to reproducibility between laboratories. In childhood ALL, MRD monitoring of response is standard and results lead to alteration of treatment. MRD monitoring has become standard in assessment of response in CML and APL. In NHL, studies are most advanced in patients with t(14;18). In these patients, conventional-dose chemotherapy does not appear to be capable of depleting PCR-detectable lymphoma cells, although lymphoma cells were detectable in peripheral blood in only half of the patients studied. Following ASCT, the persistence or reappearance of PCR-detectable lymphoma cells in the bone marrow is associated with an

increased likelihood of relapse. In lymphomas that do not express t(14;18), it is not yet clear whether failure to detect MRD in peripheral blood and bone marrow will predict which patients will relapse since other subtypes of lymphoma may relapse in nodal sites without detectable lymphoma cells in the circulation.

From the available data, there are clearly diseases in which the persistence of PCR-detectable disease following treatment predicts relapse and others in which it does not. The full relevance of these findings will become clearer as we understand more about the biology of the diseases and additional data are generated as part of ongoing major clinical trials.

## Further reading

### Polymerase chain reaction

Kwok S, Higuchi R. (1989) Avoiding false positives with PCR. *Nature*, **339**, 237–238.

Saiki RK, Gelfand DH, Stoffel S *et al.* (1988) Primer-directed enzymatic amplification of DNA with a thermostable DNA polymerase. *Science*, **239**, 487–491.

### Antigen receptor genes

Aisenberg AC. (1993) Utility of gene rearrangements in lymphoid malignancies. *Annual Review of Medicine*, **44**, 75–84.

Griesser H, Tkachuk D, Reis MD *et al.* (1989) Gene rearrangements and translocations in lymphoproliferative diseases. *Blood*, **73**, 1402–1415.

Tonegawa S. (1983) Somatic generation of antibody diversity. *Nature*, **302**, 575–581.

Toyonaga B, Mak TW. (1987) Genes of the T-cell antigen receptor in normal and malignant T cells. *Annual Review of Immunology*, **5**, 585–620.

van Dongen JJ, Langerak AW, Brüggemann M *et al.* (2003) Design and standardization of PCR primers and protocols for detection of clonal immunoglobulin and T-cell receptor gene recombinations in suspect lymphoproliferations: report of the BIOMED-2 Concerted Action BMH4-CT98-3936. *Leukemia*, **17**, 2257–2317.

### Acute leukemias

Cave H, van der Werff ten Bosch J, Suciu S *et al.* (1998) Clinical significance of minimal residual disease in childhood acute lymphoblastic leukemia. European Organization for Research and Treatment of Cancer Childhood Leukemia Cooperative Group. *New England Journal of Medicine*, **339**, 591–598.

Diverio D, Rossi V, Avvisati G *et al.* (1998) Early detection of relapse by prospective reverse transcriptase-polymerase chain reaction analysis of the PML/RARα fusion gene in patients with acute promyelocytic leukemia enrolled in the GIMEMA-AIEOP multicenter AIDA trial. *Blood*, **92**, 784–789.

Gameiro P, Moreira I, Yetgin S *et al.* (2002) Polymerase chain reaction (PCR)- and reverse transcription PCR-based minimal residual disease detection in long-term follow-up of childhood acute lymphoblastic leukaemia. *British Journal of Haematology*, **119**, 685–696.

Grimwade D, Jovanovic JV, Hills RK *et al.* (2009) Prospective minimal residual disease monitoring to predict relapse of acute promyelocytic leukemia and to direct pre-emptive arsenic trioxide therapy. *Journal of Clinical Oncology*, **27**, 3650–3658.

Mancini M, Nanni M, Cedrone M *et al.* (1995) Combined cytogenetic, FISH and molecular analysis in acute promyelocytic leukemia at diagnosis and in complete remission. *British Journal of Haematology*, **91**, 878–884.

Marcucci G, Livak KJ, Bi W *et al.* (1998) Detection of minimal residual disease in patients with AML1/ETO-associated acute myeloid leukemia using a novel quantitative reverse transcription polymerase chain reaction assay. *Leukemia*, **12**, 1482–1489.

Sykes PJ, Brisco MJ, Hughes E *et al.* (1998) Minimal residual disease in childhood acute lymphoblastic leukemia quantified by aspirate and trephine: is the disease multifocal? *British Journal of Haematology*, **103**, 60–65.

van Dongen JJ, Seriu T, Panzer-Grumayer ER *et al.* (1998) Prognostic value of minimal residual disease in acute lymphoblastic leukaemia in childhood. *Lancet*, **352**, 1731–1738.

Yamada M, Wasserman R, Lange B *et al.* (1990) Minimal residual disease in childhood B-lineage lymphoblastic leukemia. *New England Journal of Medicine*, **323**, 448–455.

Zhou J, Goldwasser MA, Li A *et al.* (2007) Quantitative analysis of minimal residual disease predicts relapse in children with B-lineage acute lymphoblastic leukemia in DFCI ALL Consortium Protocol 95-01. *Blood*, **110**, 1607–1611.

## Chronic leukemias

Bose S, Deininger M, Gora-Tybor J *et al.* (1998) The presence of typical and atypical BCR-ABL fusion genes in leukocytes of normal individuals: biologic significance and implications for the assessment of minimal residual disease. *Blood*, **92**, 3362–3367.

Khouri IF, Keating MJ, Vriesendorp HM *et al.* (1994) Autologous and allogeneic bone marrow transplantation for chronic lymphocytic leukemia: preliminary results. *Journal of Clinical Oncology*, **12**, 748–758.

Nowell PC, Hungerford DA. (1960) A minute chromosome in human granulocytic leukemia. *Science*, **132**, 125–132.

Provan D, Bartlett-Pandite L, Zwicky C *et al.* (1996) Eradication of polymerase chain reaction-detectable chronic leukemia cells is associated with improved outcome after bone marrow transplantation. *Blood*, **88**, 2228–2235.

Radich JP, Gehly G, Gooley T *et al.* (1995) Polymerase chain reaction detection of the BCR-ABL fusion transcript after allogeneic marrow transplantation for chronic myeloid leukemia: results and implications in 346 patients. *Blood*, **85**, 2632–2638.

Rawstron AC, Villamor N, Ritgen M *et al.* (2007) International standardized approach for flow cytometric residual disease monitoring in chronic lymphocytic leukaemia. *Leukemia*, **21**, 956–964.

## Non-Hodgkin lymphoma

Corradini P, Tarella C, Olivieri A *et al.* (2002) Reduced-intensity conditioning followed by allografting of hematopoietic cells can produce clinical and molecular remissions in patients with poor-risk hematologic malignancies. *Blood*, **99**, 75–82.

Gribben JG, Neuberg D, Freedman AS *et al.* (1993) Detection by polymerase chain reaction of residual cells with the bcl-2 translocation is associated with increased risk of relapse after autologous bone marrow transplantation for B-cell lymphoma. *Blood*, **81**, 3449–3457.

Gribben JG, Neuberg DN, Barber M *et al.* (1994) Detection of residual lymphoma cells by polymerase chain reaction in peripheral blood is significantly less predictive for relapse than detection in bone marrow. *Blood*, **83**, 3800–3807.

Lopez-Guillermo A, Cabanillas F, McLaughlin P *et al.* (1998) The clinical significance of molecular response in indolent follicular lymphomas. *Blood*, **91**, 2955–2960.

Sharp JG, Joshi SS, Armitage JO *et al.* (1992) Significance of detection of occult non-Hodgkin's lymphoma in histologically uninvolved bone marrow by culture technique. *Blood*, **79**, 1074–1080.

Taniwaki M, Nishida K, Ueda Y *et al.* (1995) Interphase and metaphase detection of the breakpoint of 14q32 translocations in B-cell malignancies by double-color fluorescence *in situ* hybridization. *Blood*, **85**, 3223–3228.

Weiss LM, Warnke RA, Sklar J *et al.* (1987) Molecular analysis of the t(14;18) chromosomal translocation in malignant lymphomas. *New England Journal of Medicine*, **317**, 1185–1189.

Yuan R, Dowling P, Zucca E *et al.* (1993) Detection of bcl-2/JH rearrangement in follicular and diffuse lymphoma: concordant results of peripheral blood and bone marrow analysis at diagnosis. *British Journal of Cancer*, **67**, 922–925.

Zwicky CS, Maddocks AB, Andersen N *et al.* (1996) Eradication of polymerase chain reaction detectable immunoglobulin gene rearrangement in non-Hodgkin's lymphoma is associated with decreased relapse after autologous bone marrow transplantation. *Blood*, **88**, 3314–3322.

## Quantitation

Cross NC, Feng L, Chase A *et al.* (1993) Competitive polymerase chain reaction to estimate the number of BCR-ABL transcripts in chronic myeloid leukemia patients after bone marrow transplantation. *Blood*, **82**, 1929–1936.

Donovan JW, Ladetto M, Poor C *et al.* (2000) Immunoglobulin heavy chain consensus probes for real-time PCR quantification of residual disease in acute lymphoblastic leukemia. *Blood*, **95**, 2651–2658.

Mensink E, van de Locht A, Schattenberg A *et al.* (1998) Quantitation of minimal residual disease in Philadelphia chromosome positive chronic myeloid leukemia patients using real-time quantitative RT-PCR. *British Journal of Haematology*, **102**, 768–774.

Pongers-Willemse MJ, Verhagen OJ, Tibbe GJ *et al.* (1998) Real-time quantitative PCR for the detection of minimal residual disease in acute lymphoblastic leukemia using junctional region specific TaqMan probes. *Leukemia*, **12**, 2006–2014.

# Chapter 7 Chronic myelogenous leukemia

## Alfonso Quintás-Cardama, Jorge Cortes, Hagop Kantarjian & Susan O'Brien

*Department of Leukemia, University of Texas M.D. Anderson Cancer Center, Houston, TX, USA*

## Introduction

Chronic myeloid leukemia (CML) is a clonal myeloproliferative neoplasm that arises from a pluripotent stem cell. The Philadelphia (Ph) chromosome, which results from a reciprocal translocation between chromosomes 9 and 22, constitutes the cytogenetic hallmark of CML and can be detected in myeloid, erythroid, megakaryocytic, B, and sometimes T, lymphoid cells, but not in marrow fibroblasts. A critical milestone in CML research was the demonstration that this translocation involved the *ABL1* (v-abl Abelson murine leukemia viral oncogene homolog 1) gene on chromosome 9 and the *BCR* (breakpoint cluster region) gene on chromosome 22 and resulted in the formation of the chimeric *BCR-ABL1* fusion transcript that encodes the constitutively active BCR-ABL1 tyrosine kinase. The discovery that BCR-ABL1 plays a pivotal role in the pathogenesis of CML set the stage for the development of therapeutic strategies aimed specifically at inhibiting this kinase. In this chapter, we summarize the current knowledge regarding the molecular biology of CML, the most relevant treatment modalities, including novel BCR-ABL1 kinase inhibitors, and the mechanisms of resistance to these targeted agents.

## Epidemiology

CML is a rare disease worldwide, with an annual incidence of 1.6 per 100 000 adults, being slightly more frequently diagnosed in male patients (male to female ratio 1.4 : 1).

*Molecular Hematology*, 3rd edition. Edited by Drew Provan and John Gribben.
© 2010 Blackwell Publishing.

CML represents approximately 14% of all leukemias and accounts for up to 20% of all cases of adult leukemia in Western societies. The median age of onset of CML is 65 years and the incidence increases with age. In the majority of patients with CML a clear etiology is absent and therefore the disease is neither preventable nor inherited. However, it is well documented that ionizing radiation is leukemogenic and CML has been observed in individuals exposed to the radiation emitted by the atomic bomb explosions in Japan in 1945. In these patients, the incidence of CML was 50-fold higher than that of non-exposed subjects and it peaked approximately 10 years after the explosion, although patients younger than 15 years of age developed CML earlier than those 30 years of age or older. Nonetheless, in most cases of CML no antecedent radiation exposure is discernible.

## Clinical presentation and natural history of CML

CML evolves typically in three phases. Approximately 90% of patients with CML are diagnosed in chronic phase (CP), characterized by overproduction of immature myeloid cells and mature granulocytes in the bone marrow and peripheral blood. At this stage, the leukemic burden is approximately $10^{12}$ cells, which replace the normal hematopoietic tissue in the bone marrow. Patients in CP are typically asymptomatic, but if symptoms are present these usually relate to the presence of splenomegaly (e.g., abdominal fullness, early satiety, pain). Other signs and symptoms that may occur are anorexia, weight loss, fever, fatigue, or anemia, which is usually normochromic and normocytic. Leukocytosis, frequently with white blood cell counts exceeding $100 \times 10^9$/L, is a common finding at this stage but only occasionally leads to signs and symptoms of hyperviscosity (priapism, cerebrovascular accidents, dizziness, confusion) or retinal hemorrhage. In CP, CML cells retain their ability to differentiate and produce morphologically normal blood elements, capable of carrying out the physiological functions of normal counterparts. In up to 50% of cases, CP CML is diagnosed after a routine blood test done for unrelated reasons. The peripheral blood smear of patients in CP is characterized by the presence of the full spectrum of myeloid cells with blasts comprising less than 5% of the white blood cell differential. Basophilia is almost invariably present and the leukocyte alkaline phosphatase activity is reduced, both in intensity and in the number of neutrophil band forms that stain positive for this enzyme. The bone marrow aspirate and biopsy are hypercellular and demonstrate granulocytic and megakaryocytic hyperplasia, basophilia, and a blast percentage of 5% or less. Historically, the median survival of patients with CP CML was 4–5 years. Left untreated, most patients in CP progress to blast phase (BP), characterized by a peripheral blood or bone marrow blast percentage of 30% or more, frequently preceded by an accelerated phase (AP). The estimated risk of transformation from CP to BP was approximately 3–4% per year. Both AP and BP are characterized by increasing arrest of maturation. Moreover, as CML evolves into AP or BP, dysplastic changes become more apparent and consist mainly of hypersegmention, hyposegmentation, or abnormal lobulation of polymorphonuclear leukocytes, the presence of both eosinophilic and basophilic granules in the same cell, Pelger-like leukocytes, karyorrhexis of the erythroblasts, and microforms of the megakaryocytes. In addition, structural studies have demonstrated that myeloid maturation is faulty, with the cytoplasm generally maturing more rapidly than the nucleus.

The transition from CP to AP is usually subclinical and laboratory monitoring is necessary for detection of disease progression. A variety of classification schemas have been use to define AP based on a series of hematological and cytogenetic parameters. One classification, proposed by investigators at the M.D. Anderson Cancer Center, defines AP as the presence of any of the following features: cytogenetic clonal evolution, 15% or more blasts, 30% or more blasts plus promyelocytes, 20% or more basophils, or platelets lower than $100 \times 10^9$/L unrelated to therapy (Table 7.1). Although other classification systems have been proposed for defining AP and BP, they have not been clinically validated. Patients in AP may be symptomatic and present with fever, night sweats, weight loss, or bleeding associated with thrombocytopenia. The average survival of patients in AP was 1–2 years.

Historically, the estimated risk of transformation to BP was 5–10% per year during the first 2 years after diagnosis but increased to 20–25% per year thereafter. A diagnosis of BP CML requires the demonstration of at least 30% blasts in the peripheral blood and/or the bone marrow, or the presence of extramedullary blastic foci. The World Health Organization (WHO) classification has proposed that the blast percentage that defines BP be changed from ≥30% to ≥20%. Immunophenotypically, BP CML can display either myeloid or lymphoid features. In rare instances, blast cells can be biphenotypic and exhibit a mixed lymphoblastic–myeloblastic lineage. BP with a lymphoid phenotype occurs in 20–30% of patients, whereas 50% exhibit a myeloid phenotype, and in the remaining 25% of patients the phenotype is undifferentiated. Cells from patients with lymphoid BP CML exhibit high levels of the enzyme terminal deoxynucle-

**Table 7.1** Diagnostic criteria of accelerated phase according to M.D. Anderson Cancer Center (MDACC), International Bone Marrow Transplant Registry (IBMTR), and the World Health Organization (WHO).

| | MDACC | IBMTR | WHO |
|---|---|---|---|
| Blasts | 15–29% | 10–29% | 10–19%* |
| Blasts + promyelocytes | ≥30% | ≥20% | NA |
| Basophils | ≥20% | ≥20%† | ≥20% |
| Platelets (×10⁹/L) | <100 | Unresponsively high or persistently low | <100 or >1000 Unresponsive |
| Cytogenetics | CE | CE | CE not at diagnosis |
| WBC | NA | Difficult to control, or doubling < 5 days | NA |
| Anemia | NA | Unresponsive | NA |
| Splenomegaly | NA | Increasing | NA |
| Other | NA | Chloromas, myelofibrosis | Megakaryocyte proliferation, fibrosis |

*In the WHO criteria, blast phase is defined as a blast percentage of 20% or higher. For MDACC and IBMTR a definition of blast phase requires the presence of at least 30% blasts.
†Basophils plus eosinophils.
CE, clonal evolution; NA, not applicable; WBC, white blood cell count.

otidyltransferase (TdT), which catalyzes the polymerization of deoxynucleoside triphosphates. TdT is found mainly in poorly differentiated normal and malignant lymphoid cells of T-cell and B-cell origin and its expression progressively diminishes as lymphocytes differentiate. Most cases of lymphoid BP arise from progenitors of the B-cell lineage, and express CD10, CD19, and CD22. T-cell BP CML has been rarely described. The phenotype of myeloid BP cells resembles that of acute myeloid leukemia cells, with blasts staining with myeloperoxidase and expressing CD13, CD33, and CD117. Clinically, BP CML is characterized by prominent hypercatabolic symptoms, related to increasing tumor burden, and a remarkable resistance to conventional chemotherapeutic agents. The median survival of patients in BP prior to the introduction of imatinib therapy was 18 weeks.

## Prognostic tools in CML

The different CML phases predict for very different survivals. However, the prognosis is highly variable even among patients in the same phase of the disease. Several patient characteristics have been found to be prognostically useful and have been used to generate prognostic systems. In 1984, Sokal and colleagues studied 813 patients with CML collected from six European and American series in the 1960s and 1970s. The following hazard ratio function for death was derived from baseline patient and disease characteristics:

$$\lambda^i(+)/\lambda_0(t) = \text{Exp } 0.0116\,(\text{age} - 43.4) + 0.0345\,(\text{spleen} - 7.51) + 0.188\left[(\text{platelets}/700)^2 - 0.563\right] + 0.0887\,(\text{blasts} - 2.10)$$

This function segregated patients into three prognostic groups with hazard ratios of <0.8, 0.8–1.2, and >1.2, and median survivals of 2.5, 3.5, and 4.5 years, respectively. Given that the Sokal prognostic score system was developed in the era before interferon (IFN)-α, the Hasford score, which takes into account age, platelet count, peripheral blast count, spleen size, eosinophils and basophils, was developed to identify risk groups in patients with CML treated with IFN-α.

Genome-wide analyses of gene expression profiles have been broadly used as prognostication tools in multiple malignancies. In a recent analysis, in which DNA microarrays were used to compare gene expression in 91 patients with CML in all phases of the disease, patients in CP or BP revealed marked differences in gene expression. Interestingly, there was a strong correlation in expression levels between AP and BP ($r = 0.81$), suggesting that the progression from CP to advanced phase (AP and BP) CML could be a two-step process rather than a triphasic process. Gene-expression profiling may facilitate a comprehensive stratification of CML capable of segregating genetically defined subgroups with an adverse prognosis.

## Molecular biology of CML

### BCR-ABL1 oncogene

The fusion of the *ABL1* and the *BCR* genes resulting from the reciprocal translocation t(9;22)(q34;q11) gives rise to the *BCR-ABL1* oncogene that encodes for the constitutively active BCR-ABL1 protein kinase. Several experimental models, such as *BCR-ABL1*-expressing CD34$^+$ cells in culture or retrovirally transduced *BCR-ABL1*-positive mouse cells, have established a causal relationship between *BCR-ABL1* and human leukemia. Notably, *BCR-ABL1* can transform hematopoietic stem cells, but not committed progenitors lacking self-renewal capacity.

Different breakpoints within *ABL1* at 9q34 have been described, located either upstream of exon Ib, downstream of exon Ia, or more frequently between the two (Figure 7.1). Breakpoints within *BCR* localize to three main breakpoint cluster regions (*bcr*). In most patients with CML and in one-third of those with Ph-positive acute lymphoblastic leukemia (ALL), the breakpoint maps to the major breakpoint cluster region (M-*bcr*), which spans *BCR* exons 12–16 (formerly called b1–b5), giving rise to a fusion transcript with either b2a2 or b3a2 junctions that translates into a 210-kDa protein (p210$^{BCR-ABL1}$). In two-thirds of patients with Ph-positive ALL and rarely in CML, the breakpoints within *BCR* localize to an area of 54.4 kb between exons e2′ and e2, termed the minor breakpoint cluster region (m-*bcr*), which translates to a 190-kDa protein (p190$^{BCR-ABL1}$). A third breakpoint cluster region (μ-*bcr*) has been identified giving rise to a 230-kDa fusion protein (p230$^{BCR-ABL1}$) associated with some cases of chronic neutrophilic leukemia.

### BCR-ABL1 kinase signaling pathways

BCR-ABL1 signals through an intricate network of molecular pathways to promote inhibition of growth-factor/adhesion dependence, decreased apoptosis, and enhanced proliferation (Figure 7.2). Phosphorylation of BCR Tyr177 provides a high-affinity docking site for the SH2 domain of growth factor receptor-bound protein 2 (GRB2), which in turn recruits SOS (a guanine-nucleotide exchanger of *RAS*), thus activating RAS and the adapter GRB2-associated binding protein 2 (GAB2). BCR-ABL1-induced GAB2 phosphorylation activates the phosphatidylinositol 3-kinase (PI3K)/AKT and the RAS/ERK pathways. BCR-ABL1 also phosphorylates the SRC family kinases (SFKs) HCK, LYN, and FGR, which is conducive to activation of STAT5 (signal

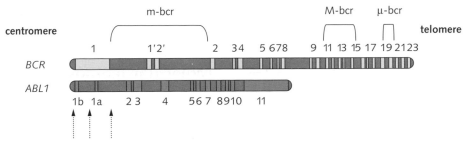

**Fig. 7.1 Schematic representation of the *BCR* and *ABL1* genes**
Exons are numbered. *BCR* spans 130 kb and is situated in a 5′ to 3′ orientation with the 5′ end closer to the centromere. The entire gene contains 23 exons. Exons 1′ and 2′ of *BCR* are alternative exons contained within the first intron. The three main breakpoint cluster regions in *BCR* are shown. The *ABL1* gene contains two alternative first exons (1b and 1a). Breakpoints within the *ABL1* gene are represented by the dashed arrows. The combination of breakpoints within *BCR* and *ABL1* genes gives rise to a series of fusion transcripts that encode for protein products with different molecular weight.

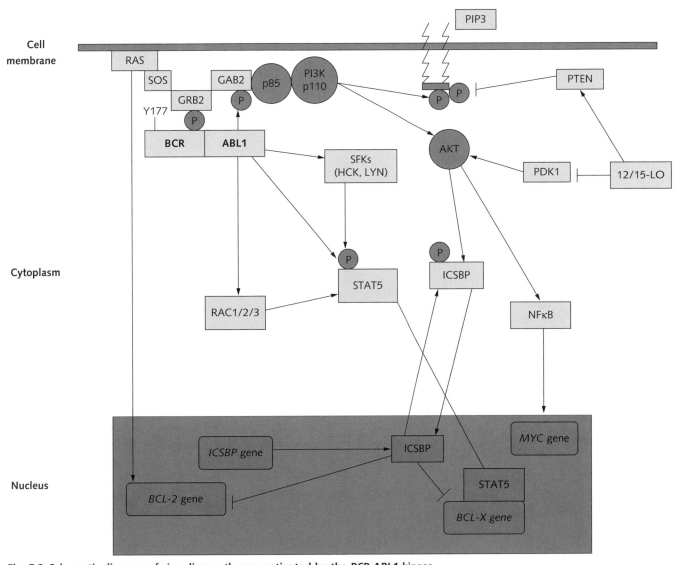

**Fig. 7.2 Schematic diagram of signaling pathways activated by the BCR-ABL1 kinase**
See text for definition of abbreviations.

transducer and activation of transcription 5), which upon dimerization translocates to the nucleus and binds to cognate DNA sequences to modulate gene transcription. Moreover, STAT5 upregulates the anti-apoptotic protein $BCL_{XL}$, which is repressed by the tumor suppressor and negative regulator of granulocyte differentiation ICSBP (transcription factor interferon consensus sequence binding protein). Recently, the RAC subfamily of guanosine triphosphatases (GTPases) RAC1, RAC2, and RAC3 as well as the enzyme 12/15-lipoxygenase (12/15-LO) have also been identified as important elements in BCR-ABL1 downstream signaling. In spite of the fact that BCR-ABL1 signals through a multitude of downstream elements, the kinase activity of this oncogenic enzyme is key to the genesis and maintenance of the CML phenotype. This realization provides the rationale for the development of therapeutic strategies to abrogate the activation of BCR-ABL1.

## Therapy for patients with CML

In recent years, the treatment of patients with CML has changed dramatically. Conventional chemotherapeutic agents such as busulfan or hydroxycarbamide (hydroxyurea) are no longer used, except as a means to achieve initial hematological control. The emergence of imatinib mesylate has brought about a change in the therapeutic algorithm for CML, to the point that IFN-α has been superseded by imatinib as frontline therapy, and imatinib has spurred the development of an array of tyrosine kinase inhibitors (TKIs) with higher potency against BCR-ABL1 kinase. Allogeneic stem cell transplantation (SCT) remains a curative modality and a valid option for patients who fail TKI therapy.

### Interferon-α

The use of recombinant IFN-α in CML was developed in the early 1980s; this agent showed significant activity, particularly in patients in early CP, but modest activity in advanced-phase CML. IFN-α therapy resulted in complete hematological response (CHR) and major cytogenetic response (MCR; i.e., <35% Ph chromosome-positive cells) in 80% and 38% of patients, respectively. Furthermore, complete cytogenetic response (CCR; i.e., 0% Ph chromosome-positive cells) was reported in 30–35% of patients. By multivariate analysis, bone marrow basophilia ($P < 0.01$) and splenomegaly ($P < 0.01$) were identified as independent poor prognostic factors for survival, whereas achievement of MCR was associated with improved survival ($P < 0.001$). In a meta-analysis involving seven large, prospective, randomized trials, IFN-α produced a significantly better survival than either hydroxycarbamide ($P = 0.001$) or busulfan

($P = 0.00007$). The 5-year survival rates were 57% with IFN-α and 42% with chemotherapy ($P < 0.00001$). Cytarabine was added to IFN-α in an attempt to improve on the response rates of single-agent IFN-α. Although associated with a higher incidence of gastrointestinal toxicity and myelosuppression, this combination resulted in improved cytogenetic response rates. Cytogenetic response to IFN-α-based therapy was associated with improved survival, with 78% of patients who achieved a CCR alive at 10 years. Interestingly, 30% of patients in CCR had undetectable BCR-ABL1 transcript levels and none of them had relapsed after more than 10 years of follow-up, suggesting that these patients might indeed be cured. These striking results are believed to be a consequence of the immunomodulatory effect of IFN-α. This is best illustrated by the presence of IFN-α-induced cytotoxic T lymphocytes specific for PR1, a peptide derived from proteinase 3 which is overexpressed in CML cells. These cytotoxic T lymphocytes have been isolated from patients in CCR after IFN-α therapy and SCT but not in those who failed to achieve CCR or were treated with chemotherapy.

### Stem cell transplantation

Allogeneic SCT remains an important therapeutic modality, particularly for younger patients with human leukocyte antigen (HLA)-identical siblings. Results after allogeneic SCT are significantly better for patients transplanted in CP than for those in advanced-phase CML. Despite initial reports of improved outcomes when allogeneic SCT was performed within 12 months from CML diagnosis, similar outcomes have been reported when SCT was performed during the first 24 months, or even within the first 36 months from diagnosis. The influence of pre-SCT therapy on outcomes after SCT has been a subject of intense debate. It was initially suggested that prior IFN-α therapy negatively impacted the outcome of SCT. Subsequent studies could not demonstrate such effect, and recent evidence suggests that this might also be true for the use of imatinib prior to SCT. The mortality during the first year post-SCT for patients younger than 40 years transplanted in early CP from an HLA-identical sibling is 10–20% due to regimen-related toxicity, graft-versus-host disease (GVHD), veno-occlusive disease, and infectious complications. After a follow-up of 10 years, patients with CML undergoing allogeneic SCT have an overall survival of 60% and an event-free survival of 50%, although at 15 years these decrease to 47% and 52%, respectively. The European Group for Blood and Marrow Transplantation (EBMT) has reported on 2628 patients who received transplants between 1980 and 1990. The overall survival rate at 20 years was 34% for all patients and 41% for those who received transplants in first CP from an HLA-

Chronic myelogenous leukemia **81**

identical sibling. However, only one-third of patients have a suitable HLA-matched sibling and the use of stringent inclusion criteria in modern transplantation protocols limits the applicability of this approach to a minority of patients. A means to overcome this hurdle is the use of matched unrelated donors. However, matched unrelated donor SCT is associated with a higher incidence of viral infections, extensive chronic GVHD, and engraftment failure compared with HLA-matched sibling donor SCT. The long-term disease-free survival rate after matched unrelated donor SCT for young patients in early CP is 57% compared with 67% in patients receiving grafts from HLA-matched siblings. Progress in molecular DNA typing of HLA alleles has decreased the rate of GVHD and improved the probability of long-term survival in patients undergoing matched unrelated donor SCT. Although these outcomes are likely to be improved by using more stringent molecular typing protocols, this will be invariably linked to a lower probability of finding suitable donors.

It has been shown that patients with minimal residual disease detected by polymerase chain reaction (PCR) 12 months from SCT have a risk of relapse of 30–40%, whereas in those with undetectable *BCR-ABL1* transcripts it is less than 5%. However, overt relapse can be frequently abrogated by donor lymphocyte infusion in a high percentage of patients when this is administered at the time of molecular relapse. Alternatively, imatinib can also be used in the post-SCT relapse setting, and induces CCR in over 40% of patients treated in CP.

Since a large proportion of patients with CML are older than 50 years of age, reduced intensity conditioning regimens are being investigated. This approach takes advantage of the ability of the T cells harbored in the graft to attack the CML cells (graft-versus-leukemia effect) instead of relying entirely on an ablative regimen to obtain this effect. The EBMT has reported on 187 patients with a median age of 50 years who received reduced intensity conditioning allogeneic SCT between 1994 and 2002, mainly from HLA-matched related donors. Notably, the 3-year overall survival was 70% for those patients with a favorable EBMT score and 30% for those with the highest scores, supporting the use of this modality in older patients. Long-term outcomes cannot yet be evaluated.

## Imatinib mesylate (Gleevec, formerly STI-571)

Imatinib mesylate is an orally bioavailable 2-phenylaminopyrimidine relatively selective for and moderately potent against the constitutively active tyrosine kinase of the BCR-ABL1 fusion protein (Figure 7.3). In addition to BCR-ABL1, imatinib also inhibits other kinases such as KIT, platelet-derived growth factor receptor (PDGFR)α and PDGFRβ, and ABL-related gene (ARG). Seminal work by Buchdunger and colleagues and Druker and colleagues demonstrated the selective activity of imatinib against *BCR-ABL1*-expressing cells lines *in vitro* and *in vivo*. Based on these promising preclinical data, imatinib was tested in Phase I and Phase II trials where it demonstrated exceptional activity in patients with CML, particularly in CP, and a safe toxicity profile when administered at a daily dose of 400 mg. It was ultimately the Phase III, randomized, multinational IRIS

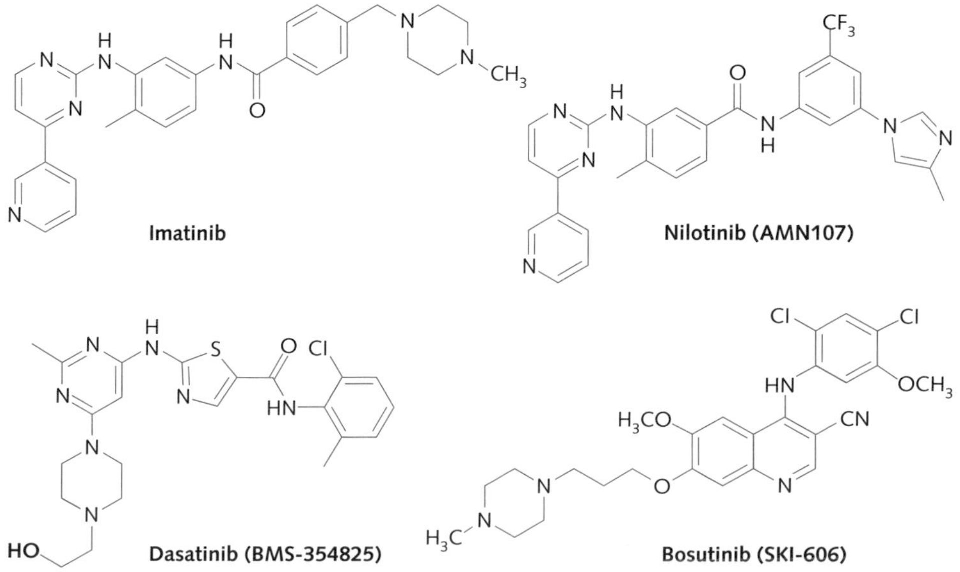

Fig. 7.3 Chemical structures of imatinib and second-generation tyrosine kinase inhibitors currently under development in CML

(International Randomized Study of IFN-α plus Ara-C versus STI571) study, comparing imatinib 400 mg orally daily with IFN-α in combination with cytarabine in newly diagnosed patients with CML in CP, which established imatinib as the standard frontline therapy for CML. In this study, 1106 patients were randomized between June 2000 and January 2001, with the possibility to cross over to the alternate therapy if treatment failure or intolerance was demonstrated (Figure 7.4). Baseline patient and disease characteristics were well balanced for all features evaluated, including age, white blood cell count, Sokal and Hasford score, and time from diagnosis to imatinib therapy. Imatinib therapy was superior to IFN-α plus low-dose cytarabine in all aspects including hematological and cytogenetic responses, tolerability, and progression to advanced-phase

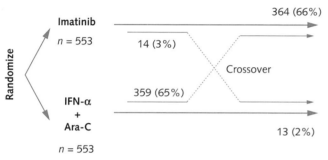

**Fig. 7.4 Design of the IRIS study**
A total of 1106 patients were randomized to receive either imatinib 400 mg daily or the combination of IFN-α and cytarabine (Ara-C). Crossover was allowed due to lack of response, loss of response or treatment intolerance. The data presented have been updated after 6 years of follow-up. To date, 181 (33%) patients have discontinued imatinib therapy.

CML. After a median follow-up of 60 months, the projected rates of CHR and CCR were 98% and 87%, respectively. Notably, the estimated 5-year survival rate was approximately 90% and the rate of progression from CP to either AP or BP during the sixth year of therapy was 0% (Figure 7.5).

The prognostic implications of achieving a major molecular response (MMR; i.e., 3-log reduction in *BCR-ABL1* transcript levels) have led to a reappraisal of the main goals of imatinib therapy for patients with CML. The depth of the response achieved after 12 months of imatinib therapy has been shown to have important implications regarding long-term outcome and, as a consequence, the emphasis in CML therapy has been placed on the achievement of not only CCR but also MMR or, ideally, of complete molecular response (CMR; i.e., undetectable *BCR-ABL1* transcripts). The importance of achieving molecular responses during imatinib therapy has been borne out by results from the IRIS trial, which demonstrated that patients who attained MMR within the first 12 months of therapy had a transformation-free survival of 100%. For that reason, once CCR is obtained, monitoring by quantitative RT-PCR in peripheral blood samples at 3–6 month intervals is recommended during the first 12 months of therapy and every 6–12 months thereafter. In this regard, results from Phase II studies suggest that imatinib at higher doses (600–800 mg daily) might result in higher rates of cytogenetic and molecular response and therefore improved long-term outcomes compared with the standard dose of 400 mg daily. Results from ongoing randomized studies will determine whether high-dose imatinib provides higher response rates or simply hastens their achievement.

Currently, there is no evidence that patients receiving imatinib can safely discontinue therapy, as most patients

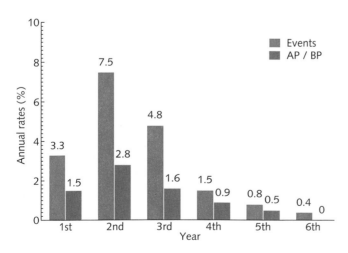

**Fig. 7.5 Disease progression during imatinib therapy in the IRIS trial after 6 years of follow-up**
Events denote loss of complete hematological response, loss of major cytogenetic response, progression to accelerated or blast phase, or death.

who have withdrawn therapy have experienced rapid molecular and cytogenetic relapse. Moreover, it appears that the most primitive quiescent leukemic progenitors are insensitive to imatinib *in vitro*, which suggests that this subset of CML cells may be responsible for CML relapse upon imatinib discontinuation. However, in a recent report, 12 patients with CML and undetectable residual molecular disease for a median of 32 months (range 24–46 months) discontinued imatinib therapy. Six patients had a molecular relapse between 1 and 5 months from imatinib interruption. In six (50%) other patients, *BCR-ABL1* transcripts remained undetectable after a median follow up of 18 months (range 9–24 months).

## Second-generation TKIs

Because only a small fraction of patients receiving imatinib therapy achieve CMR and because 20–30% of patients will eventually develop resistance to imatinib, several other TKIs are in clinical development. The common denominator of most of these agents is their superior potency relative to imatinib and their activity against a wide spectrum of imatinib-resistant BCR-ABL1 kinase mutations, which represent the most common mechanism of resistance encountered in patients with CML undergoing TKI therapy. Therapy with either nilotinib or dasatinib, the two agents furthest along in clinical development, has been shown to render a better 2-year survival than allogeneic SCT in patients in CP CML after imatinib failure.

Nilotinib (Tasigna, formerly AMN107) is a phenylaminopyrimidine derived from the crystal structure of imatinib in complex with ABL1 kinase (Figure 7.3). Nilotinib has 20- to 30-fold improved affinity and inhibitory activity against unmutated BCR-ABL1 and inhibits the tyrosine kinase activity of 32 of 33 *BCR-ABL1* mutants tested, the exception being T315I. The maximum tolerated dose of nilotinib in a

**Table 7.2** Response to the second-generation tyrosine kinase inhibitors nilotinib and dasatinib in Phase II studies* of patients with imatinib-resistant or -intolerant CML.

| ABL kinase inhibitor | CML phase | Number of patients | Response rate (%) | | |
|---|---|---|---|---|---|
| | | | | Cytogenetic | |
| | | | CHR | Complete response | Partial response |
| Nilotinib | Chronic | 321 | 77 | 41 | 16 |
| | Accelerated | 129 | 26 | 19 | 12 |
| | Blastic (myeloid) | 22 | 11 | 29 | 9 |
| | Blastic (lymphoid) | 19 | 13 | 32 | 16 |
| Dasatinib | Chronic | 387 | 91 | 53 | 9 |
| | Accelerated | 174 | 50 | 33 | 7 |
| | Blastic (myeloid) | 109 | 26 | 27 | 7 |
| | Blastic (lymphoid) | 48 | 29 | 46 | 6 |

CHR, complete hematological response (normalization of peripheral blood counts and disappearance of all signs and symptoms related to leukemia for at least 4 weeks); partial cytogenetic response, 1–35% Ph-positive cells; complete cytogenetic response, 0% Ph-positive cells.

* Gambacorti C, Cortes, J, Kim, D *et al.* (2007) Efficacy and safety of dasatinib in patients with chronic myeloid leukemia in blast phase whose disease is resistant or intolerant to imatinib: 2-year follow-up data from the START Program. *Blood*, **110**, (abstract 472).

Giles F, Larson RA, Kantarjian K *et al.* (2007) Nilotinib in patients (pts) with Philadelphia chromosome-positive (ph+) chronic myelogenous leukemia in blast crisis (CML-BC) who are resistant or intolerant to imatinib. *Blood*, **110**, (abstract 1025).

Guilhot F, Apperley JF, Kim D *et al.* (2007) Efficacy of dasatinib in patients with accelerated-phase chronic myelogenous leukemia with resistance or intolerance to imatinib: 2-year follow-up data from START-A (CA180-005). *Blood*, **110**, (abstract 470).

Kantarjian H, Hochhaus A, Cortes J *et al.* (2007) Nilotinib is highly active and safe in chronic phase chronic myelogenous leukemia (CML-CP) patients with imatinib-resistance or intolerance. *Blood*, **110**, (abstract 735).

le Coutre P, Giles FJ, Apperley J *et al.* (2007) Nilotinib is safe and effective in accelerated phase chronic myelogenous leukemia (CML-AP) patients with imatinib resistance or intolerance. *Blood*, **110**, (abstract 471).

Stone R, Kantarjian H, Baccarani M *et al.* (2007) Efficacy of dasatinib in patients with chronic-phase chronic myelogenous leukemia with resistance or intolerance to imatinib: 2-year follow-up data from START-C (CA180-013). *Blood*, **110**, (abstract 734).

Phase I study in imatinib-resistant CML and Ph-positive ALL was 600 mg twice daily. In the Phase II pivotal trial, nilotinib was administered at 400 mg twice daily to 321 patients with CP CML, producing a CHR rate of 77% and complete and partial cytogenetic response rates of 41% and 16%, respectively (Table 7.2); 84% of patients maintained an MCR after 18 months, and the progression-free survival for the total population of patients was 64% at 18 months. The most frequent grade 3–4 hematological toxicity included thrombocytopenia (27%), neutropenia (30%), and anemia (9%). Asymptomatic serum lipase elevation was observed in 15% of patients. Nilotinib can potentially prolong the QTc interval but in all these studies this occurrence was infrequent, mild, and clinically irrelevant. The activity of nilotinib in patients with advanced disease was more modest and responses were sustained for shorter periods of time (Table 7.2). Nilotinib has been recently approved by the US Food and Drug Administration (FDA) for the treatment of patients with CML in CP or AP who have developed resistance or intolerance to imatinib.

Dasatinib (Sprycel, formerly BMS-354825) is a sub-nanomolar inhibitor of BCR-ABL1 and SFKs, with potent activity against KIT ($IC_{50}$ 13 nmol/L), PDGFRβ ($IC_{50}$ 28 nmol/L), and ephrin receptor EPHA2 ($IC_{50}$ 17 nmol/L) tyrosine kinases (Figure 7.3). Like nilotinib, dasatinib inhibits multiple imatinib-resistant *BCR-ABL1* mutant isoforms, except for T315I. In a dose-finding study conducted in 84 patients with CML in all phases resistant or intolerant to imatinib or with Ph-positive ALL, dasatinib proved very active across a wide spectrum of *BCR-ABL1* mutations. The maximum tolerated dose was not determined and no patient withdrew from the study as a result of toxic effects. However, non-malignant pleural effusion was a distinct side effect associated with dasatinib therapy. In the Phase II

international multicenter trial START-C, 387 patients with CP CML received dasatinib 70 mg twice daily (Table 7.2). The CHR rate was 91%, whereas complete and partial cytogenetic response rates were 53% and 9%, respectively; 27% of patients developed pleural effusions, being grade 3–4 in 6% of cases. Responses in patients with either AP CML (study START-A) or BP CML (study START-B) were less satisfactory, with CCR in 33%, 27%, and 46% of patients in AP, myeloid BP, or lymphoid BP, respectively (Table 7.2).

Dasatinib administered at 70 mg twice daily to patients with CP CML resistant to imatinib 400–600 mg daily appears superior to imatinib dose escalation (800 mg daily) as shown in a randomized study (START-R). After a median follow-up of 24 months, CHR, MCR and CCR rates, as well as progression-free survival, significantly favored dasatinib therapy. Notably, dasatinib 100 mg once daily is equally effective as 50 mg twice daily, 140 mg once daily, and 70 mg twice daily, but results in a significantly lower rate of myelo-suppression, pleural effusions, and dose modifications. Dasatinib is FDA-approved for the treatment of adults with CML in all phases with resistance or intolerance to prior therapy, including imatinib mesylate. The currently approved dose for patients in CP is 100 mg once daily whereas for patients in AP or BP it is 70 mg twice daily.

The prognosis of patients with CML post imatinib failure is believed to be poor but data on clinical outcomes derived from the different therapeutic strategies currently available in this setting are lacking. Preliminary data suggest that the prognosis of patients in CP who received therapy with either nilotinib or dasatinib is better than that of patients who underwent allogeneic SCT or other treatment modalities (Figure 7.6). Longer follow-up is required to confirm these findings.

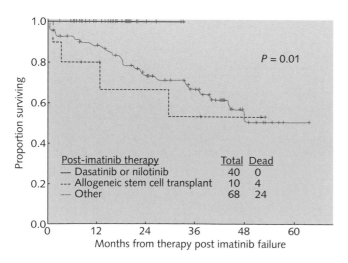

**Fig. 7.6 Overall survival of patients with CML in chronic phase after failure of imatinib therapy according to the treatment modality subsequently employed**

## Other second-generation TKIs

Besides nilotinib and dasatinib, other second-generation TKIs are currently in clinical development, of which bosutinib (SKI-606) and INNO-406 are two of the most promising. Bosutinib is a potent dual SFK and ABL1 kinase inhibitor with negligible activity against KIT or PDGFR, which may result in an improved toxicity profile (Figure 7.3). In a Phase I/II study, bosutinib showed a remarkably benign toxicity profile among 152 patients enrolled in all phases of the disease; a dose of 500 mg daily was selected for testing in the ongoing Phase II portion of the study. The CHR rate among 115 patients in CP CML who had failed prior therapy with imatinib was 89%, with MCR and CCR rates of 41% and 30%, respectively; 33% of patients had an MMR and 19% a CMR. A total of 37 patients had failed treatment with nilotinib or dasatinib in addition to imatinib; 10 of 13 (77%) evaluable patients had a CHR and 2 of 10 (20%) an MCR. Reponses were observed in patients with and without *BCR-ABL1* mutations. Grade 3–4 adverse events were infrequent; thrombocytopenia was reported in 14% of patients, neutropenia in 9%, and diarrhea and rash in 7% each. Notably, no pleural effusions were noted.

INNO-406 is another potent BCR-ABL1 inhibitor with activity against BCR-ABL1, ARG and FYN kinases, capable of reaching high enough concentrations in the central nervous system to inhibit the growth of *BCR-ABL1*-positive leukemic cells expressing multiple *BCR-ABL1* mutant isoforms. Preliminary data on 32 patients in CP CML enrolled in a Phase I study of INNO-406 have been recently reported. A cytogenetic response was observed in 42% of patients who had failed prior imatinib therapy and in 38% of those who had failed imatinib and dasatinib therapy. The dose selected for ongoing Phase II studies is 240 mg twice daily.

## Clinical resistance to imatinib therapy

Imatinib resistance can be categorized as primary (also dubbed "refractoriness"), in which patients fail to respond to this TKI from the onset of therapy, and secondary (or "acquired resistance"), which ensues after the initial achievement of some degree of response to imatinib durable for a variable period of time. Mutations within the kinase domain of *BCR-ABL1* are regarded as the most frequent mechanism involved in TKI resistance in CML. The frequency of *BCR-ABL1* mutations in imatinib-resistant patients ranges from 40 to 90%, depending on the definition of resistance, the methodology of detection, and CML phase. More than 100 different *BCR-ABL1* point mutations encoding for single amino acid substitutions have been reported in patients with CML, conferring different degrees of imatinib resistance (Table 7.3). The most frequently reported mutations in

**Table 7.3** Activity of imatinib on kinase- and cell-based assays against a selection of clinically relevant *BCR-ABL1*.

| *BCR-ABL1* (construct) | Imatinib | |
|---|---|---|
| | Autophosphorylation | Proliferation |
| *BCR-ABL1* p210 + IL-3 | NA | >7700 |
| WT p210 | 221 ± 31 | 678 ± 39 |
| G250E | 2287 ± 826 | 3329 ± 1488 |
| G250V | 489 | 624 |
| Q252H | 1080 ± 119 | 851 ± 436 |
| Y253H | >10000 | >7000 |
| E255K | 4856 ± 482 | 5567 |
| E255K | 2455 ± 433 | 7161 ± 970 |
| E255V | 6353 ± 636 | 6111 ± 854 |
| D276G | 1284 | 2486 |
| E292K | 275 ± 81 | 1552 |
| T315I | >10000 | >7000 |
| F317C | 1090 | 694 |
| F317L | 797 ± 92 | 1528 ± 227 |
| F317V | 544 ± 47 | 549 ± 173 |
| M351T | 593 ± 57 | 1682 ± 233 |
| E355G | 601 | 1149 |
| F359V | 1528 | 595 |
| F486S | 1238 ± 110 | 3050 ± 597 |

All concentrations are shown in nmol/mL. Cell-based assays were carried out in Ba/F3 cells.
IL-3, interleukin-3.

clinical specimens are those that map to the P-loop region of the kinase domain, which serves as a docking site for phosphate moieties of ATP. However, mutations also frequently map to the activation loop, which impair the achievement of the inactive conformation of the kinase to which imatinib binds, the catalytic domain, and the gatekeeper T315 residue. Of particular concern is the development of the T315I mutation, which causes steric hindrance to TKI binding and confers resistance to all TKIs currently approved for CML therapy. Moreover, some patients with CML failing sequential therapy with imatinib and dasatinib carry more than one mutation within the same *BCR-ABL1* molecule ("compound" mutations or "polymutants"), which was associated with increased oncogenic potency compared with each single mutation.

It is worth emphasizing that *BCR-ABL1* mutations do not explain all cases of clinical resistance to TKI therapy. In recent years a variety of mechanisms have been investigated as potential causes of imatinib resistance in CML. *BCR-ABL1*-independent mechanisms have been found to be most common in patients with primary resistance. For instance, imatinib plasma levels have been shown to be associated with cytogenetic and molecular responses to standard-dose imatinib. It has been proposed that excessive binding of imatinib to the plasma protein $\alpha_1$-acid glycoprotein 1 (AGP1), overexpression of the ABCB1 (MDR-1) transmembrane protein, which regulates imatinib efflux from the cell, polymorphisms of the human organic cation transporter (hOCT1), which regulates imatinib influx, clonal evolution, SFK or BCR-ABL1 overexpression, and the intrinsic low TKI sensitivity of quiescent CML stem cells (Lin⁻CD34⁺BCR-ABL1-positive cells) account for most cases of TKI resistance in patients in whom *BCR-ABL1* mutations are not present. Each of these mechanisms of resistance suggests that different therapeutic interventions may be necessary to overcome TKI resistance, whereas the resistance imposed by most *BCR-ABL1* mutations has been shown to be overcome by using high-dose imatinib (800 mg daily) or second-generation TKIs. Novel agents with activity against the highly resistant T315I mutation or with activity against quiescent CML stem cells are under development.

## Monitoring of patients with CML during imatinib therapy

Consensus statements on standardization of monitoring of patients with CML receiving TKI therapy, response and failure definitions at specific time-points during therapy, and alternative therapeutic approaches for patients who fail imatinib have been issued by the National Comprehensive Cancer Network and the European Leukemia Net. Both panels of experts recommend imatinib 400 mg daily as first-line therapy for patients with newly diagnosed CML. Although most patients on imatinib achieve a cytogenetic response, a subset will develop acquired resistance that results in clinical failure. For patients who fail to obtain a cytogenetic response on imatinib, the current recommendations from the European Leukemia Net include the use of higher imatinib doses (600 or 800 mg daily), an alternative TKI, allogeneic SCT, or enrollment in clinical trial of an experimental therapy (Table 7.4). Patients with suboptimal response need close monitoring, and dose escalation from 400 to 800 mg is also justified. The effectiveness and timing of switching to a second-generation TKI in this setting is currently being assessed in ongoing trials.

Cytogenetic analysis is critical to define failure or suboptimal response to TKI therapy and not only provides invaluable information as to whether a given patient is responding appropriately to therapy but also detects the presence of clonal cytogenetic abnormalities in Ph-negative cells. It is estimated that 5–10% of patients receiving imatinib will develop such changes. The most frequent cytogenetic abnormalities encountered are trisomy 8, monosomy 5 or 7, and 20q–. Although typically transient, these abnormalities have

**Table 7.4** Criteria for failure and suboptimal response for patients with CML in early chronic phase receiving imatinib therapy at 400 mg daily.*

| Time after diagnosis | Failure | Suboptimal response | Warnings |
|---|---|---|---|
| 0 months | NA | NA | High risk, del der(9), ACAs in Ph⁺ cells |
| 3 months | No HR (stable disease or progression) | Less than CHR | NA |
| 6 months | Less than CHR, no cytogenetic response | Less than PCR | NA |
| 12 months | Less than PCR | Less than CCR | Less than MMR |
| 18 months | Less than CCR | Less than MMR | NA |
| Anytime | Loss of CHR or CCR, mutation | ACA in Ph⁺ cells, loss of MMR, mutation | Rise in transcript level; other chromosomal abnormalities in Ph⁻ cells |

*Failure suggests that imatinib therapy must be switched whenever available, whereas suboptimal response suggests that further therapeutic benefit may still be attained with continuation of imatinib although long-term outcome is not likely to be optimal. Warnings indicate that patients must be closely monitored and may be eligible for other therapies. High risk is defined according to the Sokal or the Hasford scores.

NA, not applicable; del der(9), deletion of derivative chromosome 9; HR, hematological response; CHR, complete hematological response; CCR, complete cytogenetic response; PCR, partial cytogenetic response; MMR, major molecular response; ACA, additional chromosomal abnormality.

been occasionally associated with progression to myelodysplasia or acute myeloid leukemia, most frequently in patients with monosomy 7. The fact that these abnormalities cannot be detected by conventional fluorescence *in situ* hybridization or PCR analyses reinforces the importance of repeat bone marrow cytogenetic examinations in patients receiving TKI therapy.

## Concluding remarks

CML is one of the most extensively studied diseases and the first human cancer to be consistently associated with a cytogenetic abnormality, the Ph chromosome. This discovery led to the recognition that the BCR-ABL1 tyrosine kinase drives the pathogenesis of CML. In turn, this resulted in the development of imatinib mesylate, a targeted inhibitor of the activity of the BCR-ABL1 oncoprotein, whose clinical efficacy in CML represents one of the greatest accomplishments in cancer history. Indeed, imatinib therapy has radically changed the natural history of CML, significantly prolonging the survival of patients who previously survived only 5–6 years from diagnosis. Not only did the development of imatinib validate the emerging paradigm of targeted therapy in cancer, but it also raised awareness of a series of potential shortcomings inherent to targeted agents of its kind. Issues such as the lack of effectiveness of imatinib against quiescent CML stem cells or the development of mutations within the kinase domain of BCR-ABL1 that impair the ability of imatinib to block the oncogenic signaling stemming from this kinase remain unsolved problems and certainly constitute challenges for the near future. These pitfalls notwithstanding, the unprecedented results obtained with TKI therapy in CML have brought to the fore the importance of understanding the molecular and genetic events that govern the growth and survival of a specific cancer. Undoubtedly, future discoveries will further our understanding of the molecular biology of CML and will translate into even better therapeutics for CML with potential to further improve the outlook of patients with this malignancy.

## Further reading

### Molecular biology of CML

Daley GQ, Van Etten RA, Baltimore D. (1990) Induction of chronic myelogenous leukemia in mice by the P210bcr/abl gene of the Philadelphia chromosome. *Science*, **247**, 824–830.

Deininger MW, Goldman JM, Melo JV. (2000) The molecular biology of chronic myeloid leukemia. *Blood*, **96**, 3343–3356.

Groffen J, Stephenson JR, Heisterkamp N, de Klein A, Bartram CR, Grosveld G. (1984) Philadelphia chromosomal breakpoints are clustered within a limited region, bcr, on chromosome 22. *Cell*, **36**, 93–99.

Heisterkamp N, Jenster G, ten Hoeve J, Zovich D, Pattengale PK, Groffen J. (1990) Acute leukemia in bcr/abl transgenic mice. *Nature*, **344**, 251–253.

Huntly BJ, Shigematsu H, Deguchi K *et al.* (2004) MOZ-TIF2, but not BCR-ABL, confers properties of leukemic stem cells to committed murine hematopoietic progenitors. *Cancer Cell*, **6**, 587–596.

Melo JV. (1996) The diversity of BCR-ABL fusion proteins and their relationship to leukemia phenotype. *Blood*, **88**, 2375–2384.

Neviani P, Santhanam R, Trotta R *et al.* (2005) The tumor suppressor PP2A is functionally inactivated in blast crisis CML through the inhibitory activity of the BCR/ABL-regulated SET protein. *Cancer Cell*, **8**, 355–368.

Ren R. (2005) Mechanisms of BCR-ABL in the pathogenesis of chronic myelogenous leukemia. *Nature Reviews. Cancer*, **5**, 172–183.

Shtivelman E, Lifshitz B, Gale RP, Canaani E. (1985) Fused transcript of abl and bcr genes in chronic myelogenous leukemia. *Nature*, **315**, 550–554.

Thomas EK, Cancelas JA, Chae HD *et al.* (2007) Rac guanosine triphosphatases represent integrating molecular therapeutic targets for BCR-ABL-induced myeloproliferative disease. *Cancer Cell*, **12**, 467–478.

### Prognostic scores

Gratwohl A, Hermans J, Goldman JM *et al.* (1998) Risk assessment for patients with chronic myeloid leukemia before allogeneic blood or marrow transplantation. Chronic Leukemia Working Party of the European Group for Blood and Marrow Transplantation. *Lancet*, **352**, 1087–1092.

Hasford J, Pfirrmann M, Hehlmann R *et al.* (1998) A new prognostic score for survival of patients with chronic myeloid leukemia treated with interferon alfa. Writing Committee for the Collaborative CML Prognostic Factors Project Group. *Journal of the National Cancer Institute*, **90**, 850–858.

Sokal JE, Cox EB, Baccarani M *et al.* (1984) Prognostic discrimination in "good-risk" chronic granulocytic leukemia. *Blood*, **63**, 789–799.

### Interferon-$\alpha$

Guilhot F, Chastang C, Michallet M *et al.* (1997) Interferon alfa-2b combined with cytarabine versus interferon alone in chronic myelogenous leukemia. *New England Journal of Medicine*, **337**, 223–229.

Hochhaus A, Reiter A, Saussele S *et al.* (2000) Molecular heterogeneity in complete cytogenetic responders after interferon-alpha therapy for chronic myelogenous leukemia: low levels of minimal residual disease are associated with continuing remission. *Blood*, **95**, 62–66.

Kantarjian HM, Smith TL, O'Brien S, Beran M, Pierce S, Talpaz M. (1995) Prolonged survival in chronic myelogenous leukemia after cytogenetic response to interferon-alpha therapy. *Annals of Internal Medicine*, **122**, 254–261.

Talpaz M, Kantarjian HM, McCredie K, Trujillo JM, Keating MJ, Gutterman JU. (1986) Hematologic remission and cytogenetic improvement induced by recombinant human interferon alpha A in chronic myelogenous leukemia. *New England Journal of Medicine*, **314**, 1065–1069.

### Allogeneic stem cell transplantation

Crawley C, Szydlo R, Lalancette M *et al.* (2005) Outcomes of reduced-intensity transplantation for chronic myeloid leukemia: an analysis of prognostic factors from the Chronic Leukemia Working Party of the EBMT. *Blood*, **106**, 2969–2976.

Gratwohl A, Hermans J, Niederwieser D *et al.* (1993) Bone marrow transplantation for chronic myeloid leukemia: long-term results. Chronic Leukemia Working Party of the European Group for Bone Marrow Transplantation. *Bone Marrow Transplantation*, **12**, 509–516.

Hansen JA, Gooley TA, Martin PJ et al. (1998) Bone marrow transplants from unrelated donors for patients with chronic myeloid leukemia. New England Journal of Medicine, 338, 962–968.

Oehler VG, Gooley T, Snyder DS et al. (2007) The effects of imatinib mesylate treatment before allogeneic transplantation for chronic myeloid leukemia. Blood, 109, 1782–1789.

Weisdorf DJ, Anasetti C, Antin JH et al. (2002) Allogeneic bone marrow transplantation for chronic myelogenous leukemia: comparative analysis of unrelated versus matched sibling donor transplantation. Blood, 99, 1971–1977.

## Imatinib

Buchdunger E, Zimmermann J, Mett H et al. (1996) Inhibition of the Abl protein-tyrosine kinase in vitro and in vivo by a 2-phenylaminopyrimidine derivative. Cancer Research, 56, 100–104.

Cortes J, Giles F, O'Brien S et al. (2003) Result of high-dose imatinib mesylate in patients with Philadelphia chromosome-positive chronic myeloid leukemia after failure of interferon-alpha. Blood, 102, 83–86.

Druker BJ, Tamura S, Buchdunger E et al. (1996) Effects of a selective inhibitor of the Abl tyrosine kinase on the growth of Bcr-Abl positive cells. Nature Medicine, 2, 561–566.

Druker BJ, Sawyers CL, Kantarjian H et al. (2001) Activity of a specific inhibitor of the BCR-ABL tyrosine kinase in the blast crisis of chronic myeloid leukemia and acute lymphoblastic leukemia with the Philadelphia chromosome. New England Journal of Medicine, 344, 1038–1042.

Druker BJ, Guilhot F, O'Brien SG et al. (2006) Five-year follow-up of patients receiving imatinib for chronic myeloid leukemia. New England Journal of Medicine, 355, 2408–2417.

Ghanima W, Kahrs J, Dahl TG III, Tjonnfjord GE. (2004) Sustained cytogenetic response after discontinuation of imatinib mesylate in a patient with chronic myeloid leukemia. European Journal of Haematology, 72, 441–443.

Graham SM, Jorgensen HG, Allan E et al. (2002) Primitive, quiescent, Philadelphia-positive stem cells from patients with chronic myeloid leukemia are insensitive to STI571 in vitro. Blood, 99, 319–325.

Kantarjian H, Sawyers C, Hochhaus A et al. (2002) Hematologic and cytogenetic responses to imatinib mesylate in chronic myelogenous leukemia. New England Journal of Medicine, 346, 645–652.

Lowenberg B. (2003) Minimal residual disease in chronic myeloid leukemia. New England Journal of Medicine, 349, 1399–1401.

O'Brien SG, Guilhot F, Larson RA et al. (2003) Imatinib compared with interferon and low-dose cytarabine for newly diagnosed chronic-phase chronic myeloid leukemia. New England Journal of Medicine, 348, 994–1004.

## Second generation tyrosine kinase inhibitors

Kantarjian H, Giles F, Wunderle L et al. (2006) Nilotinib in imatinib-resistant CML and Philadelphia chromosome-positive ALL. New England Journal of Medicine, 354, 2542–2551.

O'Hare T, Walters DK, Stoffregen EP et al. (2005) In vitro activity of Bcr-Abl inhibitors AMN107 and BMS-354825 against clinically relevant imatinib-resistant Abl kinase domain mutants. Cancer Research, 65, 4500–4505.

Quintas-Cardama A, Kantarjian H, Cortes J. (2007) Flying under the radar: the new wave of BCR-ABL inhibitors. Nature Reviews. Drug Discovery, 6, 834–848.

Shah NP, Tran C, Lee FY, Chen P, Norris D, Sawyers CL. (2004) Overriding imatinib resistance with a novel ABL kinase inhibitor. Science, 305, 399–401.

Talpaz M, Shah NP, Kantarjian H et al. (2006) Dasatinib in imatinib-resistant Philadelphia chromosome-positive leukemias. New England Journal of Medicine, 354, 2531–2541.

Weisberg E, Manley PW, Breitenstein W et al. (2005) Characterization of AMN107, a selective inhibitor of native and mutant Bcr-Abl. Cancer Cell, 7, 129–141.

## Mechanisms of resistance to tyrosine kinase inhibitors

Azam M, Latek RR, Daley GQ. (2003) Mechanisms of autoinhibition and STI-571/imatinib resistance revealed by mutagenesis of BCR-ABL. Cell, 112, 831–843.

Azam M, Nardi V, Shakespeare WC et al. (2006) Activity of dual SRC-ABL inhibitors highlights the role of BCR/ABL kinase dynamics in drug resistance. Proceedings of the National Academy of Sciences of the United States of America, 103, 9244–9249.

Donato NJ, Wu JY, Stapley J et al. (2003) BCR-ABL independence and LYN kinase overexpression in chronic myelogenous leukemia cells selected for resistance to STI571. Blood, 101, 690–698.

Gorre ME, Mohammed M, Ellwood K et al. (2001) Clinical resistance to STI-571 cancer therapy caused by BCR-ABL gene mutation or amplification. Science, 293, 876–880.

Shah NP, Nicoll JM, Nagar B et al. (2002) Multiple BCR-ABL kinase domain mutations confer polyclonal resistance to the tyrosine kinase inhibitor imatinib (STI571) in chronic phase and blast crisis chronic myeloid leukemia. Cancer Cell, 2, 117–125.

Shah NP, Skaggs BJ, Branford S et al. (2007) Sequential ABL kinase inhibitor therapy selects for compound drug-resistant BCR-ABL mutations with altered oncogenic potency. Journal of Clinical Investigation, 117, 2562–2569.

# Chapter 8 Myelodysplastic syndromes

**M Mansour Ceesay, Wendy Ingram & Ghulam J Mufti**

*Department of Haematological Medicine, King's College Hospital, London, UK*

## Introduction

The myelodysplastic syndromes (MDS) are a heterogeneous group of clonal bone marrow stem cell disorders characterized by ineffective dysplastic hematopoiesis with propensity to transformation to acute myeloid leukemia (AML). Clinically, it manifests as peripheral cytopenias of varying degree despite a hypercellular bone marrow. MDS is predominantly a disease of the elderly with a median age of 70 years and affects approximately 1 in 500 people over the age of 60. The vast majority of MDS cases are primary but the disease may occur following exposure to radiation and/or chemotherapy. One of the first descriptions can be traced to Rhoades and Barker in 1938 who described 60 cases with refractory anemia. Dreyfus made a seminal observation in the 1970s that the blast count at presentation was a key determinant of clinical deterioration. Van Den Berghe and colleagues in 1974 described, for the first time, a distinct cytogenetic abnormality in MDS in what is now referred to as the 5q– syndrome. In 1976 the French, American and British Cooperation Group (FAB) proposed a unified diagnostic criteria. The initial diagnostic groups described were refractory anemia with excess of blasts and chronic myelomonocytic leukemia. The classification was revised in 1982 and three additional subtypes were added to complete the current FAB classification. The most recent modification, which is now widely used, is the World Health Organization (WHO) classification that seeks to further strengthen the prognostic usefulness of the morphological classification system.

In recent years there have been significant advances in our understanding of the pathogenesis of MDS, leading to improved prognostic stratification of patients and more targeted therapeutic options.

## Etiology

The vast majority of MDS cases are primary; that is, they have no known predisposing event and occur in a sporadic fashion. Familial MDS/AML cases are rare but may provide useful information for the investigation of predisposing mutations that underpin MDS. Two genes, *RUNX1* and *CEBPA*, have been implicated. *RUNX1* (or *AML1* or *CBFA2*), located on chromosome 21q22, encodes the α subunit of core-binding factor (CBF), a transcription factor that regulates several hematopoietic genes. Germline mutation in *RUNX1* leads to familial platelet disorder with a propensity to develop MDS/AML. The *CEBPA* gene encodes the CCAAT enhancer binding α protein, a transcription factor that regulates genes involved in myeloid differentiation. Germline mutations of *CEBPA* are implicated in the development of familial AML with high degree of penetrance.

Familial MDS/AML cases are younger than those with sporadic MDS and the pattern of inheritance is mostly single gene mutations inherited in an autosomal dominant manner. These mutations are most frequently associated with genetic syndromes such as Diamond–Blackfan anemia, severe congenital neutropenia, Shwachman–Diamond syndrome and dyskeratosis congenita. MDS/AML is also common in cases with defective DNA repair mechanisms such as Fanconi anemia, where 35–50% of cases develop MDS/AML by the age of 40 years. It must be pointed out that these genetic lesions in syndromic MDS/AML have not been identified in sporadic cases, suggesting that there is a different underlying

*Molecular Hematology*, 3rd edition. Edited by Drew Provan and John Gribben.
© 2010 Blackwell Publishing.

pathophysiology. Although these familial cases present at a relatively young age, most overt cases present in adulthood. This would suggest that a long latency period is required for acquisition of secondary events/mutations for the full phenotypic expression.

Therapy-related (t)-MDS/AML accounts for 10–20% of sporadic/acquired cases. Two broad groups are recognized: alkylating agents/radiation related and topoisomerase II inhibitor related. In the former group MDS/AML develops 5–6 years following exposure to the leukemogenic agents and the risk is related to the total cumulative exposure dose. In the latter group there is shorter latency period (12–130 months), frequently associated with balanced translocations and frank AML with little preceding dysplastic phase. Three classes of mutations have been described in t-MDS/AML. Class 1 mutations involve genes in the tyrosine kinase RAS/ BRAF signal transduction pathway such as FLT3, c-KIT, c-FMS or JAK2, or genes further downstream in the RAS– BRAF–MEK ERK signal transduction pathway, such as N-RAS, K-RAS, BRAF or PTPN11. These class 1 mutations lead to constitutive activation of cell cycling and proliferation. Class 2 mutations involve inactivating mutations of genes of hematopoietic transcription factors such as RUNX1, NPM, or RARA leading to disturbed differentiation. Mutations involving the tumor-suppressor gene p53 (class 3) have been extensively studied in solid tumors and de novo MDS and AML. This represents the most frequent single genetic mutation, detected in 20–30% of t-MDS/AML. Patients with p53 mutation commonly present with complex cytogenetic abnormalities and have a distinctly poor prognosis. Cooperation exists between class 1 and 2 mutations but not within each class.

High-dose therapy with autologous stem cell transplantation can induce long-term disease-free survival especially in lymphoma patients. However, in long-term survivors there is a significant risk of developing therapy-related MDS or AML. The incidence is variable but may reach 20% at 10 years follow-up from registry and single institution experiences.

## Clinical and laboratory features

Most MDS patients present with symptoms related to cytopenia, most commonly macrocytic (but may be normocytic) anemia and less commonly neutropenia or thrombocytopenia. Diagnosis is made by careful inspection of the peripheral blood film and confirmed by bone marrow examination showing dysplastic features to a varying degree and frequently associated with a hypercellular bone marrow. Conventional cytogenetics and fluorescence in situ hybridization (FISH) are crucial for both diagnostic and prognostic

purposes, although only about 50% of the cases have demonstrable abnormalities. The various subtypes have their distinct characteristic features (Table 8.1). Most cases are elderly, although secondary MDS may present at any age consequent on chemotherapy or radiotherapy for a primary malignancy. Overall, the sex ratio of patients with MDS is equal; however, 5q– syndrome has a strong female preponderance.

## Classification

The diagnosis and classification of MDS are achieved chiefly through the morphological examination of peripheral blood and bone marrow. Cytogenetics and increasingly molecular diagnostics provide important prognostic information. The application of whole-genome scanning using comparative genomic hybridization (CGH) arrays and single-nucleotide polymorphism (SNP) arrays for analysis of somatic and clonal unbalanced chromosomal defects is not routinely employed in diagnosis but may come to play an important role in the future.

The current FAB classification of MDS, published in 1982, evolved from the initial two broad categories of "dysmyelopoietic syndrome." It is based on the number of blasts in the peripheral blood and bone marrow, number of monocytes in the peripheral blood, and presence or absence of significant sideroblastic erythropoiesis. There are five subtypes, as determined by peripheral blood and bone marrow morphology:
- refractory anemia (RA);
- refractory anemia with ring sideroblasts (RARS);
- refractory anemia with excess blasts (RAEB);
- refractory anemia with excess blasts in transformation (RAEB-T);
- chronic myelomonocytic leukemia (CMML).

The FAB classification has allowed physicians to communicate about a very heterogeneous group of disorders and allow comparisons to be made of clinical trials. It also predicts survival and risk of AML transformation (Figure 8.1).

In 1999 the WHO published a revised classification of MDS, revised again in 2001, which comprises eight subtypes (Table 8.1). The WHO abolished RAEB-T and defined AML as having 20% or more bone marrow blasts. CMML is now classified as myelodysplastic/myeloproliferative disorder. The WHO group also makes a distinction between cases of RA and RARS with or without involvement of other hematopoietic cell lineages since this has prognostic relevance. More importantly, cytogenetic features have been recognized to have prognostic importance and this is exemplified by the recognition of the 5q– syndrome as a separate entity of MDS.

**Table 8.1** World Health Organization classification of MDS.

| Disease | Peripheral blood | Bone marrow |
|---|---|---|
| Refractory anemia (RA) | Anemia<br>No or rare blasts | Erythroid dysplasia only<br><5% blasts<br><15% ringed sideroblasts |
| Refractory anemia with ringed sideroblasts (RARS) | Anemia<br>No blasts | ≥15% ringed sideroblasts<br>Erythroid dysplasia only<br><5% blasts |
| Refractory cytopenia with multilineage dysplasia (RCMD) | Cytopenias (bicytopenia or pancytopenia)<br>No or rare blasts<br>No Auer rods<br><1 × 10⁹/L monocytes | Dysplasia in ≥10% of the cells of two or more myeloid cell lines<br><5% blasts in marrow<br>No Auer rods<br><15% ringed sideroblasts |
| Refractory cytopenia with multilineage dysplasia and ringed sideroblasts (RCMD-RS) | Cytopenias (bicytopenia or pancytopenia)<br>No or rare blasts<br>No Auer rods<br><1 × 10⁹/L monocytes | Dysplasia in ≥10% of the cells of two or more myeloid cell lines<br>≥15% ringed sideroblasts<br><5% blasts in marrow<br>No Auer rods |
| Refractory anemia with excess blasts I (RAEB-I) | Cytopenia<br><5% blasts<br>No Auer rods<br><1 × 10⁹/L monocytes | Unilineage or multilineage dysplasia<br>5–9% blasts<br>No Auer rods |
| Refractory anemia with excess blasts II (RAEB-II) | Cytopenia<br>5–9% blasts<br>Auer rods ±<br><1 × 10⁹/L monocytes | Unilineage or multilineage dysplasia<br>10–19% blasts<br>Auer rods ± |
| Myelodysplastic syndrome unclassified (MDS-U) | Cytopenias<br>No or rare blasts<br>No Auer rods | Unilineage dysplasia: one myeloid cell line<br><5% blasts<br>No Auer rods |
| MDS associated with isolated del(5q) | Anemia<br>Usually normal or increased platelets count<br><5% blasts | Normal to increased megakaryocytes with hypolobated nuclei<br><5% blasts<br>Isolated del(5q) cytogenetic abnormality<br>No Auer rods |

*Source*: Jaffe ES, Harris NL, Stein H, Vardiman JW (eds). (2001) *WHO Classification of Tumors, Pathology and Genetics of Tumours of Haematopoetic and Lymphoid Tissues*. Lyon: IARC.

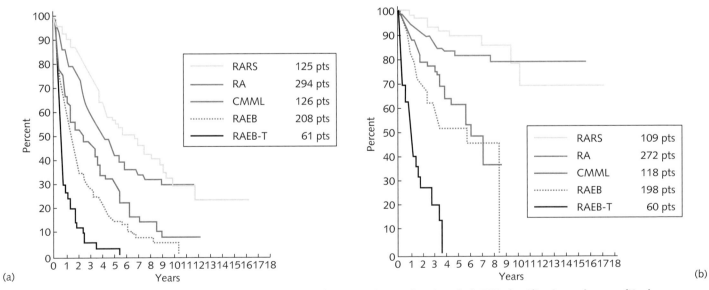

**Fig. 8.1 Survival (a) and freedom from AML evolution (b) of MDS patients related to their FAB classification subgroup (Kaplan–Meier curves)**

See text for definition of abbreviations. From Greenberg P, Cox C, Le Beau MM *et al.* (1997) International scoring system for evaluating prognosis in myelodysplastic syndromes. *Blood*, 89, 2079–2088, with permission. ©American Society of Hematology.

**Table 8.2** International Prognostic Scoring System for MDS.

| Prognostic variable | Score value | | | | |
| --- | --- | --- | --- | --- | --- |
| | 0 | 0.5 | 1.0 | 1.5 | 2.0 |
| Bone marrow blasts (%) | <5 | 5–10 | – | 11–20 | 21–30 |
| Karyotype* | Good | Intermediate | Poor | – | – |
| Cytopenias† | 0 or 1 | 2 or 3 | – | – | – |

Scores for risk groups are as follows: low, 0; intermediate-1, 0.5–1.0; intermediate-2, 1.5–2.0; high > 2.5.
\* Karyotype: Good indicates normal, −Y, del(5q), del(20q); Poor indicates complex (more than three abnormalities), or chromosome 7 anomalies; Intermediate indicates other abnormalities.
† Cytopenias defined as hemoglobin < 10 g/dL, absolute neutrophil count < $1.5 \times 10^9$/L and platelet count < $100 \times 10^9$/L.
*Source*: Greenberg P, Cox C, Le Beau MM *et al.* (1997) International scoring system for evaluating prognosis in myelodysplastic syndromes. *Blood*, **89**, 2079–2088, with permission. © American Society of Hematology.

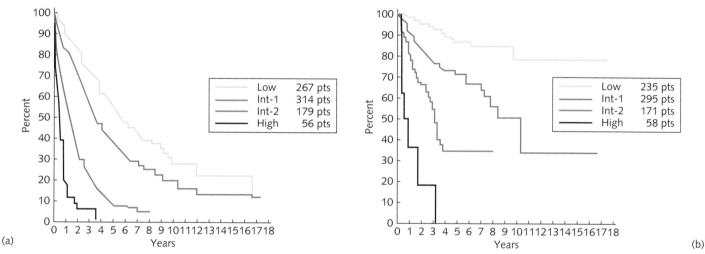

(a)                                                          (b)

**Fig. 8.2 Survival (a) and freedom from AML evolution (b) of MDS patients related to their classification by the IPSS for MDS: Low, INT-1, INT-2, and High (Kaplan–Meier curves)**
From Greenberg P, Cox C, Le Beau MM *et al.* (1997) International scoring system for evaluating prognosis in myelodysplastic syndromes. *Blood*, 89, 2079–2088, with permission. ©American Society of Hematology.

The International Prognostic Scoring System (IPSS) was developed in 1997 using cytogenetic, morphological and clinical data from patients with primary MDS. IPSS is a risk-based classification system in which scores are given for marrow blast percentage, cytogenetic features and number and degree of cytopenias (Table 8.2). Using these variables patients could be separated into four distinct subgroups based on risk of transformation to AML and median survival: low, int-1, int-2, and high (Figure 8.2).

More recently, a classification system that combines the WHO classification and transfusion requirement has emerged. Transfusion dependency is associated independently with decline in both overall survival and time to progression to AML. This recognition led to the development

of the WHO classification-based prognostic scoring system (WPSS), which uses WHO subtype, karyotype and transfusion requirement (Table 8.3). The WPSS is able to classify patients into five risk groups correlating with survival (median survival 12–103 months) and probabilities of leukemic evolution (Figure 8.3). Transfusion dependency is the key difference between the IPSS and WPSS. The degree of transfusion dependency is a good surrogate clinical marker for the degree of maturation defect in MDS. The negative impact of transfusion dependency is restricted to low-risk MDS patients, namely those with RA, RARS, refractory cytopenia with multilineage dysplasia (RCMD), refractory cytopenia with multilineage dysplasia and ringed sideroblasts (RCMD-RS) and 5q− syndrome. Moreover, the frequency

**Table 8.3** WHO classification-based prognostic scoring system (WPSS).

| Variable | 0 | 1 | 2 | 3 |
|---|---|---|---|---|
| WHO category | RA/RARS/5q– | RCMD/RCMD-RS | RAEB-1 | RAEB-2 |
| Karyotype* | Good | Intermediate | Poor | – |
| Transfusion requirement† | No | Regular | – | – |

Risk groups: very low (score 0), low (score 1), intermediate (score 2), high (score 3–4), very high (score 5–6).

* Karyotype: Good indicates normal, –Y, del(5q), del(20q); Poor indicates complex (more than three abnormalities), or chromosome 7 anomalies; Intermediate indicates other abnormalities.

† Transfusion dependency: ≥1 unit red cells in 8 weeks over a period of 4 months.

*Source*: Malcovati L, Germing U, Kuendgen A *et al.* (2007) Time-dependent prognostic scoring system for predicting survival and leukemic evolution in myelodysplastic syndromes. *Journal of Clinical Oncology*, **25**, 3503–3510, with permission. © 2008 American Society of Clinical Oncology. All rights reserved.

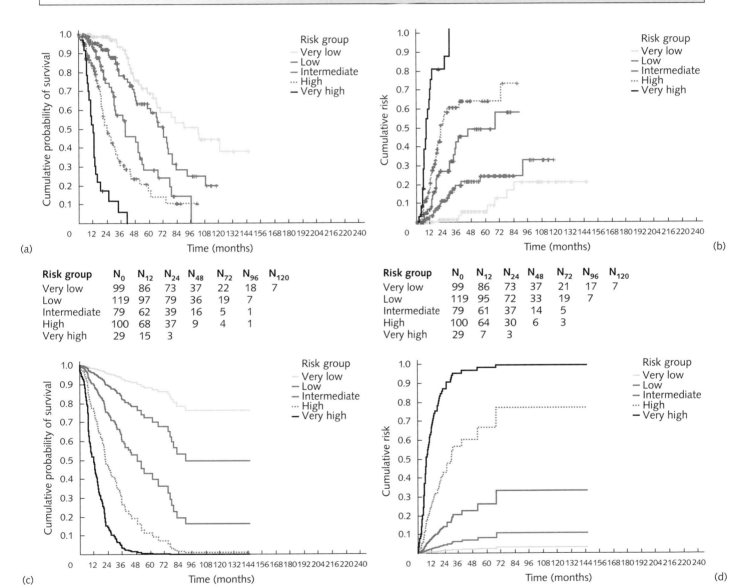

**Fig. 8.3 Overall survival and risk of acute leukemia among MDS patients classified (a, b) into WHO classification-based prognostic scoring system (WPSS) groups at diagnosis and (c, d) into time-dependent WPSS groups**

From Malcovati L, Germing U, Kuendgen A *et al.* (2007) Time-dependent prognostic scoring system for predicting survival and leukemic evolution in myelodysplastic syndromes. *Journal of Clinical Oncology*, **25**, 3503–3510, with permission. © 2008 American Society of Clinical Oncology. All rights reserved.

and number of red cell transfusions directly correlated with lower overall survival and leukemia-free survival. The negative impact of iron loading with increased ferritin levels contributes to the morbidity and mortality associated with transfusion dependency. WPSS may be a dynamic prognostic scoring system that can provide an accurate prediction of survival and risk of leukemic transformation in MDS patients at any time during the course of their disease, which may be particularly useful in lower-risk patients.

## Management

The heterogeneity of MDS suggests that no common management strategy can be adopted. Until recently the only available treatment option was supportive care. However, there has been a phenomenal increase in the number of agents now available to patients, including the following.
• Best supportive care.
• Growth factors: granulocyte colony-stimulating factor, erythropoietin.
• Transcriptional modification therapy: azacitidine, decitabine, histone deacetylase inhibitors.
• Immunomodulatory agents: lenalidomide, antithymocyte globulin, cyclosporin.
• Conventional chemotherapy.
• Allogeneic stem cell transplantation.
The goal of therapy must be defined at the beginning, tailored to each patient. The factors that govern the choice of therapy include age, performance status, and the IPSS/WPSS score. The options range from management of cytopenias in low-risk MDS to altering the natural history of disease in higher-risk MDS by, for instance, chemotherapy and allogeneic stem cell transplantation. Various treatment guidelines exist in both the USA and UK to aid therapeutic decision-making.

### Lenalidomide

Lenalidomide is an analog of thalidomide with a better side-effect profile. The US Food and Drug Administration (FDA) approved its use in low to intermediate risk, transfusion-dependent MDS with del(5q) abnormality in December 2005.

The MDS-001 Phase I study included 43 patients with symptomatic anemia. Overall, 56% of patients experienced durable erythroid responses: 83% 5q–, 57% normal cytogenetics and 12% other chromosomal abnormalities. This was followed by two multicenter Phase II trials: MDS-002 (non 5q–, 214 patients) and MDS-003 (5q–, 148 patients). In the MDS-002 trial, the overall transfusion response rate was 43%, with 26% of patients achieving transfusion independ-

ence sustained for a median of 43 weeks. Cytogenetic remission was uncommon (19%). In patients with 5q– treated on the MDS-003 trial, an erythroid response was reported in 76% of patients with 67% achieving transfusion independence. Cytogenetic response was achieved in 73% of cases and correlated with achievement of transfusion independence. Interestingly, there was no significant difference between isolated 5q– (71%), 5q– and one additional chromosomal abnormality (65%), and 5q– and more than one additional chromosomal abnormality (75%) but the numbers were small. The disappearance of non-5q– cytogenetic abnormalities consistently accompanied disappearance of the 5q– clone.

Lenalidomide's precise mechanism of action is not fully understood. It possesses potent immunomodulatory and anti-angiogenic properties not associated with vascular endothelial growth factor or its receptor (KDR) downregulation. It is thought to specifically target the 5q– clone as evidenced by the complete hematological and cytogenetic responses seen in some patients. In responders, its well-known transient period of profound neutropenia and thrombocytopenia after initiation of treatment supports this theory, i.e., disruption of clonal hematopoiesis to allow normal residual clone to expand. *In vitro* studies have also shown that lenalidomide can inhibit the growth of cell lines with 5q–.

The cytogenetic-dependent lenalidomide sensitivity has not been fully explained. However, this is an active area of ongoing research. Inhibition of two candidate genes, *Cdc25C* and *PP2A$_{C\alpha}$*, located on 5q31 and which produce phosphatases that regulate the cell cycle, have been implicated.

## Modifying the epigenome in MDS

It is well recognized that classical genetics alone cannot explain the phenotypic variation at population level. Epigenetics refers to a number of heritable biochemical modifications of chromatin without DNA sequence alteration and offers a partial explanation to this phenotypic variation. The main epigenetic modifications are DNA promoter hypermethylation and histone modification (deacetylation and methylation), both of which are potentially reversible (Figure 8.4). Methylation, mediated by DNA methyltransferases, involves incorporation of a methyl group into position 5 of the cytosine ring that precedes a guanine (dinucleotide CpG; the 'p' refers to a phosphodiester bond between cytosine and guanine). CpG-rich regions (CpG islands) cluster around the 5′ end of the regulatory region of many genes and in a normal cell are usually unmethylated. Methylation of promoter-associated CpG islands is a way of silencing gene expression. This can be either physiological, as in genetic imprinting, or pathological, where aberrant

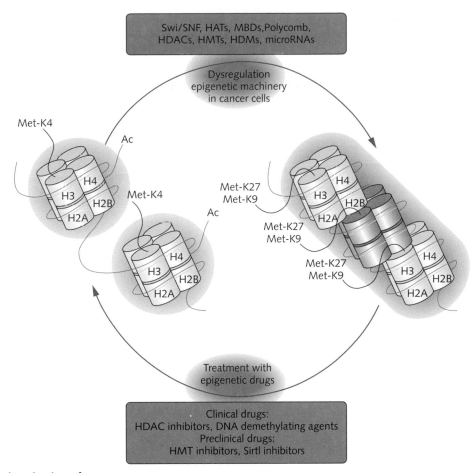

**Fig. 8.4 Epigenetic inactivation of tumor-suppressor genes**
Gray cylinders indicate octamers of histones, consisting of histones H2A, H2B, H3, and H4. They form the nucleosomes, and the double strand of DNA is wrapped around them. A combination of selection and targeted disruption of the DNA methylation and histone-modifier proteins disrupts the epigenetic circumstances in the cancer cell. Epigenetic inactivation of tumor-suppressor genes is associated with dense CpG-island promoter hypermethylation and the appearance of repressive histone markers such as methylation of lysines 9 and 27 of H3. Epigenetic drugs can partially restore the distorted epigenetic picture by removing inactivation markers (e.g., DNA methylation) and inducing the presence of active markers (e.g., histone acetylation). AC, acetylation; DNMTs, DNA methyltransferases; HATs, histone acetyltransferases; HDAC, histone deacetylase; HDMs, histone demethylases; HMTs, histone methyltransferases; MBDs, methyl-CpG-binding domain proteins; Met-K4, methylation of lysine 4; Met-K9, methylation of lysine 9; Met-K27, methylation of lysine 27; Sirt1, sirtuin 1; Swi/SNF, switching/sucrose non-fermenting chromatin-remodeling complex. From Esteller M. (2008) Epigenetics in cancer. *New England Journal of Medicine*, 358, 1148–1159. Copyright © 2008 Massachusetts Medical Society. All rights reserved.

methylation of promoter regions of tumor-suppressor genes are functionally equivalent to gene silencing by deletion, or inactivating mutations.

The pattern of CpG island hypermethylation in tumor-suppressor genes is specific to the type of malignancy. In MDS, the genes that are frequently hypermethylated include *p15*, *RIL* (a LIM gene on 5q31) and the calcitonin gene, among others. Most of the studies have concentrated on *CDKN2B*, which encodes the cyclin-dependent kinase inhibitor p15^INK4b, an important checkpoint protein that prevents quiescent cells from entering the cell cycle. Hypermethylation

of the *CDKN2B* promoter is not only important in the pathogenesis of MDS but also in disease progression.

Histones are DNA packaging proteins that also play an important role in the regulation of gene expression. DNA methylation occurs in the context of chemical modification of histone proteins such as lysine acetylation and methylation, arginine and serine phosphorylation (Figure 8.4). What emerges is a multitude of biochemical alterations that can be imposed on the histone tails, referred to as the "histone code," which can have a permissive or repressive effect on gene expression. Histone acetylation is controlled by two sets of enzymes: histone acetyltransferases and histone deacetylases (HDACs). HDACs are recruited to regulatory DNA sequences and in the process inhibit access to activating transcription factors to the DNA by oncogenes such as *AML1-ETO*, *PML/RARα*. Histone methylation is catalyzed by lysine or arginine methyltransferases.

## Hypomethylating agents

Currently, the two hypomethylating agents approved in MDS are azacitidine and 5-aza-2′-deoxycytidine (decitabine) (Figure 8.5). Azacitidine is a pyrimidine analog where the ring carbon 5 is replaced by nitrogen. It incorporates into both RNA and DNA where it binds DNA methyltransferases irreversibly, thereby preventing genomic methylation (Figure 8.6). At high doses it is cytotoxic, whereas at lower doses it induces differentiation and demethylation. It is a prodrug of decitabine, which is 10 times as potent in inhibiting DNA methyltransferases. In contrast, decitabine incorporates into DNA alone.

In a Phase III Cancer and Leukemia Group B (CALGB) 9221 randomized trial with crossover design involving 191 subjects, Silverman and colleagues compared daily azacitidine 75 mg/m² subcutaneously for 7 days every 28 days with

best supportive care. Patients treated with azacitidine showed durable clinical and symptomatic improvements in bone marrow function [complete response (CR) 7%, partial response (PR) 16%, hematological response 37%], a reduction in the risk of leukemic transformation, and significant improvement in the quality of life compared with best supportive care. This study led to its FDA approval for all FAB MDS subtypes in 2004. Subsequent trials have confirmed

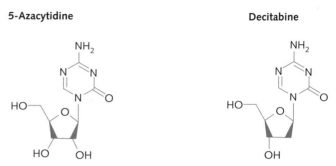

**Fig. 8.5 Ring structure of 5-azacytidine (azacitidine) and 5-aza-2′-deoxycytidine (decitabine) showing substitution of N at position 5**
Azacitidine is attached to a ribose sugar whereas decitabine is attached to a deoxyribose sugar.

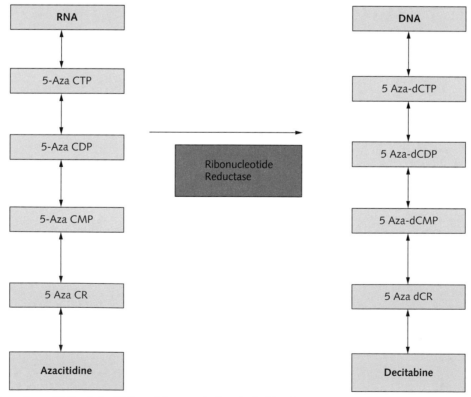

**Fig. 8.6 Incorporation of azacitidine into RNA and its metabolite decitabine into DNA**

these findings. Patients with trisomy 8 and monosomy 7, who have poor prognosis, tend to experience highest response rates. Best responses were observed between courses 4 and 6 of therapy, with a plateau after that. Azacitidine is well tolerated and may be safely given to patients with cytopenia. In our own institution several patients have continued on azacitidine for over 1 year with stable disease and excellent quality of life.

Decitabine is approved for int 1 or higher-risk MDS based on the IPSS. In a Phase III randomized controlled trial of decitabine versus supportive care, decitabine-treated patients showed increased response rates (overall 35%, CR 9%, PR 8%, hematological improvement 18%), reduced transfusion requirement and a trend toward a longer median time to AML transformation or death but no overall survival benefit. However, it is important to note that a significant number of the randomized patients in that study received less than two cycles of the drug. We now know that responders require a median of 3.3 cycles.

### Modifying histone acetylation and methylation

Valproic acid is the only HDAC inhibitor that has been extensively studied in MDS. The most frequent response is that of partial morphological or hematological response, with very small reported complete responses. Often the toxicity associated with doses required to achieve significant HDAC inhibition precludes use in most patients. Several others have been tested as single agents in MDS or AML, such as phenylbutyrate, depsipeptide, MS-275, MGCD-0103 and SAHA.

Combination epigenetic therapy such as a hypomethylating agent plus HDAC inhibitor appears to achieve better response rates and many such combination studies are ongoing.

## Molecular basis of MDS

Precisely what is responsible for transformation from a highly organized and effective hemopoiesis to a dysplastic and ineffective one is not entirely clear. It is likely to be a combination of genetic, epigenetic and receptor signaling abnormalities, and microenvironmental factors (Figure 8.7). Peripheral blood cytopenias arise as a consequence of abnormal regulation of survival and differentiation programs affecting proliferation, apoptosis, and differentiation of hematopoietic progenitors. The homeostatic balance between proliferation and apoptosis shifts during disease progression such that apoptosis predominates in early stages of the disease process, whereas in patients with higher-risk MDS the proliferative fraction may escalate as a result of

inhibition of apoptosis. Upregulation of molecular survival signals such as NF-κB, phospho-Akt, Bim-1, Bcl-2, Bcl-XL, and heat-shock protein chaperones are linked to suppression of apoptosis and consequent propagation and evolution of the malignant clone.

The identification of recurrent cytogenetic/molecular abnormalities and, more recently, epigenetic changes are an important mechanistic basis for MDS. However, these changes are not specific to MDS as some can be found in AML and myeloproliferative disorders (MPDs). The non-hematopoietic milieu, which supports the MDS process, has been the subject of intensive research. Negative microenvironmental signals may be mediated through increased macrophage function with increased production of cytokines, immune dysregulation (often found in aplastic anemia, Diamond–Blackfan syndrome, etc.), and changes in microvessel density. The importance of T-regulatory cells (CD4$^+$CD25$^{high}$Foxp3$^+$) has recently been shown to be a feature of high-risk MDS.

## Cytogenetic abnormalities

The importance of cytogenetic studies in MDS cannot be over-emphasized. The aim is to detect a clonal abnormality. A clone is defined conventionally as either (i) two cells with exactly the same structural abnormality or the same additional chromosome or (ii) three cells with the same missing chromosome. These may occur singly or as complex abnormalities (more than three chromosomal abnormalities). These clones give rise to fusion genes and unbalanced aberrations. In MDS the typical abnormalities are partial and complete chromosome loss, most commonly −5, 5q−, −7, 7q−, 11q−, 13q−, 20q− and −Y. Gain of chromosomal material is less common and is mostly +8. The preponderance of chromosomal loss would suggest loss of tumor-suppressor genes or haploinsufficiency of genes necessary for normal hematopoiesis. Such abnormalities are present in approximately 30–50% of primary MDS and 80% of secondary MDS. Since MDS can progress to AML, all the cytogenetic abnormalities found in MDS are also found in AML, although their incidence is different. However, certain balanced translocations found in AML, such as t(15;17), inv(16) and t(8;21), are quite rare in MDS.

### 5q− syndrome

Del(5q) is the most commonly reported deletion in *de novo* MDS and is found in 10–15% of all patients. The 5q− syndrome was first described by Van den Berghe and colleagues in 1974. It occurs primarily in elderly women (unlike other MDS subtypes) and is associated with macrocytic anemia (usually marked), absent or mild leukopenia, a normal or

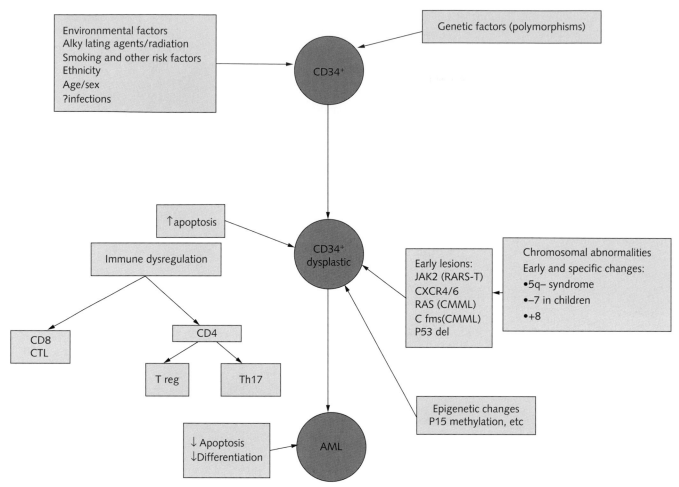

**Fig. 8.7 Pathogenesis of MDS**
The normal stem cell undergoes a series of genetic and epigenetic modifications in a dysregulated milieu that produces MDS and progression to AML.

elevated platelet count, and increased megakaryocytes with characteristic morphological abnormalities such as abnormal large monolobulated megakaryocytes with eccentric nuclei and bone marrow blast percentage below 5%. Del(5q) is the sole cytogenetic abnormality and has a favorable prognosis with low risk of transformation to AML.

However, the median survival of patients is still shorter than the age- and sex-matched control population. Survival is further reduced in MDS patients with isolated 5q– and bone marrow blast count above 5% as a result of risk of AML transformation. Similarly, the risk of AML transformation dramatically increases and median survival is shortened when additional chromosomal abnormalities are present.

The deletion in the long arm of chromosome 5 is an interstitial deletion of a large segment of variable size on 5q13–33. However, a common deleted region (CDR) has been variously defined by different groups using different

techniques. The current accepted CDR is mapped to a 1.5-Mb interval on 5q32 using FISH. However, using high-resolution SNP arrays on 5q– syndrome patients, the CDR extends from 5q23.3 to 5q33.1 (Figure 8.8). It is likely that the CDR is quite heterogeneous and that multiple CDRs exist, with several genes involved in the pathogenesis and progression of 5q– syndrome. This deletion is generally present in pluripotent hematopoietic stem cells (CD34$^+$CD38$^-$).

The CDRs contains many genes and the ones that have attracted most attention include *SPARC*, *NPM1*, *CTNNA1* (α-catenin) and *EGR1*. However, the culprit putative tumor-suppressor gene eluded researchers for 30 years. As a result the pathogenesis of this unique syndrome with a sole chromosomal abnormality remained unknown. This failure to identify the tumor-suppressor gene appears to run contrary to an important cornerstone of modern cancer biology,

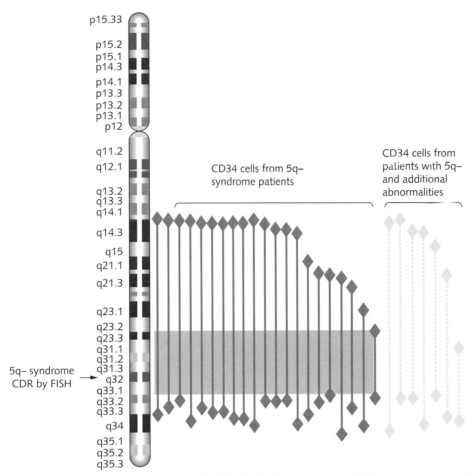

**Fig. 8.8 Heterogeneity of proximal and distal breakpoints in CD34⁺ cells from patients with 5q– syndrome and those with 5q– and additional cytogenetic abnormalities determined using 250K SNP arrays**
The shaded area represents the common deleted region (CDR) using SNP arrays.

Knudson's two-hit hypothesis, which postulates that inactivation of both copies (alleles) of a tumor-suppressor gene has an essential role in cancer development. However, no patients with the 5q– syndrome have been reported to have biallelic deletions within the CDR, and no point mutations have been reported in the remaining allele of any of the 40 genes in this region. A paradigm shift was required: 5q– syndrome may be caused by haploinsufficiency (inactivation of a single allele).

Recently, the Golub laboratory used an RNA-mediated interference (RNA-i)-based approach to individually shut down each of the 40 genes on the CDR of chromosome 5q. The gene found to recapitulate the 5q– phenotype was *RPS14*, a gene that encodes a structural protein of the 40S ribosomal subunit. In addition, these authors also showed that expressing *RPS14* in CD34⁺ cells from patients with 5q– syndrome restores normal differentiation. Moreover, by reducing the *RPS14* expression of normal CD34⁺ cells they

induced a gene expression profile that correlates with responsiveness to lenalidomide. Taken together, these results provide strong evidence that *RPS14* functions as a haploinsufficient tumor-suppressor gene in the 5q– syndrome.

The protein encoded by *RPS14* is an essential part of the 33-protein complex associated with the 18S rRNA forming the 40S subunit of the ribosome where protein synthesis occurs. The RPS14 protein is essential for efficient RNA–protein complex. Several bone marrow failure syndromes have now been linked to a ribosomal gene mutation. Many ribosomal proteins, such as RPS17, RPS19, RPS24 and more recently Rpl35A, have been implicated in Diamond–Blackfan anemia, functionally equivalent to the block in the processing of pre-ribosomal RNA in RPS14-deficient cells, thus linking the molecular pathophysiology of a congenital anemia with 5q– syndrome. Similarly, defects in ribosomal genes have been linked with Shwachman–Diamond syndrome, cartilage hair hypoplasia and dyskeratosis congenita.

How the reduced levels of these ribosomal proteins impair the formation of red cells is not precisely known. The increased demand of hemoglobin production on erythroid progenitor cells places an enormous burden on the translational machinery of the cell and any impairment such as haploinsufficiency or mutation could trigger apoptosis or dysregulated differentiation.

### Monosomy 7/7q–

Loss of chromosome 7 (monosomy 7) or deletion of the long arm (7q–) is a recurring abnormality in myeloid malignancies and is found in 5–10% of adult patients with *de novo* MDS and in approximately 50% of all therapy-related cases. It is often found in children with juvenile myelomonocytic leukemia, MDS/AML arising from those with bone marrow failure syndromes such as Fanconi anemia, Shwachman–Diamond syndrome, severe congenital neutropenia, and familial –7 MDS. The loss of chromosomal material and the development of MDS would suggest loss of a tumor-suppressor gene(s) as the underlying pathophysiology. The deletion is interstitial and there are two distinct common deleted regions: 7q11–22 and 7q31–36. A total of 14 candidate genes including *MLL5*, a homolog of the *trithorax* gene of *Drosophila*, have been localized to the common deleted segment on 7q22. Knockdown of the *MLL5* gene by RNA-i leads to cell cycle arrest.

Monosomy 7 is not a germline mutation but represents a "second hit" in the development of MDS/AML. It is usually associated with poor response to chemotherapy and high risk of transformation to AML.

### Other cytogenetic abnormalities

The del(20q) abnormality is found in 3–5% of patients with primary MDS. The cytopenia generally involves the erythroid and megakaryocytic lineages and may be confused with idiopathic thrombocytopenic purpura clinically. As a sole cytogenetic abnormality it carries a good prognosis. It is seen in all subtypes of MDS and MPD. The critical genes that are deleted in 20q– are unknown but the Nimer laboratory has identified a polycomb group gene, *L(3)MBTL1*, a human homolog of *Drosophila L(3)MBT* (lethal malignant brain tumor) on 20q12, which functions as a transcriptional repressor.

Trisomy 8 (+8) is the commonest chromosomal gain in MDS. Its prognostic value or indeed its contribution to the pathogenesis of MDS is unknown. Patients with +8 as well as those with –7 respond well to hypomethylating agents such as azacitidine.

Less common chromosomal abnormalities seen in MDS include isochromosome 17, der(1;7)(q10;q10), +6, +14, isochromosome 14q, del(13q), inv(3) and del(11q).

## Molecular abnormalities

### Mutations of *RAS*, *NF1* and *PTPN11* genes

The *RAS* gene encodes proteins that regulate signal transduction by cycling between an active GTP-bound state and an inactive GDP-bound state. These proteins regulate cellular proliferation and differentiation. *RAS* gene mutations (mostly N-*RAS*) are the most common molecular abnormalities in MDS. When mutated in codon 12, 13, or 61, the *RAS* genes encode a protein that remains in the active state and continuously transmits signals by linking tyrosine kinases to downstream serine and threonine kinases. This constitutive activation induces continuous cell growth. Mutation of oncogenes in the RAS family have been associated with exposure to environmental carcinogens. The reported incidence of *RAS* mutations in MDS has varied but is perhaps 10% of MDS cases overall, with a relatively high incidence in CMML. Often N-*RAS* mutations are found at diagnosis but have also been found to occur during disease progression. Their real significance remains unknown, although most studies report them as unfavorable prognostic markers.

Neurofibromin is the protein encoded by the neurofibromatosis type 1 gene (*NF1*), a tumor-suppressor gene. It contains a domain with sequence homology to GTPase-activating proteins. The binding of neurofibromin to RAS protein accelerates the conversion of RAS-GTP to RAS-GDP. In the majority of children with neurofibromatosis type 1 and MDS, both alleles of *NF1* are inactivated.

### Mutations of the *p53* gene

Abnormalities of *p53* are relatively uncommon in hematological malignancies compared with solid tumors. As in solid tumors, mutations tend to occur in exons 5–8 of the *p53* gene. They are found principally in RAEB, RAEB-T and CMML. Interestingly, they generally occur in association with a deletion of the other allele. The cases harboring *p53* mutations generally have complex karyotypic abnormalities, making it difficult to assess the contribution of *p53* abnormalities to MDS. These *p53* mutations are associated with the pseudo-Pelger–Huët anomaly and vacuoles in neutrophils giving rise to the 17p– syndrome.

### Other gene mutations

The *FLT3* internal tandem duplication is a rare mutation in MDS, occurring in about 5% of patients and almost always in patients with advanced/high-risk MDS. Similarly, mutations of the *AML1* gene are rare in primary MDS.

The *JAK2* V617F mutation has become an important diagnostic tool in MPDs, where over 90% of cases of polycythemia vera and 50% of primary myelofibrosis and essential thrombocythemia have been found to carry the mutation. The overlap between MPD and MDS is well recognized. Some cases of 5q– syndrome have a significant proliferative component, with raised platelet and leukocyte counts. In such patients the *JAK2* V617F mutation is common (10%). In RARS with thrombocytosis (RARS-T) the prevalence of this mutation is even higher, where about 66% of cases carry the mutation. The *JAK2* mutation identifies a subgroup of MDS patients with a significant proliferative marrow where it may provide a proliferative signal to the dysplastic clone.

## Genome-wide scanning

There is no doubt about the diagnostic and prognostic significance of cytogenetic abnormalities in MDS recognized by both the IPSS and WPSS. However, using metaphase cytogenetics, chromosomal abnormalities are found in about half of MDS patients. Low-risk MDS accounts for at least 50% of all MDS patients, and up to 80% of these patients may have a normal karyotype.

Advances in microarray technology using CGH and SNP can be used for analysis of somatic or clonal unbalanced chromosomal defects. Cryptic deletions and duplications can be detected due to higher resolution. Moreover, this technology can identify loss of heterozygosity (LOH), which occurs without concurrent changes in gene copy number and might be an early event in the development of the neoplastic clone. However, LOH can also occur by uniparental disomy (UPD), where an individual acquires a duplicated copy of an entire or partial chromosome derived from one parent attributed to errors in mitotic recombination in somatic cells, resulting in LOH without copy number changes. UPD cannot be detected by metaphase cytogenetic techniques and FISH, as there is no net loss/gain of genetic material.

Mohamedali and colleagues studied 119 low-risk MDS patients using SNP microarrays to seek chromosomal markers not detected by conventional cytogenetics. UPD was found in 46%, deletions in 10% and amplification in 8% of cases. There was a high incidence of constitutional UPD in these patients, which may suggest a predisposition to genomic instability. Other researchers have also found previously unrecognized lesions as well as UPDs. There is no doubt that this technology will redefine what is "normal."

## Animal models

The first animal model of MDS was a mouse model developed by Buonamici and colleagues using a retrovirus to overexpress EVI-1 in murine stem cells and then transplant-

ing these cells into irradiated recipients. They achieved 70% engraftment of the transduced cells but the MDS phenotype only developed after 7–8 months in the transplanted mice. This delay may suggest that EVI-1 induces defects such as hyperproliferation and impaired differentiation due to decreased erythropoietin receptor and Mpl expression. However, at a later stage (10–12 months post transplant) additional defects developed, resulting in bone marrow failure leading to severe cytopenias and death. None of the mice developed AML.

Nucleophosmin (NPM) is a nuclear protein that plays an important role in ribosome biogenesis and the p53 pathway, and regulates centrosome duplication. Little wonder therefore that it has been implicated in cancer pathogenesis. Grisendi and colleagues developed the second MDS model by generating NPM mutant series in mice. Absence of NPM (NPM1$^{-/-}$) resulted in abnormal organogenesis and death between embryonic day E11.5 and E16.5. However, heterozygotes (NPM$^{+/-}$) survived and developed features of MDS.

The third model is the NUP98/HoxD13 transgenic mouse developed by Lin and colleagues This model uses the t(2;11)(q31;p15) associated fusion protein containing nucleoporin protein, which mediates transport of protein and RNA across the nuclear membrane fused to HoxD13 protein. The mice developed MDS by 4–7 months and by 10 months they either transformed to AML or developed progressive cytopenias and all died by 14 months. This model accurately recapitulates all the key features of MDS and is currently being used to evaluate therapeutic approaches.

## Conclusions

The last few years have seen tremendous developments in our understanding of the molecular pathogenesis of MDS. Although bone marrow examination remains the pivotal diagnostic tool, advances in recognizing cryptic molecular aberrations by SNP arrays are an important advance, which may soon be incorporated into routine clinical practice. The interesting area of epigenetics will undoubtedly further our understanding of MDS and add to our armamentarium for treatment. Stem cell transplantation remains the only curative option available and the emergence of reduced intensity transplants has opened the door to more treatment possibilities for what is essentially a disease of the elderly.

## Further reading

### MDS and its etiology

Bennett JM, Catovsky D, Daniel MT *et al.* (1982) Proposals for the classification of the myelodysplastic syndromes. *British Journal of Haematology*, **51**, 189–199.

Deguchi K, Gilliland DG. (2002) Cooperativity between mutations in tyrosine kinases and in hematopoietic transcription factors in AML. *Leukemia*, **16**, 740–744.

Dreyfus B. (1976) Preleukemic cases I. Definition and classification. II. Refractory anemia with an excess of myeloblasts in the bone marrow (smoldering acute leukemia). *Nouvelle Revue Francaise D'Hematologie: Blood Cells*, **17**, 33–55.

Hake CR, Graubert TA, Fenske TS. (2007) Does autologous transplantation directly increase the risk of secondary leukemia in lymphoma patients? *Bone Marrow Transplantation*, **39**, 59–70.

Kutler DI, Singh B, Satagopan J et al. (2003) A 20-year perspective on the International Fanconi Anemia Registry (IFAR). *Blood*, **101**, 1249–1256.

Owen C, Barnett M, Fitzgibbon J. (2008) Famililal myelodysplasia and acute myeloid leukaemia: a review. *British Journal of Haematology*, **140**, 123–132.

Pedersen-Bjergaard J, Andersen MT, Andersen MK. (2007) Genetic pathways in the pathogenesis of therapy-related myelodysplasia and acute myeloid leukemia. *Hematology. American Society of Hematology Education Program*, 392–397.

Rhoades CP, Barker WH. (1938) Refractory anemia: an analysis of one hundred cases. *JAMA*, **110**, 794–796.

Smith ML, Cavenagh JD, Lister TA, Fitzgibbon J. (2004) Mutation of CEBPA in familial acute myeloid leukemia. *New England Journal of Medicine*, **351**, 2403–2407.

Song WJ, Sullivan MG, Legare RD et al. (1999) Haploinsufficiency of CBFA2 causes familial thrombocytopenia with propensity to develop acute myelogenous leukaemia. *Nature Genetics*, **23**, 166–175.

Van den Berghe H, Cassiman JJ, David G et al. (1974) Distinct haematological disorder with deletion of long arm of no. 5 chromosome. *Nature*, **251**, 437–438.

Vardiman JW. (2002) The World Health Organisation (WHO) classification of the myeloid neoplasms. *Blood*, **100**, 2292–2302.

## Laboratory features and classification

Greenberg P, Cox C, Le Beau MM et al. (1997) International scoring system for evaluating prognosis in myelodysplastic syndromes. *Blood*, **89**, 2079–2088.

Malcovati L, Della Porta MG, Cazzola M. (2006) Predicting survival and leukemic evolution in patients with myelodysplastic syndrome. *Haematolgica*, **91**, 1588–1590.

Malcovati L, Germing U, Kuendgen A et al. (2007) Time-dependent prognostic scoring system for predicting survival and leukemic evolution in myelodysplastic syndromes. *Journal of Clinical Oncology*, **25**, 3503–3510.

## Management

Bowen D, Culligan D, Jowitt S et al. (2003) Guidelines for the diagnosis and therapy of adult myelodysplastic syndromes. *British Journal of Haematology*, **120**, 187–200.

Gandhi AK, Kang J, Naziruddin S et al. (2006) Lenalidomide inhibits proliferation of Namalwa CSN.70 cells and interferes with Gab1 phosphorylation and adaptor protein complex assembly. *Leukemia Research*, **30**, 849–858.

Greenberg PL, Baer MR, Bennett JM et al. (2006) Myelodysplastic syndromes clinical practice guidelines in oncology. *Journal of the National Comprehensive Cancer Network*, **4**, 58–77.

Kelaidi C, Eclache V, Fenaux P. (2008) The role of lenalidomide in management of myelodysplasia with del 5q. *British Journal of Haematology*, **140**, 267–278.

List A, Kurtin S, Roe DJ et al. (2005) Efficacy of lenalidomide in myelodysplastic syndromes. *New England Journal of Medicine*, **352**, 549–557.

List A, Dewald G, Bennett J et al. (2006) Lenalidomide in the myelodysplastic syndrome with chromosome 5q deletion. *New England Journal of Medicine*, **355**, 1456–1465.

Pellagatti A, Jädersten M, Forsblom AM et al. (2007) Lenalidomide inhibits the malignant clone and up-regulates the *SPARC* gene mapping to the commonly deleted region in 5q– syndrome patients. *Proceedings of the National Academy of Sciences of the United States of America*, **104**, 11406–11411.

Raza A, Reeves JA, Feldman EJ et al. (2008) Phase 2 study of lenalidomide in transfusion-dependent, low-risk, and intermediate-1 risk myelodysplastic syndromes with karyotypes other than deletion 5q. *Blood*, **111**, 86–93.

Wei S, Rocha K, Williams A et al. (2007) Gene dosage of the cell cycle regulatory phosphatases Cdc25C and PP2A determines sensitivity to lenalidomide in del(5q) MDS. *Blood*, **110**, Abstract 118.

## Epigenetics

Esteller M. (2008) Epigenetics in cancer. *New England Journal of Medicine*, **358**, 1148–1159.

Garcia-Manero G. (2007) Modifying the epigenome as a therapeutic strategy in myelodysplasia. *Hematology. American Society of Hematology Education Program*, 405–411.

## Novel therapies

Christman JK. (2002) 5-Azacytidine and 5-aza-2'-deoxycytidine as inhibitors of DNA methylation: mechanistic studies and their implications for cancer therapy. *Oncogene*, **21**, 5483–5495.

Dao MA, Taylor N, Nolta JA. (1998) Reduction in levels of the cyclin dependent kinase inhibitor p27(kip-1) coupled with transforming growth factor beta neutralization induces cell-cycle entry and increases retroviral transduction of primitive human hematopoietic cells. *Proceedings of the National Academy of Sciences of the United States of America*, **95**, 13006–13011.

Jones PA, Baylin SB. (2007) The epigenomics of cancer. *Cell*, **128**, 683–692.

Kantarjian H, Issa JP, Rosenfeld CS et al. (2006) Decitabine improves patient outcomes in myelodysplastic syndromes: results of a phase III randomized study. *Cancer*, **106**, 1794–1803.

Kuendgen A, Strupp C, Aivado M et al. (2004) Treatment of myelodysplastic syndromes with valproic acid alone or in combination with all-trans retinoic acid. *Blood*, **104**, 1266–1269.

Nimer SD. (2008) Myelodysplastic syndromes. *Blood*, **111**, 4841–4851.

Raj K, Mufti GJ. (2006) Azacytidine (Vidaza®) in the treatment of myelodysplastic syndromes. *Therapeutics and Clinical Risk Management*, **2**, 377–388.

Silverman LR, Demakos EP, Peterson BL *et al.* (2002) Randomized controlled trial of azacitidine in patients with the myelodysplastic syndrome: a study of the Cancer and Leukemia Group B. *Journal of Clinical Oncology*, **20**, 2429–2440.

## Molecular basis of MDS

Aoki Y, Niihori T, Narumi Y *et al.* (2008) The RAS/MAPK syndromes: novel roles of the RAS pathway in human genetic disorders. *Human Mutation*, **29**, 992–1006.

Boultwood J, Fidler C, Strickson AJ *et al.* (2002) Narrowing and genomic annotation of the commonly deleted region of the 5q– syndrome. *Blood*, **99**, 4638–4641.

Buonamici S, Li D, Chi Y *et al.* (2004) EVI1 induces myelodysplastic syndrome in mice. *Journal of Clinical Investigation*, **114**, 713–719.

Ceesay MM, Lea NC, Ingram W *et al.* (2006) The JAK2 V617F mutation is rare in RARS but common in RARS-T. *Leukemia*, **20**, 2060–2061.

Cmejla R, Cmejlova J, Handrkova H *et al* (2007) Ribosomal protein S17 gene (RPS17) is mutated in Diamond–Blackfan anemia. *Human Mutation*, **28**, 1178–1182.

Ebert BL, Pretz J, Bosco J *et al.* (2008) Identification of RPS14 as a 5q– syndrome gene by RNA interference screen. *Nature*, **451**, 335–339.

Farrar JE, Nater M, Caywood E *et al.* (2008) Abnormalities of the large ribosomal subunit protein, Rpl35A, in Diamond–Blackfan anemia. *Blood*, **112**, 1582–1592.

Fenaux P, Kelaidi C. (2006) Treatment of the 5q– syndrome. *Hematology. American Society of Hematology Education Program*, 192–198.

Fidler C, Watkins F, Bowen DT *et al.* (2004) NRAS, FLT3 and TP53 mutations in patients with myelodysplastic syndrome and a del(5q). *Haematologica*, **89**, 865–866.

Gazda HT, Sieff CA. (2006) Recent insights into the pathogenesis of Diamond–Blackfan anaemia. *British Journal of Haematology*, **135**, 149–157.

Gondek LP, Tiu R, O'Keefe CL *et al.* (2008) Chromosomal lesions and uniparental disomy detected by SNP arrays in MDS, MDS/MPD, and MDS-derived AML. *Blood*, **111**, 1534–1542.

Grisendi S, Bernardi R, Rossi M *et al.* (2005) Role of nucleophosmin in embryonic development and tumorigenesis. *Nature*, **437**, 147–153.

Haase D, Germing U, Schanz J *et al.* (2007) New insights into the prognostic impact of the karyotype in MDS and correlation with subtypes: evidence from a core dataset of 2124 patients. *Blood*, **110**, 4385–4395.

Ingram W, Lea NC, Cervera J *et al.* (2006) The JAK2 V617F mutation identifies a subgroup of MDS patients with isolated deletion 5q and a proliferative bone marrow. *Leukemia*, **20**, 1319–1321.

Jaffe ES, Harris NL, Stein H, Vardiman JW (eds). (2001) *WHO Classification of Tumors, Pathology and Genetics of Tumours of Haematopoetic and Lymphoid Tissues.* Lyon: IARC.

Knudson AG. (2001) Two genetic hits (more or less) to cancer. *Nature Reviews. Cancer*, **1**, 157–162.

Kordasti SY, Ingram W, Hayden J *et al.* (2007) CD4$^+$CD25$^{high}$Foxp3$^+$ regulatory T cells in myelodysplastic syndrome (MDS). *Blood*, **110**, 847–850.

Lea NC, Mohamedali A, Twine N *et al.* (2006) Kinesin family member 20A (KIF20A) is specifically down regulated in 5q– CD34$^+$ and CD61$^+$ cells and uniparental disomy is not a feature of 5q– syndrome. *ASH Annual Meeting Abstracts*, **108**, 2611.

Le Beau MM, Espinosa R III, Davis EM *et al.* (1996) Cytogenetic and molecular delineation of a region of chromosome 7 commonly deleted in malignant myeloid diseases. *Blood*, **88**, 1930–1935.

Lin YW, Slape C, Zhang Z, Aplan PD. (2005) NUP98-HOXD13 transgenic mice develop a highly penetrant, severe myelodysplastic syndrome that progresses to acute leukemia. *Blood*, **106**, 287–295.

Maciejewski JP, Mufti GJ. (2008) Whole genome scanning as a cytogenetic tool in hematologic malignancies. *Blood*, **112**, 965–974.

Mohamedali A, Gaken J, Twine NA *et al.* (2007) Prevalence and prognostic significance of allelic imbalance by single nucleotide polymorphism analysis in low risk myelodysplastic syndromes. *Blood*, **110**, 3365–3373.

Padua RA, Guinn BA, Al-Sabah AI *et al.* (1998) RAS, FMS and p53 mutations and poor clinical outcome in myelodysplasias: a 10-year followup. *Leukemia*, **12**, 887–892.

Parker J, Mufti G, Rasool F *et al.* (2000) The role of apoptosis, proliferation, and the Bcl-2-related proteins in the myelodysplastic syndromes and acute myeloid leukemia secondary to MDS. *Blood*, **96**, 3932–3938.

Shannon KM, Le Beau MM. (2008) Hay in a haystack. *Nature*, **451**, 252–253.

Szpurka H, Tiu R, Murugesan G *et al.* (2006) Refractory anemia with ringed sideroblasts associated with marked thrombocytosis (RARS-T), another myeloproliferative condition characterized by JAK2 V617F mutation. *Blood*, **108**, 2173–2181.

# Chapter 9 Myeloproliferative disorders

## Anthony J Bench[1], George S Vassiliou[2,3] & Anthony R Green[3]

[1] Haemato-Oncology Diagnostics Service, Department of Haematology, Addenbrooke's Hospital, Cambridge, UK
[2] Wellcome Trust Sanger Institute, Cambridge, UK
[3] Cambridge University Department of Haematology, Cambridge Institute for Medical Research and; Addenbrooke's Hospital, part of Cambridge University Hospitals NHS Foundation Trust, Cambridge, UK

## Introduction

The classical myeloproliferative disorders (MPDs) comprise polycythemia vera (PV), essential thrombocythemia (ET) and idiopathic myelofibrosis (IMF). These disorders share many features including altered stem cell behavior, overproduction of myeloid lineages and, rarely, transformation to acute myeloid leukemia (AML). They were originally grouped together by Dameshek along with chronic myeloid leukemia (CML) in 1951. The World Health Organization groups the MPDs along with CML and rarer clonal disorders including chronic neutrophilic leukemia (CNL), chronic eosinophilic leukemia (CEL) and clonal mast cell diseases (MCD) under the heading of myeloproliferative neoplasms. This chapter focuses on PV, ET and IMF but will also depict recent advances in our understanding of rarer myeloproliferative neoplasms including CEL and MCD.

Evidence that the MPDs represent clonal disorders was derived from two sources: analysis of karyotypic abnormalities and X-chromosome inactivation patterns in female patients. Recurrent abnormal karyotypes were reported in approximately one-third of PV and IMF patients. In normal females, X-chromosome inactivation occurs randomly so that approximately half of all cells carry an active maternal X chromosome with the remainder carrying an active paternal X chromosome. In contrast, tumor cells, being clonally derived from a single cell, all carry either an active maternal X chromosome or an active paternal X chromosome. Using assays based on X-linked polymorphisms, the majority of PV and IMF patients and a proportion of ET patients demonstrate clonally derived blood cells. However, X inactivation-based clonality assays are inherently insensitive and many cases classified as "polyclonal" hide small clones not detectable by this method.

The biology of the MPDs was initially investigated through hematopoietic progenitor cell assays. Within semisolid media, progenitors from normal individuals only give rise to erythroid colonies in the presence of exogenous erythropoietin (EPO). In 1974, Prchal and Axelrad demonstrated that erythroid progenitors from the bone marrow of PV patients could be grown without the addition of EPO, termed endogenous erythroid colonies (EECs), and this attribute has become an important diagnostic tool in PV. Subsequently, it became clear that hematopoietic progenitors from MPD patients are hyperreactive to a range of growth factors.

Much of the biological behavior of these diseases became clearer with the demonstration of an acquired mutation within JAK2 (Janus kinase 2) in MPD patients. In 2005, several groups identified an acquired valine to phenylalanine change at codon 617 of JAK2 (V617F) (Figure 9.1) in the majority of PV patients and in approximately 50% of ET and IMF patients.

## The role of JAK2 in cytokine signaling

JAK2 belongs to a family of tyrosine kinases including JAK1, JAK2, JAK3 and TYK2 that form a link between cytokine receptors and intracellular signaling pathways. JAK2 is crucial for effective signaling through cytokine receptors including the erythropoietin receptor (EPOR) and receptors for thrombopoietin, interleukin-3 (IL-3), granulocyte colony-stimulating factor (G-CSF) and granulocyte macrophage colony-stimulating factor (GM-CSF). Homozygous

Molecular Hematology, 3rd edition. Edited by Drew Provan and John Gribben.
© 2010 Blackwell Publishing.

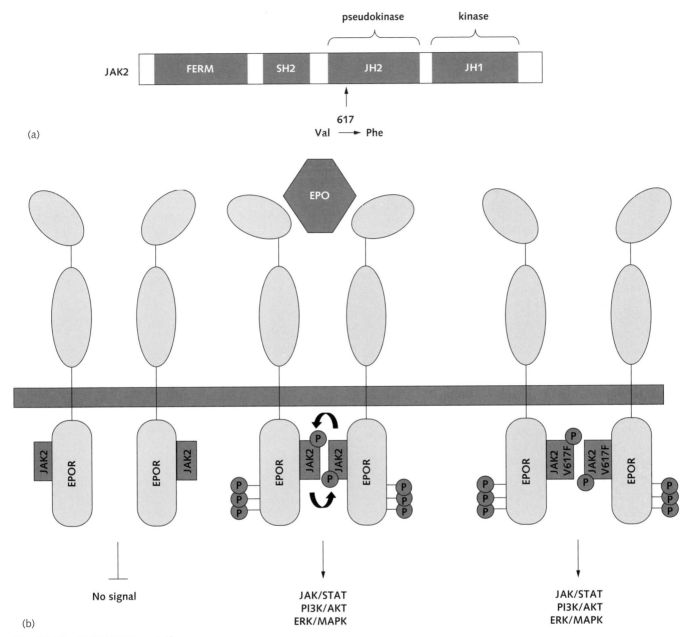

**Fig. 9.1 The JAK2 V617F mutation**

(a) JAK2 protein showing the valine to phenylalanine substitution at codon 617. (b) Role of JAK2 in cytokine signaling. The cytokine receptor EPOR binds JAK2 as a homodimer (left). On ligand binding, a conformational change within EPOR brings the two JAK2 molecules into close proximity, initiating a cascade of phosphorylation events and activation of downstream pathways (middle). The JAK2 V617F molecule is constitutively active, leading to EPO-independent activation of signaling pathways (right).

knockout of murine *Jak2* results in embryonic lethality due to complete absence of erythropoiesis. In the unstimulated state, EPOR forms a transmembrane homodimer, the cytoplasmic domain of which is bound to two JAK2 molecules (Figure 9.1). Ligand binding to the extracellular domain results in a conformational change within the receptor which brings together the two receptor-bound JAK2 molecules leading to their transphosphorylation and activation (Figure 9.1). Activated JAK2 then phosphorylates tyrosine residues within EPOR which, in turn, promotes recruitment and subsequent JAK2-mediated phosphorylation of other JAK2 substrates such as STAT5 and phosphatidylinositol 3-kinase (PI3K). Activation of various intracellular signaling pathways ensues (Figure 9.1). JAK2 possess two JAK homology

(JH) domains (Figure 9.1); the JH1 domain possesses tyrosine kinase activity while the JH2 or pseudokinase domain is homologous to JH1 but lacks kinase activity. Instead JH2 plays an autoinhibitory role by directly interacting with and stabilizing the activation loop within JH1 in the inactive form.

## JAK2 mutations in MPD

The valine at codon 617 of JAK2 lies at an evolutionarily conserved position within the JH2 domain (Figure 9.1) and is important for the interaction between the JH1 and JH2 domains. Substitution of valine 617 with the much bulkier phenylalanine residue, as found in MPD, is thought to interfere with JH2-mediated autoinhibition leading to constitutive activation of the tyrosine kinase (Figure 9.1). JAK2 binding is also important for trafficking of both EPOR and the thrombopoietin receptor (MPL) to the cell surface and the JAK2 V617F mutation may lead to reduced cell surface levels of MPL.

Biochemical studies have shown that most JAK2 targets are affected by the V617F mutation. The JAK2 V617F possesses much greater kinase activity than wild-type JAK2. Expression of JAK2 V617F results in increased autophosphorylation, increased phosphorylation of STAT5, ERK and AKT and altered transcription of cell cycle regulators. These experiments demonstrate a direct link between mutant JAK2 V617F and the activation of JAK/STAT, PI3K/AKT and MAPK/ERK pathways observed in PV progenitor cells.

Altered expression of many other genes in MPD is likely also a consequence of the JAK2 V617F mutation. The anti-apoptotic protein BCL2L1 (BCLX), which is upregulated in PV erythroid progenitors, is a target of STAT5 and its overexpression may underlie the generation of EPO-independent erythroid colonies. PV erythroid progenitors also display increased levels of another inhibitor of apoptosis, FLIPshort, due to upregulated PI3K/AKT and MAPK/ERK signaling. *SOCS3*, also transcriptionally regulated by STAT5, is overexpressed in PV and other JAK2 V617F-positive MPDs. SOCS3 is a negative regulator of JAK2 and targets it for proteasome-mediated degradation. However, in contrast to its effect on wild-type JAK2, SOCS3 is unable to inhibit transphosphorylation of mutant JAK2 V617F and may even enhance its kinase activity. Overexpression of NFE2, an inducer of erythroid differentiation, in PV is probably another consequence of increased STAT5 signaling. Taken together, these observations indicate that acquisition of the JAK2 V617F mutation underlies many of the changes observed in MPDs.

Further evidence for a direct link between the JAK2 V617F mutation and MPD was derived using murine models. Transduction of murine bone marrow with retroviruses carrying JAK2 V617F, but not wild-type JAK2, induces an MPD phenotype. These mice develop erythrocytosis, often leukocytosis and eventually myelofibrosis, and their bone marrow displays features found in human MPD. Thrombocytosis, on the other hand, is only seen in mice expressing a lower level of JAK2 V617F.

## Lineage specificity of JAK2 V617F

The MPDs arise in a multipotent hematopoietic stem cell. Hence, it would be expected that any pathogenetic mutation would also arise in a stem cell. Indeed, erythroid, myeloid and megakaryocytic progenitors from PV, ET and IMF patients carry the JAK2 V617F mutation as do CD34+CD38− cells, a population enriched for pluripotent progenitors. Surprisingly, the JAK2 V617F mutation is also detectable in highly purified B cells, natural killer cells and even T cells of some IMF and, more rarely, PV patients. Clonal involvement of B and T cells has also been demonstrated in IMF using cytogenetic markers. Taken together, these results suggest that the JAK2 V617F mutation arises in a progenitor cell with both lymphoid and myeloid potential but that its effect is predominantly manifested within the myeloid lineage as a consequence of the requirement for type I cytokine receptor expression within this lineage (e.g., EPOR, MPL, G-CSFR) as a scaffold for JAK2 V617F transforming ability.

## Cooperating mutations

The JAK2 V617F mutation is sufficient to cause a myeloproliferative phenotype in mice, suggesting that it represents an initiating lesion. However, it has been suggested that in some patients one or more unknown mutations arise prior to mutation within JAK2. Firstly, in some patients, especially ET or IMF, the percentage of clonal cells calculated using X-inactivation assays is greater than the percentage of JAK2 V617F-positive cells, suggesting that a pre-JAK2 aberration initiates clonal proliferation. However, care must be taken interpreting such results since many normal elderly females display a skewed X-inactivation pattern leading to an overestimation of the number of clonal granulocytes within MPD patients. To avoid such inherent flaws, Kralovics *et al.* also assessed two patients who carried a 20q deletion. In both cases, the percentage of cells carrying a 20q deletion was greater than those carrying a JAK2 V617F mutation, implying that acquisition of the 20q deletion preceded the JAK2 V617F mutation. Secondly, in rare situations of familial MPD, an inherited allele distinct from JAK2 V617F predisposes to an MPD phenotype. Thirdly, under some culture conditions, *in vitro* differentiation of JAK2 V617F-positive progenitor cells leads to reduced frequency of the mutant allele and JAK2 V617F-negative EECs from some JAK2

V617F-positive PV patients have been isolated. These data suggest that an additional mutation may arise prior to the JAK2 V617F mutation that is able to confer EPO independence, with the JAK2 V617F mutation being responsible for terminal erythroid differentiation. Finally, in a proportion of JAK2 V617F-positive MPD patients who transformed to AML, the leukemia cells no longer carried the JAK2 V617F mutation. Although treatment-related leukemia cannot be ruled out in all cases, this observation is consistent with transformation from a pre-JAK2 V617F clonal MPD.

## Disease association of JAK2 V617F mutation

The JAK2 V617F mutation can be detected by a number of different molecular genetic techniques (Figure 9.2). Due to its reduced sensitivity, sequencing is not usually the method

of choice and tends to underestimate the frequency of the mutation. Combining data from a number of studies employing sensitive allele-specific approaches to detect V617F, the true frequency of the mutation is 98% in PV, 57% in IMF and 57% in ET. A biallelic V617F mutation, arising as a result of mitotic recombination between the short arms of the two copies of chromosome 9, is seen in 30% of PV and 20% of IMF. The V617F mutation is also detected, albeit uncommonly, in other MPDs including CNL, CEL and atypical MPD/CML.

The JAK2 V617F mutation is not found in lymphoid malignancies and is only infrequently detected in patients with AML, myelodysplastic syndromes (MDS) and chronic myelomonocytic leukemia (CMML). Although rare cases of JAK2 V617F-positive, *BCR-ABL* positive CML have been reported, these cases appear to represent coexistence of two separate diseases and most CML patients do not carry a

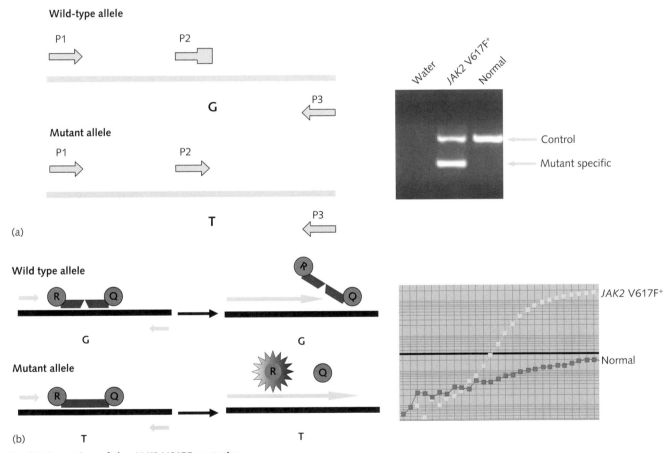

**Fig. 9.2 Detection of the *JAK2* V617F mutation**
(a) Allele-specific PCR. Amplification with primers P1 and P3 yields a product of 364 bp (control) whereas amplification with primers P1 and P2 yields a 203-bp PCR product from the mutant allele only. (b) Real-time PCR using a dual labeled probe specific for the mutant allele. Amplification from the wild-type allele results in displacement but not destruction of the probe, resulting in no release of fluorescence. In contrast, amplification from the mutant allele results in *Taq*-dependent destruction of the probe releasing the reporter (R) whose fluorescence can then be detected.

JAK2 V617F mutation. Hence, the JAK2 V617F mutation is uncommon in most myeloid malignancies other than PV, ET and IMF. An interesting exception is the MPD/MDS disorder refractory anemia with ringed sideroblasts with thrombocytosis (RARS-T), in which the mutation is detectable in approximately half of patients. Whether this disease represents a variant of ET is not clear.

## Clinical significance of the JAK2 V617F mutation

Since a significant proportion of ET and IMF patients do not carry the JAK2 V617F mutation, they may constitute a distinct disorder with different clinical, hematological and prognostic features. ET patients carrying a JAK2 V617F mutation tend to have more PV-like characteristics at diagnosis – higher hemoglobin level, higher white cell count and increased granulocytic and erythroid features within the bone marrow. Patients without a JAK2 V617F mutation often present with isolated thrombocytosis with a higher platelet count that requires higher doses of hydroxycarbamide (hydroxyurea) to control. JAK2 V617F-positive patients are also at higher risk of thrombosis, which is particularly associated with those patients with a higher level of JAK2 V617F.

The clinical importance of JAK2 V617F in IMF is not clear, possibly due to the different effects of biallelic mutations. Patients carrying a JAK2 V617F mutation tended to have a higher white count and/or hemoglobin level particularly if the mutation was biallelic. The mutation was associated with a poorer survival in one study, increased risk of leukemia transformation in another, but neither of these in a third. In another study, IMF patients with a low mutant allele burden demonstrated a shorter survival compared with JAK2 V617F-negative patients and those with a high allele burden. The investigators postulate that a low JAK2 V617F allele burden represents a surrogate marker for the presence of another mutation associated with a poorer prognosis.

PV patients with a high allele burden or for whom a biallelic mutation can be inferred tend to have a more progressive disease. This includes increased erythrocytosis and myelopoiesis, higher risk of splenomegaly and myelofibrotic transformation and increased requirement for chemotherapeutic intervention.

## Modulation of the V617F phenotype

The similarities between JAK2 V617F-positive ET and PV suggest that they represent a continuum within a single disorder (Figure 9.3). The different degrees of erythrocytosis, leukocytosis and thrombocytosis are thought to be influenced by a number of variables including gender, iron levels, effect of EPO, additional acquired mutations and inherited genetic modifiers.

Acquisition of a second JAK2 V617F allele by mitotic recombination is implicated in the pathogenesis of PV. Loss of heterozygosity of chromosome 9p (9p LOH) is observed in approximately 30% of PV patients. This recombination results in replacement of the wild-type *JAK2* allele with the mutant V617F allele. The presence of biallelic mutation within a proportion of cells can be indirectly inferred from an allele burden of greater than 50%, an observation which is much more frequent in PV than ET. Furthermore, high levels of mutant JAK2 V617F lead to erythrocytosis and myelofibrosis in mouse models whereas lower levels lead to thrombocytosis. The vast majority of PV patients but only rare cases of ET carry erythroid colonies with biallelic JAK2 V617F mutation, indicating that mitotic recombination occurs in progenitor cells and leads to erythrocytosis. Erythroid progenitors carrying a biallelic V617F mutation are more sensitive to low levels of EPO than cells carrying a single mutant allele. An additional consequence of mitotic recombination is loss of the wild-type *JAK2* allele which may lead to reduction of inhibition of JAK2 V617F.

Two lines of evidence indicate that inherited polymorphisms modify the phenotype associated with an acquired JAK2 V617F mutation. Firstly, different strains of mice

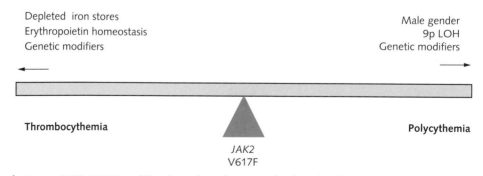

Depleted iron stores
Erythropoietin homeostasis
Genetic modifiers

Male gender
9p LOH
Genetic modifiers

Thrombocythemia

Polycythemia

*JAK2*
V617F

**Fig. 9.3 Continuum between JAK2 V617F-positive thrombocythemia and polycythemia**
Adapted from Campbell PJ, Scott LM, Buck G *et al.* (2005) Definition of subtypes of essential thrombocythaemia and relation to polycythaemia vera based on JAK2 V617F mutation status: a prospective study. *Lancet*, 366, 1945–1953, with permission.

expressing the same JAK2 V617F allele yield different myelo-proliferative phenotypes. Secondly, inherited single-nucleotide polymorphisms (SNPs) within *JAK2* and *EPOR* have been associated with PV and/or ET. In fact, a particular common SNP within the *JAK2* locus itself is associated with an increased risk of acquiring a JAK2 V617F mutation and thus of developing an MPD. The explanation for the latter is not well understood but it is likely that the SNP is found within a haplotype that affects the transcriptional regulation of JAK2.

## Other mutations within myeloproliferative disorders

Approximately 2% of well-characterized PV patients do not carry a JAK2 V617F mutation. Many of these patients carry a mutation within *JAK2* exon 12. These mutations cluster within a small region spanning codons 537–547, most of

which affect Leu539 or Glu543 (Figure 9.4). This region lies just upstream of the JH2 pseudokinase domain (Figure 9.4) and is thought to affect the interaction between the JH1 and JH2 domains. The *JAK2* exon 12 mutations lead to a higher degree of cytokine independence and phosphorylation of JAK2 substrates than does JAK2 V617F. In murine models, the JAK2 K539L mutation leads to elevated hematocrit, leukocytosis and thrombocytosis but the leukocytosis and thrombocytosis are less dramatic than with the V617F mutation. Similarly, patients carrying a *JAK2* exon 12 mutation tend to display isolated erythrocytosis within the bone marrow, in contrast to JAK2 V617F-positive patients who characteristically show hyperplasia of all three myeloid lineages. In fact, *JAK2* exon 12 mutations are often detected in patients previously diagnosed with idiopathic erythrocytosis, while the JAK2 V617F mutation is uncommon in such patients. *JAK2* exon 12 mutations have not been detected within JAK2 V617F-negative ET or IMF patients. Hence, mutations within *JAK2* exon 12 lead to increased kinase

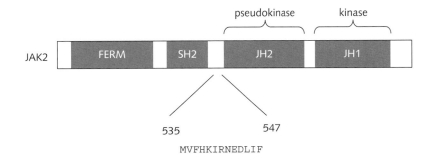

| Mutation | Sequence | Number of cases |
|---|---|---|
| F537-K539delinsL | MV--LIRNEDLIF | 7 |
| H538QK539L | MVFQLIRNEDLIF | 1 |
| H538-K539delinsL | MVF-LIRNEDLIF | 3 |
| K539L | MVFHLIRNEDLIF | 4 |
| I540-E543delinsMK | MVFHKMK-DLIF | 3 |
| R541-E543delinsK | MVFHKIK-DLIF | 9 |
| N542-E543del | MVFHKIR-DLIF | 17 |
| E543-D544del | MVFHKIRN-LIF | 7 |
| V536-I546dup11 | MVFHKIRNEDLIV | 1 |
| F537-I546dup10+F547L | MVFHKIRNEDLIL | 1 |
| | | 53 |

**Fig. 9.4 *JAK2* exon 12 mutations and reported frequencies (at March 2008)**
Three types of mutation can be described: leucine to lysine substitution at codon 539 (shaded); deletion of glutamic acid at codon 543 (shaded); duplication (underlined) and substitution of phenylalanine at codon 547.

activity that drives the hematopoietic stem cell toward erythropoiesis but not other hematopoietic lineages.

JAK2 V617F-negative MPD patients often display features associated with an MPD, such as EEC formation, abnormal megakaryocyte morphology and clonal granulopoiesis. It is therefore likely that mutations within other components of signaling pathways play a role in some JAK2 V617F-negative ET and IMF patients. Large multigene sequencing projects failed to identify mutations within tyrosine kinases other than *JAK2* or within *EPOR* and *GCSFR* but did identify mutations within *MPL*, which encodes the thrombopoietin receptor. *MPL* mutations have been demonstrated in approximately 7% of IMF and 3% of all ET patients. ET and IMF cases carrying both a *MPL* exon 10 mutation and a JAK2 V617F mutation have been described, although it is not clear if the two mutations are clonally related.

MPL W515 mutations confer cytokine-independent growth and phosphorylation of JAK2 targets and are particularly associated with abnormal megakaryopoiesis. Clinically, MPL W515 IMF patients tend to be more anemic and ET patients carrying an *MPL* mutation tend to present with lower hemoglobin, a higher platelet count and lower cellularity compared with JAK2 V617F-positive patients.

Mutations within the *TET2* gene have been detected in 10–20% of MPD patients, including both JAK2 V617F-positive and -negative patients. Similar mutations are also found in other myeloid malignancies, including AML, MDS and CMML. The acquisition of a *TET2* mutation preceded a JAK2 V617F mutation in patients carrying both mutations, indicating that *TET2* mutations may well be the initiating event discussed earlier. The function of TET2 is not clear, although a related molecule, TET1, plays a role in the demethylation of methylated cytosine molecules, suggesting a role for epigenetic regulation by the TET proteins.

# Tyrosine kinases in other myeloproliferative disorders

## KIT mutations in mast cell disease

KIT is a class III receptor tyrosine kinase that is activated by the cytokine, stem cell factor (SCF) (Figure 9.5). Cytokine binding leads to KIT homodimerization, autophosphorylation, tyrosine kinase activation and activation of the PI3K/AKT, ERK/MAPK and JAK/STAT pathways. An aspartate to valine substitution at position 816, within the active loop of the tyrosine kinase domain (Figure 9.5), is detected in more than 90% of patients with systemic mastocytosis.

The KIT D816V mutation, or its murine equivalent, leads to growth factor independence in murine cell lines and hematopoietic progenitor cells probably via pathways

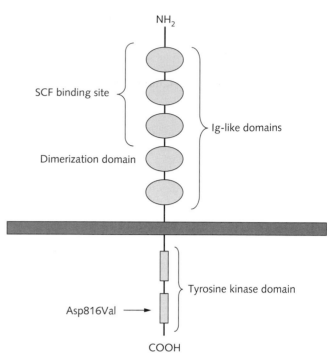

**Fig. 9.5 The KIT receptor showing the aspartic acid to valine substitution at codon 816 in mast cell disease**

involving PI3K and STAT molecules. As for JAK2 V617F, the KIT D816V mutation probably arises in a hematopoietic progenitor cell with lymphoid and myeloid potential. Wild-type KIT but not KIT D816V is inhibited by imatinib mesylate, but other inhibitors of KIT, such as dasatinib, or inhibitors of downstream targets, such as NF-κB, may be potential therapeutic agents.

## *FIP1L1–PDGFRA* rearrangement in CEL

Submicroscopic deletion of chromosome 4q12 leading to the generation of a novel fusion gene, *FIP1L1–PDGFRA*, has been identified in many cases previously labeled as idiopathic hypereosinophilic syndrome (HES) and now reclassified as CEL. Approximately 10–15% of patients with apparent HES carry the *FIP1L1–PDGFRA* fusion gene, many of whom display features characteristic of systemic mastocytsosis.

Unlike other fusion proteins involving tyrosine kinases such as TEL–PDGFRB and BCR–ABL, FIP1L1 does not contain a dimerization domain and is completely dispensable for activation of platelet-derived growth factor receptor alpha (PDGFRA). Rather, disruption of the PDGFRA juxtamembrane domain affects its autoinhibitory function, leading to constitutive activation of the kinase domain. Consistent with this, *PDGFRA* breakpoints cluster within exon 12, which encodes the juxtamembrane domain whereas

*FIP1L1* breakpoints span exons 7–10 (Plate 9.1). In contrast to other MPDs, the *FIP1L1–PDGFRA* fusion gene may arise in myeloid progenitors rather than a hematopoietic stem cell. Furthermore, the full development of CEL may require elevated IL-5 signaling in addition to the *FIP1L1–PDGFRA* fusion gene.

The *FIP1L1–PDGFRA* fusion transcript is expressed at very low levels within unfractionated peripheral blood and bone marrow but can be detected by nested reverse transcriptase polymerase chain reaction (RT-PCR) (Plate 9.1). Alternatively, the 4q12 deletion can be detected by fluorescence *in situ* hybridization (FISH) using a probe (*CHIC2*) within the 800-kb deleted region (Plate 9.1). Identification of *FIP1L1–PDGFRA*-positive patients is of clinical importance since such patients respond well to imatinib and the disease is now classified as "myeloid neoplasm with *PDGFRA* rearrangement".

### *FGFR1* rearrangements in 8p11 myeloproliferative syndrome

The 8p11 myeloproliferative syndrome (EMS) is a rare atypical MPD characterized by both myeloid and lymphoid malignancies with an aggressive clinical course. Balanced translocations involving chromosome 8p11 result in a novel fusion gene containing the fibroblast growth factor receptor 1 (FGFR1) receptor tyrosine kinase. The most common translocation is t(8;13), which yields a *ZNF198–FGFR1* fusion gene. The fusion protein contains a ZNF198-derived oligomerization domain and this leads to ligand-independent dimerization and activation of the ZNF198-FGFR1 tyrosine kinase. A number of other partner genes of FGFR1 have

been identified and all are thought to result in a constitutively active fusion protein. The activated FGFR1 kinase is unaffected by imatinib but other tyrosine kinase inhibitors are under investigation.

## Other chromosomal changes in myeloproliferative disorders

Visible chromosomal abnormalities, detected by G-banding, occur in approximately one-third of patients with PV or IMF but are rare in ET. This frequency increases when FISH techniques are used, indicating that submicroscopic or cryptic rearrangements are a common feature. The most common visible chromosomal abnormalities in MPD are deletions of the long arms of chromosome 20, del(20q), and chromosome 13, del(13q), trisomies of chromosomes 8 and 9, and duplication of part of the long arm of chromosome 1. Within IMF, del(20q) and del(13q) are associated with a more indolent course whereas other cytogenetic changes, in particular trisomy 8, chromosome 12 abnormalities and deletion of chromosome 7, confer a poorer prognosis.

### Deletion of chromosome 20q

Deletion of the long arm of chromosome 20 is observed in approximately 10% of patients with PV or IMF and in some with MDS or AML. It can arise within a multipotent progenitor with both myeloid and lymphoid potential. It shows a close association with the JAK2 V617F mutation and may arise prior to it, suggesting that the 20q deletion marks the site of one or more genes that cooperate with the JAK2 V617F mutation.

Molecular and cytogenetic mapping of patients with a 20q deletion has enabled the definition of a common deleted region (CDR). Based on simple deletions, the MPD CDR spans 3 Mb and overlaps the MDS CDR by 2 Mb (Figure 9.6). Among the genes within this region with a putative pathogenetic role in MPD, *L3MBTL* offers an attractive candidate. This gene encodes a polycomb-like protein that functions as a transcriptional repressor. No acquired mutations in *L3MBTL* have been detected in patients with a 20q deletion or a normal karyotype. Within normal hematopoietic cells, two of the gene's four CpG islands show monoallelic methylation due to maternal imprinting and this is associated with transcriptional silencing. Deletion of 20q results in loss of either the methylated or unmethylated allele and *L3MBTL* mRNA expression levels in patients with a 20q deletion do not correlate with methylation status. Hence, the role of *L3MBTL* in myeloid malignancies associated with a 20q deletion remains unclear.

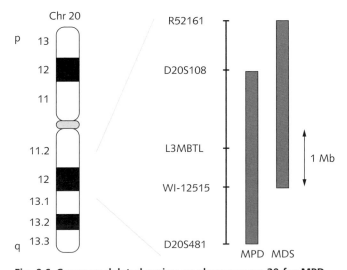

**Fig. 9.6 Common deleted region on chromosome 20 for MPD and MDS**

## Deletion of chromosome 13q

Unlike del(20q), deletion of the long arm of chromosome 13 is not associated with the JAK2 V617F mutation, suggesting that it may represent an alternative pathogenetic mechanism. The region of loss in MPD patients is less well characterized than the 20q deletion, although it does encompass the 13q deleted region in lymphoid malignancies.

## Abnormalities of chromosome 12q

Translocations and other aberrations involving the long arm of chromosome 12 are an uncommon but consistent feature of IMF and sometimes PV. These aberrations result in overexpression of *HMGA2*, a member of the high mobility group A proteins with important roles in gene regulation via chromatin modifications. HMGA2 is also disrupted in other myeloid malignancies and in non-hematopoietic tumors, although the molecular consequences of this are unclear. *HMGA2* is also overexpressed in many IMF patients without chromosome 12q abnormalities through mechanisms that may involve downregulation of microRNAs, miR-150 and miR-149, which putatively target *HMGA2* mRNA.

## Other translocations

Balanced translocations are rare in classical MPD (PV, ET, IMF) but may provide useful information. Within atypical CML/MPD, analysis of rare translocations has identified many fusion transcripts involving tyrosine kinases that form targets for novel drug development.

## A new classification for myeloproliferative disorders

It is now clear that clinical classification schemes can be greatly enhanced in their ability to aid diagnosis, prognosis and therapy by the incorporation of their relevant molecular features. In some cases, the impact of newly identified mutations is so significant that schemes have had to change dramatically to accommodate them. This is particularly true for the MPDs.

Classification of the MPDs, first attempted by the Polycythemia Vera Study Group (PVSG), was a tool for distinguishing these disorders from phenotypically similar clonal and non-clonal blood disorders. The identification of the JAK2 V617F mutation offers a highly specific diagnostic test for the MPDs. New simplified classification systems have been devised that incorporate the molecular changes underlying the MPDs (Tables 9.1 and 9.2). As shown in these

**Table 9.1** The 2008 World Health Organization (WHO) diagnostic criteria for polycythemia vera, essential thrombocythemia and primary myelofibrosis.*

**Polycythemia vera**
*Major criteria*
1  Hb > 18.5 g/dL (men), > 16.5 g/dL (women) *or*
   Hb or Hct > 99th percentile of reference range for age, sex or altitude of residence *or*
   Hb > 17 g/dL (men), > 15 g/dL (women) if associated with a sustained increase of ≥2 g/dL from baseline that cannot be attributed to correction of iron deficiency *or*
   Elevated red cell mass > 25% above mean normal predicted value
2  Presence of JAK2 V617F or similar mutation

*Minor criteria*
1  Bone marrow trilineage myeloproliferation
2  Subnormal serum erythropoietin level
3  EEC growth

**Essential thrombocythemia**
*Major criteria*
1  Platelet count ≥450 × 10⁹/L
2  Megakaryocyte proliferation with large and mature morphology. No or little granulocyte or erythroid proliferation
3  Not meeting WHO criteria for CML, PV, PMF, MDS or other myeloid neoplasm
4  Demonstration of JAK2 V617F or other clonal marker *or* no evidence of reactive thrombocytosis

**Primary myelofibrosis**
*Major criteria*
1  Megakaryocyte proliferation and atypia accompanied by either reticulin and/or collagen fibrosis, *or*
   In the absence of reticulin fibrosis, megakaryocyte changes accompanied by increased marrow cellularity, granulocytic proliferation and often decreased erythropoiesis (i.e., pre-fibrotic PMF)
2  Not meeting WHO criteria for CML, PV, MDS or other myeloid neoplasm
3  Demonstration of JAK2 V617F or other clonal marker *or* No evidence of reactive marrow fibrosis

*Minor criteria*
1  Leukoerythroblastosis
2  Increased serum LDH
3  Anemia
4  Palpable splenomegaly

*Diagnosis of polycythemia vera (PV) requires both major criteria and one minor criterion or major criterion **1** and two minor criteria. Diagnosis of essential thrombocythemia requires all four major criteria. Diagnosis of primary myelofibrosis (PMF) requires all three major criteria and two minor criteria.
CML, chronic myeloid leukemia; EEC, endogenous erythroid colony; Hb, hemoglobin; Hct, hematocrit; LDH, lactate dehydrogenase.
*Source:* Adapted from Tefferi A, Vardiman JW. (2008) Classification and diagnosis of myeloproliferative neoplasms: the 2008 World Health Organization criteria and point-of-care diagnostic algorithms. *Leukemia,* **22,** 14–22, with permission.

**Table 9.2** Proposed diagnostic criteria for myeloproliferative diseases.

*JAK2* **mutation positive**
*JAK2*-positive polycythemia (**A1** and **A2** required)
**A1** High hematocrit (men > 52%, women > 48%) or an increased red cell mass (>25% above predicted value)
**A2** Mutation in *JAK2*

*JAK2*-positive thrombocythemia (**A1, A2** and **A3** required)
**A1** Platelet count > 450 × 10⁹/L
**A2** Mutation in *JAK2*
**A3** No other myeloid malignancy especially *JAK2*-positive polycythemia, myelofibrosis or MDS

*JAK2*-positive myelofibrosis (**A1, A2** plus two **B** criteria required)
**A1** Reticulin grade 3 or higher (on a 0–4 scale)
**A2** Mutation in *JAK2*
**B1** Palpable splenomegaly
**B2** Otherwise unexplained anemia (hemoglobin: men < 11.5 g/dL, women < 10 g/dL)
**B3** Teardrop red cells on peripheral blood film
**B4** Leukoerythroblastic blood film
**B5** Systemic symptoms (drenching night sweats, weight loss > 10% over 6 months or diffuse bone pain)
**B6** Histological evidence of extramedullary hematopoiesis

*JAK2* **mutation negative**
*JAK2*-negative polycythemia vera (**A1, A2, A3** plus **A4** or **A5** or two **B** criteria required)
**A1** High hematocrit (men ≥ 60%, women > 56%) or an increased red cell mass (>25% above predicted value)
**A2** Absence of mutation in *JAK2*
**A3** No causes of secondary erythrocytosis (normal arterial oxygen saturation and no elevation of serum EPO)
**A4** Palpable splenomegaly
**A5** Presence of acquired genetic abnormality (excluding *BCR-ABL*) in hematopoietic cells
**B1** Thrombocytosis (platelets > 450 × 10⁹/L)
**B2** Neutrophilia (neutrophils > 10 × 10⁹/L; > 12.5 × 10⁹/L in smokers)
**B3** Splenomegaly on radiography
**B4** Endogenous erythroid colonies or low serum EPO

*JAK2*-negative essential thrombocythemia (**A1–A5** required)
**A1** Platelet count > 600 × 10⁹/L on two occasions at least 1 month apart
**A2** Absence of mutation in *JAK2*
**A3** No reactive cause for thrombocytosis
**A4** Normal ferritin (>20 μg/L)
**A5** No other myeloid disorder especially CML (*BCR-ABL* negative), myelofibrosis, polycythemia or MDS

*JAK2*-negative idiopathic myelofibrosis (**A1, A2, A3** plus two **B** criteria required)
**A1** Reticulin grade 3 or higher (on a 0–4 scale)
**A2** Absence of mutation in *JAK2*
**A3** Absence of *BCR-ABL* fusion gene
**B1** Palpable splenomegaly
**B2** Otherwise unexplained anemia (hemoglobin: men < 11.5 g/dL, women < 10 g/dL)
**B3** Teardrop red cells on peripheral blood film
**B4** Leukoerythroblastic blood film (presence of at least two nucleated red cells or immature myeloid cells in peripheral blood film)
**B5** Systemic symptoms (drenching night sweats, weight loss > 10% over 6 months or diffuse bone pain)
**B6** Histological evidence of extramedullary hematopoiesis

CML, chronic myeloid leukemia; EPO, erythropoietin.
*Source*: Campbell PJ, Green AR. (2006) The myeloproliferative disorders. *New England Journal of Medicine*, **355**, 2452–2466, with permission.

tables, both approaches emphasize the importance of the demonstration of an acquired mutation (either V617F or exon 12) within *JAK2*, but differ in the significance attached to it.

Assessment of JAK2 V617F (and exon 12) status is now a frontline test in patients with erythrocytosis and thrombocytosis. To avoid false-negative results, sensitive detection methods are required. Examples of such technologies include allele-specific PCR, melting curve analysis, pyrosequencing and real-time PCR (see Figure 9.2). Furthermore, the demonstration of a JAK2 V617F mutation in a patient not otherwise meeting appropriate diagnostic criteria suggests an underlying MPD, for example those presenting with an unexplained splanchnic thrombosis.

## Conclusions and future directions

Identification of *JAK2* and *MPL* mutations within PV, ET and IMF has reinforced Dameshek's dictum that these disorders are closely linked. It has also revolutionized all aspects of the MPDs, including our understanding of pathogenetic mechanisms, clarification of diagnostic criteria and, importantly, development of new therapies. Indeed, a number of drugs have been identified that are able to inhibit growth of JAK2 V617F-positive cell lines *in vitro*, limit EEC formation and rescue the JAK2 V617F-induced murine disease. Some therapies are now entering Phase I clinical trials in poor-performing MPDs such as myelofibrosis. Quantification of the JAK2 V617F burden will enable the response to these novel therapies to be assessed in a fashion similar to *BCR-ABL* transcript quantification in CML.

High-throughput technologies are now being used to identify new alterations within MPD patients. Gene expression profiling studies have identified genes whose expression is altered within the MPDs, often as a result of the JAK2 V617F mutation and thus represent secondary changes. Differences in the gene expression profile between PV and IMF may help to explain the processes controlling myelofibrotic transformation. Finally, differentially expressed microRNA molecules in MPD represent a novel mechanism of regulating gene expression.

## Acknowledgments

The authors thank Dr Philip Beer, Dr Elaine Boyd, Dr Peter Campbell, Dr Wendy Erber, Andrea Goday and Bridget Manasse for assistance with figures.

## Further reading

### Introduction

Bench AJ, Pahl HL. (2005) Chromosomal abnormalities and molecular markers in myeloproliferative disorders. *Seminars in Hematology*, **42**, 196–205.

Campbell PJ, Green AR. (2006) The myeloproliferative disorders. *New England Journal of Medicine*, **355**, 2452–2466.

Kralovics R, Prchal JT. (1998) Haematopoietic progenitors and signal transduction in polycythaemia vera and primary thrombocythaemia. *Baillieres Clin Haematology*, **11**, 803–818.

Prchal JF, Axelrad AA. (1974) Letter: Bone-marrow responses in polycythemia vera. *New England Journal of Medicine*, **290**, 1382.

### JAK2 and its role in MPD

Baxter EJ, Scott LM, Campbell PJ *et al.* (2005) Acquired mutation of the tyrosine kinase JAK2 in human myeloproliferative disorders. *Lancet*, **365**, 1054–1061.

Garcon L, Rivat C, James C *et al.* (2006) Constitutive activation of STAT5 and Bcl-xL overexpression can induce endogenous erythroid colony formation in human primary cells. *Blood*, **108**, 1551–1554.

Hookham MB, Elliott J, Suessmuth Y *et al.* (2007) The myeloproliferative disorder-associated JAK2 V617F mutant escapes negative regulation by suppressor of cytokine signaling 3. *Blood*, **109**, 4924–4929.

James C, Ugo V, Le Couedic JP *et al.* (2005) A unique clonal JAK2 mutation leading to constitutive signalling causes polycythaemia vera. *Nature*, **434**, 1144–1148.

Kralovics R, Passamonti F, Buser AS *et al.* (2005) A gain-of-function mutation of JAK2 in myeloproliferative disorders. *New England Journal of Medicine*, **352**, 1779–1790.

Lacout C, Pisani DF, Tulliez M *et al.* (2006) JAK2V617F expression in murine hematopoietic cells leads to MPD mimicking human PV with secondary myelofibrosis. *Blood*, **108**, 1652–1660.

Levine RL, Wadleigh M, Cools J *et al.* (2005) Activating mutation in the tyrosine kinase JAK2 in polycythemia vera, essential thrombocythemia, and myeloid metaplasia with myelofibrosis. *Cancer Cell*, **7**, 387–397.

Silva M, Richard C, Benito A *et al.* (1998) Expression of Bcl-x in erythroid precursors from patients with polycythemia vera. *New England Journal of Medicine*, **338**, 564–571.

Tefferi A, Gilliland DG. (2007) Oncogenes in myeloproliferative disorders. *Cell Cycle*, **6**, 550–566.

Tiedt R, Hao-Shen H, Sobas MA *et al.* (2008) Ratio of mutant JAK2-V617F to wild type JAK2 determines the MPD phenotypes in transgenic mice. *Blood*, **111**, 3931–3940.

Walz C, Crowley BJ, Hudon HE *et al.* (2006) Activated Jak2 with the V617F point mutation promotes G1/S phase transition. *Journal of Biological Chemistry*, **281**, 18177–18183.

Wernig G, Mercher T, Okabe R *et al.* (2006) Expression of Jak2V617F causes a polycythemia vera-like disease with associated myelofibrosis in a murine bone marrow transplant model. *Blood*, **107**, 4274–4281.

Zeuner A, Pedini F, Signore M *et al.* (2006) Increased death receptor resistance and FLIPshort expression in polycythemia vera erythroid precursor cells. *Blood,* **107,** 3495–3502.

Zhao R, Xing S, Li Z *et al.* (2005) Identification of an acquired JAK2 mutation in polycythemia vera. *Journal of Biological Chemistry,* **280,** 22788–22792.

## Lineage specificity of JAK2 V617F

Delhommeau F, Dupont S, Tonetti C *et al.* (2007) Evidence that the JAK2 G1849T (V617F) mutation occurs in a lymphomyeloid progenitor in polycythemia vera and idiopathic myelofibrosis. *Blood,* **109,** 71–77.

Ishii T, Bruno E, Hoffman R, Xu M. (2006) Involvement of various hematopoietic-cell lineages by the JAK2V617F mutation in polycythemia vera. *Blood,* **108,** 3128–3134.

Jamieson CH, Gotlib J, Durocher JA *et al.* (2006) The JAK2 V617F mutation occurs in hematopoietic stem cells in polycythemia vera and predisposes toward erythroid differentiation. *Proceedings of the National Academy of Sciences of the United States of America,* **103,** 6224–6229.

Lu X, Levine R, Tong W *et al.* (2005) Expression of a homodimeric type I cytokine receptor is required for JAK2V617F-mediated transformation. *Proceedings of the National Academy of Sciences of the United States of America,* **102,** 18962–18967.

## Cooperating mutations

Bellanne-Chantelot C, Chaumarel I, Labopin M *et al.* (2006) Genetic and clinical implications of the Val617Phe JAK2 mutation in 72 families with myeloproliferative disorders. *Blood,* **108,** 346–352.

Campbell PJ, Baxter EJ, Beer PA *et al.* (2006) Mutation of JAK2 in the myeloproliferative disorders: timing, clonality studies, cytogenetic associations, and role in leukemic transformation. *Blood,* **108,** 3548–3555.

Kralovics R, Teo SS, Li S *et al.* (2006) Acquisition of the V617F mutation of JAK2 is a late genetic event in a subset of patients with myeloproliferative disorders. *Blood,* **108,** 1377–1380.

Levine RL, Belisle C, Wadleigh M *et al.* (2006) X-inactivation-based clonality analysis and quantitative JAK2V617F assessment reveal a strong association between clonality and JAK2V617F in PV but not ET/MMM, and identifies a subset of JAK2V617F-negative ET and MMM patients with clonal hematopoiesis. *Blood,* **107,** 4139–4141.

## Disease association and clinical significance of JAK2 V617F

Barosi G, Bergamaschi G, Marchetti M *et al.* (2007) JAK2 V617F mutational status predicts progression to large splenomegaly and leukemic transformation in primary myelofibrosis. *Blood,* **110,** 4030–4036.

Campbell PJ, Griesshammer M, Dohner K *et al.* (2006) V617F mutation in JAK2 is associated with poorer survival in idiopathic myelofibrosis. *Blood,* **107,** 2098–2100.

Campbell PJ, Scott LM, Buck G *et al.* (2005) Definition of subtypes of essential thrombocythaemia and relation to polycythaemia vera based on JAK2 V617F mutation status: a prospective study. *Lancet,* **366,** 1945–1953.

Jones AV, Kreil S, Zoi K *et al.* (2005) Widespread occurrence of the JAK2 V617F mutation in chronic myeloproliferative disorders. *Blood,* **106,** 2162–2168.

Kittur J, Knudson RA, Lasho TL *et al.* (2007) Clinical correlates of JAK2V617F allele burden in essential thrombocythemia. *Cancer,* **109,** 2279–2284.

Levine RL, Loriaux M, Huntly BJ *et al.* (2005) The JAK2V617F activating mutation occurs in chronic myelomonocytic leukemia and acute myeloid leukemia, but not in acute lymphoblastic leukemia or chronic lymphocytic leukemia. *Blood,* **106,** 3377–3379.

Schmitt-Graeff AH, Teo SS, Olschewski M *et al.* (2008) JAK2V617F mutation status identifies subtypes of refractory anemia with ringed sideroblasts associated with marked thrombocytosis. *Haematologica,* **93,** 34–40.

Scott LM, Beer PA, Bench AJ *et al.* (2007) Prevalance of JAK2 V617F and exon 12 mutations in polycythaemia vera. *British Journal of Haematology,* **139,** 511–512.

Steensma DP, Dewald GW, Lasho TL *et al.* (2005) The JAK2 V617F activating tyrosine kinase mutation is an infrequent event in both "atypical" myeloproliferative disorders and myelodysplastic syndromes. *Blood,* **106,** 1207–1209.

Tefferi A, Lasho TL, Huang J *et al.* (2008) Low JAK2V617F allele burden in primary myelofibrosis, compared to either a higher allele burden or unmutated status, is associated with inferior overall and leukemia-free survival. *Leukemia,* **22,** 756–761.

Vannucchi AM, Antonioli E, Guglielmelli P *et al.* (2007) Clinical profile of homozygous JAK2 617V→F mutation in patients with polycythemia vera or essential thrombocythemia. *Blood,* **110,** 840–846.

## Modulation of the V617F phenotype

Pardanani A, Fridley BL, Lasho TL *et al.* (2008) Host genetic variation contributes to phenotypic diversity in myeloproliferative disorders. *Blood,* **111,** 2785–2789.

Scott LM, Scott MA, Campbell PJ, Green AR. (2006) Progenitors homozygous for the V617F mutation occur in most patients with polycythemia vera, but not essential thrombocythemia. *Blood,* **108,** 2435–2437.

Tiedt R, Hao-Shen H, Sobas MA *et al.* (2008) Ratio of mutant JAK2-V617F to wild type JAK2 determines the MPD phenotypes in transgenic mice. *Blood,* **111,** 3931–3940.

Campbell PJ. (2009) Somatic and germline genetics at the *JAK2* locus. *Nature Genetics* **41,** 385–386.

## Other mutations within MPDs

Beer PA, Campbell PJ, Scott LM *et al.* (2008) *MPL* mutations in myeloproliferative disorders: analysis of the PT-1 cohort. *Blood,* **112,** 141–149.

Delhommeau F, Dupont S, Della Valle V *et al.* (2009) Mutation in *TET2* in myeloid cancers. *New England Journal of Medicine,* **360,** 2289–2301.

Pardanani AD, Levine RL, Lasho T *et al.* (2006) MPL515 mutations in myeloproliferative and other myeloid disorders: a study of 1182 patients. *Blood,* **108,** 3472–3476.

Scott LM, Tong W, Levine RL *et al.* (2007) JAK2 exon 12 mutations in polycythemia vera and idiopathic erythrocytosis. *New England Journal of Medicine*, **356**, 459–468.

## Tyrosine kinases in other MPDs

Cools J, DeAngelo DJ, Gotlib J *et al.* (2003) A tyrosine kinase created by fusion of the PDGFRA and FIP1L1 genes as a therapeutic target of imatinib in idiopathic hypereosinophilic syndrome. *New England Journal of Medicine*, **348**, 1201–1214.

Garcia-Montero AC, Jara-Acevedo M, Teodosio C *et al.* (2006) KIT mutation in mast cells and other bone marrow hematopoietic cell lineages in systemic mast cell disorders: a prospective study of the Spanish Network on Mastocytosis (REMA) in a series of 113 patients. *Blood*, **108**, 2366–2372.

Jovanovic JV, Score J, Waghorn K *et al.* (2007) Low-dose imatinib mesylate leads to rapid induction of major molecular responses and achievement of complete molecular remission in FIP1L1-PDGFRA-positive chronic eosinophilic leukemia. *Blood*, **109**, 4635–4640.

Orfao A, Garcia-Montero AC, Sanchez L, Escribano L. (2007) Recent advances in the understanding of mastocytosis: the role of KIT mutations. *British Journal of Haematology*, **138**, 12–30.

Stover EH, Chen J, Folens C *et al.* (2006) Activation of FIP1L1-PDGFRalpha requires disruption of the juxtamembrane domain of PDGFRalpha and is FIP1L1-independent. *Proceedings of the National Academy of Sciences of the United States of America*, **103**, 8078–8083.

Xiao S, McCarthy JG, Aster JC, Fletcher JA. (2000) ZNF198-FGFR1 transforming activity depends on a novel proline-rich ZNF198 oligomerization domain. *Blood*, **96**, 699–704.

Xiao S, Nalabolu SR, Aster JC *et al.* (1998) FGFR1 is fused with a novel zinc-finger gene, ZNF198, in the t(8;13) leukaemia/lymphoma syndrome. *Nature Genetics*, **18**, 84–87.

## Other chromosomal changes in MPDs

Andrieux J, Demory JL, Dupriez B *et al.* (2004) Dysregulation and overexpression of HMGA2 in myelofibrosis with myeloid metaplasia. *Genes Chromosomes and Cancer*, **39**, 82–87.

Bench AJ, Cross NC, Huntly BJ *et al.* (2001) Myeloproliferative disorders. *Best Pract Res Clin Haematol.* **14**, 531–551.

Bench AJ, Li J, Huntly BJ *et al.* (2004) Characterization of the imprinted polycomb gene L3MBTL, a candidate 20q tumour suppressor gene, in patients with myeloid malignancies. *British Journal of Haematology*, **127**, 509–518.

De Keersmaecker K, Cools J. (2006) Chronic myeloproliferative disorders: a tyrosine kinase tale. *Leukemia*, **20**, 200–205.

Odero MD, Grand FH, Iqbal S *et al.* (2005) Disruption and aberrant expression of HMGA2 as a consequence of diverse chromosomal translocations in myeloid malignancies. *Leukemia*, **19**, 245–252.

Strasser-Weippl K, Steurer M, Kees M *et al.* (2005) Chromosome 7 deletions are associated with unfavorable prognosis in myelofibrosis with myeloid metaplasia. *Blood*, **105**, 4146.

## A new classification for MPD

Campbell PJ, Green AR. (2006) The myeloproliferative disorders. *New England Journal of Medicine*, **355**, 2452–2466.

McMullin MF, Reilly JT, Campbell P *et al.* (2007) Amendment to the guideline for diagnosis and investigation of polycythaemia/erythrocytosis. *British Journal of Haematology*, **138**, 821–822.

Tefferi A, Vardiman JW. (2008) Classification and diagnosis of myeloproliferative neoplasms: the 2008 World Health Organization criteria and point-of-care diagnostic algorithms. *Leukemia*, **22**, 14–22.

Vannucchi AM, Barbui T. (2007) Thrombocytosis and thrombosis. *Hematology. American Society of Hematology Education Program*, 363–370.

## Future directions

Bruchova H, Yoon D, Agarwal AM *et al.* (2007) Regulated expression of microRNAs in normal and polycythemia vera erythropoiesis. *Experimental Hematology*, **35**, 1657–1667.

Kralovics R, Teo SS, Buser AS *et al.* (2005) Altered gene expression in myeloproliferative disorders correlates with activation of signalling by the V617F mutation of Jak2. *Blood*, **106**, 3374–3376.

Pardanani A. (2008) JAK2 inhibitor therapy in myeloproliferative disorders: rationale, preclinical studies and ongoing clinical trials. *Leukemia*, **22**, 23–30.

# Chapter 10 Lymphoma genetics

## Anthony G Letai[1] & John G Gribben[2]

[1] *Harvard Medical School, Dana-Farber Cancer Institute, Boston, MA, USA*
[2] *Centre for Experimental Cancer Medicine, Institute of Cancer, Barts and The London School of Medicine & Dentistry, London, UK*

## Introduction

As with all cancers, lymphomas were originally categorized based primarily on morphology and clinical behavior. The use of antibodies against cell surface markers allowed the study of lymphoma specimens with antibody panels that could, along with morphological criteria, usually place a given lymphoma into a diagnostic category. Even within a given lymphoma category, however, there is considerable heterogeneity of clinical behavior. A prominent example is the category of diffuse large B-cell lymphomas, in which approximately 50% are cured with chemotherapy, but 50% die of disease, usually within a few years of diagnosis. In this case, as with many of the lymphomas, a prognostic index (the International Prognostic Index or IPI) based on a few pretreatment criteria is able to further subdivide the category, and provide very useful prognostic information. However, even within IPI classes, significant clinical heterogeneity persists. Furthermore, it is likely that the IPI defines subclasses of lymphomas based on biological differences among these lymphomas. Studies of genetic abnormalities are proving important tools for the improved classification and prognostication of diseases. In addition, a better understanding of the molecular pathophysiology of the disease will likely lead to improvements in treatment of lymphoma.

*Molecular Hematology*, 3rd edition. Edited by Drew Provan and John Gribben.
© 2010 Blackwell Publishing.

## Techniques

The techniques for studying genetic abnormalities in tumor specimens have undergone a revolution in the past 5–10 years (Table 10.1). Initial genetic analyses were based on the technique of Giemsa-trypsin banding of chromosomes. In these studies, cells are grown in short-term culture, usually in the presence of mitogens. Colcemid treatment results in cell accumulation in metaphase, at which point the cells are fixed and dropped on glass slides. The slides are treated with trypsin followed by Giemsa to give a banding pattern. An experienced cytogenetic technician can then identify normal chromosomes, translocations, numerical abnormalities, and sometimes more subtle deletions. The technique can identify only genetic changes large enough to disrupt a Giemsa-stained band, requiring a change of many megabases.

More modern techniques are able to detect abnormalities with greater sensitivity. Southern hybridization starts with the electrophoretic separation of tumor DNA on a gel, followed by transfer to a membrane. This membrane is then probed with radioactively labeled polynucleotide probes specific for certain genes of interest. Changes in the expected size or intensity of the band of interest can indicate mutation, translocation, amplification, or deletion of the gene of interest. It can also be used to evaluate the presence of clonal rearrangements of the immunoglobulin loci in B cells or the T-cell receptor locus in T cells.

Polymerase chain reaction (PCR) technology has allowed the detection of genetic abnormalities using only a small amount of tumor DNA. PCR for detection of lymphoma cells is discussed in more detail in Chapter 6. Using primers designed to flank the genomic region of interest, repetitive cycles of annealing, DNA polymerization, and thermal melting eventually yield a PCR product. The presence and size of this product may be analyzed by gel electrophoresis to determine the presence of a translocation. Furthermore, a PCR product may be sequenced to look for point mutations. Like Southern blotting, PCR can also be used to evaluate the presence of clonal rearrangements of the immunoglobulin loci in B cells or the T-cell receptor locus in T cells.

Fluorescence *in situ* hybridization (FISH) uses fluorescently labeled DNA probes to bind to specific regions of genomic DNA. Images are then analyzed under a fluorescent microscope. Numerical chromosomal abnormalities may be detected by simply counting the number of signals per cell:

greater than 2 indicates the addition of a chromosome, whereas less than 2 indicates a deletion (Plate 10.1). To investigate a potential translocation, two probes are used, one to detect the genomic DNA on each side of the known translocation. If the two probes are consistently approximated, this indicates the presence of a translocation (Plate 10.2). FISH may be performed on interphase cells, so that growth in culture is not a requirement for this type of analysis as it is for conventional cytogenetics. Tests for small deletions or other more subtle abnormalities may be better performed on metaphase cells. FISH requires knowledge of the area to be labeled.

Since they rely on the annealing of a labeled specific DNA probe or primer, Southern hybridization, PCR, and FISH are techniques for determining the presence or absence of a *known* genetic abnormality. Modern techniques that can provide a genome-wide scan for abnormalities but which require no prior suspicion of a particular abnormality include comparative genomic hybridization (CGH), gene expression profiling (GEP), single-nucleotide polymorphism (SNP) arrays, and microRNA arrays. These are beginning to have a clinical impact.

In original CGH techniques (Figure 10.1), DNA is isolated from the tumor sample and a normal control sample. The DNA in each is labeled with a different fluorescent dye, for example green for the tumor DNA and red for the normal DNA. These samples are then mixed and hybridized onto slides of metaphase spreads of normal cells. Images of met-

---

**Table 10.1** Techniques for studying lymphoma genetics.

Cytogenetic analysis
Southern blot analysis
Polymerase chain reaction
Fluorescence *in situ* hybridization
Comparative genomic hybridization (CGH)
CGH microarray
Gene expression profiling
Proteomic profiling
Single-nucleotide polymorphism array
Micro-RNA expression profiling

---

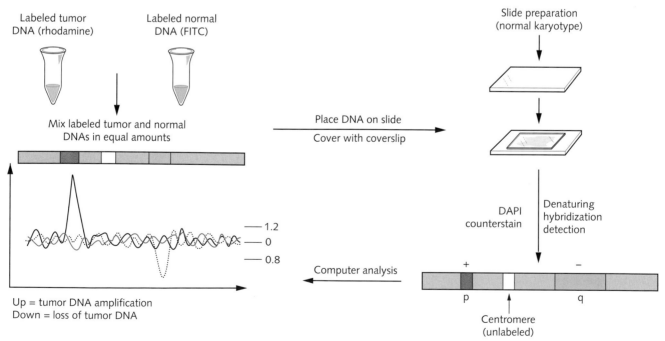

Up = tumor DNA amplification
Down = loss of tumor DNA

**Fig. 10.1 Comparative genomic hybridization**

aphase spreads are then analyzed for green to red color ratio. Regions of chromosomes that have a high green to red ratio contain a putative area of amplification. Regions that have a low green to red ratio contain a putative deletion. In this way, the entire genome may be examined for abnormalities. Other techniques, generally beyond what is performed in clinical laboratories, are required to determine the critical genes involved in areas of amplification and deletion. Small abnormalities and balanced translocations cannot be observed using this technique. Currently in more common use is a variation of the CGH technique (known as array CGH) that hybridizes the DNA to defined arrays of genomic DNA fragments (Figure 10.2). These arrays can cover the genome and improve resolution to the size of the DNA fragments within the microarray, currently down to the level of 1 Mb.

GEP is described in more detail in Chapter 27. This technique allows a comprehensive quantitative examination of the mRNA transcripts of a tumor sample, a group of molecules that has been termed the *transcriptome*. In this technique, mRNA is purified from a fresh or frozen tumor sample. Formalin-fixed tissue cannot be used. It is important that when a group of samples is being compared, tissue acquisition, mRNA preparation, and all subsequent steps are performed as identically as possible. When possible, steps should be performed on all samples in parallel, with identical reagents, and simultaneously. Techniques exist to amplify very small amounts of mRNA to obtain usable quantities;

while some have reported that this may be done without bias to the relative quantities of transcripts, this may not be universally true. The mRNA is reverse transcribed, then transcribed with fluorescently labeled nucleotides to develop a fluorescently labeled complementary RNA (cRNA) representation of the original mRNA mixture. The labeled cRNA is then used for hybridization to immobilized, indexed oligonucleotide or cDNA probes. The signals at each of the loci on the slide or "gene chip" may then be quantitated by microscopy and image analysis software. The strength of fluorescent signal may then be related to the abundance of a particular mRNA in the original sample. Comparison of different tumor samples, and comparison with wild type, can then allow the determination of transcripts that are over- or under-represented in certain conditions or tumors. Tumors may be categorized using these profiles, and subgroups of messages may be used to create predictors of clinical behavior. This powerful technique has the potential to analyze an entire transcriptome of tens of thousands of genes simultaneously. However, it cannot determine the genomic abnormalities that lead to the differences in expression pattern. Given the amount of data this technique can encompass, it is possible that it will some day be part of the routine pathological analysis of cancers, providing, like conventional pathology today, categorical and prognostic information, and possibly even directing therapeutic decision-making.

The whole-genome analysis of SNPs has been greatly facilitated by the development of SNP arrays. To use an SNP

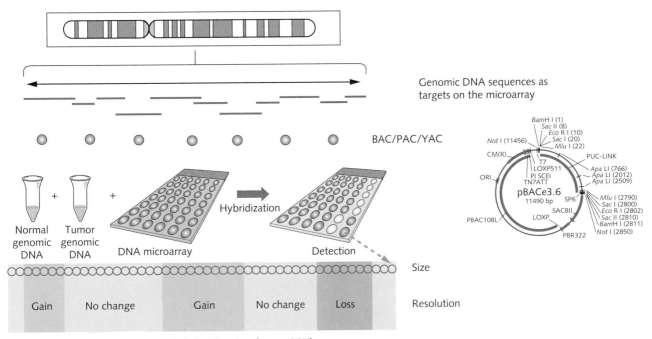

Fig. 10.2 Array comparative genomic hybridization (array CGH)

array, DNA from a cell of interest is digested with an endonuclease. To the exposed ends of the DNA are annealed oligonucleotide linkers. These DNA fragments are then amplified via PCR, end labeled, and finally hybridized to an SNP array chip. Hundreds of thousands of oligonucleotides, representing all known SNPs in the genome, as determined by whole-genome sequencing, are covalently attached to the chip. The fluorescent signal at each SNP location is measured by a dedicated reader. Two kinds of data can be obtained from an SNP array. Perhaps most obviously, one can simply determine what SNPs are present in a given tumor sample. One can then ask related questions, such as "Is there loss of heterozygosity at certain SNP locations compared to somatic tissues?" or "Are certain SNPs preferentially present in this tumor type, or selected for after a particular therapy?" In addition, however, one can also obtain data similar to that obtained by CGH. Because the genomic location of all the SNPs is known, one can orient the SNP results according to the geography of the chromosomes. Consistent loss of all SNPs along a region indicates a region of chromosomal loss, whereas consistent increase in SNP signal at a particular region indicates amplification. Software programs are available for the ready analysis of such data.

The field of microRNA biology is relatively young compared with other genetic studies of cancer. MicroRNAs are small non-coding RNA transcripts that act primarily by modulating expression of other genes. MicroRNAs exert this function by annealing to mRNAs, the consequence of which can be shortened mRNA half-life or decreased translation. Any single microRNA can modulate the expression at many different genes. It has been difficult, however, to use the primary sequence of the microRNA to predict the genes at which it acts. Recently, several studies have demonstrated that by measuring the levels of the hundreds of known microRNAs in the genome, one can segregate cancers into different groups. Furthermore, such segregation may provide information about prognosis, progression, and response to therapy. Supporting the concept that microRNAs play an important role in determining cancer behavior, non-coding regions of the genome that are frequently deleted in cancer often contain microRNA genes.

Chronic lymphocytic leukemia (CLL) is an example of a lymphoid cancer for which microRNA biology has been informative. For instance, it has been found that in many cases of CLL, particularly those of indolent behavior, there is downregulation or deletion of the *mir-15-A* and *mir-16-1*, located at 13q14.3. Both of these microRNAs have the ability to decrease BCL-2 levels, so their deletion may explain the high levels of BCL-2 found in nearly all CLL cells. In addition, expression levels of a limited number of microRNAs may distinguish between indolent and aggressive clinical subtypes in CLL.

## Types of genetic abnormality

The types of genetic abnormalities found in lymphoma may be crudely divided into two main classes: those that foster increased proliferation and those which inhibit programmed cell death, or apoptosis. The classical gene in lymphomagenesis that induces proliferation is c-*myc*. Burkitt lymphoma, one of the most rapidly dividing lymphomas, is the archetype of a lymphoma that overexpresses c-*myc* due to the t(8;14) translocation. c-MYC is a helix–loop–helix leucine zipper transcription factor that requires heterodimerization with the protein MAX to activate transcription and induce proliferation. Targets of this dimer include genes controlling cell cycle progression, cell growth, metabolism, differentiation, and apoptosis. The net effect of c-*myc* expression is generally an increase in proliferation; however, this effect is context-specific. In some cells, c-*myc* overexpression can induce cell-cycle arrest or apoptosis via p53. Therefore, it may require an apoptotic defect to permit c-*myc* overexpression.

*BCL-2* is an oncogene that does not directly foster increased proliferation, but rather opposes apoptosis. It does this at least in part by binding and sequestering pro-apoptotic BCL-2 family members, preventing them from communicating or executing death signals, especially at the mitochondrion. It is classically overexpressed in the indolent follicular lymphoma due to t(14;18) translocation. Other apoptotic defects often found in lymphoma include those allowing for activation or stabilization of NF-κB transcription factors.

A frequent hallmark of translocations found in B-cell lymphomas is their exploitation of immunoglobulin gene regulatory elements to drive expression of an oncogene in a malignant B-cell or B-cell precursor. Burkitt lymphoma is an example of a lymphoma characterized by the overexpression of c-*myc*. While the most common translocation is t(8;14), which puts c-*myc* under the control of the immunoglobulin heavy chain (IgH) transcription elements, the less common t(2;8) and t(8;22) are also found, putting c-*myc* transcription under the control of the light-chain κ and λ transcription elements, respectively. The t(14;18) found in follicular lymphoma drives BCL-2 expression using IgH transcription elements. The BCL-6 expression found in many cases of diffuse large B-cell lymphomas (DLBLs) is often driven by IgH, Igκ, and Igλ elements in t(3;14), t(2;3) and t(3;22) respectively. PAX5 expression in lymphoplasmacytoid lymphoma and cyclin D1 expression in mantle cell lymphoma are likewise driven by the t(9;14) and t(11;14) translocations, which exploit the IgH locus.

Improved techniques of genetic study have allowed the identification of a large number of chromosomal transloca-

**Table 10.2** Chromosomal translocations in non-Hodgkin lymphoma (NHL).

| NHL histological type | Translocation | Per cent of cases involved | Proto-oncogene | Function | Mechanism of activation of oncogene |
|---|---|---|---|---|---|
| Burkitt lymphoma | t(8;14) | 80% | c-myc | Cell proliferation and growth | Transcriptional deregulation |
| | t(2;8) | 15% | | | |
| | (t8;22) | 5% | | | |
| Diffuse large-cell lymphoma | der(3) | 35% | BCL-6 | Transcriptional repressor, required for GC formation | Transcriptional deregulation |
| Mantle cell lymphoma | t(11;14) | >70% | BCL-1 | Cell cycle regulator | Transcriptional deregulation |
| Follicular lymphoma | t(14;18) | 90% | BCL-2 | Anti-apoptotic | Transcriptional deregulation |
| Lymphoplasmacytic lymphoma | t(9;14) | 50% | PAX-5 | Transcription factor regulating B-cell proliferation | Transcriptional deregulation |
| MALT lymphoma | t(11;18) | 50% | API-2–MLT | API-2 is anti-apoptotic | Fusion protein |
| | t(1;14) | Rare | BCL-10 | ?Anti-apoptotic | Transcriptional deregulation |
| Anaplastic large T-cell lymphoma | t(2;5) | 60% in adults, 85% in children | NPM/ALK | ALK is a tyrosine kinase | Fusion protein |

tions, the most common of which are shown in Table 10.2. The most common abnormalities, or those which have been demonstrated to have the greatest impact on prognosis or treatment, are described. Figure 10.3 shows the molecular pathogenesis, the putative cell of origin within B-cell development in the lymph node and germinal center, and immunophenotype of the most common types of lymphomas. The molecular pathogenesis of CLL/small lymphocytic lymphoma remains unknown.

## Burkitt lymphoma

Burkitt lymphoma is a very high grade B-cell malignancy. Pathologically, it is characterized by small non-cleaved cells. The presence of many apoptotic malignant cells gives rise to tingible body macrophages and "starry sky" appearance characteristic of this and other very rapidly dividing tumors. Frequent mitotic figures demonstrate the rapid cell division characteristic of this tumor. Though rapidly dividing, it is one of the most curable lymphomas, with more than 90% of adults enjoying long-term survival when treated with a regimen similar to that proposed by MacGrath. Because the MacGrath regimen is quite different and yields much improved results compared with the CHOP (cyclophosphamide, doxorubicin, vincristine, prednisone) regimen used for other aggressive B-cell lymphomas, it is important to make the diagnostic distinction between Burkitt and large B-cell lymphoma.

Genetic testing plays a key role in making the diagnosis of Burkitt lymphoma. The genetic hallmark of Burkitt lym-

phoma is overexpression of the c-myc oncogene due to a translocation that places c-myc transcription under the control of elements at an immunoglobulin locus. The most common translocation, t(8;14), is a chromosomal rearrangement involving c-myc and the immunoglobulin heavy chain locus. Other translocations involve c-myc with the κ [t(2;8)] or λ [t(8;22)] light-chain loci. It is difficult to make the diagnosis of Burkitt lymphoma in the absence of evidence for a c-myc translocation by cytogenetics, FISH, or PCR. The c-myc (myelocytomatosis) oncogene encodes a helix–loop–helix, zinc finger-containing transcription factor. The expression of the transcriptional targets of c-MYC is associated with a proliferative phenotype.

There is a type of lymphoma that lies histologically and clinically between Burkitt lymphoma and the DLBLs. These Burkitt-like lymphomas lack c-myc translocations; 30% possess rearrangements involving the BCL-2 gene. The prognosis of these tumors is generally inferior to that of the true Burkitt lymphomas.

Evidence for latent Epstein–Barr virus infection is found in nearly all African endemic Burkitt lymphomas but in only 20% of the sporadic form found outside Africa. It has been suggested that Epstein–Barr virus plays a causative role by opposing apoptosis.

## Diffuse large B-cell lymphoma

The DLBLs are a heterogeneous group of lymphomas of aggressive clinical behavior. The majority likely derive from follicular center cells, and roughly one-fifth of large B-cell

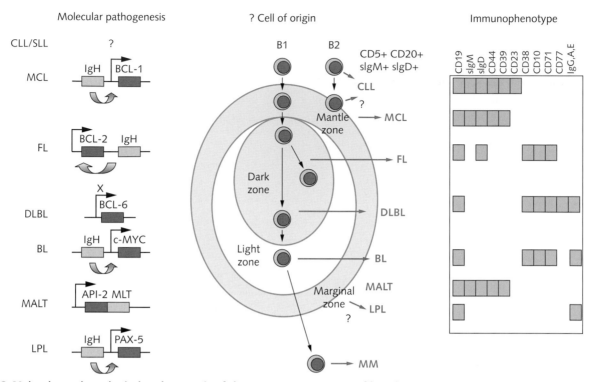

**Fig. 10.3 Molecular and cytological pathogenesis of the most common types of lymphomas**
BL, Burkitt lymphoma; CLL/SLL, chronic lymphocytic leukemia/small-cell lymphoma; DLBL, diffuse large B-cell lymphoma; FL, follicular lymphoma; LPL, lymphoplasmacytoid lymphoma; MALT, mucosa-associated lymphoid tissue lymphoma; MCL, mantle cell lymphoma.

lymphomas derive from transformation of a pre-existing follicular lymphoma. As the name suggests, DLBL has a diffuse histological pattern of large lymphoid cells. Approximately 40% of patients with this disease will be cured. The mainstay of therapy is combination chemotherapy including doxorubicin. Some relapsing patients may be rescued by autologous stem cell transplantation following high-dose therapy.

Numerous heterogeneous genetic abnormalities have been reported for DLBL. These lymphomas are not characterized by a single archetypical translocation, as with the t(14;18) in follicular lymphoma or the t(8;14) of Burkitt lymphoma. Of the abnormalities that have been identified, those involving the *BCL-6* gene at 3q27 are the most common.

*BCL-6* was initially described as the gene involved in translocations involving the 3q27 locus in a group of follicular and large B-cell lymphomas. Its expression is often deregulated via translocation with heterologous promoters, including immunoglobulin promoters. While only 10% of large B-cell lymphomas demonstrate the 3q27 translocation by cytogenetics, gene rearrangements involving 3q27 can be found by Southern hybridization analysis in 40% of large B-cell lymphomas. Additionally, somatic mutation of 5′ non-coding sequences has been shown. Overall, *BCL-6*

expression is found in more than 80% of DLBLs. BCL-6 is required for germinal center formation. Expression of BCL-6 is now used in clinical pathology laboratories as a marker for germinal center origin. Containing six zinc fingers, BCL-6 functions as a transcriptional repressor, at least partially by recruiting histone deacetylases. Likely gene targets of BCL-6 repression include chemokines, cell cycle proteins, and other transcriptional effectors. How repression of the heterogeneous BCL-6 targets leads to oncogenesis is unclear.

Approximately 20% of DLBLs have the t(14;18) resulting in BCL-2 expression, which confers a worse prognosis. A significant proportion of these tumors likely arise via transformation of a follicular cell lymphoma. Overexpression of BCL-2 by amplification of the *BCL-2* allele has been observed by quantitative Southern hybridization and by CGH in 11–31% of DLBL cases tested. Other genes which have demonstrated amplification by these techniques include *REL*, *MYC*, *CDK4*, and *MDM2*.

## Expression profiling

Pathological diagnosis is perhaps most important to the oncologist to the extent that it can inform prognosis and treatment choice. Current diagnostic categorization of a lymphoma as DLBL relies on a fairly small amount of data, including cell surface markers, nuclear and cytoplasmic appearance, and tissue morphology. When these data lead to the diagnosis of DLBL, the oncologist is left with a diagnostic grouping that combines those who will die of unresponsive disease in the first 6 months after diagnosis despite the most aggressive treatment approaches, and those who will rapidly obtain and maintain a durable complete remissions following administration of anthracycline-based combination chemotherapy. It seems odd to call two diseases that behave so differently by the same name.

In an attempt to better divide the heterogeneous group of diseases encompassed by the label DLBL, Shipp and colleagues developed the IPI. The IPI uses data from just four clinical and laboratory parameters to further subclassify DLBL into four groups. While this formulation does provide a useful refinement of prognosis, it still falls short of the ideal predictor, namely one that would definitively determine, prior to a particular therapy, whether that therapy would work.

While the ideal predictor may be unattainable in practice, attempts are being made to improve prognostic prediction using the massive amount of molecular data provided by GEP. Two groups, one based at the National Cancer Institute and the other at the Dana-Farber Cancer Institute, have published results of applying GEP to lymphoma samples for which clinical data were available. In both cases, predictors generated by GEP were able to identify new subclasses of lymphomas and also to further refine prognosis even within IPI subgroups. Furthermore, when prognosis is predicted by a molecular signature, the molecules involved in that signature can be immediately identified as potential targets of anticancer therapy, a feat not possible when prognosis is determined by purely clinical criteria. The Dana-Farber group identified protein kinase C (PKC)-β as such a target, and clinical trials incorporating a PKC-β inhibitor in DLBL are underway. Recent work has assessed the impact of the addition of rituximab to CHOP chemotherapy and has identified the importance of the stromal signature in determining outcome.

GEP potentially places a huge mass of data at the disposal of the pathologist and oncologist. As the field's experience with this fascinating technology grows, its use in prognosis and therapeutic development will only improve.

## Mantle cell lymphoma

Mantle cell lymphoma is a B-cell lymphoma thought to be the malignant counterpart of the memory B cells found in the mantle zone of lymphoid follicles. It has characteristic cell surface markings of CD5$^+$CD10$^-$CD23$^-$. Clinically, it is characterized by a moderate rate of growth. While it often

responds to cytotoxic chemotherapy, it has frustrated attempts at cure with chemotherapy, although there are reports of long-term survivors following allogeneic bone marrow transplantation. The median survival is generally 3–5 years.

Mantle cell lymphoma is almost uniformly characterized via classical cytogenetics or PCR by a t(11;14) translocation which puts the cyclin D1, also known as *BCL-1* (B-cell leukemia/lymphoma 1), gene under control of the immunoglobulin heavy chain transcription control elements. Cyclin D1 binds to and activates cyclin-dependent kinases. An important target of this activated cyclin-dependent kinase complex is the retinoblastoma (RB) gene product. In its hypophosphorylated state, RB inhibits entry into S phase of the cell cycle by binding the transcription factor E2F. When RB is phosphorylated, E2F is freed to activate the transcription of genes that propel the cell into S phase. Therefore, overexpression of cyclin D1 acts to overcome this late G$_1$ phase checkpoint and maintain continuous proliferation.

## Follicular lymphoma

Follicular lymphoma is an indolent lymphoma. The cell of origin is thought to be the follicular center B cell. While it can be cured by local therapy in very localized stages, it is more usually diagnosed in an advanced stage where cure is exceedingly rare. It is generally quite responsive to chemotherapy, but almost always relapses. The clinical course is commonly marked by a series of chemotherapy-induced remissions followed by relapses, with the interval between these decreasing over time. The end stage of the disease may be characterized by insuperable resistance to chemotherapy or by transformation to an aggressive large B-cell phenotype. Despite the very low cure rate, many patients nonetheless survive more than a decade due to the indolent nature of the disease.

Histologically, it is characterized by a follicular pattern in the lymph node. The appearance can be similar to that of the non-malignant follicular hyperplasia. Light-chain restriction can be useful in suggesting the clonality of the tumor, which distinguishes it from benign hyperplasia.

### Genetics

A t(14;18) translocation (Plate 10.2; Figure 10.4) is found in more than 85% of follicular lymphomas. This rearrangement puts the *BCL-2* gene under the transcriptional control of elements from the immunoglobulin heavy chain locus. The BCL-2 protein functions to oppose programmed cell death. It is presumed that BCL-2 expression in malignancies such as follicular lymphoma permits survival of the cancer

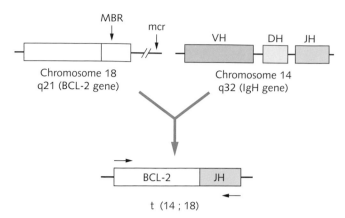

**Fig. 10.4 Detection of t(14;18) by PCR amplification**

cells under conditions (cell cycle checkpoint violation, meta-static location, genomic instability) that would otherwise trigger programmed cell death. The cloning of *BCL-2* led to the identification of a family of related proteins. While some are anti-apoptotic like BCL-2, many are pro-apoptotic, but all function in the control of apoptosis.

Follicular lymphoma can transform into a higher-grade lymphoma with DLBL morphology. Numerous genetic changes have been associated with this transformation including trisomy 7, loss of *p53*, and *c-myc* rearrangements.

## Lymphoplasmacytoid lymphoma

Lymphoplasmacytoid lymphoma is an indolent lymphoma. The cells of this lymohoma have a phenotype that lies midway between mature lymphocytes and plasma cells, for which reason they are often nicknamed "plymphocytes." This lymphoma commonly expresses IgM, which can lead to the syndrome of Waldenström macroglobulinemia. Waldenström macroglobulinemia is characterized by IgM expression, hyperviscosity, bleeding, Raynaud phenomenon, visual disturbances, and other neurological symptoms.

Roughly half of all lymphoplasmacytoid lymphoma cases will demonstrate t(9;14), which juxtaposes the *PAX-5* gene and the IgH locus. *PAX-5* encodes the B-cell specific activator protein, which is a transcription factor. Its expression is associated with increased expression of genes important in early B-cell development and decreased expression of the *p53* tumor suppressor.

## Mucosa-associated lymphoid tissue lymphoma

The mucosa-associated lymphoid tissue (MALT) lymphomas are thought to arise from the extranodal counterpart to

post-follicular memory B cells found in the marginal zone of lymph node follicles. These tumors are often localized, and their behavior is generally indolent. At least some have a dependence on continued antigen stimulation for survival, as demonstrated by the prolonged complete responses that are seen when early-stage gastric MALT lymphoma is treated with an antibiotic regimen to eradicate chronic *Helicobacter pylori* infection.

The translocation t(11;18)(q21;q21) is found in more than half of all low-grade MALT lymphomas, with a preference for gastric lymphomas. The translocation is not typically found in high-grade MALT lymphomas. API-2–MALT-1 fusion protein is expressed from the mutant locus. API-2 (also known as IAP-2) belongs to a family of inhibitors of apoptosis that prevent death, likely due to their direct inter-action with caspases, the proteases activated by programmed cell death. The physiological function of the MALT-1 protein is less well understood, though it possesses a caspase-like domain at its C-terminus. The function of the fusion protein is unclear, although there is some evidence that it activates NF-κB, perhaps leading to inhibition of apoptosis.

BCL-10 is overexpressed in a minority of MALT lymphoma cases via t(1;14)(p22;q32), putting the coding region of *BCL-10* under the influence of the immunoglobulin heavy chain enhancer. The function of this protein is unclear, but some have suggested an interaction between BCL-10 and MALT-1, leading to NF-κB activation. Others have shown that API-2–MALT-1 correlates with the nuclear location of BCL-10. These findings suggest that these two translocations may be involved in activating the same pathway.

Trisomy 3 is observed in 20–60% of all MALT lymphomas. The oncogenic properties of this numerical chromosomal abnormality are not understood.

## Anaplastic large cell lymphoma

Anaplastic large cell lymphoma (ALCL) is characterized by strong surface expression of the CD30 (Ki-1) antigen, a cytokine receptor in the tumor necrosis factor receptor family. The majority of ALCLs demonstrate T-cell surface markers and/or clonal rearrangements of the T-cell receptor locus. There are two main clinical forms, systemic and cuta-neous. The cutaneous form is particularly indolent. While it is clinically aggressive, systemic ALCL is generally sensitive to chemotherapy. Approximately 30% of those diagnosed die of the disease.

Approximately 50% of systemic ALCLs carry t(2;5), which confers good prognosis. Long-term survival of t(2;5)-positive patients is 80%, while that of t(2;5)-negative patients is 25%. The t(2;5)(p23;q35) results in a chimeric gene encoding a fusion of the nuclephosmin (NPM) and anaplastic lymphoma kinase (ALK) proteins. NPM is a multifunctional protein that has been implicated in ribosome assembly, control of centrosome duplication, and nuclear transport as a shuttle protein; it also possesses chaperonin and ribonuclease activities. ALK is a member of the insulin family of receptor tyrosine kinases. Its natural ligand is unknown. The NPM–ALK fusion contains the oligomerization domain of NPM and the tyrosine kinase domain of ALK. It results in a self-oligomerizing, constituitively active tyrosine kinase with transforming properties. NPM–ALK can activate numerous downstream effectors, including phospholipase C-γ, phosphatidylinositol 3-kinase, and RAS.

**Table 10.3** Abnormal genes in CLL.

| Abnormality | Frequency (%) | Median survival (months) |
|---|---|---|
| 13q deletion | 50 | 133 |
| 11q deletion | 18 | 79 |
| 12 trisomy | 16 | 114 |
| 17p deletion | 7 | 7 |
| Normal karyotype | 18 | 111 |

## Chronic lymphocytic leukemia

CLL is a low-grade lymphoma marked by a peripheral lymphocytosis of CD5$^+$CD20$^+$CD23$^+$ small lymphocytes similar in morphology to normal lymphocytes. BCL-2, which is expressed at low levels in normal lymphocytes, is expressed at high levels in more than 70% of CLL cases, but this is rarely if ever due to t(14;18). Staging based on presence of lymphadenopathy, organomegaly, anemia or thrombocytopenia can provide prognositic information, with those in the best prognostic groups enjoying normal mean survival times.

Prognosis can also be estimated by purely molecular criteria. In about half of CLL cases, lymphocytes are CD38$^-$IgD$^-$, and contain V$_H$ genes which exhibit somatic hypermutation. In the other half of CLL cases, the malignant lymphocytes resemble a naive B cell, with surface marking CD38$^+$IgD$^+$, and lack V$_H$ mutations. CLL with immunoglobulin V$_H$ genes that exhibit more than 2% somatic hypermutation has significantly better survival than those that are unmutated.

Other B-cell malignancies are characterized by chromosomal translocations, but there are no chromosomal translocations that characterize a significant subset of CLL. However, there are several important genetic abnormalities in the absence of translocations. Whereas conventional Giemsa–trypsin banding analysis of chromosomes from CLL cells detected cytogenetic abnormalities in about half of CLL cases, the higher sensitivity of FISH has allowed the detection of genomic aberrations in 82% of cases. As FISH is a directed rather than a screening technique, conventional banding techniques had previously demonstrated these abnormalities, including del(13q) (50%), del(11q) (18%), +12q (16%), del(17p) (7%) and del(6q) (7%) (Table 10.3). Regression analysis allowed the assignment of 90% of these cases to one of five prognostic classes based on genetic abnormalities. The best prognostic group included those who had 13q deletion as their sole abnormality, with a median survival of 133 months. The worst prognostic group contained those with a 17p deletion, with a mean survival of 32 months. CLL cases with 17p and 11q deletions were more likely to have extensive lymphadenopathy, splenomegaly, cytopenias and B symptoms. Examples of chromosome 13q deletion and trisomy 12 detected by FISH and CGH microarray are shown in Plates 10.3 and 10.4 respectively. These data raise the question of whether the classical clinical staging, which can be used to predict survival, is partly just a surrogate for particular genetic abnormalities, and it is the genetic abnormalities and resulting expression patterns that are more important in determining prognosis.

The specific genes affected by these abnormalities that are important for CLL oncogenesis are not known. The critical tumor suppressor lost in the 13q deletion is probably not RB, but rather a gene that lies telomeric and has so far defied definitive identification. As described above, it is possible that the deletion of two microRNA genes, *mir-15-A* and *mir-16-1*, which downregulate BCL-2 levels, may be important in selecting for this deletion. Tumor suppressor *p53* is involved in 17p deletions. Overall, *p53* abnormalities have been found in at least 15% of patients, and are associated with increased percentage of prolymphocytes and a poorer outcome.

Molecular details of CLL may now be yielding specific therapeutic benefit as well. Nearly all CLL cases demonstrate high levels of BCL-2 expression. Furthermore, data are emerging to suggest that many, if not most, CLL cells are dependent on BCL-2 for survival. It appears that this dependence is largely due to the requirement for BCL-2 to tonically sequester the large amounts of the pro-death molecule BIM that are generated in CLL cells. When BCL-2 function is abrogated, BIM is released, the mitochondria are permeabilized and the cell dies. Exciting new selective inhibitors of CLL are currently in early phase clinical trials in CLL, among other cancers.

## Conclusions

Identification of the genes involved in lymphoma pathogenesis has allowed better characterization of the disease. A fuller understanding of the mechanisms causing specific subgroups of lymphomas should provide us the means to develop specific therapies that will provide rational targets for improved therapies in these diseases.

## Further reading

### Burkitt lymphoma

Battey J, Moulding C, Taub R et al. (1983) The human c-myc oncogene: structural consequences of translocation into the IgH locus in Burkitt lymphoma. Cell, 34, 779–787.

### Diffuse large B-cell lymphoma

Alizadeh AA, Eisen MB, Davis RE et al. (2000) Distinct types of diffuse large B-cell lymphoma identified by gene expression profiling. Nature, 403, 503–511.
Houldsworth J, Mathew S, Rao PH et al. (1996) REL proto-oncogene is frequently amplified in extranodal diffuse large cell lymphoma. Blood, 87, 25–29.
Lenz G, Wright G, Dave SS et al. (2008) Stromal gene signatures in large-B-cell lymphomas. New England Journal of Medicine, 359, 2313–2323.
Monni O, Joensuu H, Franssila K et al. (1997) BCL2 overexpression associated with chromosomal amplification in diffuse large B-cell lymphoma. Blood, 90, 1168–1174.
Pasqualucci L, Migliazza A, Basso K et al. (2003) Mutations of the BCL-6 proto-oncogene disrupt its negative autoregulation in diffuse large B-cell lymphoma. Blood 101, 2914–2923.
Shipp MA, Ross KN, Tamayo P et al. (2002) Diffuse large B-cell lymphoma outcome prediction by gene-expression profiling and supervised machine learning. Nature Medicine, 8, 68–74.
Ye BH, Lista F, Lo Coco F et al. (1993) Alterations of a zinc finger-encoding gene, BCL-6, in diffuse large-cell lymphoma. Science, 262, 747–750.

### Follicular lymphoma

Bernell P, Jacobsson B, Liliemark J et al. (1998) Gain of chromosome 7 marks the progression from indolent to aggressive follicle centre lymphoma and is a common finding in patients with diffuse large B-cell lymphoma: a study by FISH. British Journal of Haematology, 101, 487–491.
Cheng EH, Wei MC, Weiler S et al. (2001) BCL-2, BCL-X(L) sequester BH3 domain-only molecules preventing BAX- and BAK-mediated mitochondrial apoptosis. Molecular Cell, 8, 705–711.
Lo Coco F, Gaidano G, Louie DC et al. (1993) p53 mutations are associated with histologic transformation of follicular lymphoma. Blood, 82, 2289–2295.
McDonnell TJ, Korsmeyer SJ. (1991) Progression from lymphoid hyperplasia to high-grade malignant lymphoma in mice transgenic for the t(14;18). Nature, 349, 254–256.
McDonnell TJ, Deane N, Platt FM et al. (1989) bcl-2-immunoglobulin transgenic mice demonstrate extended B cell survival and follicular lymphoproliferation. Cell, 57, 79–88.

Sander CA, Yano T, Clark HM et al. (1993) p53 mutation is associated with progression in follicular lymphomas. Blood, 82, 1994–2004.
Tsjimoto Y, Yunis J, Onorato-Showe L et al. (1984) Molecular cloning of the chromosomal breakpoint of B-cell lymphomas and leukemias with the t(11;14) chromosome translocation. Science, 224, 1403–1406.
Vaux DL, Cory S, Adams JM. (1988) Bcl-2 gene promotes haemopoietic cell survival and cooperates with c-myc to immortalize pre-B cells. Nature, 335, 440–442.

### Lymphoplasmacytoid lymphoma

Iida S, Rao PH, Nallasivam P et al. (1996) The t(9;14)(p13;q32) chromosomal translocation associated with lymphoplasmacytoid lymphoma involves the PAX-5 gene. Blood, 88, 4110–4117.

### MALT lymphoma

Lucas PC, Yonezumi M, Inohara N et al. (2001) Bcl10 and MALT1, independent targets of chromosomal translocation in malt lymphoma, cooperate in a novel NF-kappa B signaling pathway. Journal of Biological Chemistry, 276, 19012–19019.
Maes B, Demunter A, Peeters B, De Wolf-Peeters C. (2002) BCL10 mutation does not represent an important pathogenic mechanism in gastric MALT-type lymphoma, and the presence of the API2-MLT fusion is associated with aberrant nuclear BCL10 expression. Blood, 99, 1398–1404.
Uren AG, O'Rourke K, Aravind LA et al. (2000) Identification of paracaspases and metacaspases: two ancient families of caspase-like proteins, one of which plays a key role in MALT lymphoma. Molecular Cell, 6, 961–967.

### Chronic lymphocytic leukemia

Calin GA, Ferracin M, Cimmino A et al. (2005) A microRNA signature associated with prognosis and progression in chronic lymphocytic leukemia. New England Journal of Medicine, 353, 1793–1801.
Damle RN, Wasil T, Fais F et al. (1999) Ig V gene mutation status and CD38 expression as novel prognostic indicators in chronic lymphocytic leukemia. Blood, 94, 1840–1847.
Del Gaizo Moore V, Brown J, Certo M et al. (2007) Chronic lymphocytic leukemia requires BCL2 to sequester prodeath BIM, explaining sensitivity to BCL2 antagonist ABT-737. Journal of Clinical Investigation, 117, 112–121.
Dohner H, Stilgenbauer S, Benner A et al. (2000) Genomic aberrations and survival in chronic lymphocytic leukemia. New England Journal of Medicine, 343, 1910–1916.

### Anaplastic large cell lymphoma

Kutok JL, Aster JC. (2002) Molecular biology of anaplastic lymphoma kinase-positive anaplastic large-cell lymphoma. Journal of Clinical Oncology, 20, 3691–3702.
Morris SW, Kirstein MN, Valentine MB et al. (1994) Fusion of a kinase gene, ALK, to a nucleolar protein gene, NPM, in non- Hodgkin's lymphoma. Science, 263, 1281–1284.

# Chapter 11 The molecular biology of multiple myeloma

## Wee Joo Chng[1] & P Leif Bergsagel[2]

[1] National University Cancer Institute, National University Health System of Singapore and; University of Singapore, National University Hospital, Singapore
[2] Division of Hematology-Oncology, Comprehensive Cancer Center, Mayo Clinic Arizona, Scottsdale, AZ, USA

## Introduction

Multiple myeloma (MM) is an incurable post-germinal center B-cell malignancy. In 2009, it is estimated that 20 580 new cases will be diagnosed, with 10 580 patients succumbing to the disease. In many instances it is preceded by a premalignant tumor called *monoclonal gammopathy of undetermined significance* (MGUS), which is the most common lymphoid tumor in humans, occurring in approximately 3% of individuals over the age of 50. The prevalence of both MM and MGUS increases with age, and is about twofold higher in African-Americans than in Caucasians, although the rate of progression from MGUS to MM is similar in these two populations.

### MM is a plasmablast/plasma-cell tumor of post-germinal center B cells

Post-germinal center B cells that have undergone productive somatic hypermutation, antigen selection, and IgH switching can generate plasmablasts, which typically migrate to the bone marrow where the microenvironment enables differ-

entiation into long-lived plasma cells. Importantly, MGUS and MM are monoclonal tumors that are phenotypically similar to plasmablasts/long-lived plasma cells, including a strong dependence on the bone marrow microenvironment for survival and growth. In contrast to normal long-lived plasma cells, MGUS and MM tumors retain some potential for an extremely low rate of proliferation, usually with no more than a few percent of cycling cells until advanced stages of MM.

## Stages of MM

Based on the current diagnostic criteria proposed by the International Myeloma Working Group, four stages of MM can be identified based on the presence of disease-defining symptoms (hypercalcemia, renal impairment, anemia, bone lesions), level of bone marrow plasma cell differentiation and serum or urine monoclonal immunoglobulins, and extramedullary involvement. The stages include MGUS, smoldering myeloma (SMM), symptomatic myeloma, and plasma cell leukemia (PCL) (Table 11.1). MGUS can progress sporadically to MM expressing the same monoclonal immunoglobulins with a probability of about 0.6–3% per year. Through the analysis of several large prospective cohort studies, three predictive factors for progression of MGUS to MM were identified, including M-protein greater than 15 g/L, IgM or IgA M-protein and presence of an abnormal

*Molecular Hematology*, 3rd edition. Edited by Drew Provan and John Gribben.
© 2010 Blackwell Publishing.

**Table 11.1** Features used to diagnose monoclonal gammopathy of undetermined significance (MGUS), smoldering myeloma (SMM) and multiple myeloma (MM).

|  | Serum M-protein | Bone marrow plasma cells | Symptoms |
| --- | --- | --- | --- |
| MGUS | <30 g/L | <10% | None |
| SMM | ≥30 g/L | ≥10% | None |
| MM | Any | Any | Hypercalcemia, anemia, renal impairment and/or bone lesions |

free light chain ratio. In the presence of all three risk factors, the risk of progression at 20 years is 58% compared with 5% in the absence of any of these risk factors. The risk of progression to MM is higher for SMM than MGUS, with a median time to progression ranging from 1 to 5 years. In one study, M-protein in excess of 30 g/L, presence of IgA subtype, and urinary M-protein excretion above 30 g/L were factors associated with early progression to MM. Extramedullary MM is a more aggressive tumor that can present as secondary or primary PCL, depending on whether or not preceding intramedullary MM has been recognized. Human MM cell lines (HMCLs), which are presumed to include most oncogenic events involved in tumor initiation and progression of the corresponding tumor, have been generated mainly from a subset of extramedullary MM tumors.

## Immunoglobulin translocations are present in the majority of MM tumors

Like other post-germinal center B-cell tumors, translocations involving the IgH locus (14q32) or one of the IgL loci (κ, 2p12 or λ, 22q11) are common. In general, these events are mediated by errors in one of the three B-cell specific DNA modification mechanisms: VDJ recombination, IgH switch recombination, or somatic hypermutation. With rare exceptions, these translocations result in dysregulated or increased expression of an oncogene that is positioned near one or more of the strong immunoglobulin enhancers on the translocated derivative chromosome 14. However, translocations involving an IgH switch region uniquely dissociate the intronic from one or both 3′ IgH enhancers, so that an oncogene might be juxtaposed to an IgH enhancer on either or both of the derivative chromosomes, as first demonstrated for *FGFR3* on der(14) and *WHSC1* on der(4) in MM. These IgH translocations are efficiently detected by fluorescence *in situ* hybridization (FISH) analyses. Large studies

from several groups show that the prevalence of IgH translocations increase with disease stage: about 50% in MGUS or SMM, 55–70% for intramedullary MM, 85% in PCL, and above 90% in HMCLs. Limited studies indicate that IgL translocations are present in about 10% of MGUS/SMM tumors, and in about 15–20% of intramedullary MM tumors and HMCL. Translocations involving an Igκ locus are rare, occurring in only 1–2% of MM tumors and HMCLs.

## Marked karyotypic complexity in MM

The karyotypes of MM are characterized by complex abnormalities including both structural and numerical abnormalities. Numerical chromosomal abnormalities are present in virtually all MM tumors and most, if not all, MGUS tumors. There is non-random involvement of different chromosomes in different myeloma tumors, and often heterogeneity among cells within a tumor. A recent large array comparative genomic hybridization (aCGH) analysis of 182 MM patients showed that the median number of aberrations per tumor, as a measure of karyotypic complexity, is significantly higher than other B-cell malignancies such as Waldenström macroglobulinemia, chronic lymphocytic leukemia, and mucosa-associated lymphoid tissue (MALT) lymphoma. The mechanism underlying this karyotypic instability is not fully understood. Centrosome abnormalities, one of the mechanisms mediating chromosomal instability in solid tumors, have been identified in MGUS and about one-third of MM. However, mutations of genes involved in the mitotic spindle checkpoint, another mechanism leading to genomic instability in solid tumors, have not been identified in MM. It is thought that karyotypic complexity increases during tumor progression, although karyotypic progression has not been well documented.

## Chromosome content seems to be associated with at least two different pathogenic pathways

There is a clear consensus that chromosome content reflects at least two pathways of pathogenesis. Approximately half of tumors are hyperdiploid (HRD) (48–75 chromosomes), and typically have multiple trisomies involving chromosomes 3, 5, 7, 9, 11, 15, 19, and 21, but only infrequently (<10%) have one of the recurrent IgH translocations. Non-hyperdiploid (NHRD) tumors (<48 and/or >75 chromosomes) usually (~70%) have one of the recurrent IgH translocations. These patterns of genetic aberration are already present in MGUS, suggesting that the HRD/non-HRD dichotomy is established early during disease pathogenesis, probably at disease initiation, and is dictated by initial oncogenic events. Tumors that have a t(11;14) translocation may represent a distinct category of NHRD tumors as they are often diploid or pseudodiploid, sometimes with this translocation as the only karyotypic abnormality detected by conventional cytogenetics. This turns out to be true for a proportion of t(11;14) MM even when assessed by high-resolution aCGH. In contrast to the selective occurrence of recurrent IgH translocations in NIIRD tumors, other genetic events (17p loss or *TP53* (gene product p53) mutations, *RAS* mutations, secondary immunoglobulin translocations, *MYC* translocations) often occur with a similar prevalence in HRD and NHRD tumors. Extramedullary MM tumors and IIMCLs nearly always have an NHRD phenotype, consistent with the hypothesis that HRD tumors are more stromal cell dependent than NHRD tumors. We have virtually no information about the timing, mechanism, or molecular consequences of hyperdiploidy. We do not know if the extra chromosomes are accumulated one at a time in sequential steps, or as one catastrophic event. For tumors that are HRD but which have one of the recurrent translocations [most often t(4;14)], we do not know if hyperdiploidy occurred before or after the translocation.

## Seven recurrent IgH translocations and the recurrent trisomies of chromosomes 3, 5, 7, 11, 15, 19 and 21 appear to represent primary oncogenic events

There are now seven recurrent chromosomal partners and oncogenes that are involved in IgH translocations in approximately 40% of MM tumors. These translocations lead to the overexpression of three classes of genes: cyclin D, MAF and MMSET/FGFR3 (Table 11.2). The recurrent translocation breakpoints usually occur within or near switch regions, but sometimes within or near VDJ sequences, suggesting that

these translocations are mediated by errors in IgH switch recombination or somatic hypermutation. Since there is no evidence that IgH switch recombination or somatic hypermutation mechanisms are active in normal plasma cells or plasma cell tumors, it is presumed that these translocations usually represent primary, perhaps initiating, oncogenic events as normal B cells pass through germinal centers. In addition, the most common of these translocations, t(4;14), t(11;14) and t(14;16), are already detected in MGUS, further highlighting their early role in disease pathogenesis. With the exception of *FGFR3* (especially with an activating mutation) and possibly *MAF*, the consequences of these translocations have not been adequately confirmed as essential for maintenance of the tumor and/or as therapeutic targets.

In HRD MM, the recurrent trisomies of chromosomes 3, 5, 7, 9, 11, 15, 19, and 21 appear to be the earliest events. In a karyotypic analysis of a large number of HRD myelomas, the presence of these trisomies is associated with the simplest karyotypes, often occurring as the only abnormalities, suggesting that they are the earliest acquired genetic abnormalities in these tumors. The pattern of acquisition of these chromosomal trisomies seems to be random. Furthermore, FISH studies have shown that this pattern of trisomies already exists in MGUS, therefore representing early events.

## Universal cyclin D dysregulation

Analysis of gene expression data suggests that almost all cases of plasma cell neoplasm starting from the MGUS stage express one or more of the cyclin D genes in an aberrant fashion. Therefore, It has been proposed that dysregulation of a cyclin D gene provides a unifying, early oncogenic event in MGUS and MM. MGUS and MM appear closer to normal, non-proliferating plasma cells than to normal proliferating plasmablasts, for which 30% or more of the cells can be in S phase, yet the expression level of cyclin D1, cyclin D2 or cyclin D3 mRNA in MM and MGUS is distinctly higher than in normal plasma cells, in fact at a level comparable to that of cyclin D2 mRNA expressed in normal proliferating plasmablasts. About 25% of MM tumors have an IgH translocation that directly dysregulates a cyclin D gene or a MAF gene encoding a transcription factor that markedly upregulates cyclin D2. Although MM tumors with t(4;14) express moderately high levels of cyclin D2, the cause of increased cyclin D2 expression remains unknown. Although normal bone marrow plasma cells express little or no detectable cyclin D1, the majority of HRD tumors express cyclin D1 biallelically, while most other tumors express increased levels of cyclin D2 compared with normal bone marrow plasma cells, both by unknown mechanism. Only a few percent of MM tumors do not express increased levels of a cyclin D gene compared

**Table 11.2** Recurrent primary IgH translocation partners in MM.

| Gene partner | Genomic locus | Class of gene dysregulated | Frequency |
|---|---|---|---|
| *CCND1* | 11q13 | *CCND* | 15% |
| *CCND2* | 12p13 | *CCND* | <1% |
| *CCND3* | 6p21 | *CCND* | 2% |
| *MAF* | 16q23 | *MAF* | 5% |
| *MAFB* | 21q12 | *MAF* | 2% |
| *MAFC* | 8q24.3 | *MAF* | <1% |
| *MMSET/FGFR3* | 4p16 | *MMSET* and usually *FGFR3* | 15% |

with normal plasma cells, but many of these tumors appear to represent samples that are substantially contaminated by normal cells and another large fraction of these tumors express little or no *RB1*, eliminating the necessity of expressing a cyclin D gene.

## Molecular classification of MM

The advent of microarray technologies has facilitated the global examination of mRNA expression in a highly paralleled fashion. The use of such high-dimension data has allowed the identification of novel disease subtypes. In myeloma, the use of supervised and unsupervised methods has led to the development of two molecular classifications. Interestingly, although the approaches are different, there are significant overlaps between the two classification systems, with the subcategories anchored by known recurrent primary genetic abnormalities, providing strong validation that the primary genetic events drive most of the subsequent changes in cellular transcription in MM.

One of these classifications, the translocation/cyclin D (TC) classification, is based on the spiked expression of genes deregulated by primary IgH translocations and the universal overexpression of cyclin D genes either by these translocations or other mechanisms. The resultant classification identifies eight groups of tumors: those with primary translocations (designated 4p16, 11q13, 6p21, Maf), those that overexpress *CCND1* and *CCND2* either alone or in combination (designated D1, D1+D2, D2), and the rare cases that do not overexpress any cyclin D genes (designated "None"). Most of the patients with HRD MM fall within the D1 and D1+D2 groups. This classification system therefore focuses on the different kinds of mechanism that dysregulate a cyclin D gene as an early and unifying event in pathogenesis.

Recently, the group from the University of Arkansas for Medical Sciences (UAMS) derived another MM classification using an unsupervised approach and identified seven tumor groups characterized by the coexpression of unique gene clusters. Interestingly, these clusters also identify tumors with t(4;14), MAF translocations, t(11;14) and t(6;14), corresponding to the MS, MF and CD-1 and/or CD-2 groups respectively. In this analysis, t(11;14) and t(6;14) can belong to either the CD-1 or CD-2 group depending on expression of CD20 and other B-cell-related genes. This is consistent with the finding that t(11;14) and t(6;14) have very similar expression profiles, clinical profiles and outcome. In contrast to the TC classification, the UAMS classification identifies HRD MM as a distinct HY group. However, this may be somewhat misleading since the HY group, which is about 28% of MM tumors, includes only

about 60% of HRD tumors. The distribution of the remaining HRD tumors among the other six groups has not been clarified, although most are probably in the PR group, defined by increased expression of proliferation-related genes; and the LB group, defined by low bone disease and lower expression of genes associated with bone disease in MM such as *FRZB* and *DKK1*.

There is significant overlap between the TC classification and the UAMS molecular classification. When TC classes are assigned to the 414 MM cases assigned a UAMS molecular classification in the original dataset, the MS and MF groups correspond to the 4p16 and Maf group respectively with 100% concordance. The CD-1 and CD-2 groups together correspond to the 11q13 and 6p21 groups (88% concordance). The HY group contains most of the TC D1 and D1+D2 cases (96% concordance). The bulk of the TC D2 cases (67%) fall within the LB group. The PR group contains a mix of patients from the different TC class: 13% 4p16, 4% Maf, 9% 11q13, 21% D1, 19% D1+D2, 28% D2 and 6% None. The PR group is therefore enriched for *CCND2*-expressing tumors, consistent with the hypothesis that these tumors are more aggressive.

## Prognostic and therapeutic implications of molecular classifications

The intrinsic properties of the tumor cell are informative in predicting the prognosis and the response to existing therapies. In particular, studies over recent years have clearly established the importance of genetic abnormalities in prognosis. For example, it has been well documented that an unfavorable outcome is associated with each of the following: hypodiploidy compared with hyperdiploidy; 17p13 deletion, p53 mutation, t(4;14) and t(14;16). A recent large study from the Intergroupe Francophone du Myélome group has confirmed that t(4;14) and 17p13 deletion are independent prognostic factors in newly diagnosed MM patients undergoing high-dose therapy with stem cell transplantation, and can further dissect each of the International Staging System (ISS) categories. Furthermore, it established that most of the prognostic impact of chromosome 13 deletion is due to the concurrent presence of t(4;14), as patients with chromosome 13 deletion without t(4;14) do not have adverse prognosis. In patients treated with stem cell transplantation, the poor prognosis associated with t(4;14) appears to be due to early disease relapse. These patients derive little benefit from stem cell transplantation and alternative therapeutic strategies are needed.

Recent studies have shown that treatment with bortezomib overcomes the deleterious impact of chromosome 13 deletion on prognosis. This has led to a proposal for risk-stratified management akin to the management of acute leukemias, where genetically defined high-risk patients will be treated with upfront bortezomib- or lenalidomide-based regimen whereas standard-risk patient will receive upfront high-dose therapy with stem cell transplantation after induction therapy. In addition, the genes or pathways deregulated by the specific genetic events could be potential novel therapeutic targets. This is best exemplified by the clinical development of FGFR3 inhibitor therapy for MM with t(4;14).

As the gene expression-based classifications have a strong genetic basis, they could easily identify these high-risk genetic groups, for example the 4p16 and MAF groups in the TC classification and the PR, MS and MF groups in the UAMS classification, and identify the clinically important molecular subtypes of myeloma. In addition, new insights provided by these classifications could be exploited therapeutically. For example, the underlying cyclin D deregulation potentially has an important therapeutic implication, as differential targeting of cyclin D may be very useful and add specificity to treatment. Indeed, some potential agents targeting cyclin D2 have been identified in a drug library screen. In addition, the high CD20 expression in the CD-2 group in the UAMS classification may benefit from anti-CD20 therapy with rituximab.

## Possible events mediating transformation of MGUS to MM

Very few differences between MGUS and MM have been identified at the genetic and molecular level. All the primary genetic events, the recurrent IgH translocations and trisomies of HRD MM are already present in MGUS. By implication, additional genetic events are therefore required for transformation to MM.

## Disruption of other component of RB pathway

Chromosome 13 deletion is one of the most common genetic abnormalities in MM and is also found in MGUS at apparently similar frequency. However, a recent study in a large cohort of MGUS patients suggests that the frequency may be lower in MGUS. It is therefore conceivable that chromosome 13 deletion represents an early secondary event mediating progression to MM. A recent combined analysis of gene expression profiling and aCGH data suggest that the critically deleted gene on chromosome 13 could be *RB1*, a classical tumor-suppressor gene linked with the Knudsen two-hit hypothesis. However, in MM, chromosome 13 deletion is often monoallelic and the other allele is not altered by mutation or epigenetic mechanism. This suggests that *RB1* may be tumorigenic through a haploinsufficiency mechanism. Functional studies using siRNA or adenoviral transfection to modulate gene expression dosage of *RB1* in HMCLs lead to dosage-dependent changes in proliferation. In additional RB protein levels are correlated with DNA and mRNA levels in both HMCLs and patient samples. RB haploinsufficiency may therefore cooperate with cyclin D deregulation and lead to transformation from MGUS to MM. Chromosome 13 deletion is significantly enriched in D2-overexpressing MM (Figure 11.1), in particular those with t(4;14) and t(14;16). Such association suggests that further RB deregulation may be required for cyclin D2, but not cyclin D1, to fully exert its oncogenic potential. Indeed, it has been shown that cyclin D1 is a more potent oncogene than cyclin D2, and can interfere with RB function without both catalytic function and RB binding. Other components of the RB pathway are also commonly dysregulated in MM. The *p16INK4A* and *p15INK4A* genes are methylated in about 20–30% of MGUS and MM tumors, and in most HMCLs. Two recent studies showed that most MM tumors

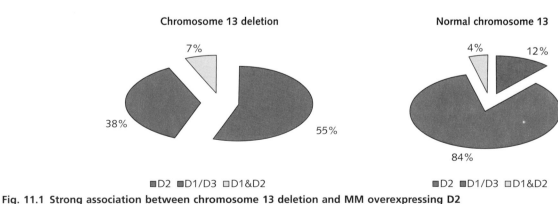

**Fig. 11.1 Strong association between chromosome 13 deletion and MM overexpressing D2**
In an analysis of the gene expression data of 101 MM patients from the Mayo Clinic, 55% of patients with chromosome 13 deletion overexpress *CCND2* whereas only 12% of patients without chromosome 13 deletion overexpress *CCND2*.

express little or no p16 regardless of whether or not the gene is methylated. This suggests that the low expression is not due to methylation, which may be an epiphenomenon. Despite one example of an individual with a germline mutation and loss of the normal p16 allele in MM tumor cells, it remains unclear if inactivation of p16 is a critical and presumably early event in the pathogenesis of MM. In contrast, it seems apparent that inactivation of *p18INK4C*, a critical gene for normal plasma cell development, is likely to contribute to increased proliferation. There is biallelic deletion of p18 in 30% of HMCLs and in nearly 10% of tumors in the highest quintile of proliferation, as determined by an expression-based proliferation index. Forced expression of *p18INK4C* by retroviral infection of HMCLs that express little or no endogenous p18 substantially inhibits proliferation. Paradoxically, about 60% of HMCLs and 60% of the more proliferative MM tumors have increased expression of p18 compared with normal plasma cells. There is evidence that the E2F transcription factor, which is upregulated in association with increased proliferation, increases the expression of p18, presumably as a feedback mechanism. Apart from the lack of a functional RB1 protein in approximately 10% of HMCLs, the mechanism(s) by which most HMCLs and proliferative tumors become insensitive to increased p18 levels is not yet understood.

## Activating *RAS* mutations

Another well-established genetic difference between MGUS and MM is activating *RAS* mutation. The prevalence of activating *N-* or *K-RAS* mutations is about 30–40% of newly diagnosed MM tumors, with only a small increase occurring during tumor progression. The prevalence is about 45% in HMCLs. Importantly, less than 5% of MGUS tumors have *RAS* mutations, consistent with the hypothesis that *RAS* mutations may mark, if not mediate, the MGUS to MM transition. Recent studies indicate that the prevalence of *RAS* mutations is substantially higher in tumors that express *CCND1* compared with tumors that express *CCND2*, with t(4;14) tumors having a particularly low prevalence of *RAS* mutations. Two recent large unpublished studies differ, in that Fonseca and colleagues find *N-RAS* and *K-RAS* mutations in 17% and 6% of tumors, respectively, whereas Kuehl and Shaughnessy find *N-RAS* and *K-RAS* mutations in 14% and 17%, respectively. The latter group also found that the prevalence of *N-RAS* mutations was substantially higher in tumors that express *CCND1*, whereas *K-RAS* mutations occurred with a similar prevalence in tumors that express *CCND1* or *CCND2*. Neither group was able to identify a specific gene expression profile or an effect on prognosis of either *N-* or *K-RAS* mutations.

## MYC activation

Previous gene expression studies have revealed little difference between MGUS and MM. Using a higher density platform with a larger sample set, investigators from UAMS have derived an MGUS signature comprising a small set of genes. However, the biological relevance of this signature, especially with regard to disease transformation, is unclear. The inability of gene expression profiling to identify differences between MM and MGUS may relate to the limitations of conventional comparative analytical methods such as SAM, *t*-test or ANOVA, with multiple testing corrections to extract subtle yet important differences, especially in the setting of the well-known molecular heterogeneity of MM. Recently, two groups using novel analytical approaches have independently identified MYC activation as a common difference between MGUS and newly diagnosed MM, suggesting that MYC activation may be an early transforming event. In one study, the use of gene-set enrichment analysis found that the difference in gene expression between MM and MGUS is strongly and consistently enriched for genes found to be associated with MYC activation in previous published studies. As MM is more proliferative than MGUS and MYC activation is associated with proliferation, a MYC activation signature, comprising MYC transcriptional targets, not related to proliferation was derived and found to be present in about 60% of MM, but not in MGUS. Among the MMs that express the MYC signature, only a percentage has high expression of MYC, suggesting that mechanisms other than IgH–MYC may mediate MYC activation. Indeed, activating RAS mutation is strongly associated with the activation of MYC signature, suggesting a link between RAS mutation and MYC activation (Figure 11.2). In another study, using Bayesian statistics to compute the probability of each sample expressing different oncogene signatures, it was found that the most significant change from MGUS to MM relates to MYC activation. These *in silico* analyses using large cohorts of MGUS and MM are therefore suggestive of MYC activation as a common transformation event. The biological validity of these *in silico* observations is provided by a recent MM mouse model, which utilizes activation induced cytidine deaminase (AID)-dependent somatic hypermutation to activate the MYC oncogene sporadically. In mice with a genetic predisposition to developing monoclonal gammopathy, the sporadic activation of MYC led to the development of MM in these mice. Recently, MYC was shown to be directly involved in DNA replication, binding and activating DNA replicative origins and regulating S-phase transition during the cell cycle through a non-transcriptional mechanism. Therefore, in MM, activation of MYC may cooperate with cyclin D/RB deregulation – which negates the early $G_1S$ cell cycle checkpoint that allows the establishment of the

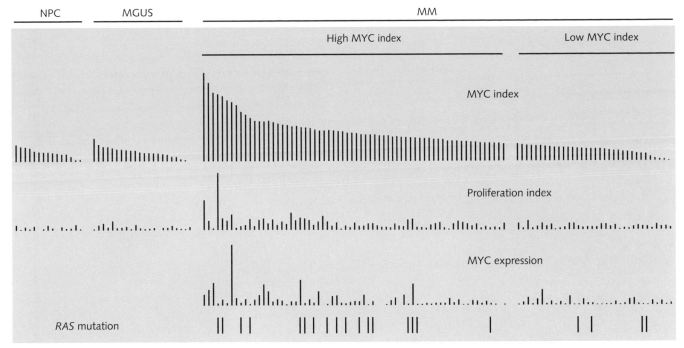

**Fig. 11.2 MYC activation is common in MM**

Almost 60% of MM express a MYC activation signature (at levels higher than normal plasma cells and MGUS), represented here as a rank order of a calculated MYC index. Of note, only some of these patients also have high MYC gene expression. Almost all the cases with an activating *RAS* mutation also express the MYC activation signature. Most patients with *RAS* mutation have low MYC gene expression, suggesting that *RAS* mutation and MYC overexpression are alternate ways to activating MYC. Additional non-overlapping mechanisms of activating MYC may be involved.

initial limited clonal plasma cell expansion (MGUS) – to overcome remaining cell cycle constraints leading to further clonal expansion and transformation to MM.

## NFκB and STAT activation represent major divergent secondary pathways

It has long been felt that activation of the NFκB pathway is important in the pathogenesis of MM, but little is known about the prevalence of NFκB activation or mechanisms that cause NFκB activation. Recently, an array of mutations that result in the constitutive activation of the NFκB pathway have been identified in about 20% of patient samples and about 50% of HMCLs. The most common event is inactivating mutations of *TRAF3* in 13% of patients. In addition inactivating mutations of *TRAF2*, *BIRC2/BIR3* (gene product cIAP1/2), and *CYLD* were identified. Chromosome translocations and amplifications resulting in activation of NFκB-inducing kinase (NIK), CD40, LTBR, TACI, NFκB1, and NFκB2 were also reported. Although activation of both the canonical and non-canonical pathways is seen, the preponderance of mutations result most directly in increased processing of NFκB2 p100 to p52 (i.e., activation of the non-

canonical pathway). Depletion of NIK with shRNAs directed against NIK results in inhibition of both the classical and alternative NFκB pathways, and also growth inhibition. Half of primary MM tumors have an expression signature of NFκB target genes, with activating mutations identified in less then half of these patients. Presumably either other mutations or ligand-dependent interactions in the bone marrow microenvironment are responsible for the NFκB activation in the remaining patients. There appears to be some segregation between the underlying genetics and the mechanism of activating NFκB. Pooling results from three large gene expression studies in MM, an analysis of the association between *TRAF3* mutations (using low *TRAF3* expression as a surrogate) and the TC subtypes showed that low *TRAF3* expression is significantly associated with t(4;14) and D2 tumors, whereas it is rare in MAF and D1 tumors (Figure 11.3a). Interestingly for the latter group, the tumors either have enhanced interaction with the microenvironment through MAF activation or are more dependent on the microenvironment and may derive their NFκB signals predominantly from the microenvironment. For the t(4;14) and D2 tumors, the acquisition of autonomous NFκB signals through gene mutations may mediate their more aggressive

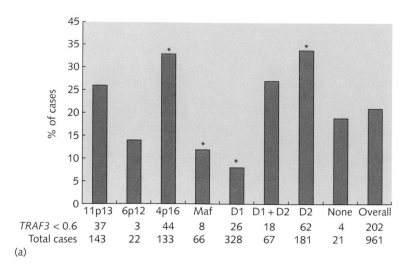

| | 11p13 | 6p12 | 4p16 | Maf | D1 | D1 + D2 | D2 | None | Overall |
|---|---|---|---|---|---|---|---|---|---|
| *TRAF3* < 0.6 | 37 | 3 | 44 | 8 | 26 | 18 | 62 | 4 | 202 |
| Total cases | 143 | 22 | 133 | 66 | 328 | 67 | 181 | 21 | 961 |

(a)

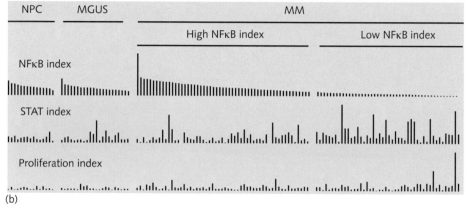

(b)

**Fig. 11.3 NFκB and STAT3 activation in MM**

(a) Analyzing gene expression data from three large published studies, *TRAF3* inactivation, using a normalized *TRAF3* mRNA expression of less than 0.6 as a surrogate, is significantly more common in t(4;14) and D2 tumors than D1 (hyperdiploid) and MAF tumors. (b) NFκB activation (high NFκB index) is present in about 50% of patients. In the other patients, the STAT3 pathway (STAT3 index) is relatively more activated. Patients with STAT3 activation also seem to be more proliferative. Unlike the NFκB pathway, which is also activated in normal plasma cells, STAT3 activation is predominantly a function of the malignant cells.

characteristics and relatively lower microenvironment dependence. Clearly we need to know more about intrinsic and extrinsic mechanisms that activate the NFκB pathway in MM, as this seems a potentially important pathway for therapeutic intervention. Further analysis of gene expression data suggests that those patients who do not express the NFκB signature overexpressed genes enriched for the interleukin (IL)-6/STAT3 pathways. Activation of NFκB and STAT3 signatures are generally mutually exclusive, with only 10% of cases expressing both (Figure 11.3b). The mechanism for STAT3 activation is probably related in large part to autocrine or paracrine IL-6. Whether mutations of genes in the STAT pathway, similar to NFκB, may contribute to constitutive signaling is current unknown.

## Late events in MM progression

### Abnormalities of *TP53* gene and chromosome 17p loss

Mutations of *TP53* are relatively rare in newly diagnosed MM, occurring in approximately 5% of tumors. However, the frequency of mutations appears to increase with disease stage, and is about 30% in PCL and 65% in HMCLs. Deletion (mainly monoallelic) of the *TP53* locus, as detected by interphase FISH, occurs in about 10% of MM and approximately 40% of PCL and HMCLs. However, it should be noted that there is no definitive evidence that the critical chromosome

17p loss is *TP53*. Certainly, *TP53* is contained within the minimal deleted region on 17p13, as found by an aCGH analysis of 67 MM patients from the Mayo Clinic. Occasionally, these deletions can be quite small, and thus not always detected by interphase FISH using BAC probes. Although almost all 17p13 deletions detected are monoallelic, there has been no definitive analysis of *TP53* mutation of the remaining allele in these patients to conclusively implicate *TP53* as the critical gene. In a large study comprising 268 MM patients entered into Eastern Cooperative Oncology Group (ECOG) combination chemotherapy studies, only 5 of 31 (16%) patients with 17p13 deletion had mutation of the remaining *TP53* allele. However, the use of whole bone marrow DNA may have resulted in markedly reduced sensitivity of the study. In a smaller study (24 newly diagnosed MM patients) using purified CD138⁺ plasma cells, no *TP53* mutations were detected, but it is unclear whether these samples also had 17p13 deletion. Therefore, current evidence does not exclude *TP53* as the critical gene deleted on 17p13. Furthermore, the actual impact of 17p13 monoallelic deletion on the p53 pathway and whether other cooperating deregulation (e.g., epigenetic silencing of p53 or increased expression of MDM2) of various components of the pathway are involved needs to be further clarified.

## Gain of chromosome 1q and loss of chromosome 1p

A number of laboratories have determined, using a combination of FISH, aCGH and gene expression profiling, that there is a gain of sequences, and corresponding increased gene expression, at 1q21 in 30–40% of tumors. These gains are concentrated substantially in those tumors that have t(4;14) or t(14;16), or which have a high proliferation expression index. It has been proposed that the increased proliferation in tumors with gain of 1q21 sequences is due to the increased expression of *CKS1B* as a result of increased copy number. One might expect to find other mechanisms, such as localized amplification or a translocation, if increased *CKS1B* expression is a cause of increased proliferation, but there is no evidence for other mechanisms to increase *CKS1B* expression. Furthermore, *CKS1B* expression correlates closely with the expression of a number of proliferation genes and therefore appears to be a consequence rather then a cause of the proliferation. So, it seems prudent to remain skeptical that *CKS1B* is the gene targeted by gain of 1q21 sequences. Furthermore, amplification of chromosome 1q tends to involve the whole q arm, and on aCGH the minimally deleted areas do not always include *CKS1B*.

Chromosome 1p loss is also common, occurring in about 46% of patients when analyzed by aCGH and in 7–36% in previous karyotype studies. Unlike 1q gain, 1p loss is usually interstitial and involves fragments of varying length. Chromosome 1p loss has been shown to be a marker of poor prognosis in cytogenetic studies.

Both 1p loss and 1q gain are therefore associated with poor prognosis. Of note, a recently developed high-risk gene expression signature from UAMS is significantly enriched for genes downregulated on 1p and upregulated on 1q in patients with the shortest survival. In addition, chromosome 1p loss and 1q gain also tend to occur in the setting of more complex karyotype and in the presence of other poor prognostic features such as adverse genetics and increased proliferation index or at relapse. Although there has been great interest in identifying important genes deleted or gained in these regions that may have functional impact on tumor progression, it is also likely that aberrations in these genomic loci represent a bystander marker of genomic instability. Indeed studies have shown that a chromosome instability signature is a predictor of poor prognosis across a broad spectrum of cancers.

## Secondary translocations dysregulate MYC

While translocations involving the recurrent translocation partners appear to be primary events, translocations of *MYC* appear to be secondary events that do not involve B-cell-specific recombination mechanisms, are often complex, and sometimes do not involve immunoglobulin loci. Using FISH analysis, rearrangements of *MYC* are reported in only 15% of MM tumors (with frequent heterogeneity within a tumor) but in nearly 40% of advanced MM tumors and 90% of HMCLs. Regarding the approximately 20% of IgH translocations not involving the recurrent partners, little is known about the multitude of partners and oncogenes. These IgH translocations, as well as most translocations involving IgL loci, share many similarities with MYC translocations and have similar frequency in HRD and NHRD tumors (whereas the recurrent or primary translocations occur predominantly in NHRD tumors). Thus, most of them are likely to represent secondary immunoglobulin translocations that can occur at any stage of tumorigenesis, including MGUS.

## Model of molecular pathogenesis of MM

Based on the results summarized above, a model for the molecular pathogenesis of MM has been proposed. Chromosome content appears to identify two different, but perhaps overlapping, pathways of pathogenesis: NHRD tumors and HRD tumors. In about 40% of the tumors, a primary chromosome translocation results in the dysregulated expression

**Table 11.3** Well-characterized genetic subtypes of MM.

| Genetics | Ploidy | Prognosis | Heavy chain | Light chain | Morphology | CD20 | RAS mutation | 13 deletion | TRAF3 mutation | Bone DKK1 | CCND |
|---|---|---|---|---|---|---|---|---|---|---|---|
| t(11;14) t(6;14) | NHRD/ diploid | Good | G | κ | Lymphoplasmacytoid | ++ | ++ | −/+ | + | ++ | D1 D3 |
| t(4;14) | NHRD | Poor | A | λ | Plasmablastic | − | − | +++ | ++ | −/+ | D2 |
| t(14;16) t(8;14) t(14;20) | NHRD | Poor | A | λ | Plasmablastic | + | − | ++ | −/+ | −/+ | D2 |
| Trisomies | HRD | Good | G | κ | Normal | − | ++ | −/+ | −/+ | ++ | D1 |

HRD, hyperdiploid; NHRD, non-hyperdiploid.

of an oncogene. These primary genetic events lead to cyclin D dysregulation either directly [cyclin D1 in t(11;14) and cyclin D3 in t(6;14)] or indirectly [cyclin D2 in t(4;14) and maf translocations] or by an as yet unknown mechanism (cyclin D1 and/or D2 in HRD MM). The dysregulation of one of three cyclin D genes may render the cells more susceptible to proliferative stimuli, resulting in selective expansion as a result of interaction with bone marrow stromal cells that produce IL-6 and other cytokines. These primary genetic events, primary IgH translocations and trisomies of chromosomes 3, 5, 7, 9, 11, 15, 19 and 21 are already present at the earliest identified stage of tumorigenesis, and define subtypes of MM with unique clinical (bone disease, heavy-chain subtypes, prognosis), molecular (types of cyclin D expressed, associated mutations), pathological (morphology, CD expression), and cytogenetic (ploidy) features (Table 11.3).

A second genetic "hit" leading to subsequent transformation from MGUS to MM may be mediated by activation of MYC or further deregulation of the RB pathway. The MYC pathway may be activated by *RAS* mutation, IgH-*MYC* translocations or other as yet unidentified mechanisms. The RB pathway may be further deregulated by RB haploinsufficiency or p18 loss. These mechanisms are not mutually exclusive and the pattern of cooperation is still not yet understood. There appears to be enrichment for some pathway deregulation depending on primary genetic abnormalities. For example, tumors with cyclin D2 overexpression are significantly enriched for chromosome 13 deletion and hence RB haploinsufficiency, whereas *RAS* mutations are significantly associated with t(11;14) tumors.

The NFκB and STAT3 pathways appear to be generally mutually exclusive secondary pathways probably important for providing the growth and survival signals for maintenance of tumor cell survival, growth and proliferation. Both pathways can be activated through external signals from the tumor microenvironment, such as IL-6 (STAT3 pathway), or signaling triggered by contact between the malignant plasma cells and the accessory cells in the bone marrow microenvironment (NFκB pathway). Alternative mechanisms intrinsic to the tumor cells such as gene mutations may also activate these pathways (e.g., mutations in the NFκB pathway).

Later events that may lead to more aggressive tumor characteristics and emancipation from dependence on the bone marrow microenvironment include mutation of *TP53* or deletion of the *TP53* locus on chromosome 17p13, and complex secondary translocations. In the future, it would be important to further interrogate how these pathways interact with each other, and differentiate the critical from noncritical pathways during tumorigenesis that should be targeted therapeutically.

## Critical role of the bone marrow microenvironment in maintaining the tumor clone and mediating drug resistance and novel therapeutic strategies targeting the bone marrow milieu

As mentioned before, different molecular pathways can be activated in the malignant plasma cells by intrinsic or extrinsic mechanisms, either through microenvironment signals derived from cytokines or via interaction between the tumor cells and accessory cells in the bone marrow microenvironment such as stromal cells, endothelial cells, osteoclasts and osteoblasts. Direct contact between MM cells and cells of the bone marrow milieu induce paracrine or autocrine release of cytokines and growth factors such as IL-6, insulin-like growth factor, hepatocyte growth factor and vascular endothelial growth factor, which provide further proliferative and survival signals by activating intracellular pathways such as PI3K/AKT/mTOR/p70S6K, IKK-α/NFκB, RAS/RAF/MAPK and JAK/STAT3.

**Table 11.4** Therapeutic compounds targeting the bone marrow microenvironment.

| Target | Pathway activated | Therapy |
|---|---|---|
| **Targeting growth factors and cytokines** | | |
| IL-6 | Ras/Raf/Mek/Erk | IL-6 antibodies |
| | JAK2/STAT3 | IL-6R antibodies |
| | PI3K/AKT | IL-6 superantagonist (SANT7) |
| IGF-1 | Ras/Raf/Mek/Erk | IGF1R kinase inhibitor (NVP-ADW742) |
| | NFκB | IGF1R antibodies |
| | PI3K/AKT | IGF-1 ligand antibodies |
| VEGF | Ras/Raf/Mek/Erk | VEGFR tyrosine kinase inhibitor (PTK787, GW654652, Pazopanib) |
| β-Catenin | Wnt | PKF115-584 |
| DKK1 | Wnt | Anti-DKK1 neutralizing antibodies |
| **Targeting interactions between MM plasma cells and accessory cells** | | |
| Adhesion molecules | | Proteasome inhibitors (bortezomib, NPI-52, PR-171) |
| Cell adherence | | Proteasome inhibitors Imids (Revlimid, thalidomide) |
| **Intracellular signaling molecules** | | |
| PI3K | | PI3 kinase inhibitor (Wartmannin, LY294002) |
| AKT | | Perifosine |
| mTOR | | Rapamycin, CCI-779 |
| MEK/ERK | | MEK1/2 inhibitor (AZD6244) |
| BCL2/ BCL-XL | | BCL2 antisense oligonucleotide BCL2/BCL-XL inhibitor (ABT-737) |

IGF, insulin-like growth factor; PI3K, phosphatidylinositol 3-kinase; VEGF, vascular endothelial growth factor.

These interactions and the activated pathways not only provide growth and survival signals but also result in the uncoupling of new bone formation from bone resorption, leading to the formation of lytic bone lesions and resistance of the tumor cells to different chemotherapeutic agents. The importance of the bone marrow microenvironment in MM biology is highlighted by the spate of new drugs being developed to target these cytokines/growth factors or contact-mediated pathways (Table 11.4). The recent

Food and Drug Administration-approved drugs thalidomide, bortezomib and lenalidomide are all thought to exert their therapeutic effect at least partly through targeting the microenvironment.

## Conclusion

Significant progress has been made in understanding the molecular pathogenesis and biology of MM. Oncogenic pathways can be activated through cell intrinsic or extrinsic mechanisms. Similar to other cancers, MM is characterized by the multistage accumulation of genetic abnormalities deregulating different pathways. Much of this knowledge is already being utilized for diagnosis, prognosis and risk stratification of patients. Importantly, from a clinical standpoint, this knowledge has led to development of novel therapeutic strategies, some of which are already in clinical use, and many others showing promise in preclinical and early clinical studies.

## Further reading

Chng WJ, Glebov O, Bergsagel PL, Kuehl WM. (2007) Genetic events in the pathogenesis of multiple myeloma. *Best Practice in Research and Clinical Hematology*, **20**, 571–96.

Cohen HJ, Crawford J, Rao MK *et al.* (1998) Racial differences in the prevalence of monoclonal gammopathy in a community-based sample of the elderly. *American Journal of Medicine*, **104**, 439–444.

Hideshima T, Mitsiades C, Tonon G, Richardson PG, Anderson KC. (2007) Understanding multiple myeloma pathogenesis in the bone marrow to identify new therapeutic targets. *Nature Reviews. Cancer*, **7**, 585–598.

Jemal A, Siegel R, Ward E, Hao Y, Xu J, Thun MJ. (2009) Cancer statistics. *CA. A Cancer Journal for Clinicians*, **59**, 225–249.

Kyle RA, Rajkumar SV. (2007) Monoclonal gammopathy of undetermined significance and smoldering multiple myeloma. *Hematology Oncology Clinics of North America*, **21**, 1093–1113

Kyle RA, Therneau TM, Rajkumar SV *et al.* (2002) A long-term study of prognosis in monoclonal gammopathy of undetermined significance. *New England Journal of Medicine*, **346**, 564–569.

Mitsiades CS, McMillin DW, Klippel S *et al.* (2007) The role of the bone marrow microenvironment in the pathophysiology of myeloma and its significance in the development of more effective therapies. *Hematology Oncology Clinics of North America*, **21**, 1007–1034.

Rajkumar SV, Kyle RA, Therneau TM *et al.* (2005) Serum free light chain ratio is an independent risk factor for progression in monoclonal gammopathy of undetermined significance. *Blood*, **106**, 812–817.

### Cytogenetics

Avet-Loiseau H, Facon T, Grosbois B *et al.* (2002) Oncogenesis of multiple myeloma: 14q32 and 13q chromosomal abnormalities are not randomly distributed, but correlate with natural history, immunological features, and clinical presentation. *Blood*, **99**, 2185–2191.

Bergsagel PL, Kuehl WM. (2001) Chromosomal translocations in multiple myeloma. *Oncogene*, **20**, 5611–5622.

Fonseca R, Bailey RJ, Ahmann GJ *et al.* (2002) Genomic abnormalities in monoclonal gammopathy of undetermined significance. *Blood*, **100**, 1417–1424.

Fonseca R, Blood E, Rue M *et al.* (2003) Clinical and biologic implications of recurrent genomic aberrations in myeloma. *Blood*, **101**, 4569–4575.

## IgH translocations

Bergsagel PL, Chesi MC, Nardini E *et al.* (1996) Promiscuous translocations into immunoglobulin heavy chain switch regions in multiple myeloma. *Proceedings of the National Academy of Sciences of the United States of America*, **93**, 13931–13936.

Chesi M, Bergsagel PL, Brents LA *et al.* (1996) Dysregulation of cyclin D1 by translocation into an IgH gamma switch region in two multiple myeloma cell lines. *Blood*, **88**, 674–681.

Chesi M, Nardini E, Brents LA *et al.* (1997) Frequent translocation t(4;14)(p16.3;q32.3) in multiple myeloma is associated with increased expression and activating mutations of fibroblast growth factor receptor 3. *Nature Genetics*, **16**, 260–264.

Chesi M, Nardini E, Lim RSC *et al.* (1998) The t(4;14) translocation in myeloma dysregulates both FGFR3 and a novel gene, MMSET, resulting in IgH/MMSET hybrid transcripts. *Blood*, **92**, 3025–3034.

Chesi M, Bergsagel PL, Shonukan OO *et al.* (1998) Frequent dysregulation of the c-maf proto-oncogene at 16q23 by translocation to an Ig locus in multiple myeloma. *Blood*, **91**, 4457–4463.

Garand R, Avet-Loiseau H, Accard F *et al.* (2003) t(11;14) and t(4;14) translocations correlated with mature lymphoplasmacytoid and immature morphology, respectively, in multiple myeloma. *Leukemia*, **17**, 2032–2035.

Hurt EM, Wiestner A, Rosenwald A *et al.* (2004) Overexpression of c-maf is a frequent oncogenic event in multiple myeloma that promotes proliferation and pathological interactions with bone marrow stroma. *Cancer Cell*, **5**, 191–199.

Shaughnessy J, Gabrea A, Qi Y *et al.* (2001) Cyclin D3 at 6p21 is dysregulated by recurrent Ig translocations in multiple myeloma. *Blood*, **98**, 217–223.

## Molecular genetic classification

Bergsagel PL, Kuehl WM, Zhan F, Sawyer J, Barlogie B, Shaughnessy J Jr. (2005) Cyclin D dysregulation: an early and unifying pathogenic event in multiple myeloma. *Blood*, **106**, 296–303.

Chng WJ, Van Wier SA, Ahmann GJ *et al.* (2005) A validated FISH trisomy index demonstrates the hyperdiploid and nonhyperdiploid dichotomy in MGUS. *Blood*, **106**, 2156–2161.

Chng WJ, Kumar S, Van Wier S *et al.* (2007) Molecular dissection of hyperdiploid multiple myeloma by gene expression profiling. *Cancer Research*, **67**, 2982–2989.

Fonseca R, Debes-Marun CS, Picken EB *et al.* (2003) The recurrent IgH translocations are highly associated with non-hyperdiploid variant multiple myeloma. *Blood*, **102**, 2562–2567.

Fonseca R, Barlogie B, Bataille R *et al.* (2004) Genetics and cytogenetics of multiple myeloma: a workshop report. *Cancer Research*, **64**, 1546–1558.

Smadja NV, Bastard C, Brigaudeau C *et al.* (2001) Hypodiploidy is a major prognostic factor in multiple myeloma. *Blood*, **98**, 2229–2238.

Tian E, Zhan F, Walker R *et al.* (2003) The role of the Wnt-signaling antagonist DKK1 in the development of osteolytic lesions in multiple myeloma. *New England Journal of Medicine*, **349**, 2483–2494.

Zhan F, Huang Y, Colla S *et al.* (2006) The molecular classification of multiple myeloma. *Blood*, **108**, 2020–2028.

Zhan F, Barlogie B, Arzoumanian V *et al.* (2007) Gene-expression signature of benign monoclonal gammopathy evident in multiple myeloma is linked to good prognosis. *Blood*, **109**, 1692–1700.

## Genetic prognostic factors

Avet-Loiseau H, Li JY, Morineau N *et al.* (1999) Monosomy 13 is associated with the transition of monoclonal gammopathy of undetermined significance to multiple myeloma. Intergroupe Francophone du Myelome. *Blood*, **94**, 2583–2589.

Avet-Loiseau H, Attal M, Moreau P, *et al.* (2007) Genetic abnormalities and survival in multiple myeloma: the experience of the Intergroupe Francophone du Myélome. *Blood*, **109**, 3489–3495.

Chng WJ, Santana-Dávila R, Van Wier SA *et al.* (2006) Prognostic factors for hyperdiploid-myeloma: effects of chromosome 13 deletions and IgH translocations. *Leukemia*, **20**, 807–813.

Facon T, Avet-Loiseau H, Guillerm G *et al.* (2001) Chromosome 13 abnormalities identified by FISH analysis and serum beta2-microglobulin produce a powerful myeloma staging system for patients receiving high-dose therapy. *Blood*, **97**, 1566–1571.

Fonseca R, Harrington D, Oken MM *et al.* (2002) Biological and prognostic significance of interphase fluorescence in situ hybridization detection of chromosome 13 abnormalities (delta13) in multiple myeloma: an Eastern Cooperative Oncology Group study. *Cancer Research*, **62**, 715–720.

Fonseca R, Van Wier SA, Chng WJ *et al.* (2006) Prognostic value of chromosome 1q21 gain by fluorescent in situ hybridization and increase CKS1B expression in myeloma. *Leukemia*, **20**, 2034–2040.

Hanamura I, Stewart JP, Huang Y *et al.* (2006) Frequent gain of chromosome band 1q21 in plasma-cell dyscrasias detected by fluorescence in situ hybridization: incidence increases from MGUS to relapsed myeloma and is related to prognosis and disease progression following tandem stem-cell transplantation. *Blood*, **108**, 1724–1732.

Moreau P, Facon T, Leleu X *et al.* (2002) Recurrent 14q32 translocations determine the prognosis of multiple myeloma, especially in patients receiving intensive chemotherapy. *Blood*, **100**, 1579–1583.

Shaughnessy JD Jr, Zhan F, Burington BE *et al.* (2006) A validated gene expression model of high-risk multiple myeloma is defined by deregulated expression of genes mapping to chromosome 1. *Blood*, **109**, 2276–2284.

## Secondary genetic events

Annunziata CM, Davis RE, Demchenko Y *et al.* (2007) Frequent engagement of the classical and alternative NF-kappaB pathways by diverse genetic abnormalities in multiple myeloma. *Cancer Cell*, **12**, 115–130.

Avet-Loiseau H, Gerson F, Margrangeas F *et al.* (2001) Rearrangements of the c-myc oncogene are present in 15% of primary human multiple myeloma tumors. *Blood*, **98**, 3082–3086.

Chesi M, Brents LA, Ely SA *et al.* (2001) Activated fibroblast growth factor receptor 3 is an oncogene that contributes to tumor progression in multiple myeloma. *Blood*, **97**, 729–736.

Chesi M, Robbiani DF, Sebag M *et al.* (2008) AID-dependent activation of a MYC transgene induces multiple myeloma in a conditional mouse model of post-germinal center malignancies. *Cancer Cell*, **13**, 167–180.

Chng WJ, Price-Troska T, Gonzalez-Paz N *et al.* (2007) Clinical significance of TP53 mutation in myeloma. *Leukemia*, **21**, 582–584.

**Dib A, Peterson TR, Raducha-Grace L *et al.* (2006) Paradoxical expression of INK4c in proliferative multiple myeloma tumors: bi-allelic deletion vs increased expression. *Cell Division*, **1**, 23.

Fonseca R, Price-Troska T, Blood E *et al.* (2003) Implication of N-ras and K-ras mutation in clinical outcome and biology of multiple myeloma. *Blood*, **102**, 113a.

Gonzalez-Paz N, Chng WJ, McClure RF *et al.* (2007) Tumor suppressor p16 methylation in multiple myeloma: biological and clinical implications. *Blood*, **109**, 1228–1232.

Keats JJ, Fonseca R, Chesi M *et al.* (2007) Promiscuous mutations activate the noncanonical NF-kappaB pathway in multiple myeloma. *Cancer Cell*, **12**, 131–144.

Liu P, Leong T, Quam L *et al.* (1996) Activating mutations of N and Kras in multiple myeloma show different clinical associations: analysis of the Eastern Cooperative Oncology Group Phase III Trial. *Blood*, **88**, 2699–2706.

Neri A, Baldini L, Trecca D *et al.* (1993) p53 gene mutations in multiple myeloma are associated with advanced forms of malignancy. *Blood*, **81**, 128–135.

Rasmussen T, Kuehl M, Lodahl M, Johnsen HE, Dahl IM. (2005) Possible roles for activating RAS mutations in the MGUS to MM transition and in the intramedullary to extramedullary transition in some plasma cell tumors. *Blood*, **105**, 317–323.

Shou Y, Martelli ML, Gabrea A *et al.* (2000) Diverse karyotypic abnormalities of the c-myc locus associated with c-myc dysregulation and tumor progression in multiple myeloma. *Proceedings of the National Academy of Sciences of the United States of America*, **97**, 228–233.

## Targeting genetic abnormalities

Malumbres M, Barbacid M. (2001) To cycle or not to cycle: a critical decision in cancer. *Nature Reviews. Cancer*, **1**, 222–231.

Trudel S, Ely SA, Farooqi Y *et al.* (2004) Inhibition of fibroblast growth factor receptor 3 induces differentiation and apoptosis in t(4;14) myeloma. *Blood*, **103**, 3521–3528.

Trudel S, Li ZH, Wei E *et al.* (2005) CHIR-258, a novel, multitargeted tyrosine kinase inhibitor for the potential treatment of t(4;14) multiple myeloma. *Blood*, **105**, 2941–2948.

Trudel S, Stewart AK, Rom E *et al.* (2006) The inhibitory anti-FGFR3 antibody, PRO-001, is cytotoxic to t(4;14) multiple myeloma cells. *Blood*, **107**, 4039–4046.

## Current therapy

Adams J. (2004) The proteasome: a suitable antineoplastic target. *Nature Reviews. Cancer*, **4**, 349–360.

Attal M, Harousseau JL, Stoppa AM *et al.* (1996) A prospective, randomized trial of autologous bone marrow transplantation and chemotherapy in multiple myeloma. Intergroupe Francais du Myelome. *New England Journal of Medicine*, **335**, 91–97.

Attal M, Harousseau JL, Facon T *et al.* (2003) Single versus double autologous stem-cell transplantation for multiple myeloma. *New England Journal of Medicine*, **349**, 2495–2502.

Bartlett JB, Dredge K, Dalgleish AG. (2004) The evolution of thalidomide and its IMiD derivatives as anticancer agents. *Nature Reviews. Cancer*, **4**, 314–322.

Child JA, Morgan GJ, Davies FE *et al.* (2003) High-dose chemotherapy with hematopoietic stem-cell rescue for multiple myeloma. *New England Journal of Medicine*, **348**, 1875–1883.

Dimopoulos M, Spencer A, Attal M *et al.* (2007) Lenalidomide plus dexamethasone for relapsed or refractory multiple myeloma. *New England Journal of Medicine*, **357**, 2123–2132.

Dispenzieri A, Rajkumar SV, Gertz MA *et al.* (2007) Treatment of newly diagnosed multiple myeloma based on mayo stratification of myeloma and risk-adapted therapy (mSMART): consensus statement. *Mayo Clinic Proceedings*, **82**, 323–341.

Mulligan G, Mitsiades C, Bryant B *et al.* (2007) Gene expression profiling and correlation with outcome in clinical trials of the proteasome inhibitor bortezomib. *Blood*, **109**, 3177–3188.

Richardson PG, Sonneveld P, Schuster MW *et al.* (2005) Bortezomib or high-dose dexamethasone for relapsed multiple myeloma. *New England Journal of Medicine*, **352**, 2487–2498.

Singhal S, Mehta J, Desikan R *et al.* (1999) Antitumor activity of thalidomide in refractory multiple myeloma. *New England Journal of Medicine*, **341**, 1565–1571.

Weber DM, Chen C, Niesvizky R *et al.* (2007) Lenalidomide plus dexamethasone for relapsed multiple myeloma in North America. *New England Journal of Medicine*, **357**, 2133–2142.

# Chapter 12  The molecular basis of anemia

Lucio Luzzatto[1] & Anastasios Karadimitris[2]

[1] National Institute for Cancer Research, Istituto Scientifico Tumori, Genova, Italy
[2] Department of Haematology, Imperial College London, Hammersmith Hospital Campus, London, UK

## Introduction

The title of this chapter is quite ambitious, and in this respect we beg the reader's indulgence. In fact, as hematologists we must have the ambition to explain anemia at the molecular level; this has been done successfully in some cases but not yet in others. One major reason is that anemia is not a disease, but a vast collection of diseases, extremely heterogeneous in terms of etiology, pathophysiology and clinico-hematological manifestations, as well as in our ability to treat them effectively. Since this book focuses on molecular pathophysiology, it is particularly pertinent to blood diseases that have a genetic basis. There are three main groups of anemia that qualify in this respect: (i) hemoglobinopathies, covered in *Chapters 1 and 15*; (ii) red cell membrane cytoskeleton disorders, which are not covered in this book; and (iii) inherited hemolytic anemia due to enzyme abnormalities, covered in this chapter. In addition, considering the space allocated to this chapter, we have included several other types of inherited and acquired anemias: our main inclusion criterion was that, based on current knowledge, we could offer at least some meaningful discussion of their molecular basis. In this area, since the first edition of this book, there have been at least three breakthrough additions: (i) autosomal dominant dyskeratosis congenita is due to mutations of telomerase; (ii) the gene mutated in congenital dyserythropoietic anemia type I has been identified; and (iii) the gene encoding red cell 5'-nucleotidase has been identified, enabling at long last the molecular diagnosis of one of the commonest red cell enzymopathies.

*Molecular Hematology*, 3rd edition. Edited by Drew Provan and John Gribben.
© 2010 Blackwell Publishing.

## Megaloblastic anemia

Megaloblastic anemia is defined by a highly characteristic set of morphological changes which affect cells of the erythroid, myeloid and megakaryocytic lineages in the peripheral blood and bone marrow. These changes include macrocytosis, Howell–Jolly bodies, hypersegmented neutrophils, giant metamyelocytes and giant platelets. Despite the multitude of these signs, the one pathognomonic feature which we regard as a *sine qua non* for the diagnosis of megaloblastic anemia is the peculiarly finely stippled chromatin of erythroid cells, combined with derangement of the normally precisely ordered parallel pattern of maturation of the nucleus and of the cytoplasm. This asynchrony, whereby maturation of the nucleus lags behind that of the cytoplasm, is the morphological hallmark of what we call megaloblastic erythropoiesis.

### Etiology

Megaloblastic anemia has multiple etiologies (Table 12.1). Indeed, it is the main hematological manifestation of, on the one hand, classic inherited disorders (e.g., Lesch–Nyhan syndrome, orotic aciduria, transcobalamin deficiency) and, on the other, classic acquired disorders such as pernicious anemia and nutritional deficiency of either vitamin $B_{12}$ (cobalamin, Cbl) or folate. In this respect, the acquired (and far more common) conditions can be regarded as *phenocopies* of the much more rare inherited conditions.

### Pathophysiology

While megaloblastosis is directly defined by its morphology, the mechanism of the anemia is complex. In general, anemia due to excessive destruction of red cells is characteristically associated with a cellular marrow and a high output of

**Table 12.1** Classification of the megaloblastic anemias

**FOLATE DEFICIENCY**
**Inherited**
*Inborn errors of folate metabolism*
Congenital folate malabsorption
Dihydrofolate reductase deficiency
Methylene tetrahydrofolate reductase deficiency

**Acquired**
*Decreased intake*
Old age, alcoholism
Hemodialysis

*Impaired absorption*
Celiac disease
Tropical sprue

*Increased requirements*
Pregnancy

*Other increased cell turnover*
Chronic hemolytic anemia

*Drugs*
Inhibitors of dihydrofolate reductase deficiency
Anticonvulsants

**COBALAMIN DEFICIENCY**
**Inherited**
*Inborn errors of cobalamin transport*
Imerslund–Grasbeck disease
Congenital deficiency of intrinsic factor
Gastrectomy

*Inborn errors of cobalamin metabolism*
Methionine synthase deficiency (cblE and cblG)
cblC and cblD disease

**Acquired**
*Impaired absorption*
Gastric causes
   Pernicious anemia
Intestinal causes
   Blind loop syndrome
   Fish tapeworm
Pancreatic insufficiency

*Decreased intake*
Vegetarians
*Other*
Nitrous oxide exposure

**OTHER**
Hereditary orotic aciduria
Lesch–Nyhan syndrome
Thiamine-responsive megaloblastic anemia

*Source*: modified from Babior BM. (1995) The megaloblastic anemias. In: Beutler E, Lichtman MA, Coller BS, Kipps TJ (eds). *Williams Hematology*, 5th edn. New York: McGraw-Hill, p. 471.

reticulocytes, whereas anemia due to decreased production of red cells is characteristically associated with a hypocellular marrow and a low output of reticulocytes. In megaloblastic anemia, the marrow is hypercellular, often to an extreme degree, but the output of reticulocytes is low. This contrast is the pathophysiological hallmark of megaloblastic anemia, and it signifies that a large proportion of megaloblasts fail to mature into viable red cells; in other words, there is a vast component of *ineffective erythropoiesis*.

## Molecular pathogenesis

In view of the above, it is clear that any explanation of the pathogenesis of megaloblastic anemia at the molecular level must, on the one hand, rationalize it as the final common pathway of a variety of underlying lesions and, on the other, account for the phenomenon of ineffective erythropoiesis. Since the inherited causes of megaloblastic anemia are defects in the purine or pyrimidine biosynthetic pathways, and folate is the coenzyme of these pathways, it is natural to focus on this area of metabolism. It has been held for a long time that in megaloblastic anemia a decreased concentration of nucleotide precursors becomes rate-limiting for DNA synthesis, and as a result cell proliferation is curtailed and therefore few cells are produced. However, since cell proliferation is most active, this model can be rejected out of hand: the marrow is hypercellular rather than hypocellular, suggesting that the underlying defect may be qualitative and not merely quantitative.

Since the hematological consequences of the deficiency of either folate or Cbl are indistinguishable, it seems reasonable to surmise that there must be at least one point in common in their action, or that one depends on the other (Figure 12.1). Indeed, Cbl is required for the conversion of methyltetrahydrofolate (methyl-THF), the main form of folate in the `, to tetrahydrofolate (THF), the active form in bone marrow cells. Various derivatives of THF intervene in several steps of the biosynthesis of purine and pyrimidine nitrogen bases, but when folate is in short supply these steps can be bypassed by using preformed bases (the so-called salvage pathway). The one reaction for which folate (in the form of 5,10-methylene-THF) is irreplaceable is the conversion of dUMP to dTMP, for which it is the methyl group donor; as a result, this conversion will be impaired when either folate or Cbl is deficient. This reaction is crucially important because thymidine is, of course, the one base in which DNA normally differs from RNA. In principle, one might have expected that a block of this reaction would prevent DNA synthesis, but we have seen that this is not the case. On the other hand, it is well established that *in vitro* DNA polymerase is able to incorporate dUTP into DNA, especially if the dUTP concentration is much higher than

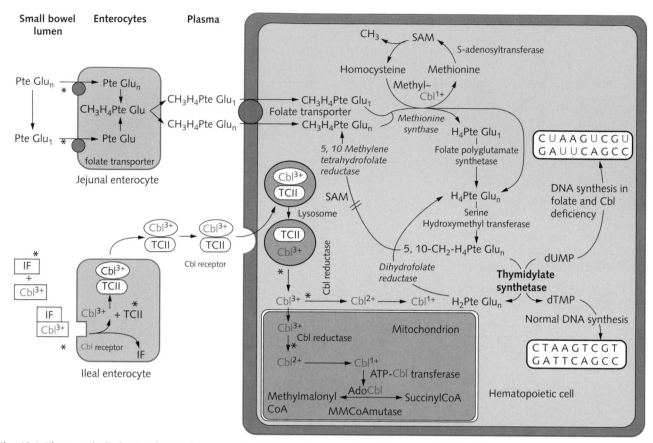

**Fig. 12.1 The metabolic basis of megaloblastosis in folate and vitamin B$_{12}$ (cobalamin, Cbl) deficiency**

The absorption of folates takes place in the proximal small bowel, while Cbl bound to intrinsic factor (IF) is absorbed in the ileum. Folate enters the cells in the form of methyltetrahydrofolate (methyl-THF). Cbl is transferred to and enters the cells bound to transcobalamin II (TCII). In the cytoplasm, Cbl is necessary for the reaction catalyzed by methionine synthase, whereby the CH$_3$ group of methyl-THF is transferred to homocysteine; THF and methionine are produced, respectively, as a result. The polyglutamated form of THF is converted to 5,10-methylene THF, which donates the single-carbon group CH$_2$ to the reaction catalyzed by thymidylate synthetase, whereby dUMP is converted to dTMP which is used in DNA synthesis. Under conditions of folate and/or Cbl deficiency, there is shortage of 5,10-methylene-THF. The result of this is, on the one hand, that dTMP is drastically reduced and not available for DNA synthesis and, on the other, that dUMP is in excess. Strong evidence exists suggesting that, under such circumstances, dUMP is misincorporated in the DNA, leading eventually to changes characteristic of megaloblastosis (*see text*). Note also that under Cbl-replete conditions the conversion of 5,10-methylene-THF to methyl-THF is inhibited by *S*-adenosylmethionine (SAM); in contrast, in Cbl deficiency SAM is in short supply and consequently this inhibition is relaxed, diverting the formation of 5,10-methylene-THF to methyl-THF, thus exacerbating further the shortage of dTMP and the accumulation of dUMP. Cbl also plays a significant role in the mitochondrial metabolic pathways necessary for the conversion of the products of propionate metabolism (i.e., methylmalonyl-CoA) into easily metabolized products. As is evident from the metabolic interrelationships of folate and Cbl, in folate deficiency homocysteine levels will increase; in Cbl deficiency, not only homocysteine but also methylmalonyl-CoA (and methylmalonic acid) will be increased: indeed, measurement of serum and urine levels of homocysteine and methylmalonic acid is used in clinical practice for the diagnosis of folate and Cbl deficiency, especially at early stages.

*Explanatory notes*

In the figure, the various forms of Cbl are shown in green. PteGlu$_1$/PteGlu$_n$, monoglutamated or polyglutamated forms of folate; CH$_3$H$_4$PteGlu$_1$, methyl-THF; 5,10-CH$_2$H$_4$PteGlu$_n$, 5,10-methylene-THF; H$_2$PteGlu$_n$, dihydrofolate. Enzymes whose hereditary deficiency causes megaloblastic anemia are shown in italics. Those steps in folate and Cbl metabolism whose defects can also cause hereditary megaloblastic anemia are indicated by asterisks.

that of dTTP, which will be the case when the conversion of the former to the latter is impeded. Several studies indicate that this also takes place *in vivo*; indeed, the major molecular lesion in megaloblastic anemia may be this misincorporation of deoxyuridine (dU) instead of thymidine into DNA. The cell's DNA replicating machinery includes an enzyme, uracil glucosidase, which has the specific function of removing dU, should it be occasionally and illegitimately incorporated into

DNA. Therefore dU will be retained in newly synthesized DNA only when the capacity of uracil glucosidase to remove it has been exceeded. For this reason, very little dU is actually found in megaloblastic DNA, but even that may have a disruptive effect on chromatin structure. Perhaps more importantly, if dU incorporation has been rampant rather than occasional, the numerous strand breaks produced by uracil glucosidase may exceed the capacity of other repair enzymes, thus causing the accumulation of damaged DNA, and eventually cell death. Surprisingly, a careful study has not detected in megaloblastic bone marrow features regarded as characteristic of apoptosis. We must therefore presume that cell death takes place by a different pathway or that phagocytosis of dead cells is rapid and highly efficient.

If shortage of dTTP is the fundamental metabolic defect underlying megaloblastic anemia, since its production is 5,10-methylene-THF dependent (the formation of which is in turn dependent on Cbl), it is clear that this same mechanism explains why megaloblastic anemia is the common manifestation not only of nutritional folate and Cbl deficiency, but also of all genetically determined lesions of the transport and metabolism of folate or Cbl (Table 12.1). It is not clear why megaloblastic anemia should occur in other inherited conditions, such as hypoxanthine-guanine phosphoribosyltransferase (HPRT) deficiency and orotic aciduria, in which it is the salvage pathway rather than the *de novo* pathway of the nitrogen bases that is compromised. At the moment we can only speculate by analogy. Perhaps the metabolic blocks in these conditions also entail serious alterations in the absolute and/or relative pool sizes of the various deoxynucleoside triphosphates. Once again, this could cause misincorporation followed by repair attempts that are not always successful. In summary, although the rate of uracil incorporation into DNA has been controversial for years, a recent review validates its role in the pathogenesis of megaloblastic anemia.

Finally, despite the significant advances in the understanding of megaloblastosis, the molecular basis of demyelination that underlies the neurological complications of advanced Cbl deficiency remains elusive.

## Congenital dyserythropoietic anemias

Congenital dyserythropoietic anemia (CDA) is the current designation for a group of rare inherited disorders that have a common feature: abnormalities in the maturation of the erythroid lineage. It is evident both from genetics and from morphology that they are heterogeneous, and it is likely that they may be even more heterogeneous at the molecular level. Of the three classical forms of CDA (Table 12.2), CDA II (or HEMPAS) is the best defined, on account of a pathognomonic serological test; CDA I is defined by characteristic ultrastructural changes in the chromatin of erythroblasts and by autosomal recessive inheritance; CDA III is defined by large, sometimes multinucleated, erythroblasts and by autosomal dominant inheritance. A variety of terms have been used to classify patients who have features of CDA but do not fit neatly in any of these three categories.

**Table 12.2** Defining features of congenital dyserythropoietic anemia types I–III.

|  | Type I | Type II | Type III |
|---|---|---|---|
| Inheritance | Autosomal recessive | Autosomal recessive | (a) Autosomal dominant<br>(b) Autosomal recessive |
| Localization of gene | 15q15.1–15.3 | 20q11.2 | 15q21–25 |
| Identity of gene | CDAN1 | Not known | Not known |
| Red cells | Macrocytes | Normocytes | |
| Erythroblasts | | | |
| (a) Light microscopy | Megaloblastic; internuclear chromatin bridges | Normoblastic; binuclearity predominates | Megaloblastic; up to 12 nuclei per cell |
| (b) Electron microscopy | "Swiss cheese" appearance of heterochromatin | Peripheral double membranes | |
| Serology | | | |
| Ham's test | Negative | Positive | Negative |
| Anti-i agglutinability | Normal/strong | Strong | Normal/strong |
| SDS-PAGE | Normal | Band 3 thinner and faster | Band 3 slightly faster |

*Source*: modified from Wickramasinghe SN. (1997) Dyserythropoiesis and congenital dyserythropoietic anaemias. *British Journal of Haematology*, **98**, 785–797, with permission.

As a result of a deranged developmental program, the mature red cells that are produced in CDA are macrocytic and abnormal in their membrane; this often entails a hemolytic component in their anemia. In addition, and most characteristically, a significant proportion of erythroid cells fail to achieve full maturity, and as a result they are destroyed in the bone marrow. Thus, the pathophysiological hallmark in CDA, just as in acquired megaloblastic anemias (*see above*), is ineffective erythropoiesis.

The biochemical basis for abnormal maturation has been well characterized in the case of CDA II. Sodium dodecyl-sulfate–polyacrylamide gel electrophoresis (SDS-PAGE) analysis of red cell membrane proteins reveals an increased sharpness of band 3, the size heterogeneity of which is normally produced by the variable size of its carbohydrate moiety. This finding has focused the attention on the enzymes required for glycosylation of membrane proteins: decreased activity of α-mannosidase and of fucosyltransferase has been reported in individual cases. Targeted inactivation of the gene encoding the latter enzyme has produced mice with features of CDA II. On the other hand, very recently it has been reported that inactivation of *AE1*, the gene encoding band 3, produces in zebrafish some features of human CDA II. However, by linkage analysis CDA II maps to 20q11.2 in a majority of families, whereas fucosyltransferase maps to 11q21 and *AE1* to 17q21–q22. Thus, the gene that is mutated in human CDA II still needs to be identified. The variability of clinical expression of CDA II could be due to different underlying genetic lesions (and of course also to different mutant alleles at the same locus). In fact, there is some indirect evidence that alleles causing mild CDA may be relatively common, because two cases have been reported as causing chronic hemolytic anemia in association with glucose 6-phosphate dehydrogenase (G6PD)-deficient variants which do not, on their own, cause this condition. We do not know whether the CDA mutations present in these patients would have caused clinical manifestations in the absence of G6PD deficiency.

The gene for CDA I has been mapped to chromosome 15 by linkage analysis in a single Swedish family (one of the first from which the concept of CDA developed). Very recently this linkage has been confirmed in Bedouin families, and this has led to the identification of a gene that is mutated in all of these families, which has been called codanin-1. Codanin-1 has a 150-residue amino-terminal domain with sequence similarity to collagens and two shorter segments that show weak similarities to the microtubule-associated proteins MAP1B (neuraxin) and synapsin.

In view of the fact that in the various forms of CDA the abnormal phenotype is almost exclusively restricted to the erythroid lineage, it is likely that the genes that are mutated in any patient with CDA serve some important role in the program of erythroid differentiation. For instance, it seems likely that in erythroid cells codanin-1 is involved in nuclear envelope integrity, conceivably related to microtubule attachments. Thus, each one of the CDA genes will be of great interest, quite out of proportion to the rarity of CDAs as clinical entities.

It has been reported that three patients with CDA I have responded to treatment with interferon (IFN)-α, with near normalization of hemoglobin values. Although the clinical data seem convincing, at the moment it is not clear by what mechanism an intrinsic erythroid molecular abnormality can benefit from this treatment.

# The sideroblastic anemias

The term "sideroblastic anemia" (SA) encompasses a diverse collection of diseases in which different causes and different mechanisms converge to produce the same rather spectacular feature: the accumulation of inorganic iron in the cytoplasm of erythroid cells in sufficient quantities to be easily demonstrated in the form of granules using Perl's Prussian Blue staining. Characteristically, the iron is found in mitochondria positioned around the nucleus, hence the term *ring sideroblast*. SAs are broadly divided into acquired and inherited forms (Table 12.3). Acquired SAs are the most common and are discussed in *Chapter 8*. Here, we discuss briefly the genetic and biochemical basis of three inherited forms of SA.

## ALAS2 deficiency

Normally, about 90% of the iron (Fe) obtained daily from the diet reaches the erythroblasts, where it is required for the final step of heme biosynthesis, namely the incorporation of iron into the tetrapyrrolic ring of protoporphyrin IX. The first and the last three of the eight steps of the heme biosynthetic pathway take place in the mitochondrion. The first and rate-limiting step consists of the condensation of glycine and succinyl-CoA to δ-aminolevulinate. This reaction is catalyzed by δ-aminolevulinate synthase (ALAS) and it requires pyridoxal 5′-phosphate (PLP) as a cofactor. Two isoforms of ALAS are known; both have a homodimeric structure, but they are encoded by different genes. *ALAS1* is a ubiquitously expressed housekeeping gene, whereas *ALAS2* is erythroid-specific.

### Genetics of ALAS2 deficiency

The first family with what is now called X-linked SA was reported by T. Cooley in 1945. Subsequently, more families with apparent X-linked SA were described. The observation that some affected males responded to pharmacological

**Table 12.3** Classification of the sideroblastic anemias.

**INHERITED**

| Mode of inheritance | Chromosomal locus | Gene | Type of mutations | Clinical manifestations other than SA |
|---|---|---|---|---|
| X-linked | Xp11.21 | ALAS2 | Missense | None |
| X-linked | Xq13.1–q13.3 | hABCB7 (Fe–S cluster transporter protein) | Missense | Cerebellar ataxia |
| Autosomal recessive | 1q23.2s–q23.3 | SLC19A2 (thiamine transporter protein) | Missense, nonsense, frameshift | Thiamine-responsive megaloblastic anemia, diabetes mellitus, sensorineural deafness |
| Autosomal dominant | Not known | Not known | | None |
| Mitochondrial (e.g., Pearson MPS) | Usually from nt 8469 to nt 13447 (see Fig.12.3) | | Deletions | Pancreatic exocrine dysfunction, cytopenia, metabolic acidosis |

**ACQUIRED**
Refractory anemia with ring sideroblasts (RARS)
Drug induced (e.g., isoniazid, chloramphenicol, ethanol)
Secondary to systemic, metabolic, malignant disorders

ALAS2, δ-aminolevulinate synthase 2; PGK1, phosphoglycerate kinase 1; SA, sideroblastic anemia; MPS, marrow–pancreas syndrome.

doses of pyridoxine focused attention on the erythroid-specific ALAS; indeed, the *in vitro* activity of this enzyme was invariably reduced. The erythroid-specific *ALAS* (*ALAS2*) gene was subsequently cloned (Figure 12.2) and mapped to Xp11.12. This locus is subject to X-chromosome inactivation and as a result female relatives of affected males may demonstrate red cell mosaicism; that is, two populations of red cells, one hypochromic and one normochromic. In general, these women do not have anemia, and therefore the disease is regarded as recessive. However, full-blown SA may develop in women, especially late in life, as a result of a skewed X-inactivation pattern: in such cases we would have to regard the same disease as dominant.

**Transcriptional and translational control of ALAS2 expression**

The expression of *ALAS2* is regulated at both the transcriptional and the translational level. Transcriptional control is effected through the programmed differentiation of the erythroid lineage, mainly through the erythropoietin-induced transcription factors which include GATA-1, EKLF and NF-E2. In contrast, as a typical example of gene expression control at the translational level, *ALAS2* is involved in the regulation of heme synthesis in relation to Fe availability. Central to this regulatory mechanism is iron regulatory protein (IRP)1, a *trans*-acting protein that requires four atoms of Fe to function and is also able to bind to an

mRNA motif called iron-responsive element (IRE). IRE has a characteristic hairpin secondary structure, present within the 5′ untranslated region of the *ALAS2* mRNA. IRP1 does not bind to IRE when it is iron replete, thus allowing the translation of *ALAS2* mRNA to proceed unimpeded. When iron is in scarce supply, the iron-depleted IRP1 binds to IRE and translation of *ALAS2* mRNA is repressed, thus decreasing the synthesis of heme and consequently of mature hemoglobin, leading to the production of hypochromic red cells. Interestingly, IRP1 can also bind to IREs present in the mRNAs of ferritin and transferrin receptor. In conditions of iron depletion, real or functional, the translational regulation is such that translation of ferritin mRNA is repressed whereas translation of the transferrin receptor is favored. Reverse effects are seen in iron-replete conditions.

**Molecular pathology of ALAS2 deficiency**

Over 20 different point mutations have been described (Figure 12.2). They all map to exons 5–11, which are highly conserved across species. Parts of these exons are thought to contribute to the formation of the catalytic site, PLP-binding site and substrate-binding site of ALAS2. The presence of only missense mutations implies that hemizygotes with *ALAS2* null mutations would not be viable. Exceptionally, a nucleotide replacement at position −206 from the transcription start of *ALAS2* has been found to cause SA; this is a rare

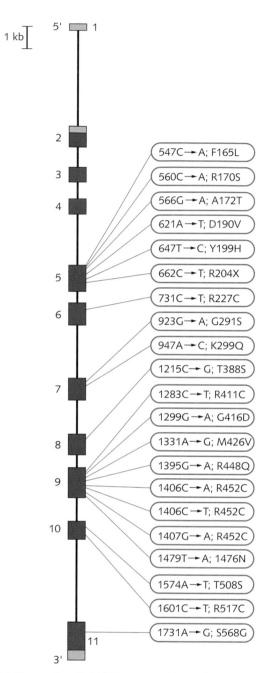

**Fig. 12.2 The erythroid *ALAS2* gene and its pathogenic mutations**

*ALAS2* spans about 22 kb and consists of 11 exons. Two mature forms of mRNA exist: one full length and one shorter as a result of alternative splicing of exon 4. The functional significance of these splicing variants is not known. Exon 1 and part of exon 2 (shown in gray) form the 5′ untranslated region and contain the iron-responsive element (*see text*). The full-length mRNA (1.95 kb) encodes a protein of 522 amino acids (64.4 kDa). The mature protein derives from the cleavage of the first 49 amino-terminal amino acids (mitochondrial signal sequence) upon entry in the mitochondrion.

example of a human disease resulting from a "promoter-down" mutation in a gene encoding an enzyme.

### Clinical aspects and treatment of ALAS2 deficiency

The clinical picture of ALAS2 deficiency is that of a hypochromic microcytic anemia with bone marrow erythroid hyperplasia as a result of ineffective erythropoiesis. The characteristic ring sideroblasts are found mainly in the late erythroid precursors. There is considerable heterogeneity in the severity of the disease, not only between individuals bearing different *ALAS2* mutations but also between related individuals with the same mutation. Patients at one extreme may present a few months after birth with severe anemia, severe microcytosis and no response to pyridoxine; at the other extreme, they may present in the ninth decade of life with anemia fully responsive to pyridoxine.

Although the anemia of pyridoxine-responsive SA is treatable, the main complication of the disease is iron overload; if left untreated, it has the same deleterious results as hereditary hemochromatosis. Iron overload can be biochemically evident as early as adolescence, does not correlate with the degree of anemia and can affect mildly anemic females. The importance of effectively treating iron overload cannot be over-emphasized for one further reason: excess iron interferes with the function of ALAS2 and patients previously unresponsive to pyridoxine, after effective iron chelation, occasionally become responsive.

The advances in the molecular aspects of X-linked SA make prenatal diagnosis and counseling feasible, especially for families with the severe, pyridoxine-resistant forms of the disease.

## X-linked sideroblastic anemia with ataxia

This pyridoxine-resistant form of SA with congenital cerebellar ataxia is due to missense mutations of the ATP-binding cassette B7 (*ABCB7*) gene which maps to Xq13.1–q13.3. ABCB7 belongs to a wider family of proteins involved in the transportation of substrates across cell and organelle membranes. Studies in yeast and mammalian systems suggest that ABCB7 is an inner mitochondrial membrane protein involved in the transportation of clusters of Fe–S (iron–sulfur) formed in the mitochondrion to the cytosol. These clusters are required for the functional maturation of a number of proteins, including those necessary for iron homeostasis. Mutations of *ABCB7* interrupt this process and lead to accumulation in the erythroid cell mitochondria of iron that is not available for heme synthesis, hence the development of microcytic SA. Interestingly, expression levels of ABCB7 were found to be considerably lower in patients with acquired SA (or refractory anemia with ring sideroblasts), a form of myelodysplastic syndrome (MDS), but not in patients with other forms of MDS or normal individuals. No genetic or epigenetic cause in *cis* was identified, raising the question of a *trans*-acting mechanism. The significance of this finding in the pathogenesis of refractory anemia with ring sideroblasts remains to be determined.

## Pearson marrow–pancreas syndrome

Pearson marrow–pancreas syndrome (PMPS) is unique among the SAs because the underlying genetic lesion is not in the nuclear DNA but in the mitochondrial DNA (mtDNA).

### Properties of mtDNA

Each somatic cell has hundreds to several thousand mitochondria, and each mitochondrion contains two to ten copies of mtDNA. mtDNA consists of a single double-stranded circular molecule, and its 16 569-nucleotide genome encodes 24 structural RNAs (22 tRNAs and two rRNAs) required for mitochondrial protein synthesis; in addition it encodes 13 protein subunits belonging to four enzyme complexes, all involved, directly or indirectly, in the generation of ATP through oxidative phosphorylation (Figure 12.3). Replication, transcription and translation of mtDNA are all quite distinct from their nuclear DNA equivalents.

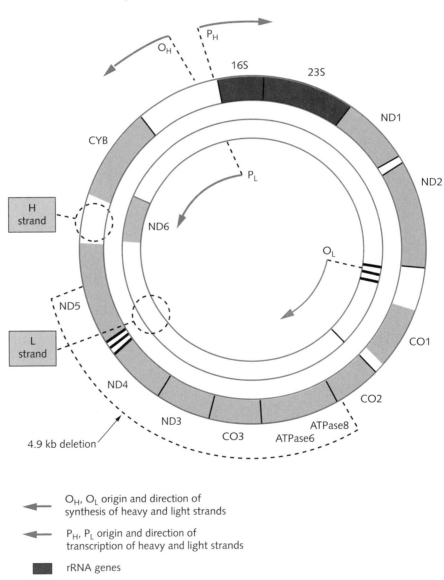

**Fig. 12.3 The human mitochondrial genome**
Both replication and transcription of the heavy (H) and light (L) strands of mtDNA run in opposite directions as indicated in the figure. The products of transcription are large and are cleaved to generate RNAs for individual genes. Note the absence of introns and close apposition of genes. *ATPase8* and *ATPase6* overlap. The approximate location of the common 4.9-kb deletion (*see text*) is indicated by the broken line. *ND1–ND6* encode NADH dehydrogenase subunits, *CO1–CO3* encode cytochrome c oxidase subunits and CYB encodes cytochrome *b*. Modified from Strachan T, Read AP. (1996) *Human Molecular Genetics*, 1st edn. New York: BIOS, with permission.

O$_H$, O$_L$ origin and direction of synthesis of heavy and light strands

P$_H$, P$_L$ origin and direction of transcription of heavy and light strands

rRNA genes

Genes encoding proteins

tRNA genes

Since mitochondria are abundant in the cytoplasm of the mature oocyte, but absent from that part of the sperm cell that enters it at the time of fertilization, the hereditary transmission of mtDNA is exclusively through the maternal germline. Consequently, a mitochondrial disease can be transmitted from a mother to all of her children, whether male or female; in other words, it is a non-Mendelian form of inheritance.

mtDNA is estimated to be at least 10 times more vulnerable than nuclear DNA to mutations and their consequences for various reasons: (i) it is constantly exposed to oxygen free radicals generated by oxidative phosphorylation; (ii) mitochondria largely lack effective DNA repair mechanisms; and (iii) because most of the mtDNA sequence is coding, many more mutations will be reflected in the structure of its protein products. On the other hand, since there are so many copies of mtDNA in each cell, mutant mtDNA may coexist with normal mtDNA, a situation called *heteroplasmy* (the opposite of *homoplasmy*). The phenotype of a particular cell or organ will depend on the relative proportions of normal and mutated mtDNA. Since, unlike nuclear chromosomes, there is no rigorous mechanism for the segregation of mtDNA molecules at either mitosis or meiosis, the inheritance of mtDNA mutations is rather unpredictable, and since heteroplasmy may exist even in oocytes, this further complicates the non-Mendelian inheritance of diseases caused by mtDNA mutations.

### Clinical aspects of PMPS

PMPS usually presents within the first few months of life with hypoproliferative SA, variable cytopenias and pancreatic exocrine dysfunction. Bone marrow examination reveals, in addition to ring sideroblasts, striking vacuolation of the erythroid and myeloid precursors (Plate 12.1). Metabolic acidosis is another frequent manifestation, and renal disease, liver failure, hypoparathyroidism and diabetes mellitus may also occur. Despite treatment with blood product support, pancreatic enzymes and various vitamins (e.g., coenzyme Q), about half of the patients do not survive beyond the third year of life. Of the patients who do survive, most develop complications in other organs, particularly ophthalmoplegia, pigmentary degeneration of the retina and cardiomyopathy, namely the features originally described as the Kearns–Sayre syndrome (KSS). The overlap between PMPS and KSS is not surprising, since similar genetic lesions are found in both conditions (*see below*).

### Molecular pathology

In all but one of the cases that have been adequately investigated, PMPS was due to deletions within mtDNA.

The size of the deletion is variable; in one study, 43% of the patients had an identical 4.9-kb deletion (Figure 12.3) that has also been found in patients with other mitochondrial diseases (such as KSS and progressive external ophthalmoplegia). In some cases, deletion dimers and/or deletion multimers were observed. There is no obvious correlation between the size or location of the deletion and the clinical severity of the disease; rather, what probably largely determines the clinical phenotype is the proportion of mutated mtDNA in a particular tissue. For example, patients with PMPS have mutated mtDNA in all tissues examined, whereas in patients with classical KSS the mutated mtDNA is restricted to muscle and is not found in blood cells. Since the mothers of PMPS patients are invariably unaffected, it can be expected that the deletion has taken place *de novo*, and this has been documented in a number of cases.

A difficult practical problem is that of genetic counseling for couples who have had the misfortune to have a child with PMPS. The risk of recurrence depends on whether the deletion is present in most or only in some of the mother's gonadal cells. At the moment there is no established methodology for determining this. At an experimental level, it could be achieved by inducing multiple ovulation and using the polymerase chain reaction (PCR) to test individual oocytes for the deletion previously detected in an affected sib. The same could be done in very early embryos after *in vitro* fertilization (preimplantation prenatal diagnosis). Because of the high copy number of mtDNA, testing for mtDNA mutations is much easier than testing for mutations in nuclear genes.

## Conditions associated with bone marrow failure

The disease entities falling under this heading are quite diverse, but they are grouped on account of a common pathogenesis: the loss of hematopoietic stem cells (HSCs). The pace of HSC depletion varies widely, from weeks (e.g., in idiopathic aplastic anemia, IAA) to years (e.g., in Fanconi anemia, FA). In fact, IAA and FA exemplify two broad categories of bone marrow failure (BMF) syndromes, acquired and inherited, respectively (Table 12.4).

## Acquired bone marrow failure syndromes

### Idiopathic aplastic anemia

IAA accounts for the majority (about 80–90%) of cases of acquired BMF syndromes, with an incidence estimated at 2 per million (twofold to threefold higher in the Orient).

**Table 12.4** Classification of the bone marrow failure (BMF) syndromes.

**INHERITED**

| Disease | Mode of inheritance | Chromosomal locus | Gene | Clinical manifestations |
|---|---|---|---|---|
| Fanconi anemia | AR | See Table 12.6 | See Table 12.6 | See text |
| Dyskeratosis congenita | X-linked | Xq28 | *DKC1* | See text |
| | AD | 3q26 | *TERC* | |
| | AD | 5p15 | *TERT* | |
| | AR | 15q14 | *NOP10* | |
| | AR | 5q35 | *NHP2* | |
| Diamond–Blackfan anemia | AD | 19q13.2 | *RPS19* | See text |
| | AD | 10q22–q23 | *RPS24* | |
| | AD | 15q | *RPS17* | |
| | AD | 3q29 | *RPL35A* | |
| | AR | 8p22–p23.31 | Not known | |
| Shwachman–Diamond syndrome | AR | 7q11 | *SBDS* | Neutropenia, exocrine pancreatic insufficiency, metaphyseal dysostosis |
| Amegakaryocytic thrombocytopenia | AR | 1p34 | *c-mpl* (thrombopoietin receptor) | Absent megakaryocytes in bone marrow, late BMF |
| Thrombocytopenia with absent radii syndrome | AR? | Not known | Not known | Bilateral radial aplasia, lower limb anomalies, cow's milk intolerance, renal anomalies, and cardiac anomalies |
| Congenital thrombocytopenia and radius–ulna synostosis | AD | 7p15–p14 | *HOXA11*? (needs confirmation) | Aplastic anemia, proximal radius–ulna synostosis, clinodactyly, syndactyly, hip dysplasia and sensorineural hearing loss |
| Pearson marrow–pancreas syndrome | Mitochondrial | Usually from nt 8469 to nt 13447 | Contiguous genes deleted | Pancreatic exocrine dysfunction, sideroblastic anemia (*see also* text) |

**ACQUIRED**
Idiopathic
Radiation
Drugs and chemicals
  Regular: cytotoxic, benzene
  Idiosyncratic: chloramphenicol, NSAIDs, antiepileptics, gold
Viruses
  Epstein–Barr virus
  Hepatitis
  Parvovirus
  Human immunodeficiency virus
Immune diseases
  Thymoma
  Pregnancy
  Paroxysmal nocturnal hemoglobinuria

AD, autosomal dominant; AR, autosomal recessive; NSAID, non-steroidal anti-inflammatory drug.

*Immunopathogenesis* The most direct evidence that IAA may be an autoimmune disorder has come from the clinical observation that patients with IAA have complete or partial reversion of their pancytopenia when they are treated with antilymphocyte globulin (ALG). Subsequently, it was shown that patients with IAA often have increased numbers of "activated" CD8$^+$C25$^+$ T cells in their blood and bone marrow. In addition, T cells from IAA patients can inhibit the growth of autologous *in vitro* hematopoietic colonies, and the growth of colonies from human leukocyte antigen

(HLA)-identical siblings. Based on these observations, a current model of the pathogenesis of IAA predicts that auto-reactive T cells attack HSCs, causing their depletion – hence the reduction of HSCs in severe IAA to about 1% of normal. The primary event that triggers this aberrant immune response remains elusive: a possible viral cause has long been sought but never proven. The identity of the putative autoantigen on HSCs also remains unknown. There is evidence, however, that the inhibitory effect of autoreactive T cells is mediated, at least in part, through IFN-γ. In addition, IFN-γ upregulates Fas receptor on the surface of HSCs, thus facilitating activation of the Fas-dependent apoptotic pathways.

As in other autoimmune diseases there is over-representation of specific HLA alleles in IAA patients compared with population controls: the HLA-DR2 allele is over-represented in patients with IAA of European ancestry, whereas another HLA class II haplotype is over-represented in Japanese patients with IAA.

Recently, a pathogenetic link between IAA and MDS has surfaced. Clinically, IAA overlaps with the hypoplastic form of MDS; in fact, the differential diagnosis between the two is often difficult. It is now recognized that 20–30% of patients with MDS, especially those who would otherwise be classified as having refractory anemia with hypocellular marrow, respond to immunosuppressive therapy with alleviation of their cytopenias, indicating that an immune process, similar to the one operating in IAA, is also involved in the pathogenesis of some forms of MDS. In addition, as in IAA, in 20% of patients with refractory anemia, small populations with paroxysmal nocturnal hemoglobinuria (PNH) are detected (*see below*). What is more, their presence is predictive of response to immunosuppressive therapy, providing further evidence of an immune process in the pathogenesis of MDS in this select group of patients, and linking them to those with IAA. The role of mutations in genes involved in telomere maintenance in the pathogenesis of IAA is discussed below (*see section Dyskeratosis congenita*).

*Clinical aspects and treatment* The clinical picture of IAA generally reflects the extent of HSC loss and the subsequent cytopenias. Typically, a patient with severe IAA presents with bruising and mucosal bleeding, anemia and septic episodes (bacterial or fungal), but without hepatosplenomegaly. The differential diagnosis of IAA, as well as hypoplastic MDS, includes inherited BMF syndromes, the aplastic form of childhood acute lymphoblastic leukemia, and infectious and malignant processes that may infiltrate the bone marrow. Thus the diagnosis of IAA is made eventually by exclusion. The contemporary treatment of IAA is dictated by its severity (as determined by the degree of pancytopenia, reticulocytopenia and bone marrow cellularity) and by the patient's age. HSC transplantation (HSCT) from an HLA-identical

sibling or from an alternative donor is the treatment of choice for younger patients with severe IAA, and offers better than 65% long-term survival. In the absence of an appropriate donor, or when the patient is older or the disease milder, immunosuppressive treatment (in particular the combination of ALG/ATG and cyclosporin) results in complete or partial response in the majority of cases. As well as PNH (*see below*), IAA bears a significant risk of late clonal disorders, especially after immunosuppressive therapy: the risk of MDS and acute myeloid leukemia (AML) is 17% at 10 years after immunosuppression, and the risk of tumors of other organs brings the total risk to 18% (compared with 3.1% after bone marrow transplantation).

### Paroxysmal nocturnal hemoglobinuria

PNH is a rare acquired hematological disorder with three main clinical features: intravascular hemolysis, tendency to thrombosis and BMF of variable severity. As in IAA, the precise cause for BMF remains unclear; in contrast, the molecular mechanism of hemolysis is well explained. For this reason, the space devoted here to this condition is out of proportion to its prevalence.

*Molecular pathogenesis* The initiating event in the pathogenesis of PNH consists of somatic mutation(s) in the X-linked gene *PIGA* (Plate 12.2) in multipotent HSC(s). The protein product of *PIGA*, although not physically isolated as yet, is thought to be the enzymatically active subunit of an *N*-acetylglucosamine transferase. This enzyme catalyzes an early step in the formation of a complex glycolipid molecule called glycosylphosphatidylinositol (GPI) (Plate 12.2). The synthesis of GPI takes place initially on the cytoplasmic surface of the endoplasmic reticulum, and is then completed on its luminal surface. Once formed, the GPI molecules (anchors) are attached through a transpeptidation reaction to the carboxy-terminus of a variety of proteins. The GPI-linked proteins, after post-translational modifications in the Golgi apparatus, emerge eventually on the cell surface, to which they remain attached through the GPI anchor. As a result of the impaired synthesis of GPI, blood cells are either completely (PNH III) or partially (PNH II) deficient in GPI-linked proteins.

*Complement activation and pathophysiology of red cell destruction* Although for the majority of GPI-linked proteins the functional consequences of their cell surface deficiency are not known, CD55 and especially CD59 are directly implicated in the pathogenesis of PNH and destruction of red cells. CD59 is a critical negative regulator of complement activation at the surface of erythrocytes. It prevents homopolymerization and pore formation by C9, the last component of the terminal membrane attack complex also comprising C6, C7 and C8; formation of this in turn depends on cleavage and activation of C5 by upstream components of the alternative and classical pathways of complement activation. When CD59 is low or absent as a result of *PIGA* mutations, red cells become susceptible to baseline or stress-induced complement activation, resulting in red cell lysis and intravascular hemolysis. The *in vitro* counterpart of this phenomenon is the Ham test, whereby the patient's red cells are lysed by either autologous or ABO-compatible donor acidified serum.

As for thrombosis, this may result in part from complement-mediated activation of platelets deficient in CD55 and CD59. Other, as yet unidentified, genetic or acquired factors affecting coagulation and/or fibrinolysis may have an additive or synergistic effect in producing thrombosis, which may be devastating especially as it tends to take place in the abdominal and cerebral vein.

Given the central role of C5 in complement activation, it would be expected that inhibition of its cleavage would prevent terminal membrane attack complex and thus destruction of red cells lacking expression of surface CD59. Eculizumab, a humanized monoclonal antibody specific for C5, is a very potent inhibitor of C5 cleavage with spectacular clinical effects (*see below*).

*Cellular pathogenesis* Since HSCs in PNH lack GPI-linked proteins, in principle they would be expected to be poorly competitive in growth with respect to normal HSCs. Instead, PNH HSCs can expand until they largely supplant normal hematopoiesis. As a first approximation, this paradox may be explained by invoking an intrinsic proliferative advantage of PNH HSCs over normal HSCs, as is the case with leukemic cells: however, the fact that patients with PNH can live for decades with normal and PNH hematopoiesis coexisting in their bone marrow militates against this notion. Lack of a competitive growth advantage by the PNH hematopoiesis has also been demonstrated experimentally in *pig-a* null mouse models.

An alternative pathogenetic model, the *escape model*, was suggested by the long known association between PNH and IAA. In this model, the link between PNA and IAA is the effect of HSC-specific T cells. It is predicted that, in PNH, such cells would selectively target normal HSCs but not PNH HSCs. Under these circumstances, PNH HSCs would expand and contribute to hematopoiesis (in some cases as much as 90% of it). Clinical evidence in support of the escape model is provided by the appearance of small PNH clones in as many as 50% of patients with bona fide IAA and by the presence of minute PNH clones (~1 in $10^5$ granulocytes) even in normal individuals. Further evidence supporting the immune model is provided by:

1 the presence of expanded T-cell clones in the blood of PNH patients at a frequency threefold higher than in appropriate controls;
2 increased frequency of CD8$^+$CD57$^+$ T cells expressing predominantly activating killer immunoglobulin and NKG2/CD94 receptors;
3 identification of exactly the same or very similar T-cell receptor (TCR)-β CDR3 clonotypic sequences in the CD8$^+$CD57$^+$ T-cell subset of different patients;
4 increased representation of the HLA-DR2 allele in PNH patients compared with population controls (as in IAA).

The molecular target of the postulated autoreactive T cells is not known. Potential targets are a surface GPI-linked protein, failure of PNH HSCs to present in the context of HLA an immunogenic peptide derived from GPI-linked protein, or the GPI molecule itself. Experimental evidence has ruled out the first mechanism; the last two are still to be tested. Although in one study natural killer cells were shown to be more effective in lysing GPI-positive than GPI-negative targets, two previous studies had found no difference; clearly, the role of natural killer cells in the pathogenesis of PNH needs further exploration.

A second mechanism of clonal expansion, at least for some cases of PNH, was suggested by a recent study of two patients who had the same t(12;12) translocation. Molecular studies revealed that in both cases, the transcription factor HMGA2 was interchromosomally rearranged in a way that resulted in truncation of its 3′ untranslated region. This may remove negative regulatory elements resulting in increased expression of HMGA2, but how increased HMGA2 could impart the cell with apparently non-malignant growth advantage is not known.

*Molecular pathology* All types of mutations have been observed in the *PIGA* gene in patients with PNH; a few are large deletions, the majority (~75%) are small insertions or deletions causing frameshifts, and the rest are nonsense and missense point mutations. Interestingly, the nonsense and frameshift mutations are spread throughout the coding sequence (exons 2–6), presumably because they cause complete inactivation of the gene product wherever they fall, whereas missense mutations are clustered mainly within exon 2, where it is presumed that amino acid residues critical for catalytic activity must be located.

*Clinical aspects and treatment* Although hemoglobinuria is by definition paroxysmal in the prototypical PNH patient, the brisk intravascular hemolysis is in fact continuous. Additionally, patients with florid PNH (Table 12.5) often experience acute exacerbations of their hemolysis during intercurrent illnesses such as infections (presumably because

**Table 12.5** Paroxysmal nocturnal hemoglobinuria (PNH): clinical heterogeneity and proposed terminology.

| Predominant clinical features | Blood findings | Size of PNH clone | Designation |
|---|---|---|---|
| Hemolysis ± thrombosis | Anemia; little or no other cytopenia | Large | Florid PNH |
| Hemolysis ± thrombosis | Anemia; mild to moderate other cytopenia(s) | Large | PNH, hypoplastic |
| Purpura and/or infection | Moderate to severe pancytopenia | Large | AA/PNH |
| Purpura and/or infection | Severe pancytopenia | Small | AA with PNH clone |
| Thrombosis | Normal or moderate cytopenia(s) | Small | Mini-PNH |

AA, aplastic anemia.
*Source*: Tremml G, Karadimitris A, Luzzatto L. (1998) Paroxysmal nocturnal hemoglobinuria: learning about PNH cells from patients and from mice. *Haema*, **1**, 12–20, with permission.

this is associated with activation of complement), other stressful events, or for no obvious reason.

Hemolytic anemia with macrocytosis (partly due to reticulocytosis and partly to BMF), different degrees of thrombocytopenia and leukopenia, iron deficiency and hemosiderinuria should raise the suspicion of PNH. The diagnosis can be confirmed by the Ham test (which only detects the PNH abnormality in erythrocytes) and/or flow cytometric analysis of erythrocytes and leukocytes; for this purpose, anti-CD59 is the most reliable antibody. The management of hemolysis has changed dramatically since the advent of eculizumab in 2004. Since then, in a series of studies it has been shown that treatment with eculizumab results in (i) almost complete abrogation of hemolysis; (ii) dramatic reduction in transfusion requirements resulting in hemoglobin stabilization or transfusion independence; (iii) significant improvement in quality of life for most patients; and (iv) a possible significant reduction in the risk of thrombosis. This is very important because in about 40% of PNH patients, venous thrombosis of small or large vessels (particularly at unusual sites, such as the abdomen or the brain) is a serious and potentially life-threatening complication. As free hemoglobin binds and reduces plasma nitric oxide, a natural vasodilator, abrogation of hemolysis by eculizumab also dramatically reduces the incidence of smooth muscle dystonias (i.e., retrosternal or abdominal pain and erectile dysfunction) that often complicate hemolytic episodes. Eculizumab should therefore be considered treatment of choice for hemolysis in PNH and patients should be vaccinated against encapsulated bacteria, especially *Neisseria meningitidis*; however, patients at risk of thrombosis (i.e., those with large PNH clones) should still be considered for prophylactic long-term anticoagulation. Venous thrombosis diagnosed within a few days from its occurrence should be treated with thrombolytic therapy, followed by short- and long-term anticoagulants.

Long-term therapeutic options for PNH include immunosuppressive agents (e.g., combination of ALG/ATG and cyclosporin, especially for patients with moderate to severe cytopenias), while in the era of eculizumab allogeneic HSCT should probably be reserved only for selected patients developing MDS.

*PNH and other clonal disorders* Patients with PNH have a small risk (<4%) of developing MDS (the reverse, i.e., patients with MDS developing PNH, is discussed above) and AML. Because a similar risk exists in IAA, it is probably the perturbed marrow environment that allows the emergence of premalignant (MDS) or malignant (AML) clones, rather than the *PIGA* mutations *per se* predisposing to MDS and AML.

*Inherited GPI deficiency* The first two families with inherited GPI deficiency have been identified. Inherited GPI deficiency is a typical autosomal recessive disorder affecting three children from consanguineous families and is characterized by spontaneous splanchnic vein thrombosis in the first year of life, absence seizures that become refractory to treatment later on but, in contrast to PNH, no significant intravascular hemolysis or BMF syndrome. In all three affected children, the same promoter mutation was identified: a C→G substitution at position −270 from the start codon of the *PIGM* gene, which encodes a mannosyltransferase that is responsible for the first and essential mannosylation reaction in the biosynthesis of GPI. The C→G mutation is hypomorphic: it allows for some transcriptional output, the extent of which varies from tissue to tissue, hence the variable degree of GPI deficiency. For example, in red cells, GPI expression is almost normal, explaining the lack of significant hemolysis; by contrast, granulocytes displayed almost complete and fibroblasts partial GPI deficiency. The C→G substitution disrupts binding of the generic transcription factor Sp1 to a GC-rich box in the core promoter of *PIGM*, resulting in reduced histone acetylation and thus transcriptional repression. However, histone hypoacetylation is reversible. Specifically, in the presence of histone deacetylase inhibitors such as

**Table 12.6** Identity of the Fanconi anemia (FA) genes and proteins.

| FA genes | Chromosome | Exons | Frequency of FA (%) | Protein size (kDa) |
|---|---|---|---|---|
| FANCA | 16q24.3 | 43 | 65 | 163 |
| FANCB | Xp22.2 | 10 | <1 | 95 |
| FANCC | 9q22.3 | 14 | 10 | 63 |
| FANCD1/BRCA2 | 13q12.3 | 27 | <1 | 380 |
| FANCD2 | 3p25.3 | 44 | <1 | 155, 162 |
| FANCE | 6p21.3 | 10 | 4 | 60 |
| FANCF | 11p15 | 1 | 4 | 45 |
| FANCG | 9p13 | 14 | 10 | 68 |
| FANCI | 15q26.1 | 35 | <1 | 140, 147 |
| FANCJ/BRIP1 | 17q23.1 | 20 | <5 | 140 |
| FANCL | 2p16.1 | 14 | <1 | 43 |
| FANCM | 14q21.3 | 23 | <1 | 250 |
| FANCN/PALB2) | 16p12.1 | 13 | <1 | 140 |

butyrate, histone acetylation, *PIGM* transcriptional activity, GPI biosynthesis and surface GPI-linked protein expression can all be restored *in vivo* as well as *in vitro*, an effect dramatically highlighted by the complete abrogation of complicated, lifelong, and treatment-refractory epilepsy in a child with inherited GPI deficiency.

## Inherited bone marrow failure syndromes

### Fanconi anemia

FA is the most common cause of hereditary BMF. Early studies indicated that FA was a genetically heterogeneous disease, a notion confirmed by the identification, through the use of somatic cell hybridization, of 13 complementation groups. All 13 FA genes have now been cloned and characterized (Table 12.6). The overall frequency of heterozygotes for FA mutant genes in the general population is estimated at 1 in 300. In Ashkenazi Jews and in the Afrikaans population of the Republic of South Africa it is much higher (1 in 100 and 1 in 89, respectively), most likely as a result of founder effects.

*Clinical aspects* Gradual onset of BMF (median age 7 years; range, birth to 31 years), skeletal abnormalities (most commonly of the radius and thumb), skin lesions (hyperpigmentation, café-au-lait spots), renal and urinary tract malformations and gonadal dysfunction are the most common clinical manifestations. However, the clinical spectrum is even wider, as it includes congenital defects of the gastrointestinal system, heart and central nervous system. BMF is often heralded by thrombocytopenia, macrocytosis and increased hemoglobin F levels. Patients with FA have an

unusually high risk of developing treatment-resistant MDS and AML, estimated at 52% in total by the age of 40 years. Furthermore, the risk of a variety of solid tumors, especially squamous cell carcinomas of the skin, is several times higher than in the general population.

*Cellular phenotype and function of the FA proteins* A wealth of recent genetic and biochemical data has shed new light on the elusive function of FA proteins. They constitute the FA pathway, a new DNA damage-response pathway responsible for repair of inter- and intra-strand DNA cross-links (ICL), either occurring spontaneously or induced by agents like mitomycin C or diexobutane (Plate 12.3). ICL lead to replication fork arrest and cell cycle arrest in late S phase. Completion of the cell cycle is not possible unless ICL are repaired. FA proteins, organized in three groups functioning in a linear fashion, are essential for the successful resolution of the stalled DNA replication at the site of the cross-link. The FA core complex (FCC), comprising eight proteins (FANCA, B, C, E, F, G and M), receives signals of DNA damage through phosphorylation by ATR, a kinase sensor of DNA damage. This promotes binding of the FCC to the damaged DNA through FANCM and FAAP24, while FANCL through its ubiquitin ligase activity monoubiquitinates FANCD2 and FANCI, the two proteins constituting group II, also called the ID complex. Ubiquitination of the ID proteins along with their phosphorylation by ATR are required for their specific localization to the site of DNA damage where they interact with group III proteins. The finding that group III proteins corresponding to FANCD1, FANCN and FANCJ complementation groups were in fact identical to BRCA2 and its associated PALB2 and BRIP1 proteins respectively was an exciting discovery linking the

FA pathway to an already established process of DNA repair. *BRCA1* and *BRCA2* are tumor-suppressor genes often mutated in familial breast cancer. In concert with a number of other proteins (e.g., the helicase RAD51) of the DNA repair machinery, they are involved in different repair processes that include nucleotide excision repair, translesional synthesis and homologous recombination, all of which are required for removal and repair of ICL and restarting of DNA replication.

*Molecular genetics* FA, with the exception of FANCB which is X-linked, is an autosomal recessive disorder. The most characteristic cellular feature of FA cells is the formation of DNA double-strand breaks on exposure to DNA inter- and intra-strand adducting agents (clastogens) such as mitomycin C and diexobutane. The *in vitro* response to clastogens has made it possible to test cells from different patients for their ability to cross-correct each other's defect by somatic cell fusion. As discussed earlier, this has led to classifying patients in 13 complementation groups.

Mutations of *FANCA* account for about 60% of FA cases and are spread throughout the gene. None of the mutant alleles is common and few have been encountered more than once. Thus, identifying mutations in newly diagnosed cases of FA is laborious, as one needs to scan the entire coding sequence (of several genes, unless the complementation group is known).

Mutations in the *FANCC* gene account for about 10–15% of FA cases. The IVS4+A→T and del322G mutations comprise more than 75% of *FANCC* mutations. The IVS4+A→T allele is found in Ashkenazi Jews at a polymorphic frequency (1 in 80), and it is responsible for 85% of the FA cases in this population. Patients with IVS4 or exon 14 mutations tend to have earlier onset of hematological complications (BMF and MDS/AML), and to have a shorter survival compared with patients with exon 1 mutations or patients with FANCA or *FANCG*-related FA. Mutations in the *FANCG* gene are found in about 10% of FA cases. The stop codon mutation E105X accounts for 44% of mutations in German FANCG patients. It is interesting that although biallelic null mutations are very frequent in FANC genes of FCC, only hypomorphic mutations have been identified in *FANCD2* (3–6% of all cases of FA), highlighting a more important role of the ID complex compared with FCC which is not restricted only to ICL correction but also the repair of ionizing irradiation-induced double-strand DNA damage. Consistent with this, FANCD2 patients, despite the hypomorphic nature of the mutations, appear to develop the most severe form of FA, with multiple developmental abnormalities and early development of BMF and malignancy. The prevalence of mutations in other FANC genes is very low (<2%).

*FA and cancer* An important role of the FA pathway in the biology of sporadic cancers is increasingly being recognized. Epigenetic silencing of FAC genes has been identified in different solid tumors and acute leukemias and in some cases correlated with their sensitivity to chemotherapeutic agents causing DNA cross-links such as cisplatin, cyclophosphamide and melphalan. In a small proportion of patients with AML, somatic mutations in *FANCA* were identified but their functional significance is unknown. Therefore, studying the functional status of the FA pathway in different tumors may offer valuable information on which therapeutic choices can be based.

*Diagnosis* The clastogen test remains the gold standard clinical diagnostic test; however, complementation studies using retroviral vectors containing all 13 genes have now entered clinical practice and allow rapid assignment of patients to a specific complementation group. This is followed by screening for pathogenic mutations in the corresponding gene. As deficiency in any of the eight proteins of the FCC impairs its ubiquitin ligase activity, immunoblotting for ubiquitinated FANCD2 can also be used as a screening test to focus the search in the FCC genes or downstream of it. With this approach, genetic counseling, prenatal and preimplantation diagnosis are now feasible for most families with affected children. In areas with a large Ashkenazi Jewish population (e.g., New York City), screening for polymorphic *FAC* alleles is feasible on a wider basis and can be offered to all couples at risk.

*Treatment* The conventional management of FA focuses on the consequences of BMF and includes hematopoietic growth factors, blood product support and androgens. About half of the patients respond to androgens initially but often suffer from significant side effects, including androgen-induced hepatic adenomas. Eventually all patients become refractory.

HSCT from an HLA-identical unaffected sibling or from alternative sources is currently the only therapeutic approach that can successfully achieve long-term correction of BMF and possible prevention of MDS and AML. Best results, with reduced short- and long-term treatment-related mortality, are obtained with fludarabine-based, reduced-intensity, non-myeloablative conditioning HSCT regimens that do not include irradiation. Unfortunately, even after HSCT the patient remains at increased risk of developing solid tumors and thus requires close long-term follow-up.

The cloning of FA genes has opened the way to gene therapy for patients with FA. There is clinical and experimental evidence that HSCs with corrected phenotype have a survival and growth advantage over uncorrected cells and can support long-term hematopoiesis. Successful transfer of

FA genes to a small number of autologous HSCs should therefore be adequate to ameliorate the severity of BMF.

### Dyskeratosis congenita

Dyskeratosis congenita (DC) is another rare, genetically heterogeneous, inherited disorder with BMF as a major feature. Lacy reticulated skin, nail dystrophy, abnormal pigmentation, and mucosal leukoplakia in the first years of life and the later development of BMF classically define DC. Leukoplakia, particularly of the oral mucosa and also of the gastrointestinal and genital tracts, is common. Other clinical manifestations include developmental delay, short stature, ocular, dental and skeletal abnormalities, hyperhidrosis, hyperkeratinization of the palms and soles, bullae on minimal trauma, hair loss, sometimes gonadal failure, and features of premature aging.

*Molecular genetics and molecular pathogenesis* In the majority of cases (~85%) the mode of inheritance is X-linked recessive, and many cases are sporadic; in the remaining cases inheritance is either autosomal dominant or autosomal recessive.

The X-linked form of DC results mostly from missense mutations in the housekeeping gene *DKC1*. Mutations in *DKC1*, which maps to Xq28, account for about 40% of all DC cases. Hoyerall–Hreidarsson syndrome, a rare disorder characterized by severe growth failure, severe immunodeficiency, cerebellar abnormalities and BMF, has been shown to be in most cases allelic to *DKC1*.

Dyskerin, the protein product of *DKC1*, is homologous to Cbf5p, a yeast protein that in conjunction with the H/ACA class of small nucleolar RNAs is involved in the pseudouridylation (i.e., conversion of uridine to pseudouridine) of pre-ribosomal RNA (rRNA), a modification essential for ribosome biogenesis. Although defective pseudouridylation and ribosome biogenesis have been observed in a hypomorphic DKC1 mouse model, other studies failed to demonstrate any qualitative or quantitative defect of rRNA in DC patients. Instead, it was shown that dyskerin binds to an H/ACA domain of the RNA component of telomerase (TERC), i.e., the template used by the reverse transcriptase component of telomerase (TERT) for telomere lengthening, linking dyskerin to the process of telomere maintenance during cell division. Telomerase is a ribonucleoprotein complex and dyskerin is among a number of proteins interacting directly or indirectly with TERC, ensuring its stability and ability to function as a template for TERT. Telomerase activity is highest in rapidly dividing cells (e.g., dividing HSCs), during organogenesis, in early life and also in tumor cells. The critical evidence that DC is a disease of telomere dysfunction was provided by the finding of heterozygous mutations in the

451-nucelotide intronless TERC in some families with the autosomal dominant form of DC (Plate 12.4) and of TERT in a disease resembling DC. More recently, homozygous mutations in NOP10 and NHP2, another two components of the telomerase complex, were identified in the autosomal recessive form of DC. Thus, the current evidence links all types of DC, X-linked, autosomal dominant and autosomal recessive, in a common molecular pathogenetic pathway, namely the maintenance of telomere length. In keeping with this notion, all types of blood cells in DC patients have significantly shorter telomeres than age-matched controls. Shortening of telomeres to a critical length can result in either growth arrest and apoptosis, hence the development of BMF or, on some occasions, neoplastic transformation, hence the increased propensity to epithelial tumors.

The study of the genetics of DC has revealed another two interesting features. First, in families with TERC and TERT mutations, more severe disease in terms of onset and clinical manifestations has been observed in succeeding generations, suggesting the possibility of genetic anticipation. Indeed, the rate of telomere length loss was higher in succeeding generations in DC families, in keeping with similar observations in *Terc*$^{-/-}$ mice. Another interesting observation is the finding of heterozygous mutations in *TERT* and *TERC* in a small minority (<5%) of patients who were initially diagnosed with IAA, although many of these mutations were not obviously deleterious for the function of telomerase *in vitro*, were not detected in the parents of index cases or did not segregate with the disease. A likely interpretation of these findings is that mild TERC and TERT mutations may predispose to BMF, which develops after a certain insult, for example an immunological attack.

*Treatment* As for FA, there is no definitive treatment for DC and most patients die before the age of 30. The main causes of death are complications of BMF, opportunistic infections, pulmonary complications and malignancy. Few patients have had successful correction of BMF by HSCT.

### Diamond–Blackfan anemia

Diamond–Blackfan anemia (DBA) is a rare inherited syndrome with isolated anemia and erythroblastopenia as the main features, although with disease progression patients may develop bilineage or trilineage hypoplasia. Clinically, it manifests itself in the first months of life with macrocytic anemia, reticulocytopenia, increased hemoglobin F and elevated erythrocyte adenosine deaminase levels; occasional patients have thrombocythemia. The bone marrow is normocellular with characteristic absence of erythroblasts (<5% of nucleated cells). Growth retardation and other developmental abnormalities (including skeletal, cardiac and urogenital defects) are seen in about one-third of patients. There is also a small risk (~2%) of transformation to MDS/AML.

*Molecular genetics and pathogenesis* Most cases of DBA are sporadic but in multiplex families both autosomal dominant and autosomal recessive patterns of inheritance have been observed. There is variable penetrance and phenotypic variability even in the same families.

In about 25% of cases, heterozygous mutations in the ribosomal protein S19 gene (*RPS19*) have been identified in familial as well as in sporadic cases. In a handful of patients, heterozygous mutations in *RPS24*, *RPS17* and *RPL35A* have been identified. The finding of whole-gene deletions of *RPS19* in some cases strongly argues that haploinsufficiency, rather than a dominant negative mechanism, is responsible for DBA. As well as being a structural component of the mature small ribosomal subunit (40S; large subunit is 60S), RPS19 is also required in the nucleolus for the correct processing and cleavage from the precursor rRNA of the 18S fragment, which is the main rRNA constituent of 40S. In the same process, which is RPS19 independent, precursor rRNA is also cleaved to 5.8S and 28S rRNA which, along with the independently transcribed 5S rRNA, are the constituents of the large ribosomal subunit. Haploinsufficiency of *RPS19* and of the other ribosomal protein genes linked to DBA results in defective formation of the ribosomal subunits and eventually defective formation of the mature ribosome. How impaired ribosome function might lead to the relatively selective phenotype of erythroid differentiation arrest is not clear. It is possible that this is related to the extraordinary demand that hemoglobin production imposes on the translational apparatus. In addition, many ribosomal proteins, including RPS19, have been shown to participate in extraribosomal functions. For example, RPS19 might affect cell cycle progression through its interaction with the serine/threonine kinase Pim-1, while RPL11 stabilizes and activates P53 through an inhibitory physical association with the P53 inhibitor HDM2.

*Treatment* Blood transfusion for moderate to severe anemia is the mainstay of treatment for DBA. Over 50% of patients respond to steroids and become blood transfusion independent. Some sustain remission after steroid withdrawal but the majority either become steroid resistant or require an unacceptably high maintenance dose. Such patients may benefit from sibling allogeneic HSCT. The median long-term survival in a small series from the North American DBA registry was 87%; in contrast, the survival of patients receiving HSCT from an alternative donor was only 14%. Recent experimental evidence has indicated that leucine can enhance ribosomal and translational activity in DBA cells

without *RPS19* mutations through activation of the rapamycin-sensitive mTOR/RPS6 pathway. Clinical studies are currently testing the clinical effectiveness of leucine supplements as treatment for DBA patients.

## Red cell enzyme deficiencies

Inherited abnormalities of red cell enzymes, *red cell enzymopathies*, are a distinct set of genetic disorders with one important clinical manifestation in common, namely chronic hemolytic anemia. Most of the enzymes involved are housekeeping enzymes present, by definition, in all cells. Therefore one might expect that a severe reduction in activity of any of these might have generalized clinical manifestations. However, we can identify at least two reasons why red cells are more severely affected. Firstly, red cells have a much more limited metabolic machinery than most other somatic cells; if a particular enzyme is deficient, other cells may cope by the use of alternative or surrogate metabolic pathways. Secondly, mature red cells are not capable of protein synthesis: therefore if a particular enzyme is made highly unstable by a mutation, other cells can compensate by increased enzyme synthesis, but red cells cannot. Nevertheless, the fact that enzymopathies are not purely red cell disorders is highlighted by the coexistence, in some cases, of clinical manifestations in other systems, particularly the muscles and the nervous system; indeed, in some enzymopathies neurological damage may dominate the clinical picture.

This section deals with those enzymopathies affecting red cell metabolism for which the molecular basis has been elucidated. We do not discuss conditions in which an enzyme abnormality is also expressed in red cells but the main clinical manifestations are elsewhere (e.g., the porphyrias, galactosemia, Lesch–Nyhan syndrome). For the sake of brevity, most of the enzymopathies are discussed in groups.

### Enzymopathies of glycolysis

#### Clinical features

All these defects are rare to very rare (Table 12.7), and all cause hemolytic anemia with varying degrees of severity. It is not unusual for the presentation to be in the guise of severe neonatal jaundice that may require exchange transfusion; if the anemia is less severe it may present later in life, or it may even remain asymptomatic and be detected incidentally when a blood count is done for unrelated reasons. The spleen is often enlarged. When other systemic manifestations occur, they involve the central nervous system, sometimes entailing severe mental retardation, or the neuromuscular system, or both.

**Table 12.7** Synopsis of red cell enzymopathies.*

| Enzyme (abbreviation) | Isoenzyme[a] characteristic of red cells | Prevalence of enzyme deficiency | Main clinical features associated with enzyme deficiency[b] | Benefit from splenectomy[c] | Chromosomal localization |
|---|---|---|---|---|---|
| Hexokinase (HK) | R (I) | Very rare | HA | Partial | 10q22 |
| Glucose 6-phosphate isomerase (GPI) | | Rare | HA, NM, CNS | Partial | 19q13.1 |
| Phosphofructokinase (PFK)[d] | M | Very rare | HA, myopathy | | 12q13 |
| | I | | | | 21q22.3 |
| Aldolase | A | Very rare | HA, myopathy | | 16q22–q24 |
| Triosephosphate isomerase (TPI) | | Very rare | HA, CNS, NM, | None | 12p13 |
| Glyceraldehyde 3-phosphate dehydrogenase (GAPD)[e] | | Very rare | HA | | 12p13.31–p13.1 |
| Diphosphoglycerate mutase (DPGM) | | Very rare | Polycythemia | | 7q31–q34 |
| Phosphoglycerate kinase (PGK) | 1 | Very rare | HA, CNS, NM | Partial | Xq13 |
| Monophosphoglycerate mutase (PGAM-B) | B | | | | 10q25.3 |
| Enolase[e] | 1 (α) | Very rare | HA | | 1pter–p36.13 |
| Pyruvate kinase (PK) | R[f] | Rare | HA | Partial | 1q21 |
| Glucose 6-phosphate dehydrogenase (G6PD) | B | Common | HA | None | Xq28 |
| Cytochrome $b_5$ reductase | | Rare | Pseudocyanosis, CNS | | 22q13.31–qter |
| Adenylate kinase (AK) | 1 | Very rare | HA, CNS | Partial | 9q34.1 |
| γ-Glutamylcysteine synthetase (GLCLC)[g] | | Very rare | HA, CNS(?) | | 6p12 |
| Glutathione synthetase (GSS) | | Very rare | HA, CNS | | 20q11.2 |
| Glutathione peroxidase (GSH-Px) | | Very rare[h] | ?[h] | | 3q11–q12 |
| Pyrimidine 5′-nucleotidase (P5′N1) | | Rare | HA | Partial | 7p15–p14 |

| | | | Number of known mutations[i] | | | | | |
|---|---|---|---|---|---|---|---|---|
| | | | | | Deletion–insertion | | | |
| Number of exons | Number of amino acids[i] | 5′ UTR | Missense | Nonsense | In-frame | With frameshift | Affecting splicing | Total |
| 19 | 916 (917)[k] | | 1 | | 3–0 | | | 4 |
| 18 | 558 | | 16 | 2 | | | 2 | 20 |
| 24 | 780 | | 7 | 1 | | 1–0 | 6 | 15 |
| 22 | 784 | | | | | | | |
| 12 | 364 | | 2 | | | | | 2 |
| 7 | 249 | 1 | 9 | 2 | | 1–0 | | 13 |
| 9 | 335 | | | | | | | |
| 3 | 259 | | 1 | | 1–0 | | | 2 |
| 11 | 417 | | 8 | | 1–0 | | 2 | 11 |
| | 254 | | | | | | | |
| | 434 | | | | | | | |
| 12 | 574[f] | 2 | 90 | 9 | 3–3 | 7–6 | 12 | 132 |
| 13 | 515 | | 122[l] | 1 | 6–0 | | 1 | 130 |
| 9 | 276[m] | | 18 | 5 | 3–0 | | 5 | 31 |
| 7 | 194 | | 2 | 1 | | | | 3 |
| 16 | 637 | | 3 | | | | | 3 |
| 12 | 474 | | 14 | | 1–0 | 1–0 | 1 | 17 |
| | 201 | | | | | | | |
| 10 | 286[n] | | 3 | 1 | | 0–1 | 2 | 7 |

**Table 12.7** *Continued*

* We have listed all enzymes in the intermediary metabolism of red cells for which, to the best of our knowledge, the corresponding cDNA/gene has been cloned.

[a] No entry in this column means that there are no known isoenzymes; therefore it is assumed that the same enzyme type is present in all tissues.

[b] CNS, central nervous system involvement; HA, hemolytic anemia; NM, neuromuscular manifestations.

[c] Data available only on some patients.

[d] PFK in normal red cells consists of a mixture of the five tetrameric species that can be formed from random association of the M (muscle) and L (liver) highly homologous subunits (i.e., M4, M3L, M2L2, ML3, L4).

[e] Since no mutations have yet been reported, there is no formal proof that HA associated with this enzyme deficiency is due to mutation of the corresponding gene.

[f] The red cell form of PK called R is produced by the gene encoding the L (liver) subunit. Because a different promoter is used, the size of liver PK is 543 amino acids.

[g] γ-Glutamylcysteine synthetase consist of two subunits, a catalytic subunit and a regulatory subunit. The data concerning the catalytic subunit are shown here.

[h] There is no clear evidence that inherited deficiency of glutathione peroxidase exists.

[i] Including N-terminal methionine which, in fact, is cleaved off in most or all cases.

[j] Each individual molecular change, if observed in more than one patient, has been counted only once.

[k] The *HK-I* gene encodes both the erythroid specific (HK-R) and ubiquitous (HK-I) isoforms. HK-R transcription starts from the erythroid specific promoter upstream exon I (exon II is missing in the erythroid HK-R mRNA). HK-I transcription starts from the ubiquitously expressed promoter upstream exon II.

[l] The 122 missense mutations include two variants with normal activity, A and São Borja. Six variants have two missense mutations each and one variant has three different missense mutations.

[m] The cytoplasmic form of this enzyme, present in red cells, differs from the microsomal form present in other cells because, as a result of an alternative splicing pathway, it lacks the first 25 N-terminal amino acids. Therefore in other cells the size of the enzyme is 301 amino acids.

[n] Two alternatively spliced forms are present in reticulocytes. The main protein is the long 286 amino-acid protein (the third exon is spliced out); a longer protein contains 11 extra amino acids at its C-terminus.

*Source*: modified from Luzzatto L, Notaro R. (1998) Red cell enzymopathies. In: Jameson JL (ed.). *Principles of Molecular Medicine*. Clifton, NJ: Humana Press, pp. 197–207, with permission.

## Diagnosis

The diagnosis of hemolytic anemia is usually not difficult, thanks to the triad of normomacrocytic anemia, reticulocytosis and hyperbilirubinemia. Enzymopathies should be considered in the differential diagnosis of any chronic Coombs-negative hemolytic anemia. In most cases of glycolytic enzymopathies, the morphological abnormalities of red cells characteristically seen in membrane disorders are conspicuous by their absence. A definitive diagnosis can be made only by demonstrating the deficiency of an individual enzyme by a quantitative assay. For the sake of economy, it is sensible to carry out these rather laborious tests in order of frequency of occurrence of the various enzymopathies: first G6PD, then pyruvate kinase (PK), then glucose 6-phosphate isomerase, and so on (Table 12.7). If a particular molecular abnormality is already known in the family, then of course one could test directly for that at the DNA level, bypassing the need for enzyme assays.

## Molecular pathophysiology

Since the main physiological significance of the glycolytic pathway (see Figure 12.4 for an overview of glycolysis) in the red cell is to produce chemical energy in the form of ATP, the main consequence of any glycolytic enzymopathy is a shortage of energy supply. Since glycolytic enzymes are apparently present in cells in considerable excess, the 50% residual enzyme activity seen in heterozygotes does not become rate-limiting; thus, heterozygotes do not have hemolytic anemia, and that is why these enzymopathies show a recessive pattern of inheritance. As seen in Table 12.7, the majority of mutations so far identified in the genes encoding glycolytic enzymes are of the missense type, causing single amino acid replacements. This is important, because the low level of residual enzyme activity can still support some metabolic flow through the glycolytic pathway, and helps explain how red cells survive in circulation, even though their lifespan is reduced. With respect to the precise

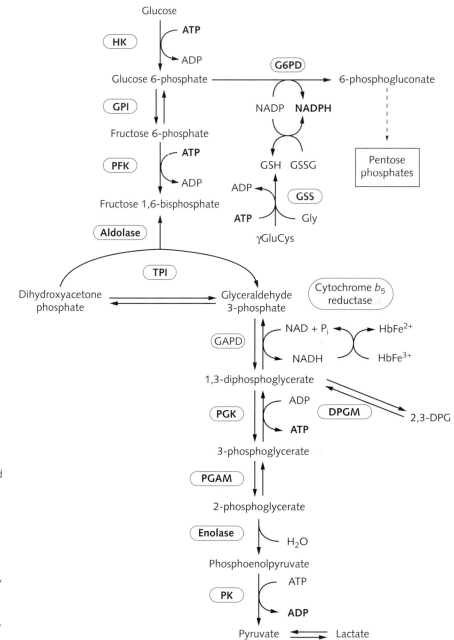

**Fig. 12.4 Intermediary metabolism in red cells**

The diagram shows the glycolytic pathway and related reactions (not the complete metabolic machinery of the red cell). Enzymes are enclosed in rounded boxes. Abbreviations as in Table 12.7. Additional abbreviations: DPG, diphosphoglycerate; GSH, reduced glutathione; GSSG, glutathione; HbFe$^{2+}$, hemoglobin; HbFe$^{3+}$, methemoglobin; γGluCys, γ-glutamylcysteine. From Luzzatto L, Notaro R. (1998) Red cell enzymopathies. In: Jameson JL (ed.). *Principles of Molecular Medicine*. Clifton, NJ: Humana Press, with permission.

reason why enzyme activity is reduced, we must consider at the protein level two basic mechanisms.

**1** In the majority of cases, loss of activity is probably due to decreased stability of the protein. In such cases we would predict that other cells might be much less affected than red cells, because the former can compensate for decreased stability through increased synthesis of the enzyme.

**2** In some cases, the amino acid replacement may affect the active center of the enzyme, which in turn may affect either substrate binding ($K_m$) or the catalytic rate of the enzyme

($K_{cat}$), or both; in this case other cells in which the rate of glycolysis is critical will be affected, as well as red cells.

**Management**

There is no specific treatment for these conditions. Patients with moderate anemia may require occasional blood transfusion when they experience exacerbations of the anemia due to increased rate of hemolysis or to decreased red cell production secondary to infection (the most extreme example being aplastic crisis from parvovirus infection). Patients with chronic severe anemia may require regular blood transfusion therapy with associated iron chelation. In some patients splenectomy has been beneficial. In severe cases bone marrow transplantation would be a rational form of treatment (for patients who have a suitable donor), provided there are no systemic manifestations other than hemolytic anemia, and provided it is carried out before there is organ damage (e.g., from iron overload).

# Glucose 6-phosphate dehydrogenase deficiency

## Epidemiology

G6PD deficiency is distributed worldwide, with a high prevalence in populations of Africa, southern Europe, the Middle East, Southeast Asia and parts of Oceania, as well as in regions to which migrations from these areas have taken place. The overall geographic distribution of G6PD deficiency and its heterogeneity, together with clinical field studies and *in vitro* culture experiments, strongly support the view that this common genetic trait has been selected by *Plasmodium falciparum* malaria, by virtue of the fact that it confers relative resistance against this highly lethal infection.

## Clinical features

Three types of clinical presentation are well characterized.
1 The vast majority of G6PD-deficient people are asymptomatic most of the time, but they are at risk of developing acute hemolytic anemia, which may be triggered by drugs, infections or fava beans.
2 The risk of developing neonatal jaundice is much greater in G6PD-deficient than in G6PD-normal newborns. This is of great public health importance, because untreated severe neonatal jaundice can lead to permanent neurological damage.
3 Chronic non-spherocytic hemolytic anemia (CNSHA): in contrast to the first two, this clinical presentation is very rare. The clinical picture is rather similar to CNSHA associated with glycolytic enzymopathies (*see above*) and again it is of variable severity. However, the hemolysis is characteristically exacerbated by the same agents that can cause acute hemolytic anemia in people with the ordinary type of G6PD deficiency.

## Diagnosis

The anemia is usually normocytic and normochromic, and its severity ranges from moderate to extremely severe. Acute hemolytic anemia is due largely to intravascular hemolysis, and hence is associated with hemoglobinemia and hemoglobinuria. The blood film may show spectacular evidence of hemolysis in the guise of anisocytosis, polychromasia, spherocytes, bite cells, blister cells and hemighosts. Supravital staining reveals the presence of Heinz bodies, consisting of precipitates of denatured hemoglobin. In CNSHA the morphology is less characteristic. The final diagnosis must rely on the direct demonstration of decreased activity of G6PD in red cells by an appropriate enzyme assay.

## Genetic basis

G6PD is a homodimeric molecule, and its single subunit is encoded by an X-linked gene. As a result of the phenomenon of X-chromosome inactivation in somatic cells, female heterozygotes are genetic mosaics, in whom approximately half of the red cells are normal and approximately half are G6PD-deficient. However, in some cases the ratio is imbalanced. Therefore clinical manifestations, such as favism, can occur in both hemizygous males and heterozygous females, but they tend to be milder in the latter, roughly in proportion to the fraction of red cells that are G6PD-deficient.

## Function of G6PD

In intermediary metabolism G6PD is aptly depicted as the first step in the pentose phosphate pathway. However, several lines of evidence indicate that its most essential role is not to produce pentose, but rather to produce reductive potential in the form of NADPH. Recently G6PD-null mouse embryos have been obtained through targeted inactivation of G6PD in embryonic stem cells. From a detailed analysis of hemizygous mutant embryos, who die by day 10.5, it was inferred that the cause of death is precisely the onset of aerobic metabolism. Interestingly, heterozygous embryos also die, somewhat later, only if their G6PD-null gene is of maternal origin: in this case the cause of death is a defective placenta, as a consequence of the selective inactivation of the paternal X chromosome in extra-embryonic tissues.

## Molecular pathophysiology

Acute hemolytic anemia is seen with variants of G6PD whereby red cells retain some 10% of normal G6PD activity, resulting in a limited capacity of these cells to withstand the oxidative action of an exogenous factor (oxidative hemolysis). In contrast, with other variants the steady-state level of G6PD is so low that it becomes limiting for red cell survival, even in the absence of any oxidant challenge: the result is CNSHA. Numerous point mutations in the *G6PD* gene

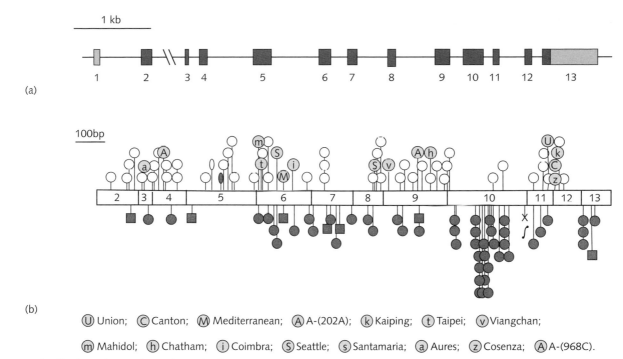

(a)

(b)

Ⓤ Union; Ⓒ Canton; Ⓜ Mediterranean; Ⓐ A-(202A); Ⓚ Kaiping; Ⓣ Taipei; Ⓥ Viangchan;

Ⓜ Mahidol; Ⓗ Chatham; Ⓘ Coimbra; Ⓢ Seattle; Ⓢ Santamaria; Ⓐ Aures; Ⓩ Cosenza; Ⓐ A-(968C).

**Fig. 12.5 Distribution of mutations along the human *G6PD* gene**
(a) Genomic structure of the human *G6PD* gene. Exons are shown as numbered rectangles (black rectangles represent coding sequences; shaded rectangles represent non-coding sequences). (b) The locations of amino acid substitutions are shown along the coding sequence of the gene, in which the exons are shown as open boxes. Substitutions giving rise to the more severe (class I) variants are shown as filled circles below. Small deletions, a nonsense mutation, and a splice site mutation are shown as filled rectangles, a cross and ≡, respectively. The milder class II and class III variants are shown as open circles above; polymorphic variants are shown as a letter in a colored circle. Class IV variants are shown as open ellipses. From Luzzatto L, Mehta A, Vulliamy T. (2001) Glucose-6-phosphate dehydrogenase deficiency. In: Scriver CR, Beaudet AL, Sly WS, Valle D (eds). *The Metabolic and Molecular Basis of Inherited Disease*, 8th edn. New York: McGraw-Hill, pp. 4517–4553, with permission.

causing CNSHA have been identified (Figure 12.5). Although we cannot explain the reason for a severe clinical phenotype in every case, a cluster of mutations causing CNSHA in exons 10 and 11 corresponds closely to the region of the molecule where the two subunits interface. It is not surprising that amino acid replacements in this region will interfere with dimer formation or cause marked instability of the dimer.

## Management

The commonest manifestations of G6PD deficiency, neonatal jaundice and acute hemolytic anemia, are largely preventable or controllable by screening, surveillance and avoidance of triggering factors, particularly fava beans, by G6PD-deficient subjects. When a patient presents with acute hemolytic anemia, and once the cause is diagnosed, no specific treatment may be needed if the episode is mild. At the other end of the spectrum, and especially in children, acute hemolytic anemia may be a medical emergency requiring immedi-

ate blood transfusion. The management of neonatal jaundice does not differ from that of neonatal jaundice due to causes other than G6PD deficiency and, in order to prevent neurological damage, treatment with phototherapy and/or exchange blood transfusion may be required. The management of CNSHA is similar to that of CNSHA due to glycolytic enzymopathies, but in addition it is important to avoid exposure to potentially hemolytic drugs. Again, although there is no evidence of selective red cell destruction in the spleen (as seen in hereditary spherocytosis), splenectomy has proven beneficial in severe cases.

Recently lifelong expression of human G6PD at therapeutic levels has been obtained in red blood cells and in white blood cells of mice through retroviral-mediated transfer into HSCs.

## 5′-Nucleotidase deficiency

This enzyme deficiency, known for some 30 years, is of interest for several reasons. First, it is probably the third most common red cell enzymopathy (trailing G6PD deficiency and PK deficiency). Second, the diagnosis can be suspected from red cell morphology because it is associated with basophilic stippling (accounted for by persistence of RNA in mature red cells). Third, although we do not really understand the precise mechanism, 5′-nucleotidase deficiency is a good example of how the red cell has virtually only one way to manifest it is suffering – almost any metabolic abnormality will lead to accelerated destruction (i.e., hemolysis). Fourth, the anemia of chronic lead poisoning (which had been known for a long time to be associated with basophilic stippling) turns out to be the consequence of the fact that lead is a powerful inhibitor of 5′-nucleotidase; thus in terms of its hematological effects, lead poisoning is a phenocopy of 5′-nucleotidase deficiency.

In 2001 a gene corresponding to a previously published 5′-nucleotidase cDNA was mapped to chromosome 7, and three different mutations in this gene were discovered in homozygosity in four subjects with 5′-nucleotidase deficiency. One was a missense mutation, one a nonsense mutation, and one a splicing mutation causing the loss of exon 9 from the mature mRNA. This important advance makes it now possible to carry out molecular diagnosis of 5′-nucleotidase deficiency. Moreover, it will be possible to explore the implications of heterozygous 5′-nucleotidase deficiency, which is of special interest in view of previous suggestions that it may interact with hemoglobin E disease to make its clinical expression more severe.

## Conclusions

Hematologists know only too well that anemia is not a diagnosis but the recognition of a sign for which we must find the cause and work out the pathogenetic mechanism, which ultimately must be explainable at the molecular level. Overall, for the majority of acquired anemias, things are by now pretty clear with respect to etiology, but not necessarily with respect to molecular mechanisms. For instance, although we do understand that iron deficiency limits heme synthesis and consequently hemoglobin synthesis, we do not know exactly how the mean cell volume is controlled by the supply of iron: for this reason we have omitted from this chapter a section on the commonest anemia of all, iron-deficiency anemia. However, it is gratifying that we can at least offer a model for the molecular basis of megaloblastic anemia, another major public health problem in many countries. With respect to the majority of congenital anemias, and certainly for the commonest among them, molecular genetics has answered not all, but most of the questions with respect to etiology and pathogenesis.

However, lest we become complacent, we must admit that, as is often the case in medicine, the time lag between fundamental discoveries and therapeutic applications too often remains too long, and that advances in knowledge are not always used wisely. On the one hand, we recently saw a patient with PNH who had massive hemoglobinuria and had become severely iron deficient as a result. He had been treated with erythropoietin but not with iron: a few weeks of daily ferrous sulfate 400 mg raised his hemoglobin from 6.7 to 10.1 g/dL. On the other hand, for patients who have, for instance, a severe chronic hemolytic disease due to PK deficiency, the outlook has only improved because we can offer better supportive treatment, not because we know the molecular basis. The latter will only become relevant once we learn to correct the PK deficiency by gene addition or by gene replacement. This is a major and worthy challenge for the next decade with respect to all the genetically determined anemias.

## Further reading

### Megaloblastic anemia and congenital dyserythropoietic anemias

Blount BC, Mack MM, Wehr CM et al. (1997) Folate deficiency causes uracil misincorporation into human DNA and chromosome breakage: implications for cancer and neuronal damage. *Proceedings of the National Academy of Sciences of the United States of America*, **94**, 3290–3295.

Chanarin I. (1979) *The Megaloblastic Anaemias*, 2nd edn. Oxford: Blackwell Scientific Publications.

Chui D, Oh-Eda M, Liao YF et al. (1997) Alpha-mannosidase-II deficiency results in dyserythropoiesis and unveils an alternate pathway in oligosaccharide biosynthesis. *Cell*, **90**, 157–167.

Dgany O, Avidan N, Delaunay J et al. (2002) Congenital dyserythropoietic anemia type I is caused by mutations in codanin-1. *American Journal of Human Genetics*, **71**, 1467–1474.

Fukuda MN. (1990) HEMPAS disease: genetic defect of glycosylation. *Glycobiology*, **1**, 9–15.

Ingram CF, Davidoff AN, Marais E, Sherman GG, Mendelow BV. (1997) Evaluation of DNA analysis for evidence of apoptosis in megaloblastic anaemia. *British Journal of Haematology*, **96**, 576–583.

Luzzatto L, Falusi AO, Joju EA. (1981) Uracil in DNA in megaloblastic anemia. *New England Journal of Medicine*, **305**, 1156.

Savage DG, Lindenbaum J. (1995) Folate–cobalamin interactions. In: Bailey L (ed.). *Folate in Health and Disease*. New York: Marcel Dekker, pp. 237–285.

Wickramasinghe SN. (1997) Dyserythropoiesis and congenital dyserythropoietic anaemias. *British Journal of Haematology*, **98**, 785–797.

Wickramasinghe SN, Fida S. (1994) Bone marrow cells from vitamin B12- and folate-deficient patients misincorporate uracil into DNA. *Blood*, **83**, 1656–1661.

# The sideroblastic anemias

## Sideroblastic anemia

Bekri S, Kispal G, Lange H et al. (2000) Human ABC7 transporter: gene structure and mutation causing X-linked sideroblastic anemia with ataxia with disruption of cytosolic iron-sulfur protein maturation. *Blood*, **96**, 3256–3264.

Bottomley SS, May BK, Cox TC, Cotter PD, Bishop DF. (1995) Molecular defects of erythroid 5-aminolevulinate synthase in X-linked sideroblastic anemia. *Journal of Bioenergetics and Biomembranes*, **27**, 161–168.

Camaschella C. (2008) Recent advances in the understanding of inherited sideroblastic anaemia. *British Journal of Haematology*, **143**, 27–38.

Cox TC, Bawden MJ, Martin A, May B. (1991) Human erythroid 5-aminolevulinate synthase: promoter analysis and identification of an iron responsive element in the mRNA. *EMBO Journal*, **10**, 1891–1902.

Rouault TA, Tong WH. (2008) Iron–sulfur cluster biogenesis and human disease. *Trends in Genetics*, **24**, 398–407.

## Pearson marrow–pancreas syndrome

Pearson HA, Lobel GS, Kocoshis SA et al. (1979) A new syndrome of refractory sideroblastic anemia with vacuolization of marrow precursors and exocrine pancreatic dysfunction. *Journal of Pediatrics*, **6**, 976–984.

Rotig A, Bourgeron T, Chretien D, Rustin P, Munnich A. (1995) Spectrum of mitochondrial DNA rearrangements in the Pearson marrow–pancreas syndrome. *Human Molecular Genetics*, **4**, 1327–1330.

# Bone marrow failure syndromes

## Aplastic anemia

Young NS. (2002) Acquired aplastic anemia. *Annals of Internal Medicine*, **136**, 534–546.

Young NS, Barrett AJ. (1995) The treatment of severe acquired aplastic anemia. *Blood*, **85**, 3367–3377.

Young NS, Maciejewski J. (1997) The pathophysiology of acquired aplastic anemia. *New England Journal of Medicine*, **336**, 1365–1372.

Young NS, Scheinberg P, Calado RT. (2008) Aplastic anemia. *Current Opinion in Hematology*, **15**, 162–168.

## Paroxysmal nocturnal hemoglobinuria

Almeida AM, Murakami Y, Layton DM et al. (2006) Hypomorphic promoter mutation in PIGM causes inherited glycosylphosphatidylinositol deficiency. *Nature Medicine*, **12**, 846–851.

Araten DJ, Nafa K, Pakdeesuwan K, Luzzatto L. (1999) Clonal populations of hematopoietic cells with paroxysmal nocturnal hemoglobinuria genotype and phenotype are present in normal individuals. *Proceedings of the National Academy of Sciences of the United States of America*, **96**, 5209–5214.

Hillmen P, Young NS, Schubert J et al. (2006) The complement inhibitor eculizumab in paroxysmal nocturnal hemoglobinuria. *New England Journal of Medicine*, **355**, 1233–1243.

Luzzatto L, Bessler M. (1996) The dual pathogenesis of paroxysmal nocturnal hemoglobinuria. *Seminars in Hematology*, **3**, 101–110.

Takeda J, Miyata T, Kawagoe K et al. (1993) Deficiency of the GPI anchor caused by a somatic mutation of the PIG-A gene in paroxysmal nocturnal hemoglobinuria. *Cell*, **73**, 703–711.

## Fanconi anemia

Alter B, Young NS. (1998) The bone marrow failure syndromes. In: Nathan DG, Orkin SH (eds). *Nathan and Oski's Hematology of Infancy and Childhood*, 5th cdn. Philadelphia: WB Saunders, pp. 237–335.

Andreassen PR, D'Andrea AD, Taniguchi T. (2004) ATR couples FANCD2 monoubiquitination to the DNA-damage response. *Genes and Development*, **18**, 1958–1963.

Cohn MA, D'Andrea AD. (2008) Chromatin recruitment of DNA repair proteins: lessons from the Fanconi anemia and double-strand break repair pathways. *Molecular Cell*, **32**, 306–312.

Garcia-Higuera I, Taniguchi T, Ganesan S et al. (2001) Interaction of the Fanconi anemia proteins and *BRCA1* in a common pathway. *Molecular Cell*, **7**, 249–262.

Howlett NG, Taniguchi T, Olson S et al. (2002) Biallelic inactivation of *BRCA2* in Fanconi anemia. *Science*, **297**, 606–609.

Joenje H, Patel KJ. (2001) The emerging genetic and molecular basis of Fanconi anaemia. *Nature Reviews. Genetics*, **2**, 446–459.

Levitus M, Waisfisz Q, Godthelp BC et al. (2005) The DNA helicase BRIP1 is defective in Fanconi anemia complementation group J. *Nature Genetics*, **37**, 934–935.

Litman R, Peng M, Jin Z et al. (2005) BACH1 is critical for homologous recombination and appears to be the Fanconi anemia gene product FANCJ. *Cancer Cell*, **8**, 255–265.

Meetei AR, Medhurst AL, Ling C et al. (2005) A human ortholog of archaeal DNA repair protein HEF is defective in Fanconi anemia complementation group M. *Nature Genetics*, **37**, 958–963.

Mosedale G, Niedzwiedz W, Alpi A et al. (2005) The vertebrate Hef ortholog is a component of the Fanconi anemia tumor-suppressor pathway. *Nature Structural and Molecular Biology*, **12**, 763–771.

Niedzwiedz W, Mosedale G, Johnson M, Ong CY, Pace P, Patel KJ. (2004) The Fanconi anaemia gene *FANCC* promotes homologous recombination and error-prone DNA repair. *Molecular Cell*, **15**, 607–620.

Pichierri P, Rosselli F. (2004) The DNA crosslink-induced S-phase checkpoint depends on ATR–CHK1 and ATR–NBS1–FANCD2 pathways. *EMBO Journal*, **23**, 1178–1187.

Strathdee CA, Gavish H, Shannon WR, Buchwald M. (1992) Cloning of cDNAs for Fanconi's anaemia by functional complementation. *Nature*, **356**, 763–767.

Venkitaraman AR. (2004) Tracing the network connecting *BRCA* and Fanconi anaemia proteins. *Nature Reviews. Cancer*, **4**, 266–276.

Wang W. (2007) Emergence of a DNA-damage response network consisting of Fanconi anaemia and BRCA proteins. *Nature Reviews. Genetics*, **8**, 735–748.

Wang X, Andreassen PR, D'Andrea AD. (2004) Functional interaction of monoubiquitinated *FANCD2* and *BRCA2/FANCD1* in chromatin. *Molecular and Cellular Biology*, **24**, 5850–5862.

Xia B, Dorsman JC, Ameziane N *et al.* (2007) Fanconi anemia is associated with a defect in the BRCA2 partner PALB2. *Nature Genetics*, **39**, 159–161.

Yamamoto K, Ishiai M, Matsushita N *et al.* (2003) Fanconi anemia FANCG protein in mitigating radiation- and enzyme-induced DNA double-strand breaks by homologous recombination in vertebrate cells. *Molecular and Cellular Biology*, **23**, 5421–5430.

### Dyskeratosis congenita

Autexier C, Lue NF. (2006) The structure and function of telomerase reverse transcriptase. *Annual Review of Biochemistry*, **75**, 493–517.

Heiss NS, Knight SW, Vulliamy JT *et al.* (1998) X-linked dyskeratosis congenita is caused by mutations in a highly conserved gene with putative nucleolar functions. *Nature Genetics*, **19**, 32–38.

Kirwan M, Dokal I. (2008) Dyskeratosis congenita: a genetic disorder of many faces. *Clinical Genetics*, **73**, 103–112.

Mitchell JR, Wood E, Collins K. (1999) A telomerase component is defective in the human disease dyskeratosis congenita. *Nature*, **402**, 551–555.

Vulliamy T, Marrone A, Goldman F *et al.* (2001) The RNA component of telomerase is mutated in autosomal dominant dyskeratosis congenita. *Nature*, **413**, 432–435.

### Diamond–Blackfan anemia

Boria I, Quarello P, Avondo F *et al.* (2008) A new database for ribosomal protein genes which are mutated in Diamond–Blackfan anemia. *Human Mutation*, **29**, E263–E270.

Draptchinskaia N, Gustavsson P, Andersson B *et al.* (1999) The gene encoding ribosomal protein S19 is mutated in Diamond–Blackfan anaemia. *Nature Genetics*, **21**, 169–175.

Farrar E, Nater M, Caywood E *et al.* (2008) Abnormalities of the large ribosomal subunit protein, Rpl35a, in Diamond–Blackfan anemia. *Blood*, **112**, 1582–1592.

Vlachos A, Ball S, Dahl N *et al.* (2008) Diagnosing and treating Diamond Blackfan anaemia: results of an international clinical consensus conference. *British Journal of Haematology*, **142**, 859–876.

### Red cell enzyme deficiencies

Beutler E. (1994) Glucose-6-phosphate dehydrogenase deficiency. *New England Journal of Medicine*, **324**, 169–174.

Hirono A, Kanno H, Miwa S, Beutler E (2001) Pyruvate deficiency and other enzymopathies of the erythrocyte. In: Scriver CR, Beaudet AL, Sly WS, Valle D (eds). *The Metabolic and Molecular Basis of Inherited Disease*, 8th edn. New York: McGraw-Hill, pp. 4637–4664.

Luzzatto L, Mehta A, Vulliamy T. (2001) Glucose-6-phosphate dehydrogenase deficiency. In: Scriver CR, Beaudet AL, Sly WS, Valle D (eds). *The Metabolic and Molecular Basis of Inherited Disease*, 8th edn. New York: McGraw-Hill, pp. 4517–4553.

Mentzer WC. (1998) Pyruvate kinase deficiency and disorders of glycolysis. In: Nathan DG, Orkin SH (eds). *Nathan and Oski's Hematology of Infancy and Childhood*, 5th edn. Philadelphia: WB Saunders, pp. 665–703.

# Chapter 13 Anemia of chronic disease

**Tomas Ganz**

*Department of Medicine, David Geffen School of Medicine at UCLA, Los Angeles, CA, USA*

## Introduction and definition

Anemia of chronic disease (more specifically referred to as anemia of inflammation) is the second most common form of anemia (after iron deficiency) and is seen in the setting of chronic infections, inflammatory disorders including rheumatological conditions and inflammatory bowel diseases, certain malignancies, and chronic kidney diseases. A related form of anemia develops within days in critically ill patients with sepsis or other acute conditions of systemic inflammation. While the prevalence of iron deficiency in the industrialized countries is now decreasing, anemia of inflammation would be expected to become more prevalent as the number of elderly with chronic inflammatory conditions continues to rise. The disorder usually presents as a mild-to-moderate anemia, with erythrocyte morphology ranging from normocytic and normochromic to microcytic and hypochromic, depending on the severity and duration of the underlying disease. Anemia of inflammation is defined by inadequate erythrocyte production in the setting of low serum iron despite preserved or even increased macrophage iron stores.

## General principles

The essential pathogenic feature of this anemia is the iron restriction of hemoglobin synthesis. Unlike iron-deficiency anemia, the restriction is due to the slow release of iron from stores rather than the absolute deficiency of total body iron. Depending on the underlying disease, the anemia is variably compounded by blood loss, decreased erythrocyte survival, decreased production of erythropoietin, true iron deficiency,

and perhaps direct suppression of the erythrocyte precursor population by inflammatory substances. Several of these factors may contribute to the pathogenesis of the extreme variant of the anemia that develops acutely in the critical care setting.

## Diagnosis

### Iron parameters

Hypoferremia, a decrease in serum iron concentration, is the defining feature of anemia of inflammation. It develops within hours of the onset of infection or severe inflammation. Synthesis of the iron-binding protein transferrin (measured directly or as total iron-binding capacity) is decreased, unlike iron-deficiency anemia where it is often increased. The decrease in transferrin concentrations develops more slowly than the decrease in serum iron levels because of the longer half-life of transferrin (8–12 days) compared with that of iron (about 90 min).

### Serum ferritin

Ferritin is found in serum as a large multimer consisting mostly of glycosylated L-ferritin subunits. Ferritin is secreted by macrophages and hepatocytes, and its serum levels are increased in response to iron loading of these cells. Systemic inflammation also increases ferritin secretion. Serum ferritin concentrations, reflecting inflammation and iron stores, are increased in anemia of inflammation and decreased in iron deficiency. Serum ferritin is thus very useful in the differential diagnosis of patients with low serum iron concentrations. However, depleted iron stores in patients with coexisting inflammation may yield intermediate ferritin values. In this situation, iron deficiency should be suspected if ferritin concentrations are below 60 µg/L. It has been

*Molecular Hematology*, 3rd edition. Edited by Drew Provan and John Gribben.
© 2010 Blackwell Publishing.

suggested that serum transferrin receptor assay may be helpful in differentiating iron-deficiency anemia from anemia of inflammation. Soluble transferrin receptor is increased in iron deficiency, reflecting the post-transcriptional stimulation of the synthesis of transferrin receptor by iron-regulatory proteins 1 and 2 during cellular iron deficiency, but it can also be increased in inflammatory disorders probably reflecting iron restriction affecting erythrocyte precursors. It is possible that the quantitative effects of inflammation and iron deficiency on serum transferrin receptor assay differ due to the differential effects of the two processes on the *in vivo* iron content of macrophages but this remains to be explored experimentally.

## Bone marrow studies

Bone marrow aspiration or biopsy is now rarely necessary for the diagnosis of anemia of inflammation. In general, the bone marrow appears normal, unless the underlying disease directly affects it. The most important information obtained from marrow examination is the content and distribution of iron, found as storage iron in the cytoplasm of macrophages or as functional iron in nucleated red cells. In normal individuals, several Prussian blue-staining particles are seen in many macrophages, and about one-third of nucleated red cells, called sideroblasts, contain blue inclusions. In iron deficiency, both sideroblasts and macrophage iron are absent. In contrast, in anemia of inflammation, sideroblasts are fewer but macrophage iron is increased. The increase in storage iron in the face of decreased plasma iron and fewer sideroblasts is characteristic of anemia of inflammation. Although the bone marrow iron stain could be considered the gold standard for the differential diagnosis of anemia of inflammation and iron deficiency, the procedure can cause patient discomfort and the serum ferritin assay has largely replaced it.

## Pathogenesis

### Hypoferremia

Within hours of the onset of systemic infection or inflammation, plasma iron concentrations markedly decrease in both humans and experimental animal models. This defensive response, hypoferremia of inflammation, is thought to restrict the availability of iron to extracellular microbes, limiting their proliferation during early phases of infection. Recent studies indicate that inflammatory cytokines, including prominently interleukin (IL)-6, increase rapidly in the first few hours of infection and induce the synthesis of the iron-regulatory hormone hepcidin. Hepcidin binds to the iron efflux channel ferroportin on iron-exporting cells (macrophages, enterocytes and hepatocytes), causing the internalization and degradation of ferroportin. Iron efflux is diminished and the continuing consumption of iron depletes the extracellular iron pool (Plate 13.1). By recycling senescent erythrocytes, macrophages in the liver and the spleen normally supply most of the extracellular iron. During infection and inflammation, macrophages retain iron, restricting its delivery to plasma and to erythrocyte precursors (Plate 13.2).

## Iron restriction of erythropoiesis

Although hypoferremia develops within hours of the onset of infection or inflammation, the effect of decreased iron and decreased hemoglobin synthesis on circulating erythrocytes is not immediately reflected in average erythrocyte hemoglobin content or size. This is because the iron restriction affects only erythrocyte precursors engaged in hemoglobin synthesis and not mature erythrocytes. New erythrocytes normally replace less than 1% of the circulating erythrocytes per day, so the average erythrocyte indices (mean corpuscular hemoglobin concentration, mean corpuscular volume) change slowly. However, some newer blood analyzers, which can measure the hemoglobin content of reticulocytes, detect the effect of iron restriction as a decrease in reticulocyte hemoglobin before there is a significant change in total hemoglobin. Iron restriction in anemia of inflammation is also detected as an increase in zinc protoporphyrin. Normally, when iron is sufficient during an intermediate step in the synthesis of heme, iron becomes incorporated into protoporphyrin IX. In iron deficiency, zinc partially replaces iron and the amount of zinc incorporated into protoporphyrin IX is increased. In anemia of inflammation, zinc protoporphyrin is also increased, indicating that insufficient iron is reaching the sites of heme synthesis in developing erythrocytes. Over the course of several weeks iron restriction results in anemia that can eventually become microcytic and hypochromic and resemble iron-deficiency anemia. The development of anemia of inflammation is accelerated by other effects of inflammation or the underlying disease that may act to shorten erythrocyte lifespan or cause blood loss.

## Effects of inflammation on iron absorption and release from stores

Inflammation-induced hepcidin also decreases the absorption of dietary iron by acting on ferroportin displayed on the basolateral membranes of enterocytes. Decreased iron absorption usually does not contribute much to the development of anemia because iron stores are generally sufficient to supply erythropoiesis for many months. However, the inflammatory blockade of iron absorption may contribute to anemia in situations where iron demand is high and inflammation is long-lasting, as is the case in growing children with inflammatory bowel diseases or juvenile rheumatological disorders. Hepcidin would also be expected to inhibit the release of iron from hepatocyte stores but the contribution of this effect to anemia of inflammation has not yet been established.

## Cytokines involved in anemia of inflammation

The contribution of specific cytokines to hypoferremia and anemia of inflammation has been difficult to delineate, mainly because cytokines interact in complex networks regulating each other's synthesis. In humans, depending on the disease, therapies targeting IL-1, IL-6 and tumor necrosis factor (TNF)-$\alpha$ have all been shown to improve anemia of inflammation along with other inflammatory manifestations. The association of IL-6 with anemia of inflammation appears to be the strongest. In both humans and mouse models, IL-6 induces hepcidin synthesis within hours by a transcriptional mechanism causing hypoferremia.

Cytokines also have direct effects on erythropoiesis. Studies in erythropoietic culture systems have demonstrated that TNF-$\alpha$, IL-1, and interferon (IFN)-$\beta$ and IFN-$\gamma$ can interfere with erythropoietin stimulation of erythroid progenitors. The role of these mechanisms *in vivo* has not yet been established.

## Inflammation and erythropoietin resistance

The normal response to anemia is an increase in erythropoietin production and subsequent compensatory increase in erythropoiesis. It has been suggested that for the same severity of anemia, erythropoietin production in anemia of inflammation is lower than it would be in other types of anemia. Indeed, in some studies of patients with anemia associated with rheumatoid arthritis or cancer, erythropoietin levels were not as high as in iron-deficiency anemia but other studies have not observed a significant difference in erythropoietin concentrations between iron deficiency and anemia of inflammation. Erythropoietin suppression by cytokines or lipopolysaccharide has been seen in some animal models of sepsis as well as in erythropoietin-producing cell lines. However, such suppression of erythropoietin production is not a major pathogenic mechanism of anemia of inflammation. If it were, the administration of relatively small amounts of erythropoietin should be sufficient to reverse the anemia of inflammation. Clinical experience and studies in animal models suggest the opposite: severe inflammation decreases the effectiveness of erythropoietin, a common clinical situation described as erythropoietin resistance. Both anemia and erythropoietin resistance have been seen in mice moderately overexpressing hepcidin, supporting the importance of the hepcidin–ferroportin axis and inflammatory iron restriction in the pathogenesis of anemia of inflammation as well as in erythropoietin resistance.

## Effects of inflammation on erythrocyte lifespan

In early studies, a small decrease in erythrocyte lifespan was noted in some animal models of inflammation, and it was suggested that inflammation activates reticuloendothelial macrophages to increase the removal of damaged or senescent erythrocytes. Other potential disease-specific mechanisms that could contribute to the decreased lifespan include the deposition of opsonic antibodies on erythrocytes and mechanical damage to erythrocytes from microvascular fibrin strands or injured endothelia. In most cases, the effects on erythrocyte lifespan are relatively small and would be compensated by a minor increase in erythropoiesis.

## Principles of treatment

Most often, the presenting symptoms of anemia of inflammation, fatigue and exercise intolerance, are difficult to distinguish from those of the underlying disease, be it an infection, inflammatory disease or malignancy. Whenever possible, the treatment should be aimed at the underlying disease. Effective treatment of the underlying disease will also lead to the resolution of anemia. Unfortunately, this is not always feasible.

Infrequently, anemia of inflammation can be severe enough to exacerbate underlying cardiac or pulmonary disease and cause cardiac ischemia. In this acute setting, erythrocyte transfusion can rapidly improve oxygen delivery and the manifestations of ischemia. More commonly, anemia is moderate and its treatment is less urgent. Erythropoietin with or without high-dose parenteral iron can be useful for anemia symptoms that cannot be reversed by treating the causative disease. High doses of parenteral iron may be required to overwhelm the hepcidin-induced retention of iron in macrophages, and possibly to expand erythrocyte precursor populations that produce a hepcidin-suppressing factor. In each patient, the potential side effects of erythropoietin and iron must be weighed against the anticipated benefits, and the clinical effectiveness of the drugs. The continued need for therapy should be evaluated regularly and critically.

## Future treatments

Improved understanding of the pathogenesis of anemia of inflammation should lead to the development of therapies targeting the cytokine pathways that mediate increased hepcidin production, hepcidin itself, its interaction with ferroportin, or the ferroportin internalization pathway. If successful, such interventions should reverse the iron block and provide sufficient iron for normal erythropoiesis.

## Further reading

### General

Weiss G, Goodnough LT. (2005) Anemia of chronic disease. *New England Journal of Medicine*, **352**, 1011–1023.

### Diagnosis

Hastka J, Lasserre JJ, Schwarzbeck A, Strauch M, Hehlmann R. (1993) Zinc protoporphyrin in anemia of chronic disorders. *Blood*, **81**, 1200–1204.

Wians FH Jr, Urban JE, Keffer JH, Kroft SH. (2001) Discriminating between iron deficiency anemia and anemia of chronic disease using traditional indices of iron status vs transferrin receptor concentration. *American Journal of Clinical Pathology*, **115**, 112–118.

### Mechanisms of hypoferremia

Kawabata H, Tomosugi N, Kanda J, Tanaka Y, Yoshizaki K, Uchiyama T. (2007) Anti-interleukin 6 receptor antibody tocilizumab reduces the level of serum hepcidin in patients with multicentric Castleman's disease. *Haematologica*, **92**, 857–858.

Kemna E, Pickkers P, Nemeth E, van der Hoeven H, Swinkels D. (2005) Time-course analysis of hepcidin, serum iron, and plasma cytokine levels in humans injected with LPS. *Blood*, **106**, 1864–1866.

Nemeth E, Rivera S, Gabayan V *et al.* (2004) IL-6 mediates hypoferremia of inflammation by inducing the synthesis of the iron regulatory hormone hepcidin. *Journal of Clinical Investigation*, **113**, 1271–1276.

Rivera S, Nemeth E, Gabayan V, Lopez MA, Farshidi D, Ganz T. (2005) Synthetic hepcidin causes rapid dose-dependent hypoferremia and is concentrated in ferroportin-containing organs. *Blood*, **106**, 2196–2199.

### Hepcidin and anemia

Nicolas G, Bennoun M, Porteu A *et al.* (2002) Severe iron deficiency anemia in transgenic mice expressing liver hepcidin. *Proceedings of the National Academy of Sciences of the United States of America*, **99**, 4596–4601.

Roy CN, Mak HH, Akpan I, Losyev G, Zurakowski D, Andrews NC. (2007) Hepcidin antimicrobial peptide transgenic mice exhibit features of the anemia of inflammation. *Blood*, **109**, 4038–4044.

Weinstein DA, Roy CN, Fleming MD, Loda MF, Wolfsdorf JI, Andrews NC. (2002) Inappropriate expression of hepcidin is associated with iron refractory anemia: implications for the anemia of chronic disease. *Blood*, **100**, 3776–3781.

### Clinical studies

Cash JM, Sears DA. (1989) The anemia of chronic disease: spectrum of associated diseases in a series of unselected hospitalized patients. *American Journal of Medicine*, **87**, 638–644.

Cazzola M, Ponchio L, de Benedetti F *et al.* (1996) Defective iron supply for erythropoiesis and adequate endogenous erythropoietin production in the anemia associated with systemic-onset juvenile chronic arthritis. *Blood*, **87**, 4824–4830.

Corwin HL, Krantz SB. (2000) Anemia of the critically ill: "acute" anemia of chronic disease. *Critical Care Medicine*, **28**, 3098–3099.

# Chapter 14 The molecular basis of iron metabolism

**Nancy C Andrews[1] & Tomas Ganz[2]**

[1] Duke University School of Medicine, Durham, NC, USA
[2] Department of Medicine, David Geffen School of Medicine at UCLA, Los Angeles, CA, USA

## Introduction

Iron is one of several metals that are essential for normal cellular processes. Its primary role in mammalian biology is to bind oxygen in hemoglobin and myoglobin, and to catalyze the enzymatic transfer of electrons by cytochromes, peroxidases, ribonucleotide reductases and catalases. When iron is deficient, the synthesis of iron-containing proteins is impaired, with adverse consequences for oxygen delivery and cellular metabolism. However, the same properties that make iron useful for these functions can also lead to cellular damage when iron is present in excess. Normally, several binding proteins constrain the activity of iron, but when their iron-binding capacity is exceeded, iron promotes the formation of reactive oxygen species that attack cellular lipids, proteins and nucleic acids. Thus, iron balance must be carefully maintained to avoid the deleterious effects of iron deficiency and iron overload. All known disorders of iron metabolism can be considered abnormalities of iron balance.

There is no physiological excretion mechanism for iron: iron losses result only from bleeding and exfoliation of skin and mucosal cells. Under normal conditions, iron enters the body exclusively by dietary absorption, and absorption is meticulously regulated to balance the small losses. Iron balance is disrupted when intake and losses are not matched. Iron deficiency occurs when the dietary iron supply is inadequate, when losses are increased (primarily because of bleeding), or when both of these circumstances are present. Iron overload results when iron absorption is inappropriately increased due to genetic defects in iron regulatory proteins,

or when repeated blood transfusions create a substantial iron burden.

Our understanding of the molecular processes of iron metabolism has advanced considerably over the last decade, as new techniques in genetics and molecular biology have been applied to problems in this field. Much of what we have learned has come from the study of patients with diseases of iron metabolism and from investigation of animals with spontaneous and induced mutations in genes important for the transport and storage of iron. Most features of iron metabolism are very similar among mammalian species, validating the use of rodent models. More recently, important insights into iron disorders in humans have also come from the study of iron metabolism in zebrafish and even yeast.

## Mechanisms of iron transport

### General principles

Iron is a large charged ion that cannot freely diffuse across cellular membranes. Transmembrane transfer requires specific carrier proteins. There are two general ways in which cells transport iron. Some cells, such as intestinal epithelial cells, hepatocytes and macrophages, are equipped both to take in (import) iron and to release (export) it. These cell types are involved in the acquisition, storage and mobilization of iron. Most other cells, and particularly erythroid precursors, import iron but do not release it unless the cells are destroyed.

Approximately 25 mg of iron are needed every day to support hemoglobin production in maturing erythrocytes. This amount is much greater than the 1–2 mg entering the body each day through the intestine. The iron for erythropoiesis is largely provided by reticuloendothelial

*Molecular Hematology*, 3rd edition. Edited by Drew Provan and John Gribben.
© 2010 Blackwell Publishing.

macrophages recycling iron from old erythrocytes and making it available to developing erythroid precursors.

Cells use at least three mechanisms to take up iron. Intestinal absorptive cells have cell surface transporters that carry ferrous ($Fe^{2+}$) ions directly across the membrane. Erythroid precursors use membrane receptors to take up iron bound to a protein carrier, concentrate the iron in a subcellular compartment, and then transfer it across the membrane of that compartment into the cytoplasm. Hepatocytes probably use both of these mechanisms. Finally, recycling macrophages acquire iron through the phagocytosis of aged or damaged erythrocytes, lysing the cells and extracting the iron from their hemoglobin.

## Intestinal iron transport

Our current understanding of intestinal non-heme iron transport is illustrated in Figure 14.1. Iron absorption takes place in an acidic environment in the proximal small intestine, just distal to the gastric outlet. Most non-heme dietary iron is in the ferric ($Fe^{3+}$) form. It is reduced to $Fe^{2+}$ by a brush border ferrireductase, most likely the duodenal cytochrome $b$ (DCYTB). The $Fe^{2+}$ ions pass through divalent metal transporter 1 (DMT1, formerly called Nramp2, DCT1), a membrane protein that allows iron to traverse the apical bilayer. DMT1 requires an acidic environment for its activity because it cotransports protons with iron atoms. Once it crosses the membrane, some of the iron is retained within the absorptive intestinal cells (enterocytes), and some is exported through the basolateral membrane through the action of a distinct transporter, ferroportin. A multicopper oxidase protein, hephaestin, facilitates basolateral transport, perhaps by oxidizing $Fe^{2+}$ to $Fe^{3+}$ to allow it to exit from ferroportin and to bind to the plasma iron carrier protein, transferrin.

The expression of ferroportin on the basolateral membrane of enterocytes is the principal mechanism controlling the rate of iron flux through this transport system. The more ferroportin on the basolateral membranes, the more iron from enterocytes is passed into the plasma. Iron retained within the enterocytes is lost from the body when these cells finish their short lifespan and slough into the gut lumen. The partitioning of iron (i.e., the process that governs how much enters the plasma and how much is retained within cells) is regulated by the hormone hepcidin through post-translational degradation of ferroportin. The hepcidin–ferroportin interaction plays an important role in determining the overall efficiency of iron absorption.

In humans and other meat-eating organisms, direct absorption of heme contributes importantly to total iron absorption. The pathways involved in heme absorption are not well understood.

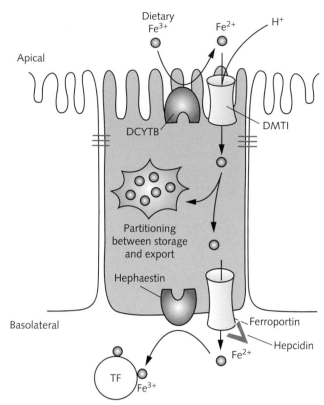

**Fig. 14.1 Intestinal non-heme iron absorption**
The cartoon shows an absorptive enterocyte from the duodenal epithelium, joined to adjacent cells by iron-impermeable tight junctions. The apical brush border is at the top and the basolateral surface is at the bottom. Dietary $Fe^{3+}$ iron is probably reduced by the ferrireductase DCYTB to produce $Fe^{2+}$ ion for transport. $Fe^{2+}$ crosses the apical membrane through the action of DMT1 to enter the cell. There, iron is partitioned between storage and export; stored iron is ultimately lost from the body when the epithelial cells senesce and exfoliate into the gut lumen. Meanwhile, a fraction of the iron is exported across the basolateral membrane by ferroportin. The iron hormone hepcidin binds to ferroportin and causes its degradation thereby inhibiting iron efflux, proportionally to hepcidin concentration. Hephaestin is a ferroxidase-like protein that aids in iron export, probably by reducing the $Fe^{2+}$ iron leaving ferroportin to the $Fe^{3+}$ form, which binds to plasma transferrin (TF).

## Other iron uptake mechanisms

Upon entry into the plasma, iron attaches to transferrin, an abundant plasma protein that binds iron with extremely high affinity. Transferrin serves three important functions. Firstly, it keeps iron in solution. In an aqueous, neutral pH environment iron exists as $Fe^{3+}$ ion, which is almost insoluble. Secondly, it renders iron non-reactive, and allows it to circulate in a safe non-toxic form. Thirdly, transferrin facilitates the delivery of iron to cells bearing transferrin receptors on their surfaces.

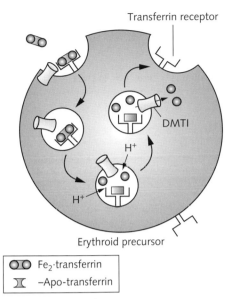

Transferrin receptor

DMTI

H⁺

H⁺

Erythroid precursor

Fe₂·transferrin
–Apo-transferrin

**Fig. 14.2 The transferrin cycle**
The transferrin cycle of receptor-mediated endocytosis is initiated by binding of diferric (Fe₂)-transferrin to a cell surface transferrin receptor. The ligand–receptor complex is internalized by invagination of clathrin-coated pits to form specialized endosomes. Influx of protons into the endosome decreases its pH to approximately 5.5, facilitating release of iron from transferrin. The iron is then transferred to the cytoplasm by DMT1. Apo-transferrin and transferrin receptor return to the cell surface for further cycles of iron uptake.

Most differentiated cell types express few, if any, transferrin receptors, but there are three important exceptions: tumor cells, activated lymphocytes and erythroid precursors. Tumor cells presumably use transferrin receptors to optimize iron uptake to support rapid proliferation. The same may be true for activated lymphocytes. However, the greatest demand for iron is by erythroid precursors, to support the large-scale production of hemoglobin. In normal adults, about two-thirds of the total body iron endowment is found in hemoglobin, distributed among erythroid precursor cells and circulating erythrocytes.

Iron-loaded transferrin binds with high affinity to transferrin receptors. Of the two forms of the receptor, transferrin receptor 1 (TFR1) appears to be critical for cellular iron uptake, but both TFR1 and transferrin receptor 2 (TFR2) are involved in systemic iron homeostasis. Transferrin receptors, carrying their iron-transferrin cargo, undergo endocytosis (Figure 14.2). Portions of the cell membrane bearing transferrin receptors invaginate into the cytoplasm, and bud off as intracellular vesicles (endosomes). Protons are pumped into the endosome to lower their internal pH, leading to the release of iron from transferrin. The liberated iron then leaves the endosome to enter the cytoplasm. This also

requires a transmembrane transport step, which is probably mediated by DMT1 and facilitated by the low endosomal pH. The process is assisted by one or more essential ferrireductases, in erythroid cells principally Steap3 (six transmembrane epithelial antigen of the prostate 3), that convert ferric to ferrous iron. Within the cytoplasm, ferrous iron is shuttled (by unknown mechanisms) to sites of use and storage. Meanwhile, transferrin and transferrin receptor proteins return to the cell surface, where transferrin is released and the receptors become available for further cycles of iron delivery.

Why should cells have evolved the complicated transferrin cycle when it is possible to take up iron directly? There are at least two likely answers. Firstly, tight binding of iron to transferrin is advantageous while iron is in the circulation, but it complicates the transport of iron into cells. The pH-dependent release of iron, occurring in a controlled intracellular environment, solves the problem of liberating the iron. Secondly, binding of iron-loaded transferrin to transferrin receptors serves to concentrate iron in the vicinity of DMT1, probably achieving much higher local iron concentrations than would be possible without such a mechanism. This allows more efficient iron uptake by cells with large needs (erythroid precursors, tumor cells, activated lymphocytes) without exposing other cells to unnecessary iron.

Undoubtedly, other cell types use these and other schemes for assimilating iron. Hepatocytes and macrophages are particularly important in iron homeostasis and their iron uptake mechanisms, though not well understood, deserve mention. Hepatocytes express both types of transferrin receptor and likely take up iron via the transferrin cycle. Hepatocytes also avidly take up non-transferrin-bound iron when the plasma iron concentration exceeds the binding capacity of transferrin. This is an abnormal situation, because there are usually about three times as many transferrin iron-binding sites as are needed (i.e., transferrin is normally about 30% saturated with iron). However, patients with iron overload may have more iron than transferrin can accommodate, and this excess iron appears to be rapidly removed from the circulation by hepatocytes. The molecular mechanism for hepatic non-transferrin-bound iron uptake has not yet been identified. Hepatocytes express ferroportin and release iron at least in part by a hepcidin-controlled ferroportin-dependent mechanism.

As discussed earlier, reticuloendothelial macrophages obtain iron by phagocytosing and breaking down erythrocytes. This process takes place in discrete phagocytic vesicles within the cells, and likely involves the action of heme oxygenase, an enzyme that catalyzes the degradation of heme. After crossing the phagosomal membranes, cytoplasmic iron is stored in ferritin. Macrophages export ferrous iron through their abundant ferroportin, assisted by the plasma ferroxidase ceruloplasmin so that ferric iron is delivered to plasma transferrin. Similar to intestinal cells and hepatocytes, reticuloendothelial macrophages partition their iron content into retained and released portions. This process is regulated in response to the iron needs of the body by the hepatic hormone hepcidin, which induces the internalization and degradation of macrophage ferroportin. While there is currently no direct way to measure how much iron is retained and how much is released, commonly used laboratory tests provide some information. The concentration of serum iron (and hence transferrin saturation) is determined by two factors: macrophage iron release and erythroid iron utilization. When erythropoiesis occurs at a steady rate, transferrin saturation is determined primarily by the rate of macrophage iron release, increasing when there is increased iron export and decreasing when iron is retained or when less iron is being recycled from erythrocytes. In contrast, the concentration of serum ferritin roughly correlates with the amount of storage iron in the body. The origin(s) of serum ferritin is not known, but it appears to be derived primarily from reticuloendothelial macrophages and hepatocytes. However, serum ferritin is not a very accurate indicator, because levels are increased by inflammation, tissue damage and rare congenital hyperferritinemia disorders. Nonetheless, a low serum ferritin value invariably indicates depleted iron stores.

## Sites of iron storage

Iron is stored within cells in the cavities of ferritin protein multimers. There are two types of ferritin subunit, L and H, both approximately 20 kDa in size. These subunits assemble in varying proportions into 24-subunit cage-like structures. Up to several thousand iron atoms can be stored in each ferritin multimer. Like transferrin, ferritin's function is to prevent iron from reacting with other cellular constituents, and allows controlled iron release in response to increased cellular needs. The molecular details of iron incorporation into and release from ferritin are not well understood. Under some circumstances, ferritin and other cellular components are partially degraded and conglomerated to form hemosiderin, a heterogeneous iron-containing substance that probably serves little purpose but to keep iron from causing harm. Both ferritin and hemosiderin accumulate in iron-overloaded tissues.

The liver serves as the primary depot for iron in excess of immediate needs. It has a very large capacity for storing iron, though this capacity is ultimately exceeded in iron overload disorders. While other tissues (myocardium, pancreas) also fill up with iron in iron overload, the liver is frequently the first site where damage from iron overload becomes appar-

ent. Hepatocytes avidly take up non-transferrin-bound iron from the plasma.

Reticuloendothelial macrophages are also important for iron storage, but their iron comes from degraded erythrocytes. Patients treated with frequent transfusions typically accumulate excess iron in macrophages first, and only later in other tissues. This pattern of iron accumulation has been referred to as "siderosis" to distinguish it from hemochromatosis, which is primary iron loading of parenchymal cells.

## Regulation of iron homeostasis

Iron homeostasis requires the coordinated regulation of iron transport and iron storage so that tissues will have adequate amounts to meet their needs but will not become overloaded with iron. Regulation must involve the control of cellular iron import, export and partitioning. Over the last few years, better understanding of regulation at each of these steps has emerged.

There are at least four known regulators of intestinal iron absorption (Plate 14.1): iron stores, erythropoietic demand, hypoxia and inflammation. The *stores regulator* modulates absorption several-fold, increasing absorption in iron deficiency and decreasing absorption in iron overload. The *erythroid regulator* is more potent: it can increase iron absorption many-fold when erythropoiesis becomes iron-restricted. The *hypoxia regulator* is not well characterized, but its effects may be at least partly distinct from those of the erythroid regulator. This regulator increases iron absorption in response to hypoxia. Finally, an *inflammation regulator* decreases iron absorption in response to inflammation from a variety of causes.

Similar influences also regulate the release of recycled iron from reticuloendothelial macrophages. During inflammation or iron sufficiency, iron is retained in macrophages but is released in response to iron deficiency or erythroid demand. The regulation of iron storage in hepatocytes is less well understood but it is clearly responsive to systemic iron requirements.

The iron-regulatory hormone hepcidin is likely to be the common effector of the stores, erythroid, hypoxia and inflammation regulators (Plate 14.1). Hepcidin (also called LEAP, HAMP) is produced by hepatocytes as a 25-amino acid peptide with four disulfide bonds that is cleaved from a larger precursor molecule. Administration of synthetic hepcidin to mice results in profound and prolonged hypoferremia. The hypoferremic effect of hepcidin is due to its ability to inhibit the major mechanisms that deliver iron to plasma: intestinal iron absorption and the release of iron from recycling compartments and stores in the spleen and the liver. Continuing consumption of iron by

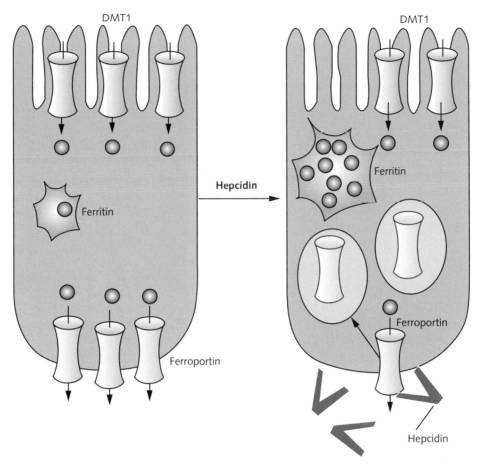

**Fig. 14.3 Regulation of cellular iron transport by hepcidin**
Hepcidin regulates the release of iron from enterocytes (shown in the figure) and macrophages by binding to ferroportin and inducing its internalization and degradation in lysosomes. Under the influence of hepcidin, iron export is decreased and iron accumulates in cytoplasmic ferritin. In enterocytes, regulatory effects of increased cellular iron may result in decreased iron uptake.

erythropoiesis and other iron-requiring processes then rapidly depletes the relatively small plasma and extracellular iron compartment.

On the cellular and molecular level, hepcidin inhibits the efflux of cellular iron into extracellular fluid or plasma, exerting its effect on the major cell types involved in iron transport: enterocytes, macrophages, hepatocytes and placental syncytiotrophoblast. Unlike other cell types, iron-exporting cells express ferroportin, the sole known cellular iron exporter. Hepcidin acts by binding to ferroportin, inducing its internalization and lysosomal degradation (Figure 14.3). The ferroportin degradation pathway is similar to that of other receptors undergoing ligand-induced endocytosis, and requires tyrosine phosphorylation in a cytoplasmic domain for internalization, and ubiquitination of a nearby lysine for degradation. The loss of ferroportin from cell membranes proportionately reduces the efflux of iron into extracellular fluid

The production of hepcidin is increased in response to dietary or parenteral iron loading, presumably as part of a compensatory mechanism to decrease iron absorption and decrease plasma iron (primarily derived from recycling macrophages). Hepcidin thus acts as the stores regulator. The production of hepcidin is decreased by iron deficiency, allowing more iron to enter the body through the intestine and more iron to enter the plasma from recycling macrophages. In addition, hepcidin is suppressed by increased erythropoietic activity, sometimes even in the face of systemic iron overload, confirming that hepcidin is the ultimate erythroid regulator. It is not yet clear how the increased erythropoietic activity in the bone marrow is communicated to the hepatocytes that make hepcidin. The production of hepcidin is also decreased in hypoxia, suggesting that it is an effector of the hypoxia regulator. Finally, hepcidin expression is induced by inflammation, probably through a direct action of the cytokine interleukin (IL)-6 and other inflammatory mediators on hepatocytes. In this case, induced hepcidin expression leads to decreased intestinal iron absorption and decreased macrophage iron release, acting as an inflammation regulator. There is growing evidence that, in response to the inflammatory regulator, increased hepcidin expression contributes to the abnormal iron homeostasis observed in the anemia of chronic disease (also known as the anemia of chronic disorders). It is likely that a useful clinical assay for hepcidin levels in serum and/or urine will soon become available.

Based on recent studies in cellular models, genetically altered mice and patients with genetic iron disorders, hepcidin synthesis in hepatocytes is regulated by iron sensors and signaling molecules assembled around the scaffold of the bone morphogenetic protein receptor (BMPR) and its signaling pathway. Two molecules that may function as iron sensors are TFR1 and TFR2. The transmembrane molecule HFE can bind to both transferrin receptors but is displaced from TFR1 when the receptor binds its main ligand, iron-transferrin. The glycosylphosphatidylinositol (GPI)-linked membrane protein hemojuvelin binds to BMPR and its BMP ligands, and may act as a co-receptor that converts the generic BMPR pathway into an iron-regulatory pathway. Although multiple BMPs, including BMP-2, BMP-4, BMP-6 and BMP-9, can stimulate hepcidin synthesis in hepatocytes and hepatocyte-derived cell lines, BMP-6 appears to be uniquely specialized for signaling in iron homeostasis. How all these molecules interact to generate the hepcidin-regulatory complex remains largely speculative but this could soon change.

# Iron disorders

In most general terms, iron disorders represent a failure of homeostatic mechanisms that match intestinal iron absorption and systemic iron distribution to the iron requirements of erythropoiesis and other iron-consuming processes. Iron homeostasis results in the maintenance of normal plasma and extracellular iron concentrations (10–30 μmol/L in humans) and normal iron stores in macrophages and hepatocytes that help buffer transient disturbances in the supply or demand for iron. Either genetic or environmental causes, and often both, can contribute to iron disorders.

## Iron-deficiency disorders

Iron deficiency is a major public health problem and the most common nutritional cause of anemia. Very rarely, iron deficiency is genetic and is manifested as hypoferremia, hypoferritinemia and iron-restricted microcytic anemia refractory to oral iron administration. Recent studies have shown that homozygous or compound mutations in a gene encoding TMPRSS6 (*Transmembrane protease, serine 6*, also called matriptase 2) are responsible for most cases of iron-refractory iron-deficiency anemia. TMPRSS6 negatively regulates hepcidin, reportedly by cleaving membrane hemojuvelin.

Most genetic disorders of iron metabolism result in iron overload rather than iron deficiency. They are attributable to mutations that affect the regulation of intestinal iron absorption and body iron distribution. The prominence of mutations that cause iron loading, rather than iron deficiency, can probably be explained by the fact that humans live in an iron-rich environment, and the body has developed strategies to limit iron absorption rather than to enhance it.

## Iron overload disorders

Several years ago, it was widely believed that there was only one major genetic disorder leading to iron overload. It is now clear that there are many genetic iron overload disorders. They can be generally classified as hemochromatosis disorders (iron deposition in parenchymal cells) or siderosis disorders (deposition of iron in reticuloendothelial macrophages). The known disorders and their genetic causes are listed in Table 14.1. Over the last few years, it has become clear that the final common mechanism for most forms of hereditary hemochromatosis is relative or absolute hepcidin deficiency or, rarely, resistance to hepcidin. The lack of hepcidin or the loss of its effect on ferroportin results in excessive or unrestrained absorption of dietary iron, as well as the depletion of the macrophage iron storage compartment. The genetically defective proteins in hereditary iron overload disease are implicated as regulators of hepcidin (HFE, TFR2, hemojuvelin), targets of hepcidin (ferroportin), or molecules that convey iron to the iron-sensing mechanism in hepatocytes (transferrin).

### HFE-associated hemochromatosis

The most common form of hemochromatosis was classically described as the triad of cirrhosis, diabetes and skin melanosis ("bronze diabetes"). It is a late-onset disorder, inherited in an autosomal recessive pattern and characterized by iron deposition in parenchymal cells of the liver, pancreas and heart. Macrophages of the reticuloendothelial system are iron-depleted or at least relatively spared. This disorder results from a small but chronic increase in intestinal iron absorption, averaging about twofold to threefold above the normal level. Over time, the presence of iron causes damage by promoting the formation of toxic oxygen radicals, which attack cellular structures and thereby cause reactive

**Table 14.1** Iron overload disorders.

| Disorder | Chromosomal location of defective genes | Gene (types of mutations) | Phenotype | Hepcidin |
|---|---|---|---|---|
| **Hemochromatosis disorders** | | | | |
| HFE-associated hemochromatosis (also called type 1 hemochromatosis) | 6p, near the HLA complex | *HFE* (missense and splicing mutations; C282Y is the most important) | Iron accumulation in the parenchymal cells of the liver, heart, pancreas; elevated transferrin saturation; relative paucity of iron in macrophages. Clinical manifestations include liver fibrosis, cirrhosis, markedly increased incidence of hepatocellular carcinoma, cardiomyopathy and diabetes | Low or inappropriately normal for iron overload |
| Juvenile hemochromatosis (also called type 2 hemochromatosis) | 1q 19q | Hemojuvelin Hepcidin (all known mutations prevent production of any hepcidin protein) | Similar to HFE-associated hemochromatosis, but greatly accelerated, leading to severe cardiac and endocrine complications in the second decade of life | Very low to absent |
| TFR2-associated hemochromatosis (also called type 3 hemochromatosis) | 7q | *TFR2* (missense and nonsense mutations) | Similar to HFE-associated hemochromatosis | Low |
| Autosomal dominant hemochromatosis (also called type 4 hemochromatosis) | 2q | Ferroportin (rare missense mutations causing resistance to hepcidin). Most other missense ferroportin mutations cause loss of function and siderosis | Iron accumulation in parenchymal cells | ? |
| Type 5 hemochromatosis | ? (Postulated to explain hemochromatosis in patients without mutations in known genes) | ? | Similar to HFE-associated hemochromatosis but apparently not due to mutations in *HFE*, *TFR2* or hepcidin | ? |
| **Siderosis disorders** | | | | |
| Autosomal dominant siderosis (also called type 4 hemochromatosis) | 2q | Ferroportin (only missense mutations) | Macrophage-predominant iron loading; in some patients parenchymal iron loading can occur later. Some patients have anemia early in their course (particularly women). Ferritin levels are markedly elevated, but serum transferrin saturation generally is not | Normal or high (few patients studied) |
| African siderosis | ? | Unknown | Similar to autosomal dominant siderosis but ferroportin mutations have not been reported. Thought to be a combination of genetic and environmental factors | ? |
| **Disorders of iron balance** | | | | |
| Atransferrinemia | 3q | Transferrin (missense mutations) | Deficiency in serum transferrin leading to tissue iron overload and severe iron-deficiency anemia | Low |
| Aceruloplasminemia | 3q | Ceruloplasmin (missense and null mutations) | Deposition of iron in the brain, liver and pancreas. Late-onset neurodegenerative disease, dementia and diabetes | ? |

fibrosis. The earliest manifestation of HFE-associated hemochromatosis is increased transferrin saturation, often approaching 100% before tissue iron deposition is noted. The treatment for hemochromatosis is phlebotomy, and this has been used effectively for more than half a century. Initially, blood is removed frequently to rapidly decrease storage iron. Later, iron balance is maintained by periodic phlebotomy, titrated to meet the needs of the individual patient. This treatment apparently produces no significant morbidity and has been shown to normalize the life expectancy of affected patients.

Hemochromatosis has been recognized as an inborn error of iron metabolism since the 1930s. In 1976 a French physician, Marcel Simon, made the important observation that the genetic predisposition to hemochromatosis was linked to the human major histocompatibility complex on chromosome 6p, and was most frequently associated with an HLA-A3 haplotype. This insight laid the groundwork for the discovery of causative mutations in the *HFE* gene 20 years later. It is now known that most patients with classical hemochromatosis are homozygous for a unique mutation (cysteine 282 to tyrosine, or C282Y) in *HFE*, perhaps originating in a northern European ancestor.

HFE is an atypical HLA class I molecule, similar to its chromosomal neighbors. Although most members of this family are involved in immune regulation, HFE has no known function in the immune system. It interacts with TFR1 on the cell surface, where its binding site overlaps with that of transferrin. Recent studies indicate that the binding of transferrin to TFR1 displaces HFE, making it active as a stimulus for hepcidin synthesis.

The C282Y mutation is highly prevalent. In typical populations of European descent, the carrier frequency has been estimated to be between about 1 in 8 and 1 in 10. This indicates that about 1 in 200 individuals are homozygous, and at risk of iron loading. However, not all C282Y homozygotes will develop clinical hemochromatosis. There is a wide range in iron loading and its complications. Some individuals will have severe manifestations by the third decade of life, whereas others may never have signs or symptoms of hemochromatosis. This variability is probably explained by gender (iron loss through menstruation), other genetic factors (modifying genes) and environmental factors (e.g., alcohol intake, dietary iron consumption). The modifying genes have not yet been identified, but their characterization is the subject of active investigation in this field.

In addition to C282Y, other mutations and polymorphisms have been identified in the *HFE* gene. The most common of these is a histidine-to-aspartic acid substitution at amino acid 63 of the protein (H63D). This polymorphism is found in about one-fifth of the world's population.

Although it may occasionally be associated with iron overload, particularly when it is found in individuals heterozygous for the C282Y mutation, its clinical significance remains poorly understood, though clinical laboratories test for it. Most other *HFE* mutations are quite rare and are not identified by routine screening tests.

In the past, the proportion of at-risk C282Y homozygous individuals who develop clinical hemochromatosis was estimated to be about 20–40%. Recently, Beutler and colleagues published the results of a large questionnaire-based study of patients seen by a health maintenance organization, in which they concluded that fewer than 1% of C282Y homozygotes would have severe disease. There is no consensus yet on laboratory parameters that identify C282Y homozygotes at risk for clinically significant organ damage but recent data indicate that few if any patients with serum ferritin levels below 1000 ng/mL develop cirrhosis, the main complication of hemochromatosis.

### Juvenile hemochromatosis

Juvenile hemochromatosis is similar to HFE-associated hemochromatosis, but very rare, and characterized by earlier onset of iron loading and its complications. The target organs are the same as those affected in HFE hemochromatosis, but cardiac and endocrine dysfunction are more problematic, and untreated patients typically die from cardiomyopathy by age 30 years. Liver cirrhosis and failure are uncommon. There are several possible explanations for this pattern. Firstly, experience with patients who develop siderosis from chronic transfusion therapy suggests that rapid iron loading is especially toxic for the heart and endocrine tissues. Secondly, pathological iron deposition in the adolescent years may be particularly bad for young hearts which are growing to meet the demands of a larger body mass; this is analogous to the problems noted with doxorubicin cardiotoxicity in this age group. Furthermore, endocrine problems are probably more apparent in adolescents because they fail to go through normal pubertal development. Juvenile hemochromatosis is a particularly lethal disorder, but it can be effectively treated by phlebotomy.

Studies of families with juvenile hemochromatosis have shown that there are at least two genetic loci responsible. Some individuals are homozygous for ablative mutations in the hepcidin gene on human chromosome 19q. However, most juvenile hemochromatosis families have homozygous or compound heterozygous mutations in hemojuvelin (also called HFE2, or repulsive guidance molecule RgmC) on chromosome 1q. Hemojuvelin is a GPI-linked membrane protein that functions as an essential regulator of hepcidin. Disruption of both copies of hemojuvelin has been shown to cause profound hepcidin deficiency. It thus appears that

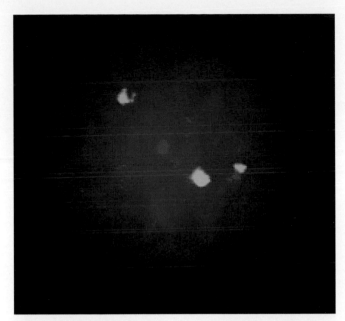

**Plate 2.1** *BCR-ABL* **rearrangement in an interphase cell**
The reciprocal t(9;22) generates two fusion signals using the Vysis dual fusion probes corresponding to the der(9) and der(22). A normal *ABL* (red) and *BCR* (green) are present.

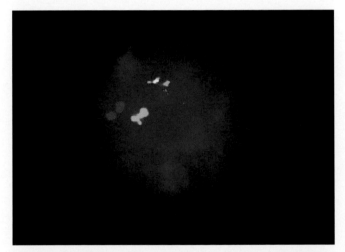

**Plate 2.2** *BCR-ABL* **dual fusion probe in a patient with deletion of sequences around the breakpoint of both the der(9) and der(22), thus generating just one fusion signal**

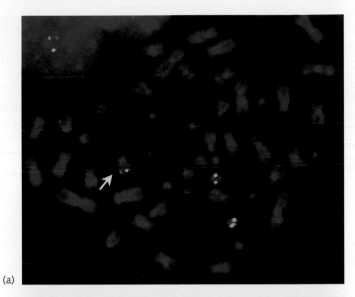

(a)

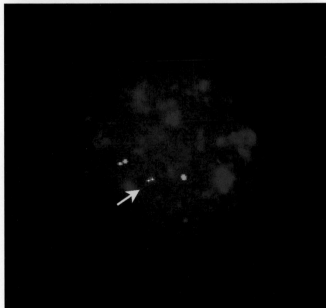

(b)

**Plate 2.3 Cryptic insertion (arrowed) of part of *RARA* (green) into the *PML* locus (red)**
The top image (a) shows FISH on metaphase chromosomes. The bottom image (b) represents an interphase cell.

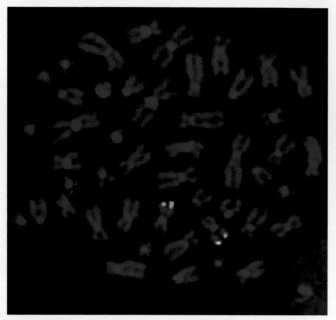

**Plate 2.4 Metaphase showing t(11;19)(q23;p13)**
The *MLL* probe mix mapping above (green) and below (red) the breakpoint is split by the translocation. The green signal remains on the der(11), the red signal is translocated to the der(19) and the normal 11 shows colocalization of both the red and green signal.

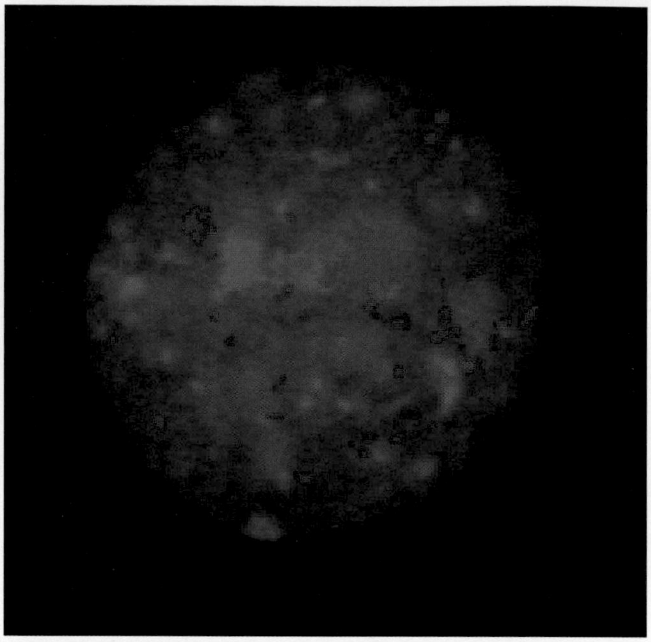

**Plate 2.5 Bone marrow aspirate from a patient with neuroblastoma**
The interphase cell shows multiple copies of N-*myc* (red).

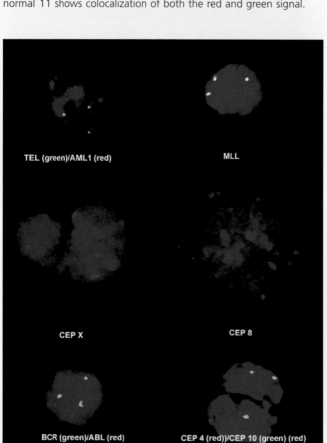

TEL (green)/AML1 (red)

MLL

CEP X

CEP 8

BCR (green)/ABL (red)

CEP 4 (red))/CEP 10 (green) (red)

**Plate 2.6 Numerous FISH probes depicting the presence of hyperdiploidy in a patient with ALL**
There are three copies of *TEL* (12p13), *MLL* (11p23), *BCR* (22q11) and centromeres 4, 8 and 10 and four copies of *AML1* (21q22) and the X centromere. The probe mapping to *ABL* (9q34) has a diploid copy number.

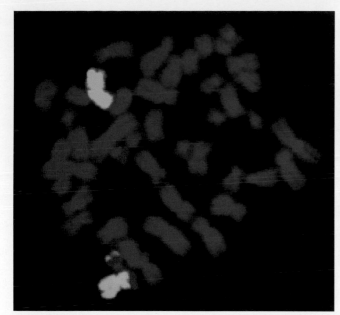

**Plate 2.7 Whole-chromosome painting**
The probes used here map to chromosomes 3 (green) and 21 (red),
showing a t(3;21) in metaphase.

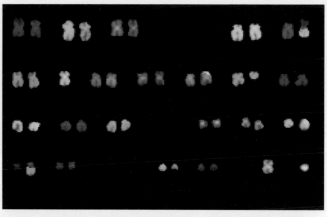

**Plate 2.8 M-FISH karyotype of a patient with secondary MDS**
In addition to structural rearrangements of chromosomes 1, 5, 11
and 19, there is loss of chromosome 7.

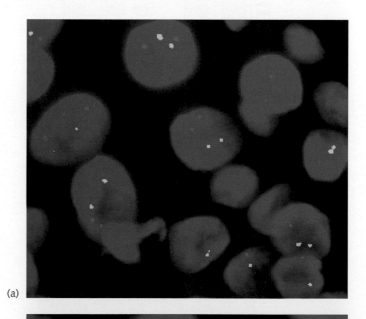

(a)

(b)

**Plate 2.9 FISH on paraffin-embedded tissue sections**
An *EWS/FLI1*-negative tumor (a: top) and an *EWS/FLI1*-positive
tumor (b: bottom), showing colocalization of an *EWS* (red) and an
*FLI1* (green) signal.

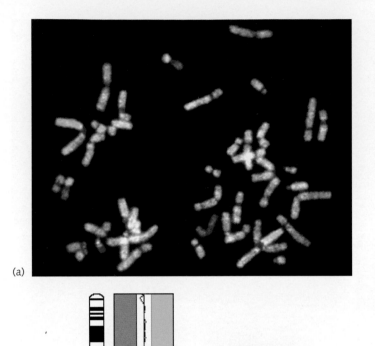

(a)

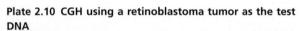

(b)

16        n=19

1        n=16

**Plate 2.10 CGH using a retinoblastoma tumor as the test DNA**
The top image (a) shows a metaphase following CGH. Green fluorescence represents gain and red loss of the region in the tumor. The CGH profile in the bottom image (b) clearly demonstrates that this corresponds to gain of 1q and loss of 16q.

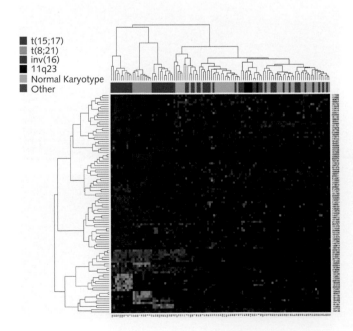

■ t(15;17)
■ t(8;21)
■ inv(16)
■ 11q23
■ Normal Karyotype
■ Other

**Plate 2.11 Hierarchical cluster analysis of expression profiles of 100 cases of AML**
The expression levels of the 100 most significant genes are illustrated.

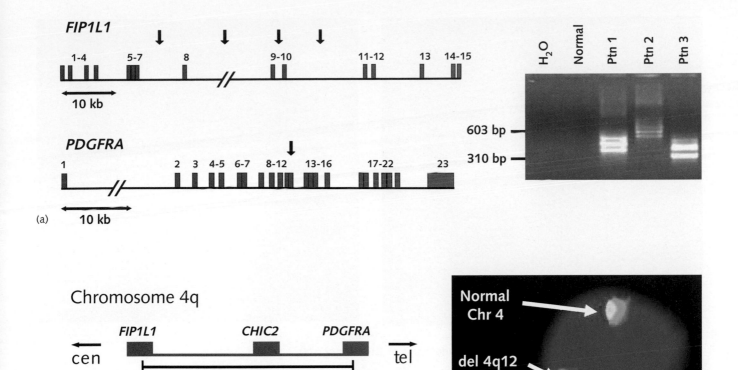

(a)

(b)

**Plate 9.1 Detection of the *FIP1L1–PDGFRA* fusion gene**
(a) *FIP1L1* and *PDGFRA* loci showing location of breakpoints (arrowed). Nested RT-PCR detects the fusion transcript in three patients with CEL. Multiple PCR products are frequently generated due to inclusion of alternatively spliced exons (not shown) from *FIP1L1*. (b) Demonstration of the 4q12 deletion in CEL by FISH.

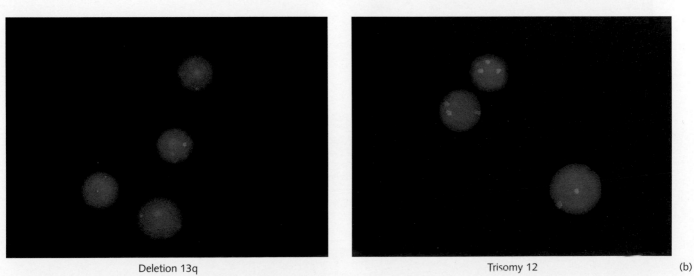

(a)                Deletion 13q                                    Trisomy 12                (b)

**Plate 10.1 FISH analysis of chromosome deletion and addition**
(a) Deletion 13q. (b) Trisomy 12.

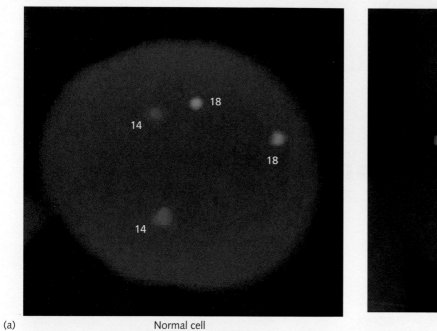
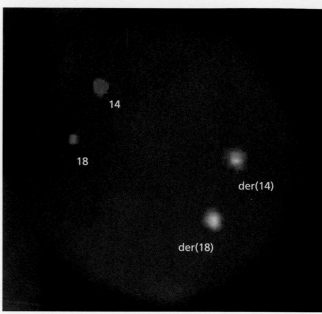

(a) Normal cell

(b)

Tumor cell

**Plate 10.2  Dual-color interphase FISH analysis for detection of t(14;18)(q32;q21)**
(a) Normal cell. (b) Tumor cell.

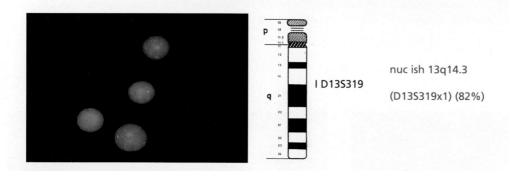

nuc ish 13q14.3

(D13S319x1) (82%)

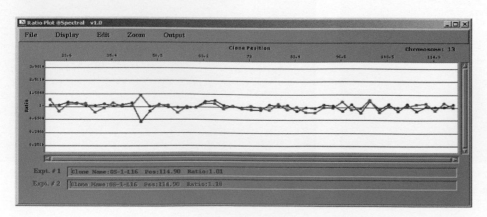

**Plate 10.3  Chromosome 13q deletion detected by FISH and array CGH**

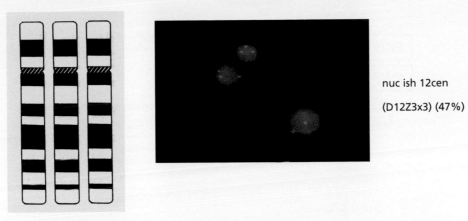

nuc ish 12cen

(D12Z3x3) (47%)

CR 12

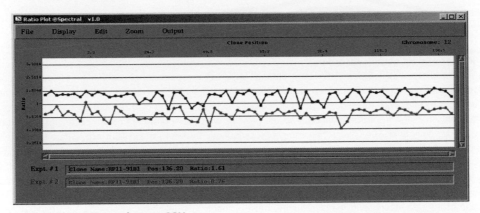

**Plate 10.4 Trisomy 12 detected by FISH and array CGH**

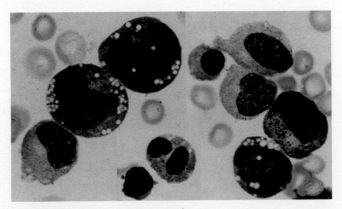

**Plate 12.1 Bone marrow findings in Pearson marrow–pancreas syndrome**
The presence of numerous vacuoles in both erythroid and myeloid precursors in an infant is virtually diagnostic of Pearson marrow–pancreas syndrome. Note also the presence of neutrophils with the Pelger anomaly of the nucleus.

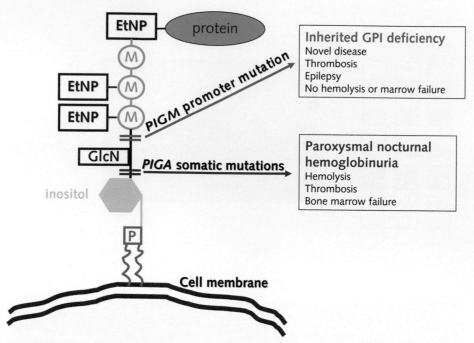

**Plate 12.2 The GPI anchor and its genetic disorders**

The structure of GPI–protein (protein–EtNP-6Manα1-2Manα1-6Manα1-4GlcNα1-6myoinositol-phospholipid) is shown. GPI biosynthesis takes place mostly in the endoplasmic reticulum. The first step involves the addition of acetylglucosamine (GlcN) to phosphatidylinositol (inositol-P). Synthesis of the GPI anchor proceeds with the serial addition of a glycan moiety consisting of three mannose (M) molecules each modified by phosphoethanolamine (EtNP). Through a transpeptidation reaction, proteins with the appropriate carboxy-terminal amino acid motif are attached covalently to the terminal EtNP. The GPI–protein complex subsequently travels to the cell surface, where the protein becomes anchored to the lipid bilayer through GPI. In PNH, PIG-A, a protein encoded by the X-linked gene *PIGA* and a member of a multi-subunit enzymatic complex that catalyzes the first step (i.e., addition of GlcN to inositol-P), is somatically mutated in one or few HSCs. As a result, very little GPI is synthesized, or none at all, with consequent severe deficiency of GPI-anchored proteins on the surface of the mutated HSCs and their progeny. In inherited GPI deficiency, a germline hypomorphic mutation in the promoter of the *PIGM* gene, an α1→4 mannosyltransferase required for the addition of the first mannose in the glycan core, causes variable GPI deficiency.

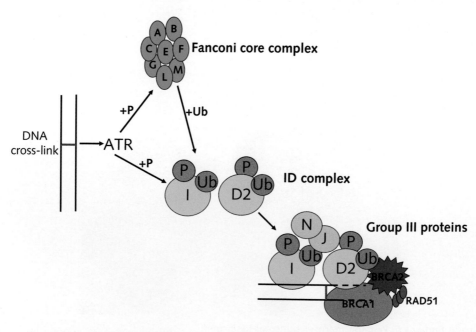

**Plate 12.3 Molecular pathogenesis of Fanconi anemia**

The FA pathway of DNA repair is activated in response to intra- or inter-strand DNA cross-links. First the DNA damage sensor ATR phosphorylates the FCC and ID complexes and subsequently FCC monoubiquitinates FANCD2 and FANCI. The ID complex is recruited to the site of DNA damage and in concert with group II FA proteins (FANCD1/BRCA2, FANCN/PALB2 and FANCJ/BRIP1) form the FA DNA repair, which also recruits other DNA repair proteins such as BRCA1 and RAD51, leading eventually to the repair of the DNA cross-link through processes that include nucleotide excision repair, translesional synthesis and homologous recombination.

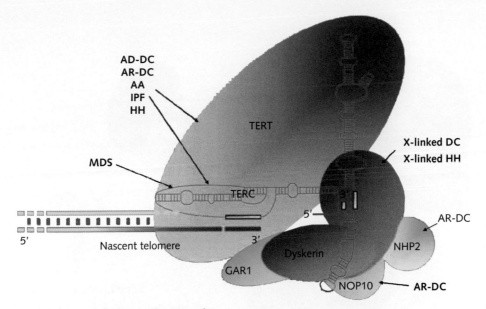

**Plate 12.4 Telomerases complex and dyskeratosis congenita**

The telomerase complex and its protein subunits TERT, dyskerin, NOP10, NHP2 and GAR1 interact with the RNA component TERC to retrotranscribe a telomeric repeat sequence. The components of the complex mutated in X-linked dyskeratosis congenita (DC), autosomal dominant (AD)-DC, autosomal recessive (AR)-DC, aplastic anemia, X-linked Hoyeraal–Hreidarsson (HH) syndrome, idiopathic pulmonary fibrosis (IPF) and myelodysplasia (MDS) are shown. From Kirwan M, Dokal I. (2008) Dyskeratosis congenita: a genetic disorder of many faces. *Clinical Genetics*, **73**, 103–112, with permission.

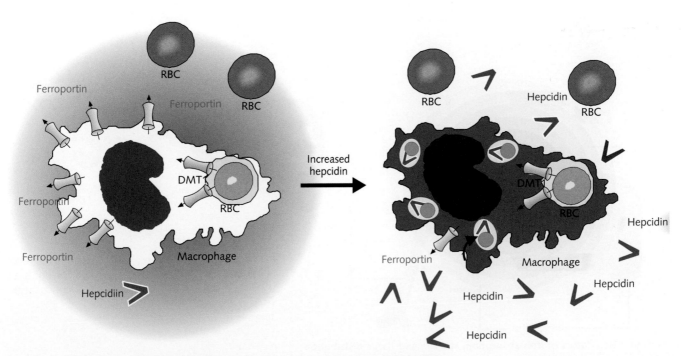

**Plate 13.1 Hepcidin–ferroportin interaction causes iron sequestration in macrophages**

(*Left*) Macrophages in the spleen and liver ingest senescent erythrocytes and extract their iron. When hepcidin is low, ferroportin molecules on macrophage cell membranes rapidly export the recycled iron (gray tint). (*Right*) During inflammation, hepcidin synthesis is increased; hepcidin binds to macrophage ferroportin and induces its internalization and degradation. Export of iron from macrophages slows, and iron remains in macrophage cytoplasm bound to ferritin.

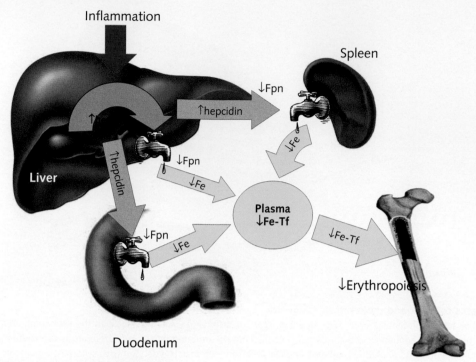

**Plate 13.2 Iron restriction in anemia of inflammation**
Under the influence of increased hepcidin concentrations, the release of stored and recycled iron from splenic and hepatic macrophages and hepatocytes is decreased, as is the absorption of dietary iron in the duodenum. Continued iron utilization depletes plasma iron, causing hypoferremia and limiting iron delivery to erythropoietic tissue. Fpn, ferroportin.

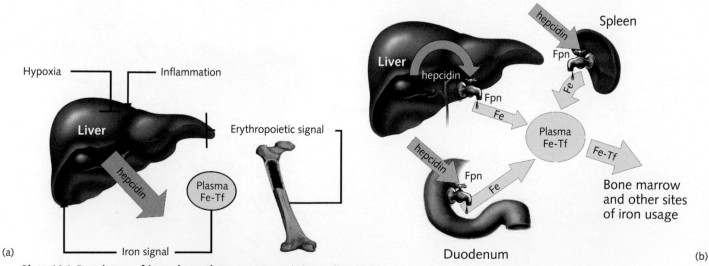

(a)      (b)

**Plate 14.1 Regulators of iron absorption, storage and tissue distribution**
(a) Iron stores, erythropoietic demand, hypoxia and inflammation modulate the hepatic production of hepcidin, an iron-regulatory hormone. Increased iron stores and inflammation both increase hepcidin expression (↑), whereas increased erythropoietic demand and hypoxia decrease hepcidin expression (⊥). (b) Hepcidin controls the major flows of iron in the body, including the efflux of iron into plasma from absorptive enterocytes, from splenic and hepatic macrophages involved in recycling of iron from erythrocytes, and from hepatocytes that store iron. Plasma iron is destined for hemoglobin synthesis by erythrocyte precursors in the bone marrow, and for other sites of iron utilization.

the greater severity of the juvenile form of the disease is due to the lower levels of hepcidin compared with the adult form of hemochromatosis.

## TFR2-associated hemochromatosis

A third form of autosomal recessive hemochromatosis (type 3) has been reported to be indistinguishable from HFE-associated hemochromatosis in its clinical manifestations, but patients have no mutations in the *HFE* gene. Instead, their disease is caused by mutations in the *TFR2* gene on chromosome 7q. TFR2 is a protein that is highly homologous to the transferrin receptor (also known as TFR1), and highly expressed by hepatocytes and hematopoietic cells. TFR2 is capable of binding transferrin and transporting it into the cell, but it does so at much lower efficiency than does transferrin receptor. TFR2 is stabilized by interaction with iron-transferrin and is also able to bind HFE. Patients and mice with homozygous TFR2 mutations have low hepcidin expression, implicating this protein in the regulation of hepcidin synthesis, possibly as a sensor of transferrin saturation. Some patients have been shown to have nonsense mutations, indicating that TFR2 is not an essential protein for survival. Type 3 hemochromatosis is effectively treated by phlebotomy.

Two siblings with combined *HFE* and *TFR2* mutations were reported to have the severe juvenile form of the disease, suggesting that HFE and TFR2 have additive effects on hepcidin expression.

## Ferroportin-associated hemochromatosis

Most reported ferroportin mutations cause the loss of ferroportin function and the clinical picture of macrophage iron overload (siderosis) with few if any clinical consequences (*see below*). A rare form of hereditary hemochromatosis is an autosomal dominant disorder (type 4 hemochromatosis) due to ferroportin mutations that confer resistance to hepcidin-induced internalization (gain of function). Such a lesion would be expected to mimic hepcidin deficiency. Its most severe form involves serine or tyrosine substitutions in C326 in the hepcidin-binding site of ferroportin. Affected patients presented with early onset of liver disease and arthritis.

## Type 5 hemochromatosis

Type 5 hemochromatosis is not yet a defined entity, but rather a disease that has been inferred to exist because there are patients with HFE-like hemochromatosis who have no apparent mutations in the *HFE*, *TFR2* or hepcidin genes. This designation probably includes a disorder due to at least

one other gene that plays a role in the regulation of iron balance.

## Autosomal dominant siderosis

Autosomal dominant siderosis, formerly also called autosomal dominant (or type 4) hemochromatosis, has a distinct clinical picture. Patients with this disorder may have iron-deficiency anemia early in life, but later present with increased serum ferritin concentration and macrophage iron accumulation. Some may eventually develop parenchymal iron deposition in addition to macrophage iron loading, probably because their specific mutations may also cause resistance to hepcidin.

This disorder has a very interesting pathogenesis. It is due to missense mutations in ferroportin, the cellular iron exporter. This seems paradoxical at first, because the mutations alter ferroportin function, and ferroportin acts as the basolateral enterocyte transporter involved in intestinal iron absorption (see Figure 14.1). However, it is important to consider that ferroportin also plays a major role in macrophage iron release. The lack of nonsense mutations in this disorder, and evidence from cellular and animal models of this disease, suggest that the mutated ferroportin exerts a dominant negative effect on the normal version of the molecule. The resulting loss of functional ferroportin is severe enough to impair macrophage iron release, resulting in accumulation of iron in macrophages and decrease in the amount of plasma iron available to developing erythroid precursors. Iron-restricted erythropoiesis probably signals for a compensatory increase in intestinal iron absorption, overcoming the genetic deficiency of ferroportin in the enterocytes. It appears that iron loading of macrophages has few if any clinical consequences.

## African siderosis

The pathology of African siderosis is strikingly similar to that of autosomal dominant siderosis due to ferroportin gene mutations, although the genetic basis of African siderosis has not been described. Once called Bantu siderosis because of the population affected, this disorder was originally attributed to excessive dietary iron intake. It is common in sub-Saharan Africans, many of whom drink a traditional alcoholic beverage brewed in non-galvanized steel drums. The iron content of the brew is substantial, resulting in massive iron ingestion. However, the observations that not all drinkers develop iron overload and that some individuals develop similar iron overload without drinking the beverage support the notion that there is a genetic component to this disorder. It is not yet known whether European and American individuals of African descent are also more susceptible to iron overload as a result of the same iron-loading gene.

## Abnormal iron distribution

There are two well-characterized (but very rare) disorders due to mutations in plasma proteins important in iron metabolism. These mutations do not directly affect intestinal iron absorption. Rather, they perturb tissue iron distribution.

### Atransferrinemia

Atransferrinemia is a severe deficiency of the plasma iron-binding protein transferrin, due to mutations that truncate or alter the coding sequence of the transferrin gene. As a result, erythroid precursors are iron-starved and severe anemia results. Paradoxically, all non-hematopoietic tissues are iron-loaded, probably because intestinal iron absorption is enhanced to try to provide more iron to erythroid precursors and because non-transferrin-bound iron is avidly taken up by many parenchymal cell types. Mice and humans with this disorder have low hepcidin, indicating that iron-transferrin is an important regulator of hepcidin synthesis. This disorder can be treated by transfusion of packed red blood cells or, more appropriately, by infusion of human transferrin.

### Aceruloplasminemia

Aceruloplasminemia is deficiency or absence of plasma ceruloplasmin. Ceruloplasmin was once thought to be a plasma copper carrier but it is now clear that its primary role is as a ferroxidase, aiding in the release of iron from macrophages, hepatocytes and cells of the central nervous system. Patients with this disorder are generally well early in life, but gradually develop tissue iron deposition in the liver, pancreas and brain. They typically present in middle age with retinal degeneration, dementia, hepatic iron deposition and diabetes. Treatment with deferoxamine is ineffectual; treatment with normal plasma may provide some benefit.

## Conclusions

Iron disorders are among the most common of human afflictions. They invariably result from abnormalities of iron balance, most often due to defects in the iron regulatory hormone hepcidin, its receptor/iron channel ferroportin or

their interaction. Iron overload is underdiagnosed because it produces signs and symptoms that are common in adult populations. However, iron overload disorders are usually easy to treat and clinicians should be vigilant in considering them.

## Further reading

### General

Aisen P, Enns C, Wessling-Resnick M. (2001) Chemistry and biology of eukaryotic iron metabolism. *International Journal of Biochemistry and Cell Biology*, **33**, 940–959.

Hentze MW, Muckenthaler MU, Andrews NC. (2004) Balancing acts: molecular control of mammalian iron metabolism. *Cell*, **117**, 285–297.

### Regulation of iron homeostasis

Andrews NC, Schmidt PJ. (2007) Iron homeostasis. *Annual Review of Physiology*, **69**, 69–85.

Nemeth E, Ganz T. (2006) Regulation of iron metabolism by hepcidin. *Annual Review of Nutrition*, **26**, 323–342.

Nemeth E, Tuttle MS, Powelson J *et al.* (2004) Hepcidin regulates cellular iron efflux by binding to ferroportin and inducing its internalization. *Science*, **306**, 2090–2093.

Nicolas G, Chauvet C, Viatte L *et al.* (2002) The gene encoding the iron regulatory peptide hepcidin is regulated by anemia, hypoxia, and inflammation. *Journal of Clinical Investigation*, **100**, 1037–1044.

### Iron overload disorders

Ajioka RS, Kushner JP. (2002) Hereditary hemochromatosis. *Seminars in Hematology*, **39**, 235–241.

Beutler E. (2006) Hemochromatosis: genetics and pathophysiology. *Annual Review of Medicine*, **57**, 331–347.

Brissot P, de Bels F. (2006) Current approches to the management of hemochromatosis. *Hematology. American Society of Hematology Educational Program*, 36–41.

Camaschella C. (2005) Understanding iron homeostasis through genetic analysis of hemochromatosis and related disorders. *Blood*, **106**, 3710–3717.

Pietrangelo A. (2007) Hemochromatosis: an endocrine liver disease. *Hepatology*, **46**, 1291–1301.

### Abnormal iron distribution

Beutler E, Gelbart T, Lee P *et al.* (2000) Molecular characterization of a case of atransferrinemia. *Blood*, **96**, 4071–4074.

Xu X, Pin S, Gathinji M *et al.* (2004) Aceruloplasminemia: an inherited neurodegenerative disease with impairment of iron homeostasis. *Annals of the New York Academy of Sciences*, **1012**, 299–305.

# Chapter 15 Hemoglobinopathies due to structural mutations

## D Mark Layton[1] & Ronald L Nagel[2]

[1] Division of Investigative Science, Imperial College London, London, UK
[2] Division of Hematology, Albert Einstein College of Medicine, New York, NY, USA

## Introduction

This chapter discusses those hemoglobin disorders that are caused by mutations in the exon (i.e., coding) portion of the α or β globin genes. Alterations of globin gene expression (thalassemias) are reviewed in *Chapter 1*. We confine ourselves mainly to the structural variants that are responsible for clinically significant hemoglobinopathies.

## Normal hemoglobin structure and function

The adult major hemoglobin molecule, Hb A, is a tetramer formed by four polypeptide chains: two α chains of 141 amino acids each and two β chains of 146 amino acids each. Each globin chain harbors a prosthetic group (heme) formed by protoporphyrin IX in a complex with a single iron atom (Figure 15.1). The heme, embedded in globin, is surrounded by a hydrophobic niche which favors maintenance of iron in the ferrous state. The heme pocket is large enough for oxygen to penetrate, but larger ligands capable of binding to the iron, such as carbon monoxide, have difficulty gaining access.

Oxygen transport to tissues, the principal function of hemoglobin, depends on blood flow, which in turn is governed by cardiac output and microcirculatory resistance and distribution, and by hemoglobin concentration. Oxygen extraction by the tissues depends on the shape of the oxygen dissociation curve of hemoglobin and on tissue $Po_2$. The shape of the oxygen equilibrium curve of hemoglobin is sigmoid. This shape is determined by the extent of cooperativity, a phenomenon whereby the hemoglobin molecule modulates its affinity for oxygen when partially saturated. The first portion of the curve has a gentle slope, reflecting hemoglobin's low affinity for oxygen at initiation of the loading process. In other words, when hemoglobin is totally deoxygenated it has a rather poor avidity for oxygen (Figure 15.2). As loading proceeds and hemoglobin binds more oxygen molecules, the slope of the curve steepens, indicating that the affinity for oxygen has increased. This occurs after two molecules of oxygen have bound to the heme of deoxyhemoglobin tetramers, a property which helps hemoglobin to rapidly become fully oxygenated. If red cells are exposed to sufficient oxygen to saturate only half of the hemes available, most molecules will either not be oxygenated at all or will be entirely oxygenated, with a very small component of partially oxygenated molecules. The sigmoid shape of the oxygen dissociation curve allows hemoglobin to release oxygen efficiently. Abnormal hemoglobins such as Hb Bart's ($\gamma_4$) which lack cooperativity are unable to deliver oxygen to the tissues efficiently.

At the molecular level, cooperativity is accounted for by the fact that hemoglobin exists stably in only two structural forms, the R (relaxed) and T (tense) states, which facilitate the switch between the oxy and deoxy state. Transition from the deoxy(T) to the oxy(R) state occurs when a molecule of hemoglobin has bound two or three molecules of oxygen. While this concept has been challenged, postulated intermediate stable states have not been generally recognized.

*Molecular Hematology*, 3rd edition. Edited by Drew Provan and John Gribben.
© 2010 Blackwell Publishing.

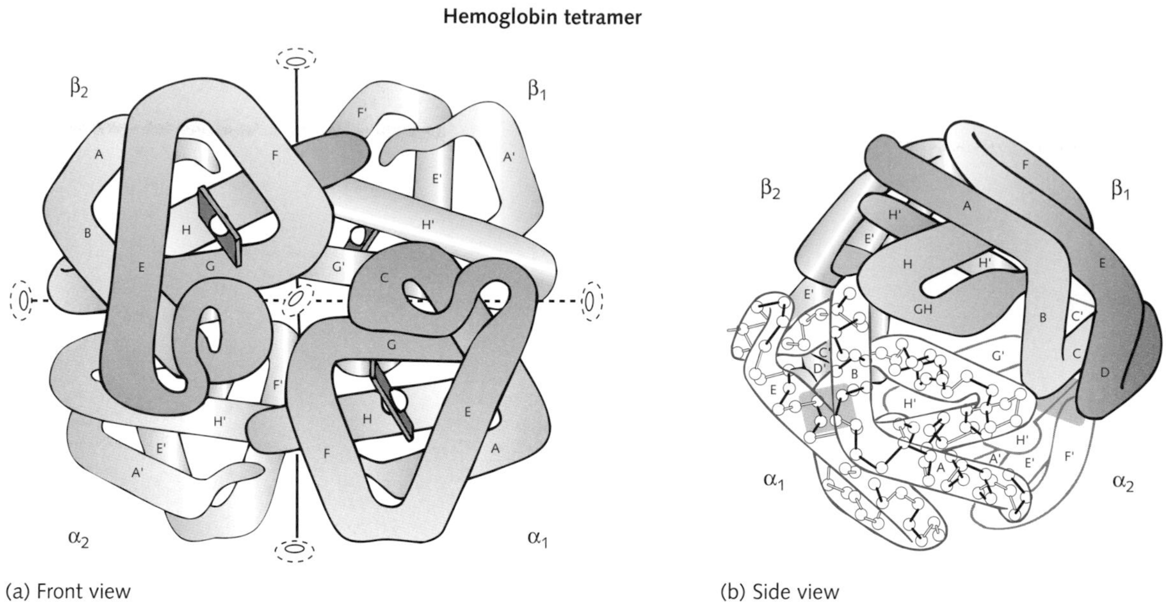

**Hemoglobin tetramer**

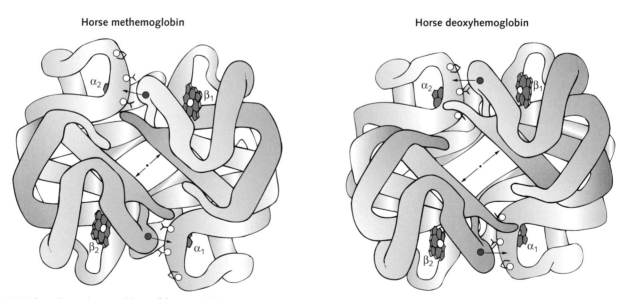

(a) Front view                                    (b) Side view

**Fig. 15.1 Hemoglobin molecule**
(a) The front view depicts the hemoglobin tetramer and the three axes of symmetry. The vertical line (marked by a solid ellipse) tracks the true twofold axis of symmetry (if you look down this axis you will see first the central cavity constituted by the $\beta$ chains). The dashed ellipses and dashed lines mark the two pseudoaxes of symmetry, since the symmetry is only approximate. Only the 21 carbons are shown, with none of the side chains. Numbers in bold type depict the residues in direct contact between the $\alpha_1$ and $\beta_2$ chains. The $\alpha_1\beta_2$ dimer (green) never dissociates and interacts with the $\alpha_2\beta_1$ dimer (light shading) to change the conformation from T to R. Alterations in this area can produce high- or low-affinity hemoglobins. (b) The side view of the tetramer depicts the stable dimer, the one that does not move or dissociate.

**Fig. 15.2 The allosteric transition of hemoglobin: R → T**
*Right*: Deoxygenated (T, tense) conformation of hemoglobin. Notice that the center cavity (space between the two $\beta$ chains, indicated in green) is larger than in the oxygenated tetramer (*left*). This space in the molecule is occupied by 2,3-diphosphoglycerate (2,3-DPG) when the tetramer is in the blue cell. The allosteric effector, 2,3-DPG, is in a little over equimolar concentration with the tetramer. The T form has low affinity for oxygen. *Left*: Oxygenated (R, relaxed) conformational state of hemoglobin. The central cavity has been reduced in size by the movement of the $\beta$ chains toward each other. This tetramer cannot bind 2,3-DPG. The R form has high affinity for oxygen. The change in conformation forms and breaks bonds between the $\beta$ chains (green) and the $\alpha$ chains (light shading) on each side of the central cavity. The title says "methemoglobin" but this hemoglobin form is identical to oxyhemoglobin. Perutz did his crystallography for reasons of convenience.

The heme triggering mechanism for conformational change has been resolved. The iron in deoxyhemoglobin is slightly out of the plane of the heme (domed configuration) because the pyrrole rings are also slightly pyramidal. When the ligand binds the sixth coordinating position of the iron, significant steric stresses are introduced, and to relieve this strain the distal histidine moves 8° to become perpendicular to the heme, significantly decreasing the doming of the iron (the angle between iron and the heme decreases to 4°). There is also the displacement of FG5 in the same direction of the histidine F8 (a conserved residue to which heme iron is covalently linked in all hemoglobins). The configuration around the heme has now changed to the oxygenated (R state), and a chain of events takes place involving the critical interactions that change the conformation of the hemoglobin tetramer.

Several heterotropic ligands within the red cell shift the oxygen dissociation curve to the right, toward lower oxygen affinity. These include $CO_2$, hydrogen ions and 2,3-diphosphoglycerate (2,3-DPG). Hemoglobin binds $CO_2$ while it is offloading oxygen and releases $CO_2$ when it binds oxygen, serving to dissipate the increase in concentration of $CO_2$ in the tissues and conveniently delivering this metabolic end product to the alveoli of the lungs. It accomplishes this particular task with ease because $CO_2$ inhibits hemoglobin's oxygen-carrying capacity by decreasing the oxygen affinity of the molecule.

Hemoglobin binds hydrogen ions more efficiently in a low-pH environment. The *Bohr effect* describes the changes in oxygen affinity secondary to pH changes within a certain range: the lower the pH, the lower the oxygen affinity or higher the $P_{50}$. This means that an increased concentration of protons favors a low-affinity state in hemoglobin. The physiological advantage this confers is twofold: in the tissues the lower pH consequent on higher $CO_2$ tension favors oxygen unloading, whereas in the lungs there is an increase in pH with $CO_2$ release which enhances oxygen uptake.

## Sickle cell anemia

### Genetics

The genetic basis of sickle cell anemia is central to the history of medical genetics. Pre-dated for generations by vernacular descriptions among West African tribes, the first account of sickle cell disease in Western medical literature is attributed to James Herrick, the Chicago physician, who in 1910 observed sickle-shaped red cells (Figure 15.3) in the blood of a dental student from Grenada who suffered from chronic hemolytic anemia. In 1947 James V. Neel concluded that with respect to the mode of inheritance sickle cell anemia

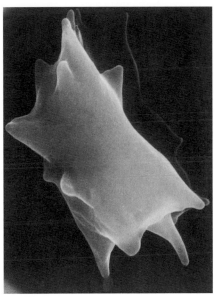

**Fig. 15.3 Sickled cell**
This is an Hb S homozygous (SS) red cell that has been deoxygenated. Notice the digitations stemming in all directions. These digitations are the product of the presence of fascicles of fibers, which are the polymerized form of deoxy Hb S.

was a homozygous state and sickle cell trait (the asymptomatic carrier state) the heterozygous state for a genetic character that had yet to be defined. Linus Pauling proposed that sickling reflected an abnormality of the hemoglobin molecule, based on the observation of Irving Sherman, then a medical student, that under the polarizing microscope sickle cells, induced by deoxygenation, exhibited birefringence. Birefringence signified to Pauling that some form of molecular alignment or orientation existed in these cells, and since the predominant molecule in the red cell is hemoglobin it had to be this that was involved in the pathology. Electrophoretic studies, which demonstrated the altered mobility of sickle hemoglobin, confirmed this interpretation and the concept of molecular disease was born.

The chemical structure of Hb S was defined by Vernon Ingram, who had developed a technique for probing the primary sequence of a protein based on its fingerprint after cleavage by trypsin. This revealed that the structure of sickle hemoglobin differed from normal hemoglobin by only one tryptic peptide, subsequently found to have a single amino acid change at position 6 of the β chain, where a polar glutamic acid residue was replaced by a non-polar valine. At the DNA level this corresponds to an A → T transversion at codon 6 (GAG → GTG) of the β chain.

The globin genes were among the first in the human genome to be cloned. The β and β-like globin genes are encoded at chromosome 11p15.5 and the α and α-like genes at chromosome 16p13.3. Utilizing 11 polymorphic sites distributed across the β globin gene cluster, it has been established that the $\beta^S$ gene is associated with three distinct chromosomal haplotypes (Benin, Bantu or Central African Republic and Senegal) in Africa, distinguishable by their array of DNA polymorphisms (haplotypes), each exclusively present in one of three separate geographical areas after which the haplotypes are named (Figure 15.4). The multicentric origin of the sickle mutation expanded further with discovery of a different haplotype linked to the $\beta^S$ gene in the eastern oasis of Saudi Arabia and among the "tribal" population of central India. It has been proposed that this Indo-European sickle mutation originated in the Harappa people of the Indus Valley, and was then dispersed, probably during the Sassanian Empire, to regions in the Middle East (now eastern Saudi Arabia, Bahrain, Kuwait and Oman). Finally, an ethnic group in southern Cameroon, the Eton, has its own unique haplotype linked to the sickle gene.

The sickle gene has thus arisen around the world on at least five separate occasions. The present-day gene frequency, which equates to carrier rates that reach 20–25% in sub-Saharan Africa, reflects heterozygote advantage that outweighs the reduced fitness in the homozygous state (balanced polymorphism). This selection pressure in favor of Hb S heterozygotes is attributable to partial protection from mortality due to *Plasmodium falciparum* malaria. The mechanism of protection has yet to be fully elucidated.

The sickle gene has also spread through gene flow; for example, the $\beta^S$ gene linked to the Benin haplotype has spread to North Africa, Sicily, Greece, Turkey, most of the Arab world and the Americas, through the vicissitudes of war (e.g., Sudanese troops in Sicily during the Arab conquest), commerce and the horrors of the Atlantic slave trade. It is estimated that worldwide approximately 250 000 children with sickle cell disorders are born annually.

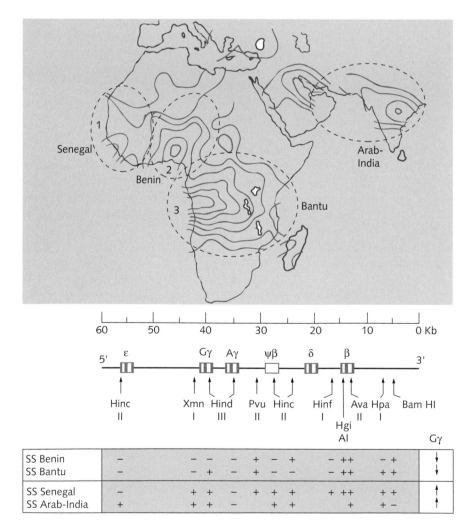

| | | | | | | | | | | | |
|---|---|---|---|---|---|---|---|---|---|---|---|
| SS Benin | – | | – | – | – | + | – | + | | – | ++ | – | + |
| SS Bantu | – | | – | + | – | + | – | – | | – | ++ | + | + |
| SS Senegal | – | | + | + | – | + | + | + | | + | ++ | + | + |
| SS Arab-India | + | | + | + | – | | + | + | | | + | + | – |

**Fig. 15.4 The β gene cluster haplotypes linked to $\beta^S$ in Africa and the Middle East/Pakistan/India**

At the top of the figure are shown the geographic distributions corresponding to the haplotypes described below. A haplotype is a particular array of polymorphic sites (i.e., sites that vary among individuals), defined here by the capacity of endonuclease enzymes to recognize the short sequence and cut the DNA.

## Clinical features

Sickle cell anemia refers to the homozygous state for the $\beta^S$ gene, in which the majority of the hemoglobin in the red cells is sickle hemoglobin (Hb S). Polymerization of Hb S when ambient oxygen tension is reduced induces sickling (marked changes in red cell shape and deformability with the formation of irreversibly sickled cells), leading to decreased pliability, lowering of rheological competence, and hemolysis. In addition, there are myriad pleiotropic effects, including increased adherence of sickle and other blood cells to endothelium, induction of red cell dehydration, procoagulability, and perturbance of vasoregulation due to reduced nitric oxide (NO) bioavailability (Figure 15.5). The primary pathophysiological events as well as the pleiotropic effects are subject to modification by epistatic genes, which may be polymorphic (i.e., differ among individuals). The combined impact of all these factors accounts for the great interindividual variability of the clinical phenotype: some patients are severely affected while others have only mild disease and the majority span these two extremes.

Anemia is present in all cases, with a mean hemoglobin concentration of around 8 g/dL (higher levels occur in Indian and some Middle Eastern populations), reticulocytosis (typically 5–20%), dense cell fraction [mean corpuscular hemoglobin concentration (MCHC) >38 g/dL or density >1.1009] of up to 40%, an elevated white cell count (mean $18 \times 10^9$/L) and commonly thrombocytosis. Anemia is tolerated

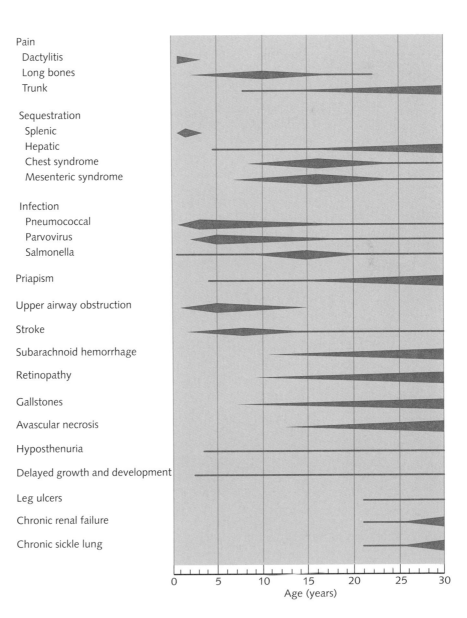

**Fig. 15.5 Age-dependency of complications in sickle cell anemia**
From Davies SC, Oni L. (1997) Management of patients with sickle cell disease. *British Medical Journal*, 315, 656–660, with permission.

relatively well due to the reduced oxygen affinity of Hb S and increased 2,3-DPG concentration within the red cell. Several hematological variables, including total hemoglobin, are modulated by the level of fetal hemoglobin (Hb F) and co-inheritance of α thalassemia (−α/−α genotype more so than −α/αα), which occurs at a significant frequency among sickle cell anemia patients (20–50% of cases, according to age). Higher levels of Hb F are associated with the Senegal and Asian β globin haplotypes. Gender also exerts an influence; for example, females with sickle cell anemia have a significantly higher Hb F level and in males hemoglobin concentration increases between 10 and 24 years, contributing to a higher frequency of vaso-occlusive crises.

The most characteristic manifestation of sickle cell anemia is the painful crisis. This commonly involves multiple sites in the extremities, joints, spine, abdomen, ribs and sternum. The onset of pain can be insidious or rapid, and may affect several sites simultaneously or extend over time from one location to others. The pathological basis of the painful crisis is infarction of the bone marrow. Systemic embolization of bone marrow or fat to the lung, brain or kidneys may occur. The site first affected in infancy is often the hands or feet (dactylitis). Necrosis of the epiphysis may lead to premature fusion with shortening of the digits. Paradoxically, painful crises are more frequent in patients with greater red cell deformability. Serial observations indicate that during painful crises a decrease in low-density cells of greater deformability precedes that of dense cells. This may be reconciled with a model whereby cells that are less dense but more adherent to the endothelium bedeck the vessels, facilitating entrapment of dense cells and ultimately vaso-occlusion. This may be an oversimplification and other mechanisms, for example reflex shunting of blood away from the bone marrow and perturbation of vasoregulation, have been invoked. Precipitating factors include cold, infection, dehydration, altitude, excessive exercise, emotional stress, sleep apnea, obstruction to the peripheral circulation (e.g., tourniquet use) and possibly cocaine abuse.

The clinical complications of sickle cell anemia are protean and involve almost every organ system. The lungs and kidneys are particularly affected. There is an increase in glomerular filtration rate as well as hyposthenuria from early childhood. Papillary necrosis with hematuria, renal insufficiency and nephrotic syndrome may occur (Plate 15.1). The lungs are the target of both acute and chronic complications. Acute chest syndrome may be associated with infection (viral, bacterial or atypical organisms) and fat embolism. The latter is associated with a more severe clinical course. Repeated episodes of acute chest syndrome predispose to the development of chronic sickle lung disease. Cerebral vasculopathy may lead to stroke and neurocognitive defects. From

infancy there is progressive splenic atrophy, against which co-inheritance of α thalassemia affords protection. The resulting loss of splenic reticuloendothelial function leads to susceptibility to infection with capsulated bacteria. Before the advent of newborn screening and prophylaxis, overwhelming *Streptococcus pneumoniae* infection was the leading cause of death in children with sickle cell disease. The prevalence of avascular necrosis of the femoral or humeral head reaches 20% in adulthood and is greater among patients whose hematocrit is higher including those with coexistent thalassemia. Peripheral retinopathy, characterized by microvascular occlusion and choroidal infarcts, is common in sickle cell disease. Abnormal arteriovenous communications develop at the border of vascular and ischemic retina and are the precursor of proliferative sickle retinopathy. In patients with sickle cell anemia, and even heterozygotes, glaucoma may occur after traumatic hyphemas since the hypoxic milieu of the anterior chamber favors sickling of red cells, which are unable to exit through the canal of Schlemm. As in other hemolytic anemias cholelithiasis is common. The prevalence of gallstones increases with age and is also correlated directly with the number of TA repeats in the promoter of the hepatic uridine diphosphate glucuronosyltranferase (*UGT1A1*) gene and inversely with the presence of α thalassemia. Hepatopathy in sickle cell anemia encompasses several entities that include intrahepatic cholestasis and hepatic sequestration. In the latter, rapid enlargement of the liver is associated with a precipitous fall in hemoglobin akin to that in acute splenic sequestration.

Congestive cardiac failure may develop in the absence of other recognized causes in sickle cell anemia. This implies that the myocardium may be the target of vaso-occlusive damage, although overt myocardial infarction is not common. The infrequency of vaso-occlusion in the heart may be the consequence of the very high perfusion pressure of coronary vessels as well as the squeezing effect of ventricular contraction. Pulmonary arterial hypertension has recently emerged as a common and serious complication. Estimated pulmonary artery pressure is increased in up to 30% of sickle cell anemia patients based on echocardiographic findings and this is associated with increased risk of premature death. Mortality among patients whose tricuspid regurgitant velocity is 2.5 m/s or higher approaches 40% at 40 months.

In sickle cell anemia, pregnancy poses a significant risk to the mother and fetus. The vogue for prophylactic transfusion during pregnancy has been superseded by a more selective approach allied to close monitoring in the context of a "high-risk" obstetric program, with generally favorable outcomes.

The basis for the striking individual variability in the clinical course and severity of sickle cell anemia has been the subject of intense study. Not surprisingly, Hb F level emerges as a major predictor of morbidity and mortality. Patients with a steady-state Hb F level of 8–9% or more have a more favorable course. Only part of the difference observed in Hb F levels is accounted for by genetic variation at the β globin locus. This has led to genome-wide association studies aimed at identification of quantitative trait loci that modulate Hb F level in *trans*. Single-nucleotide polymorphisms at the *HBS1L-MYB* and *BCL11A* loci on chromosomes 6 and 2, respectively, have been shown to be associated with variation in Hb F level in normal non-anemic populations and, more recently, sickle cell anemia patients. The mechanisms by which these quantitative trait loci act may have important implications for the future treatment of β hemoglobinopathies.

## Pathophysiology

There are five major contributors to the pathophysiology of sickle cell anemia.

### Polymerization of Hb S

The substitution of valine for glutamic acid at β6 subverts an essential property of hemoglobin, that it should maintain solubility at high concentration within the red cell. The initial step in polymerization of Hb S, known as nucleation, involves the assembly of small aggregates of deoxy Hb S molecules. Once nucleation has occurred, propagation of the polymer ensues at an exponential rate. The self-association of deoxy Hb S molecules to form a nucleus is a stochastic process, hence the reaction has a delay time. This is shortened by an increase in intracellular hemoglobin concentration, lowering the pH and an increase in temperature, which may be one reason dehydration and infection trigger vaso-occlusive events in sickle cell disorders. The final product of polymerization is a rope-like fiber composed of seven double strands twisted helically around a vertical axis. Depending on their orientation within the cell, these polymers deform the shape of the red cell to produce one of several morphological forms (Figure 15.6). The intermolecular contacts within and between the double strands have been extensively characterized. Lateral contact between adjacent tetramers in the double strand involves the mutant β6 Val, which is buried in a hydrophobic acceptor pocket formed by β88 Leu and β85 Phe, allowing ingress of water molecules which form bridging hydrogen bonds that stabilize the contact. The failure of Hb F and Hb $A_2$ (and the corresponding hybrid tetramers) to copolymerize with Hb S has been attributed to specific amino acid residues but how these disrupt axial and lateral contacts in the Hb S polymer is still not fully resolved.

### Adhesion of sickle red cells and other blood cells to the endothelium

Based purely on the kinetics of Hb S polymerization, it is predicted that the majority of red cells will not undergo sickling *in vivo* because the delay time for polymerization exceeds the time taken to traverse the microvascular and venous circulation and reach the lungs where reoxygenation occurs. From this has emerged the concept that sickle red cells are more adherent to the vascular endothelium, which has shaped our understanding of the pathophysiology of sickle cell anemia. Adhesion of sickle red cells to the vascular endothelium plays a key role in vaso-occlusion by retarding transit, thereby favoring Hb S polymerization and contributing to mechanical obstruction. In early studies Hebbel and colleagues, originally using human umbilical vein endothelial cell monolayers, established that sickle red cells were abnormally adherent to endothelial cells and postulated that this was linked to disease severity. The enhanced adherence of sickle red cells has been reproduced in more physiological systems. Young sickle red cells, which express the integrin α4β1 (VLA-4) that binds to both vascular cell adhesion molecule (VCAM)-1 and fibronectin displayed on the surface of endothelial cells, show increased adherence to the endothelium of post-capillary venules, the principal site of vaso-occlusion. This has been demonstrated both in the mesenteric circulation *ex vivo* as well as in the cremaster muscle of transgenic sickle mice *in vivo*. Obstruction of the microcirculation is preceded by adhesion of young sickle red cells, which trap dense cells and irreversibly sickled cells (ISCs) in those areas to which they are adherent. Leukocytes and platelets are also implicated in vaso-occlusion. Circulating activated leukocytes are present in sickle cell anemia and exhibit increased adhesive properties in experimental systems. Intravital microscopy in a murine sickle model has shown that following an inflammatory stimulus neutrophils are recruited to the endothelium of post-capillary venules, where they capture sickle red cells possibly through recognition of surface IgG, complement or ICAM-4 (Landsteiner–Weiner blood group antigen). Platelets may also contribute to the vaso-oclusive process. The platelets of patients with sickle cell anemia show increased expression of activation markers and adhesion via the glycoprotein IIb/IIIa receptor to fibrinogen and form heterocellular aggregates with red cells. Thrombospondin released from activated platelets and shown to be elevated in plasma during painful crisis may bridge CD36 or αvβ3 integrin expressed on microvascular endothelial cells and CD36 or sulfated glycans on sickle red cells. Increased levels of platelet-derived soluble CD40 ligand, which potentially contribute to endothelial activation and procoagulant activity, are found in patients with sickle cell anemia.

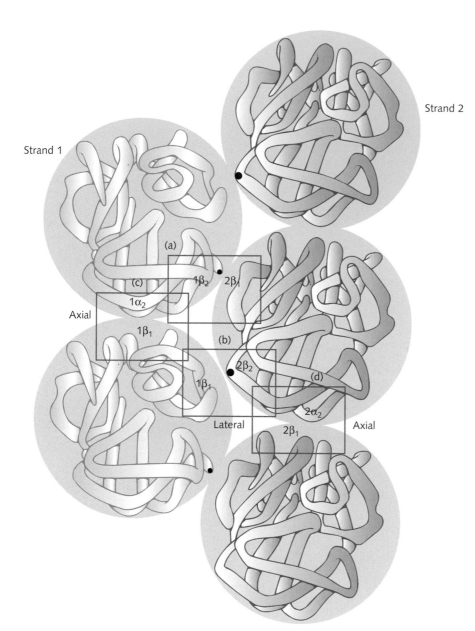

**Fig. 15.6 Polymer Hb S structure**
This is the assembly unit of the Hb S polymer: the Werner–Love double strand. This double strand is part of the Hb S crystal, but in the crystal it propagates in all directions to form a lattice. The sickle fiber wraps around to form a helical fiber. The squares depict the four different areas of contact that form the double strand.

The candidate mechanisms proposed for these adhesive interactions are complex and full discussion is beyond the scope of this chapter. Only a minority has been validated in microcirculatory preparations and not all have been proven to be relevant to the microvascular bed in which vaso-occlusion occurs. Von Willebrand factor and αvβ3 integrin appear good candidates since antibodies against both inhibit cell adhesion in living circulatory preparations. Endothelial injury, which may be mediated by sickle cells or NO depletion (*see below*), leads to activation of endothelial cells with upregulation of the transcription factor nuclear factor (NF)-κB and enhanced expression of multiple cell adhesion molecules and establishes a vicious circle that potentiates adherence of sickle red cells and vaso-occlusion.

**Red cell dehydration**

Red cell dehydration represents an integral component of the pathophysiology of sickle cell anemia because polymerization of Hb S is critically dependent on intracellular hemoglobin concentration. Although the MCHC is close to normal, sickle red cells have a wide density distribution. After they enter the circulation a proportion of young sickle red cells undergo rapid dehydration and conversion to dense cells and ultimately ISCs. Cell dehydration is due to loss of potassium accompanied by water efflux. Several membrane transport pathways have been implicated in the dehydration of sickle red cells. Probably the two most important are the $Ca^{2+}$-dependent $K^+$ (Gardos) channel and $K^+/Cl^-$ cotransport. Activation of $K^+/Cl^-$ cotransport occurs in sickle cell anemia as well as other hemoglobinopathies due to positively charged hemoglobin variants such as Hb C. It has been proposed that this may be mediated by binding of the abnormal hemoglobin to the inner surface of the cell membrane. In normal red cells $K^+/Cl^-$ cotransport is confined to reticulocytes but in sickle cell anemia activity persists in mature red cells. The $Ca^{2+}$-dependent $K^+$ (Gardos) channel is activated by intracellular accumulation of $Ca^{2+}$, which occurs on deoxygenation in sickle red cells. Cells containing Hb F are less susceptible to this effect, suggesting it is due to polymerization. When red cells undergo sickling there is increased cation permeability due to distortion of the membrane sufficient to activate the $Ca^{2+}$-dependent $K^+$ (Gardos) channel, leading to $K^+$ efflux and cell dehydration. Dense cells and ISCs have markedly shortened survival and reduced oxygen affinity.

## Anemia

Anemia is not simply a product of hemolysis in sickle cell anemia. The extent of marrow expansion is less than in thalassemia major (five as opposed to ten times normal). One explanation for this is the right-shift in the oxygen equilibrium curve, to which high red cell 2,3-DPG contributes as described above. This results in increased oxygen delivery to the tissues and explains why erythropoietin levels do not increase until the hemoglobin falls below 9 g/dL. Even below this threshold, however, the erythropoietin response is blunted (i.e., inappropriately low for the degree of anemia). The reason for this is not fully understood, but the fact that this relative deficiency of erythropoietin increases with age suggests that "silent" renal damage might be responsible.

The hemolysis is also complex because of the heterocellular nature of red cells in sickle cell anemia. There are actually three red cell populations: the most dense red cells, which survive only 4–5 days; F cells (which contain predominantly Hb F), which have close to a normal lifespan; and the remaining majority of red cells, which have an intermediate survival. Coexistent α thalassemia or high Hb F levels reduce hemolysis and consequently anemia.

Interestingly, the level of Hb F mirrors the pattern of circulating progenitors and hematopoietic cytokines seen in sickle anemia. Low-Hb F sickle cell anemia patients have an increased number of peripheral blood burst-forming units, erythroid (BFU-E), which are in active cycle. In addition, these patients have constitutively elevated levels of erythropoietin, granulocyte/macrophage colony-stimulating factor and stem cell factor and lower levels of the inhibitory cytokine transforming growth factor (TGF)-β, presumably reflecting the need to maintain a more intense erythropoietic drive. Sickle cell anemia patients are susceptible to an acute anemia superimposed on that resulting from chronic hemolysis, due to infection with parvovirus B19. This can produce a life-threatening fall in hemoglobin, which is generally self-limiting (after 7–15 days). This results from the ability of parvovirus B19 to infect BFU-E through the blood group P system that serves as its receptor.

## Nitric oxide effects

In recent years a new paradigm linking vascular dysfunction and hemolysis in the pathophysiology of sickle cell anemia has come to the fore. This is underpinned by evidence that in sickle cell anemia, even in the steady state, the bioavailability of NO is decreased, leading to perturbance of vascular homeostasis. This arises because free hemoglobin, released into the plasma as a consequence of intravascular hemolysis at a rate which exceeds haptoglobin binding capacity, reacts rapidly with NO produced by the endothelium to form methemoglobin and nitrate. This scavenging mechanism does not occur under physiological conditions because of the diffusion barriers presented by the red cell membrane and the cell-free zone adjacent to the endothelium. The release of arginase-1 contained in red cells compounds the effect on NO bioavailability through conversion of L-arginine, the substrate for NO synthase, to L-ornithine. Renal dysfunction in sickle cell anemia may further compromise the supply of arginine as the kidneys are the primary site of *de novo* synthesis. Low plasma arginine levels are found in adults with sickle cell disease and predict early mortality. The consequences of reduced NO bioavailability include vasoconstriction, activation of endothelial cells with production of endothelin-1 (a potent vasoconstrictor and inflammatory mediator), and upregulation of adhesion molecules, platelet activation, tissue factor expression and thrombin generation all of which might contribute to the complex pathophysiology of sickle cell anemia.

## Treatment

Preventive measures have proved highly effective in reducing childhood mortality in sickle cell disorders. These constitute prophylaxis against pneumococcal infection in the form of penicillin and vaccination and the early detection of splenic sequestration through training parents to monitor spleen size. The judicious use of transfusion in complications such as acute chest syndrome, stroke, splenic sequestration and aplastic crisis has also improved outcomes dramatically.

The treatment of painful crises remains a challenge. Rapid assessment of the intensity, quality and distribution of pain and presence of comorbidities coupled with prompt administration of opioid analgesia and hydration remain the mainstay of effective management. Individually tailored analgesia regimens with the adjunctive use of non-steroidal anti-inflammatory drugs are favored by many centers. As an alternative to treatment in the acute hospital setting, a daycare facility dedicated to sickle cell anemia has emerged as the best service model.

Hydroxycarbamide (hydroxyurea) lowers the incidence of painful crises and acute chest syndrome in adult and pediatric sickle cell anemia patients; in addition, hydroxycarbamide therapy leads to a reduction in transfusion requirement. Predictors of response to hydroxycarbamide include high white cell count and absence of the Bantu haplotype. The mechanism by which hydroxycarbamide, a ribonucleotide reductase inhibitor, acts involves recruitment of erythroid progenitors programmed to produce Hb F. This appears to be mediated through NO-dependent activation of soluble guanylyl cyclase. Although predicated on its action as an inducer of Hb F, it is apparent that hydroxycarbamide exerts other effects of potential relevance to its efficacy in sickle cell disease. These include reduced expression of adhesion molecules, enhanced NO production and red cell hydration, and reduction in the leukocyte, platelet and reticulocyte counts. The role of hydroxycarbamide in preservation of organ function is under investigation in ongoing clinical trials. Other agents that have been shown in small-scale studies to be effective inducers of Hb F in sickle cell anemia include the DNA hypomethylating agents azacitidine (5-azacytidine) and its analog decitabine (2-deoxy-5-azacytidine) as well as the butyrate derivatives sodium phenylbutyrate and arginine butyrate, which modify chromatin structure through inhibition of histone deacetylase and are believed to act through transcriptional derepression of the $\gamma$ globin gene.

Allogeneic bone marrow transplantation (BMT) has been performed in younger patients (up to 16 years of age) with sickle cell anemia with favorable results, including splenic regeneration in some cases. The disease-free survival at 5 years after BMT for sickle cell disease from a fully HLA-matched related donor using conventional myeloablative conditioning is currently around 90%. However, overall transplant-related mortality remains about 5% with a similar risk of graft rejection so the option of BMT is reserved for those with a severe clinical phenotype in whom these risks can be justified. Selection of patients with a history of central nervous system involvement was initially associated with a higher probability of stroke in the post-transplant period, but protocol amendment has reduced this risk. Alternative sources of donor hematopoietic stem cells including unre-lated umbilical cord blood or non-myeloablative protocols with reduced toxicity may enable the success of conventional BMT in sickle cell disease to be extended to older patients and for a broader range of indications.

Other approaches to pharmacotherapy of sickle cell anemia to emerge include prevention of red cell dehydration with imidazoles or magnesium pidolate, which inhibit the $Ca^{2+}$-activated $K^+$ (Gardos) channel and $K^+/Cl^-$ cotransport pathways respectively, and vasodilator therapies. The latter are predicated on the role that perturbation of NO metabolism plays in the pathophysiology of sickle cell disease. Plasma arginine levels are low in sickle cell anemia, particularly during vaso-occlusive crises and in the sickle transgenic mouse model ($\beta^{S+S\text{-}Antilles}$), indicating substrate depletion. In transgenic mice arginine supplementation was unexpectedly associated with a reduction in MCHC and the proportion of dense red cells. These outcomes were found to be the consequence of Gardos channel inhibition. The initial promise of arginine supplementation has yet to be borne out in clinical trials, although pilot data suggest potential benefit in the treatment of pulmonary hypertension. The successful use of inhaled NO has been reported in refractory acute chest syndrome and Phase II studies in the acute management of vaso-occlusive crisis are in progess. The phosphodiesterase 5 inhibitor sildenafil, which augments NO signaling through inhibition of cGMP hydrolysis, is the subject of clinical trials in patients with and without pulmonary hypertension and has been used to treat priapism in sickle cell disease. It is likely other mechanisms central to the pathophysiology of sickle cell disease will be future targets for therapeutic intervention. Inhibition of cell adhesion to the vascular endothelium is an attractive candidate in this respect. A recent clinical trial of tinzaparin, a low-molecular-weight heparin that emulates the inhibitory activity of unfractionated heparin in blocking P-selectin- and thrombospondin-mediated adherence of sickle red cells to the endothelium, showed significant benefit in the management of painful crisis.

The prospect of gene therapy for hemoglobinopathies has gained impetus from recent developments. Efficient transduction of hematopoietic stem cells with a lentiviral vector containing an anti-sickling globin construct at a level likely to be of clinical benefit has proved to be attainable in murine models. Long-term expression of a $\beta^A$ globin gene modified by an amino acid alteration (Gln $\rightarrow$ Thr) at position $\beta87$, which accounts for more than 90% of the anti-sickling effect of Hb F, has been achieved in syngeneic recipients. In the absence of preselection there was erythroid-specific accumulation of the anti-sickling protein in almost all circulating red blood cells which accounted for up to 52% of total hemoglobin. In two transgenic mouse models of sickle cell disease, BERK and SAD, inhibition of red blood cell dehydration and sickling was observed with correction of hematological parameters, splenomegaly and hyposthenuria. There remains a concern surrounding the risk of insertional mutagenesis due to random viral integration based on the occurrence of leukemogenic activation of LMO-2 and BCL-2A1 in clinical and non-human primate gene therapy studies. Gene replacement therapy avoids this problem but until recently has been hampered by low efficiency in hematopoietic cells. Targeted correction of the $\beta^S$ gene has been achieved by homologous recombination in murine embryonic stem cells. The discovery that induced pluripotent stem cells, which resemble embryonic stem cells, can be generated from skin fibroblasts by transduction of just four defined transcription factors (Oct3/4, Sox2, Klf4 and c-Myc) offers a potential solution to the problem of deriving sufficient corrected hematopoietic progenitors for transplantation. Notwithstanding the challenges which lie ahead, these advances give grounds for optimism that gene therapy for hemoglobinopathies may soon reach clinical application.

## Sickle/β thalassemia

This syndrome is observed in geographical regions in which both Hb S and β thalassemia are frequent, such as Africa, Sicily, Greece, Turkey, the Arab countries, and regions of the Americas with African and southern Mediterranean admixture.

There are two phenotypic forms: S/$\beta^+$ thalassemia, in which the red cells contain between 20 and 40% Hb A, the remainder comprising Hb S, Hb F and Hb $A_2$; and S/$\beta^0$ thalassemia, in which the red cells contain only Hb S, Hb F and Hb $A_2$. The latter may sometimes be difficult to distinguish from the homozygous state for the $\beta^S$ gene and this may require pedigree or genotypic analysis. The relative frequency of S/$\beta^0$ and S/$\beta^+$ thalassemia reflects the prevalence of individual β thalassemia mutations, which varies from one geographic region to another. In people of African descent S/$\beta^+$ thalassemia predominates, whereas in the Mediterranean S/$\beta^0$ thalassemia is more common.

Though similar to that of sickle cell anemia, the clinical spectrum of S/β thalassemia is broader and in its S/$\beta^+$ thalassemia form significantly milder. The hemoglobin level is higher and mean cell volume (MCV) as well as mean corpuscular hemoglobin (MCH) typically lower than in sickle cell anemia. However, retinopathy, osteonecrosis and hypersplenism are more common.

## Hemoglobin C disease

Worldwide, hemoglobin C is the third most common structural hemoglobin variant (after Hb S and Hb E). Individuals who are homozygous for Hb C display a mild hemolytic anemia that is generally asymptomatic. Splenomegaly is common but usually clinically benign. The anemia is mild to moderate in degree and accompanied by a reduced MCV. The peripheral blood film is fairly characteristic and, with some experience, diagnostic. The red cells appear hypochromic due to their flatness (rather than low MCH or MCHC; in fact, the red cells have a normal MCH and an increased MCHC). Folded and target cells are prominent. Red cells may, though infrequently in the absence of splenectomy, show intracellular tetragonal crystals of Hb C, best detected in reticulocyte preparations, where they retain their red color.

The $\beta^C$ gene (β6 Glu → Lys) has a frequency one-quarter that of the $\beta^S$ gene among African-Americans. The $\beta^C$ mutation most likely originated in Burkina Faso, where we find the highest gene frequency (up to 0.5), decreasing concentrically, and encompassing Mali, Ivory Coast and Ghana, all of which lie east of the Niger river.

The pathophysiology of Hb C disease is dominated by the reduced solubility of hemoglobin that results from replacement of β6 glutamic acid by lysine and its effect on membrane transport. The former is manifest as a tendency for oxy Hb C to form tetragonal crystals (Plate 15.2). Although less deformable, the red cells in Hb C disease do not produce vaso-occlusion even when present in significant numbers after splenectomy. This may be explained by dissolution of oxy Hb C crystals under conditions of low $Po_2$ in the microvascular circulation. The red cells are uniformly denser. This characteristic is associated with stimulation of $K^+/Cl^-$ cotransport (higher than in SS cells, despite a lower reticulocyte count), a transport system which, through efflux of $K^+$ and accompanying water loss, leads to red cell dehydration. The kinetics of $K^+/Cl^-$ cotransport are altered in Hb C disease red cells, with delayed switch-off when the stimulus for activity (cell volume increase or low pH) is removed. Whether this alteration is sufficient to explain the pathophysiology of Hb C disease and its relation to interaction of Hb C with the red cell membrane remains to be determined.

Epidemiological data from Burkina Faso reveals that individuals homozygous for Hb C are particularly resistant to death from malaria. This is congruent with previous observations that the red cells of Hb C homozygotes are less able to release merozoites than normal or heterozygote (Hb AC) red cells. By virtue of this greater protective effect, Hb C may eventually supersede the Hb S gene with respect to prevalence in those populations where the two mutants coexist. The multiplication rate of *P. falciparum* is lower in the red cells of Hb C homozygotes than in normal red cells, probably due to disintegration of ring forms and trophozoites. It appears that only a subset of red cells of Hb C homozygotes supports normal parasite replication.

The structural basis for Hb C crystallization has been elucidated. Hb C crystals form by nucleation and grow by the attachment of individual Hb C molecules from the solution. Hb C crystallization is possible because of the huge entropy gain, likely stemming from the release of up to 10 water molecules per protein intermolecular contact–hydrophobic interaction. The propensity of oxy Hb C to form crystals is attributable to increased hydrophobicity resulting from the conformational changes that accompany the β6 Lys mutation. The oxy ligand state is thermodynamically driven to a limited number of aggregation pathways, with a high propensity to form the tetragonal crystal structure. This contrasts with deoxy Hb C, which energetically favors equally multiple pathways of aggregation, not all of which will culminate in crystal formation, and which has a different crystal form.

## Hemoglobin SC disease

The compound heterozygous disorder hemoglobin SC disease combines two structural variants, Hb S and Hb C, neither of which is associated with a clinical phenotype in the simple carrier state. The clinical basis of Hb SC disease, a significant sickling disorder, therefore demands an explanation. The pathophysiology of Hb SC disease derives from two mechanisms. The relative proportion of Hb S to Hb C is 50:50, in contrast to sickle cell trait in which the ratio of Hb S to Hb A is 40:60. This reflects the variable electrostatic affinity of structurally distinct β chains for α globin which governs the proportion of different αβ subunits and hemoglobin assembly within the red cell. The red cells of Hb SC individuals have a higher MCHC, reflecting dehydration due to increased $K^+/Cl^-$ cotransport. Since polymerization is dependent on intracellular Hb S concentration, both of these factors favor polymer formation. In keeping with this, *in vitro* studies have shown that increasing the proportion of Hb S from 40 to 50% increased the rate of polymerization almost 15-fold. Hb SC red cells are denser than normal or the majority of sickle cell anemia red cells (Plate 15.3). Interestingly, Hb S favors Hb C crystallization; this explains, in addition to loss of splenic function, why crystals are generally more prominent in Hb SC than Hb C disease. However, for the reasons given above, this does not contribute to vaso-occlusion.

Hb SC disease is milder than sickle cell anemia. Virtually all patients survive to adulthood and average life expectancy is close to that of matched controls. The clinical spectrum resembles that of sickle cell anemia but the frequency and severity of most specific complications are generally less. Three exceptions show a disproportionate prevalence or severity in Hb SC disease – osteonecrosis, acute chest syndrome and retinopathy – the latter being more common than in sickle cell anemia. Splenomegaly is more frequent and functional hyposplenism delayed. Mean red cell survival is around 27 days compared with 17 days in sickle cell anemia. Hematologically, Hb SC disease is characterized by a higher hemoglobin, lower MCV, lower reticulocyte count, fewer dense red cells and lower Hb F level compared with sickle cell anemia. The blood film in Hb SC disease may be diagnostic. In addition to the red cell forms seen in Hb C disease, there are frequent dense cells, some of which resemble a broad-beamed canoe and occasionally ISCs. Intraerythrocytic crystals are best visualized with supravital stains (Plate 15.4) or after incubation of blood with 3% NaCl.

## Other sickle hemoglobinopathies

Many compound heterozygous states have been described in which Hb S is co-inherited with a second β globin variant most of which are of no clinical significance. Exceptions are Hb SO-Arab, Hb SD-Punjab (Los Angeles) and Hb SE. Hb O-Arab (β121 Glu → Lys) and Hb D-Punjab (β121 Glu → Gln) interact with Hb S to produce a severe clinical phenotype akin to sickle cell anemia. This is explained by the fact that these substitutions at the β121 residue, a contact point in the Hb S polymer, increase the nucleation rate for polymer formation. Only a small number of cases of Hb SE have been described, all of which displayed a mild phenotype. Other compound heterozygous sickling disorders due to a second structural variant are rare. Co-inheritance of Hb Quebec-Chori (β87 Thr → Ile) and Hb S is an interesting example. Since Hb Quebec-Chori is electrophoretically silent, the compound heterozygous state with Hb S mimics sickle cell trait; however, its presence can be distinguished by mass spectrometry. The proposed mechanism for the interaction between the two variant globin chains is that substitution of a bulky hydrophobic isoleucine residue at β87 creates a more favorable environment in the acceptor pocket for β6 Val which stabilizes intermolecular contacts in the polymer.

Several dominant sickle mutations in which there is a second substitution in addition to β6 Val in the same β chain have been described. This results in assembly of a "super-Hb S" which manifests with symptoms in the heterozygote. Two examples have been well characterized. Hb S-Antilles (β6 Glu → Val; 23 Val → Ile) is expressed in the heterozygote at a level of around 40% and produces a syndrome resembling a mild sickle cell anemia phenotype. The mechanism is complex; the second mutation reduces the solubility from a $C_{sat}$ of 18 g/dL for Hb S to 12 g/dL, with the result that polymerization is promoted. Hb S-Antilles also has reduced oxygen affinity. This oxygen equilibrium shift favors sickling. The other well-documented dominant sickle mutation is Hb S-Oman (β6 Glu → Val; 121 Glu → Lys). This generates an even more powerful "super-Hb S." Even at expression levels as low as 20%, resulting from concomitant inheritance of the α thalassemia genotype −α/−α, this is associated with a phenotype similar to Hb S-Antilles. Since the two dominant forms of Hb S have similar solubility in the deoxy state, the more severe phenotype of Hb S-Oman implies that the β121 mutation (identical to that in Hb O-Arab) possesses intrinsic pathophysiological properties. This hypothesis is supported by the hemolysis and perturbance of red cell cation transport evident in individuals homozygous for Hb O-Arab. Rare symptomatic Hb S heterozygotes in whom deficiency of pyruvate kinase has been identified have been described. The mechanism in these cases is attributed to the increased 2,3-DPG content of red cells, with a block in glycolysis distal to the Rapoport–Luebering shuttle that shifts the hemoglobin oxygen equilibrium in favor of deoxy Hb S.

## Homozygous Hb E and Hb E/β thalassemia

Hemoglobin E (β26 Glu → Lys), the most common structural hemoglobin variant worldwide, is prevalent across a wide geographic area from the eastern provinces of India to the Philippines. Populations living near the common border of Cambodia, Laos and Thailand (the Khmer people) have the highest incidence (gene frequency reaching 0.5) of Hb E, the selection pressure for which is resistance to infection by *P. falciparum* malaria.

In heterozygotes Hb E constitutes 25–30% of the hemoglobin. In common with the other widespread β chain variants, Hb S and Hb C, this proportion is reduced in the presence of α thalassemia. Homozygotes exhibit a benign thalassemic phenotype because the mutation responsible produces both a structurally altered β chain and reduced expression due to the generation of an alternative splice site. The clinical syndrome of homozygous Hb E disease is very mild, with no or minimal anemia (once nutritional causes of anemia are treated) and low MCV, with target cells in the smear and hypochromia. Density gradient separation reveals that although the red cells are small they have a normal MCHC, as a consequence of a diminished MCH, due to the thalassemic component of this disease. People who inherit Hb E and β thalassemia trait present with the features of thalassemia major or intermedia (*see Chapter 1*).

The protective effect of Hb E against *P. falciparum* malaria has been assessed in a mixed erythrocyte invasion assay. The parasite preferentially invaded normal red cells compared with Hb AE, Hb EE or Hb E/β thalassemia red cells. Heterozygote red cells were the worst target, showing invasion restricted to approximately 25% of the red cells. It has been postulated Hb AE red cells might have an unidentified membrane abnormality that renders the majority of the red cell population relatively resistant to invasion by *P. falciparum*, consequently reducing parasitemia and hence the lethality of infection. This is consistent with the Haldane hypothesis of heterozygote protection against severe malaria.

## Unstable hemoglobins

Cases of non-spherocytic hemolytic anemia due to a structurally unstable hemoglobin were first recognized because precipitation occurred on thermal incubation of hemolysate, a phenomenon which forms the basis of the heat stability test. In many patients Heinz bodies were present. There are over 100 mutations that render the hemoglobin molecule unstable, of which only a minority are associated with significant clinical symptoms. About 75% are β chain variants. Unstable hemoglobins are generally inherited in an autosomal dominant manner, although rare homozygous cases, for example Hb Bushwick (β74 Gly → Val) and Hb Taybe (α₁38/39 Thr deletion), have been described. In a significant number of cases there is no antecedent family history, indicating that the mutation has arisen spontaneously. The unstable variant usually accounts for 10–30% of the total hemoglobin. Structural alterations render hemoglobin unstable by four mechanisms:

- destabilization of the attachment of heme to globin;
- interference with stability of the $\alpha_1\beta_1$ contact area, which does not normally dissociate;
- introduction of either a bulky or charged side chain to the hydrophobic interior of the hemoglobin molecule;
- disruption of the secondary structure of the molecule by a side chain that is not α-helix-friendly (commonly as a result of proline substitution).

Hb Köln (β98 Val → Met) is the most common of the unstable hemoglobins and shows no ethnic predilection. Many unstable hemoglobin variants do not alter the surface charge of the hemoglobin molecule and therefore have an electrophoretic mobility identical to that of Hb A. Light bands representing dissociated globin subunits, in some cases devoid of heme, may be observed. Clinically, unstable hemoglobins are characterized by hemolytic anemia, which ranges from mild to severe depending on the causative mutation, and the presence of pigmenturia (due mostly to dipyrroles). Unstable hemoglobins due to γ chain variants, such as Hb Poole (Gγ130 Trp → Gly), are a rare cause of transient neonatal hemolysis. The mechanism of red cell destruction, much of which occurs in the bone marrow, involves displacement of heme, which destabilizes the hemoglobin tetramer and its composite globin subunits and leads to the formation of hemichrome. Globin subunits aggregate and precipitate, leading to reduced deformability and removal or entrapment of red cells which contain Heinz bodies. Febrile episodes and ingestion of oxidant drugs may accelerate hemolysis. Hemoglobin level may be modulated by altered oxygen affinity, being near normal in those unstable variants with increased oxygen affinity (e.g., Hb Köln) and much lower in those with reduced oxygen affinity (e.g., Hb Hammersmith).

In most cases treatment revolves around supportive measures that include folic acid supplementation, prompt treatment of infection and fever, and avoidance of oxidant drugs. In severe cases splenectomy has been performed and is generally, though not universally, beneficial. Hydroxycarbamide has been used to stimulate Hb F in unstable β chain variants. Some unstable hemoglobin variants result in low hemoglobin oxygen saturation measurements by pulse oximetry due to their altered absorbance spectra.

## High oxygen affinity hemoglobins

The sigmoid curve of the oxygen binding of hemoglobin reflects the transition from the low-affinity deoxy(T) to the oxy(R) state. With this molecular switch hemoglobin acquires a high affinity for oxygen. Mutations that stabilize the R state or destabilize the T state produce hemoglobins with increased oxygen affinity. In response, the oxygen-sensing mechanism in the kidney triggers an increased output of erythropoietin, which in turn stimulates red cell production. This results in erythrocytosis and an elevated hematocrit.

There are approximately 100 high-affinity hemoglobin variants most of which are rare. Almost all show a dominant mode of inheritance. Variants associated with a marked increase in hemoglobin oxygen affinity are likely to be lethal in homozygotes and the few examples of homozygous high-affinity hemoglobins reported are confined to less severe phenotypes. The first high-affinity variant to be described was Hb Chesapeake ($\alpha_2 98$ Arg → Leu), which has a $P_{50}$ on whole blood of 19 mmHg (normal 26 mmHg) and exhibits reduced cooperativity. This mutation results in substitution at a conserved residue of the $\alpha_1\beta_2$ interface between dimer subunits that is important for stability of the T conformer. The substitution of leucine stabilizes the R state.

The molecular defects responsible for high-affinity hemoglobins may be divided into those that occur at sites directly involved in the R → T transition (the $\alpha_1\beta_2$ contact area or the switch region of the molecule, particularly the C and N terminals), such as Hb Chesapeake; those which disrupt the 2,3-DPG binding site in the central cavity, such as Hb Old Dominion (β143 Val → Met); mutations at the $\alpha_1\beta_1$ interface that produce a structural change favoring the R state, such as Hb San Diego (β109 His → Tyr); and those which constrain quaternary conformational change through polymerization, such as Hb Porto Alegre (β9 Ser → Cys).

The clinical course of high-affinity hemoglobin variants is benign. The reduction in tissue oxygen delivery is compensated for by an increased red cell mass and treatment is not generally required. Maternal high-affinity hemoglobin variants do not compromise fetal well-being, arguing against a physiologically important role for the greater affinity for oxygen of Hb F than Hb A in normal pregnancy. Curiously, the degree of erythrocytosis may differ among individuals who inherit high-affinity variants with similar $P_{50}$ values, suggesting other factors influence the adaptation to hypoxia.

## Low oxygen affinity hemoglobins

Hemoglobins with low oxygen affinity deliver oxygen to the tissues more efficiently and are associated with anemia due to reduced erythropoietic drive. Relatively few hemoglobin variants with low oxygen affinity have been described. Cyanosis will be evident if the deoxyhemoglobin level exceeds 5 g/dL. This may be present at birth in low-affinity α chain variants, but its onset is delayed in low-affinity β chain variants because of the latency in β globin expression. The first low-affinity variant to be described was Hb Kansas (β102 Asn → Thr). Two other substitutions at β102 are associated with low affinity, Hb Beth Israel (β102 Asn → Ser) and Hb St Mande (β102 Asn → Tyr). This is explained by the fact that β102 Asn, a highly conserved residue, is required to stabilize the hemoglobin molecule at the $\alpha_1\beta_2$ interface in the R state. If cyanosis in the absence of overt cardiopulmonary causes and anemia are evident, the diagnosis of a low-affinity hemoglobin variant should be considered partly to avoid unnecessary investigation. However, neither cyanosis nor anemia are universal. In patients in whom the $P_{50}$ is markedly increased, anemia is not usually present. Hemoglobin separation techniques are helpful only if the amino acid substitution alters the charge of the molecule and measurement of the oxygen dissociation curve ($P_{50}$) is the gold standard. The oxygen delivery properties of high- and low-affinity hemoglobins are illustrated in Figure 15.7.

## M hemoglobins

M hemoglobins result from mutations which stabilize heme iron in the oxidized ferric ($Fe^{3+}$) state. Inheritance is autosomal dominant. Nine M hemoglobin variants have been described most of which are the product of substitution, in all but one case by tyrosine, of the proximal or distal histidine interacting with the heme group. All are rare, with the exception of Hb Iwate ($\alpha_2 87$ His → Tyr) originally described in the Iwate prefecture of Japan. The interactions between the tyrosine-substituted histidine residues and heme iron have been resolved for some M hemoglobins by X-ray crystallography and NMR spectroscopy and suggest a model whereby the side group of tyrosine acts as an internal ligand preventing interaction with the residual histidine residue. One other molecular defect, Hb M-Milwaukee 1 (β67

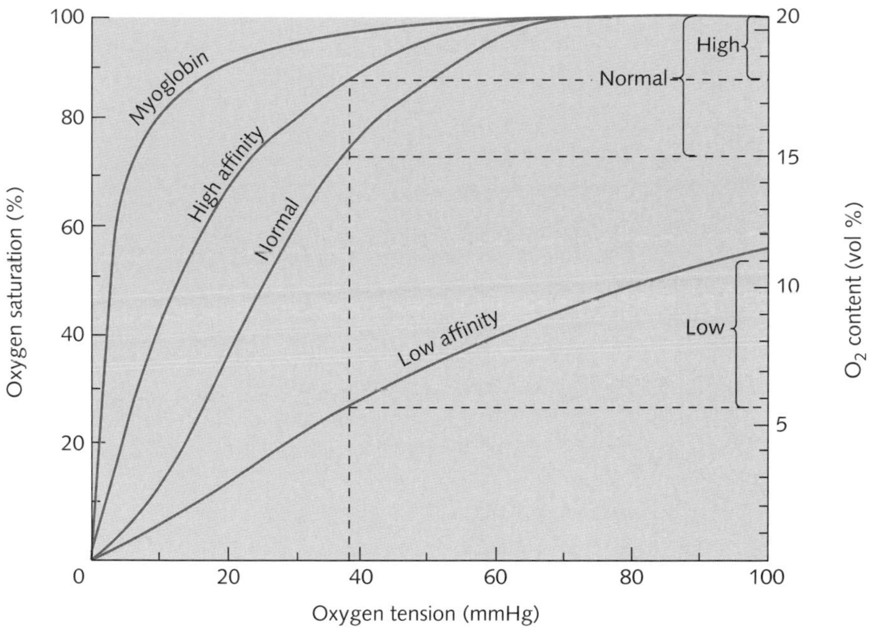

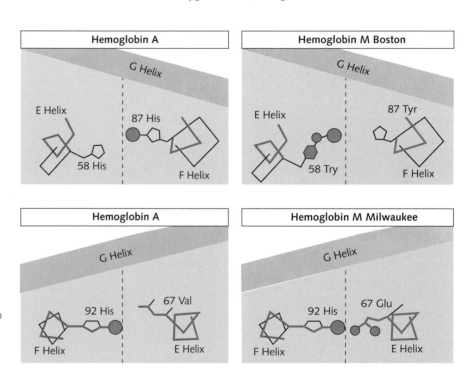

**Fig. 15.7 Oxygen binding curves of hemoglobins with high and low oxygen affinity**

Notice that the extraction of oxygen by the tissues, which is the difference between pulmonary oxygen pressure (100 mmHg) and capillary oxygen pressure (40 mmHg), is lower than normal in high-affinity hemoglobins (low $P_{50}$) and higher than normal in low-affinity hemoglobins. This is why the former have erythrocytosis and the latter (most of the time) anemia.

**Fig. 15.8 Structure of M hemoglobins**

Heme environment of two M hemoglobins compared with Hb A. Note the diverse changes in the distal and proximal tyrosines (which have replaced the normal histidines) in each of the M hemoglobins. These hemoglobins have a characteristic visible spectrum around 610 nm.

Val → Glu) has been described in which the carboxyl group of the substituted glutamic acid residue binds and stabilizes oxidized heme iron. Predictably some M hemoglobins have reduced oxygen affinity.

M hemoglobins resulting from mutation of the α, β, or $^G\gamma$ genes have been described. The latter were identified in newborns with "cyanosis" that resolved spontaneously in the first few months of life. Affected individuals appear slate gray in color due to pseudocyanosis (there may in addition be an element of true cyanosis in low-affinity M hemoglobin variants) but are otherwise asymptomatic and have a normal life expectancy. Pulse oximetry measurements are unreliable. Although standard hemoglobin separation techniques may be helpful, definitive diagnosis requires examination of the visible absorbance spectrum between 450 and 650 nm of a hemolysate, which reveals individual spectral patterns that differ from that of methemoglobin (Figure 15.8). Differential diagnosis includes enzymopathic or acquired methemoglobinemia, sulfhemoglobinemia, and unstable hemoglobin variants such as Hb Chile ($\beta$28 Leu → Met) associated with accelerated methemoglobin formation. The main value in identification of M hemoglobins lies in the avoidance of unnecessary medical intervention.

## Conclusions

Structurally abnormal hemoglobins usually present as one of several well-defined clinical syndromes.

1 Homozygous or compound heterozygous inheritance of Hb S produces a picture of chronic anemia and cumulative organ damage punctuated by intermittent painful crises and other acute manifestations.

2 Hb C in the homozygous state is associated with mild chronic hemolysis, but when co-inherited with Hb S produces a syndrome similar to but generally milder than sickle cell anemia.

3 Homozygous Hb E results in hemolysis and a mild microcytic anemia but in combination with $\beta$ thalassemia produces a phenotype of remarkable variability, ranging from mild thalassemia intermedia to transfusion-dependent thalassemia major.

4 Unstable hemoglobins lead to a hemolytic anemia of variable severity.

5 Low oxygen affinity variants and M hemoglobins are characteristically associated with cyanosis or pseudocyanosis, though if unstable may also be associated with hemolysis of mild degree.

6 High oxygen affinity mutant hemoglobins present with erythrocytosis.

This panoply of clinical syndromes can be attributed to the following alterations of the hemoglobin molecule: (i) modification of the biophysical properties of the hemoglobin molecule (e.g., polymerization of deoxy Hb S); (ii) altered ligand binding affinity; (iii) changes in the heme environment (e.g., M hemoglobins); (iv) instability of the functional tetramer; and (v) reduced globin synthesis (e.g., Hb E). Of over 1000 genetic variants of hemoglobin described, only Hb S, Hb C and Hb E have reached a high frequency in human populations as a result of the selective pressure of malaria; the others, though rare, have provided a wealth of insight into the structure and function of human hemoglobin.

## Further reading

### General

Aldrich T, Nagel RL. (1998) The pulmonary complications of sickle cell disease. In: Bone RC, Dantzker DR, George RB *et al.* (eds). *Pulmonary and Critical Care Medicine*, 5th edn. New York: Mosby.

Eaton WA, Hofrichter J. (1990) Sickle cell hemoglobin polymerization. *Advances in Protein Chemistry*, **40**, 63–279.

Henry ER, Jones CM, Hofrichter J *et al.* (1997) Can a two-state MWC allosteric model explain haemoglobin kinetics? *Biochemistry*, **36**, 6511–6528.

Henry ER, Bettati S, Hofrichter J *et al.* (2002) A tertiary two-state allosteric model of hemoglobin. *Biophysical Chemistry*, **98**, 198–164.

Nagel RL. (1995) Disorders of hemoglobin function and stability. In: Handon RI, Lux SE, Stossel TP (eds). *Blood: Principles and Practices of Hematology*. Philadelphia: J.B. Lippincott.

Nagel RL, Roth EF Jr. (1989) Malaria and red cell genetic defects. *Blood*, **74**, 1213–1221.

Steinberg M, Higgs D, Forget B *et al.* (eds). (2000) *Disorders of Haemoglobin*. Cambridge: Cambridge University Press.

Thein SL. (1998) Hematological diseases. In: Jameson JL (ed.). *Principles of Molecular Medicine*. Totowa, NJ: Humana Press.

### Sickle hemoglobin

Castro O, Hoque M, Brown BD. (2003) Pulmonary hypertension in sickle cell disease: cardiac catheterization results and survival. *Blood*, **101**, 1257–1261.

Gaziev J, Lucarelli G. (2003) Stem cell transplantation for hemoglobinopathies. *Current Opinion in Pediatrics*, **15**, 24–31.

Halsey C, Roberts IA. (2003) The role of hydroxyurea in sickle cell disease. *British Journal of Haematology*, **120**, 177–186.

Herrick JB. (1910) Peculiar elongated and sickle-shaped red blood corpuscles in a case of severe anemia. *Archives of Internal Medicine*, **6**, 517.

Imren S, Payen E, Westerman KA *et al.* (2002) Permanent and panerythroid correction of murine beta thalassemia by multiple lentiviral integration in hematopoietic stem cells. *Proceedings of the National Academy of Sciences of the United States of America*, **99**, 14380–14385.

Kaul DK, Fabry ME, Nagel RL. (1996) The pathophysiology of vascular obstruction in the sickle syndromes. *Blood Reviews*, **10**, 29–44.

Kaul DK, Liu XD, Fabry ME *et al.* (2000) Impaired nitric oxide-mediated vasodilation in transgenic sickle mouse. *American Journal of Physiology. Heart and Circulatory Physiology*, **278**, H1799–H1806.

Morris CR, Morris SM Jr, Hagar W *et al.* (2003) Arginine therapy: a new treatment for pulmonary hypertension in sickle cell disease? *American Journal of Respiratory and Critical Care Medicine*, **168**, 63–69.

Nagel RL, Fleming AF. (1992) Genetic epidemiology of the $\beta^S$ gene. In: Fleming AF (ed.). *Baillière's Clinical Haematology, Volume 5*. London: Harcourt Brace Jovanovich, pp. 331–365.

Nagel RL, Johnson J, Bookchin RM *et al.* (1980) Beta-chain contact sites in the haemoglobin S polymer. *Nature*, **283**, 832–834.

Pawliuk R, Westerman KA, Fabry ME *et al.* (2001) Correction of sickle cell disease in transgenic mouse models by gene therapy. *Science*, **294**, 2368–2371.

Prengler M, Pavlakis SG, Prohovnik I *et al.* (2002) Sickle cell disease: the neurological complications. *Annals of Neurology*, **51**, 543–552.

Reiter CD, Gladwin MT. (2003) An emerging role for nitric oxide in sickle cell disease vascular homeostasis and therapy. *Current Opinion in Hematology*, **10**, 99–107.

Romero JR, Suzuka SM, Nagel RL *et al.* (2002) Arginine supplementation of sickle transgenic mice reduces red cell density and Gardos channel activity. *Blood*, **99**, 1103–1108.

Vichinsky E. (2002) New therapies in sickle cell disease. *Lancet*, **360**, 629–631.

## Hemoglobin C

Dewan JC, Feeling-Taylor A, Puius YA *et al.* (2002) Structure of mutant human carbonmonoxyhemoglobin C (betaF6K) at 2.0 Å resolution. *Acta Crystallographica Section D, Biological Crystallography*, **58**, 2038–2042.

Fabry ME, Romero JR, Suzuka SM *et al.* (2000) Hemoglobin C in transgenic mice: effect of HbC expression from founders to full mouse globin knockouts. *Blood Cells, Molecules and Diseases*, **26**, 331–347.

Fairhurst RM, Fujioka H, Hayton K *et al.* (2003) Aberrant development of *Plasmodium falciparum* in hemoglobin CC red cells: implications for the malaria protective effect of the homozygous state. *Blood*, **101**, 3309–3315.

Lawrence C, Nagel RL. (2001) Compound heterozygosity for Hb S and Hb C coexisting with AIDS: a cautionary tale. *Hemoglobin*, **25**, 347–351.

Modiano D, Luoni G, Sirima BS *et al.* (2001) Haemoglobin C protects against clinical *Plasmodium falciparum* malaria. *Nature*, **414**, 305–308.

Nagel RL, Lawrence C. (1991) The distinct pathobiology of SC disease: therapeutic implications. *Hematology/Oncology Clinics of North America*, **5**, 433–451.

Olson JA, Nagel RL. (1986) Synchronized cultures of *P falciparum* in abnormal red cells: the mechanism of the inhibition of growth in HbCC cells. *Blood*, **67**, 997–1001.

Vekilov PG, Feeling-Taylor AR, Petsev DN *et al.* (2002) Intermolecular interactions, nucleation, and thermodynamics of crystallization of hemoglobin C. *Biophysics Journal*, **83**, 1147–1156.

## Hemoglobin E

Chotivanich K, Udomsangpetch R, Pattanapanyasat K *et al.* (2002) Hemoglobin E: a balanced polymorphism protective against high parasitemias and thus severe *P falciparum* malaria. *Blood*, **100**, 1172–1176.

Fucharoen S, Winichagoon P. (2000) Clinical and hematologic aspects of hemoglobin E beta-thalassemia. *Current Opinion in Hematology*, **7**, 106–112.

Olivieri NF, De Silva S, Premawardena A *et al.* (2000) Iron overload and iron-chelating therapy in hemoglobin E-beta thalassemia. *Journal of Pediatric Hematology Oncology*, **22**, 593–597.

Schrier SL. Pathophysiology of thalassemia. (2002) *Current Opinion in Hematology*, **9**, 1231–1226.

# Chapter 16 Molecular pathogenesis of malaria

**David J Roberts[1] & Chetan E Chitnis[2]**

[1] National Health Service Blood and Transplant (Oxford), John Radcliffe Hospital, Oxford, UK
[2] Malaria Group, International Centre for Genetic Engineering and Biotechnology, New Delhi, India

The epidemiology of malaria, 196
The life cycle of malaria, 198
Invasion of red blood cells, 199
Adhesion of infected red blood cells to host cells, 203

Malarial anemia, 204
Ineffective erythropoiesis in malaria, 205
Future prospects, 206
Further reading, 207

## Introduction

Malaria is a major global public health problem and it is estimated that it is responsible for 1–3 million deaths annually and 300–500 million infections. The vast majority of morbidity and mortality from malaria is caused by infection with *Plasmodium falciparum*, although *P. vivax*, *P. ovale*, *P. malariae* and *P. knowlesi* also cause infection and illness. The pathology of malaria is entirely related to growth and development of the parasite in red blood cells and indeed a significant proportion of the mortality and morbidity is due to anemia. Malaria could therefore quite reasonably, if somewhat unconventionally, be considered the greatest single cause of years of lost life due to a hematological disease.

The malarial parasite has a complex life cycle, alternating between humans and the female *Anopheles* mosquito, a liver and blood stage of growth, complex eukaryotic metabolic systems, and a panoply of mechanisms to evade protective host responses. The vast landscape of interactions between humans, parasites and mosquitoes has been recently illuminated by the completion of sequencing the respective genomes. A short review can only highlight some of the many key molecular processes involved in growth, pathology and prevention or treatment of malaria. Here, we examine the basic features of malaria the parasite and malaria the disease, the molecular aspects of invasion of red blood cells, and adhesion of infected red blood cells to host cells and receptors and their role in pathogenesis. We also consider the pathology of anemia, which is a prominent feature of disease, and outline drug treatment and vaccine development for malaria, and genomic approaches to the study of the parasite, pathology and prevention of disease.

## The epidemiology of malaria

Approximately 1000 million people live in areas where malaria parasites are endemic. The most recent estimates of global malaria morbidity and mortality suggest that 350 million cases and 1 million deaths occur annually when the prevalence of infection in Southeast Asia is considered (Figure 16.1). There is some evidence that the incidence of severe disease, particularly in East and West Africa, is falling, possibly substantially, due to the use of artemisinin combination treatment and impregnated bednets as part of the Gates Foundation and World Health Organization (WHO) initiatives (available at http://www.gatesfoundation.org/topics/Pages/malaria.aspx and http://rbm.who.int/). Although there is understandable and appropriate interest in the molecular aspects of the disease and new therapies, it remains true that in endemic areas the disease is associated with poverty and poor access to established treatments or simple preventive measures.

Malaria occurs when the mean temperature is above 20°C for *P. falciparum* and 15°C for other human malarias, permitting development of the mosquito stages of development (sporogony). Transmission rarely occurs above 1500 m, in arid regions or in the Central and South Pacific, where suitable vectors are absent. Moreover, *P. vivax* malaria is rare in Africa where the population frequency of the blood group Duffy negative (Fya⁻ Fyb⁻) is high. In malarious areas, the pattern of clinical malaria is determined by the number and timing of infective mosquito bites. Mosquito numbers increase after rainfall, leading to an increase in new

*Molecular Hematology*, 3rd edition. Edited by Drew Provan and John Gribben.
© 2010 Blackwell Publishing.

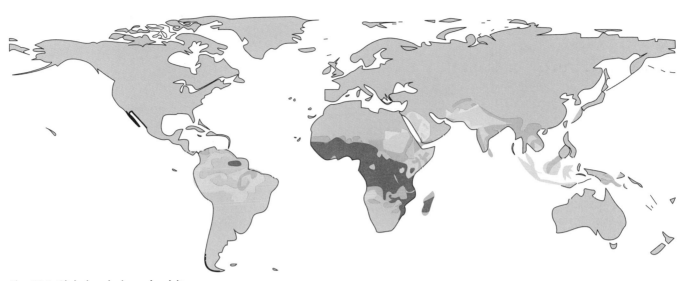

**Fig. 16.1 Global malaria endemicity**
Areas are colored according to malaria endemicity (prevalence): light green, hypoendemic (areas in which childhood infection prevalence is less than 10%); medium green, mesoendemic (areas with infection prevalence between 11 and 50%); dark green, hyperendemic and holoendemic (areas with an infection prevalence of 50% or more). Gray areas are a combined mask of areas outside of the transmission limits and areas of population density less than 1 person per km². From Snow RW, Guerra CA, Noor AM, Myint HY, Hay SI. (2005) The global distribution of clinical episodes of *Plasmodium falciparum* malaria. *Nature*, **434**, 214–217, with permission.

infections; in naive individuals, parasites can cause chronic infection lasting many months.

The intensity of transmission determines the distribution of clinical symptoms in different age groups. In general, in areas of high transmission younger children suffer from severe disease; as transmission decreases, older children suffer from severe disease. When transmission is sporadic, the population can lose much of its natural immunity and a sudden increase in mosquitoes can result in epidemics where large numbers fall ill in all age groups.

The clinical presentation of malaria infection is also wide and influenced by age, immune status, and pregnancy and by the species, genotype and perhaps the geographical origin of the parasite. In endemic areas many infections present as an uncomplicated febrile illness. In more severe forms of the disease children may present with prostration or inability to take oral fluids, or in younger children an inability to suckle. Alternatively, they may exhibit a number of syndromes of severe disease, including anemia, coma, respiratory distress and hypoglycemia and may also have a high rate of bacteremia. In most age groups, anemia is frequently accompanied by more than one syndrome of severe disease and the already substantial case fatality rate of 15–20% for severe malaria in African children rises significantly when multiple syndromes of severe disease are present.

The age distribution of anemia and other syndromes of severe disease are a consistent but puzzling feature of the epidemiology of clinical malaria. Children born in endemic areas are protected from severe malaria in the first 6 months of life by the passive transfer of maternal immunoglobulins and by fetal hemoglobin. Beyond infancy, the most common presentation of severe disease changes from anemia in children aged 1–3 years, in areas of high transmission, to cerebral malaria in older children, in areas of lower transmission. As transmission intensity declines further, severe malaria is most frequently found in older age groups.

There is scant evidence to explain the relationships between age, transmission and predominant clinical syndrome of severe malaria. One possible explanation is the age-dependent increase in expression of CR1 on red blood cells and so a parallel age-dependent increase in the capacity to inactivate complement components absorbed or deposited directly onto the surface of the red blood cell. Another explanation, by no means mutually exclusive, is that erythropoietin (EPO) has a powerful cytoprotective effect on neural, cardiac and other tissues and, indeed, increased levels of EPO are found in younger children with anemia and with malaria. A clinical study showed that there was a significant protective effect of high levels of endogenous EPO on survival after coma, particularly in children under 2 years old.

In endemic areas, even today, 1–2% of all children may die of malaria and this exerts a substantial selection for human traits that protect from infection. It is believed that selection for these protective alleles has taken place over the last 5000 years, after the widespread introduction of agriculture allowed significant increases in population density, transmission and parasite virulence. Sickle cell trait and thalassemia traits protect from infection and are truly polymorphic characteristics in many parts of the world. Understanding the genetic epidemiology has provided classic examples of the principle of genetic selection *in vivo*, for example balancing selection for sickle cell trait and negative epistasis for sickle cell trait and α thalassemia. The homozygous forms of these disorders cause significant clinical disease, such as sickle cell disease, β thalassemia and glucose 6-phosphate dehydrogenase (G6PD) deficiency. In endemic areas these genetic diseases represent major public health problems.

## The life cycle of malaria

In *P. falciparum* malaria, the infective sporozoite forms are inoculated from the salivary glands of a female *Anopheles* mosquito into the subcutaneous tissues and sometimes the bloodstream (Figure 16.2). These thin needle-shaped cells, 10–12 μm in length, circulate briefly with a half-life of approximately 30 min, traversing macrophages and several hepatocytes before residing in a single hepatocyte. Invasion depends, at least partly, on the thrombospondin domains on the circumsporozoite protein (CSP) and the thrombospondin-related adhesive protein (TRAP). CSP and TRAP bind to heparan sulfate proteoglycans on the surface of hepatocytes. Within these cells rapid multiplication takes place over 4–10 days to produce a liver schizont containing about 30 000 merozoites. When ready to leave, the parasite induces hepatocyte cell death, causing the release of merozoites in membrane-enclosed structures or "merosomes" that are extruded from the infected cell, so avoiding host-cell defense mechanisms.

The merozoites bind and then invade red blood cells (*see below*). The host plasma membrane is invaginated to form the parasitophorous vacuole. Immediately after invasion, the developing parasites appear as fine "ring forms." Between 10 and 15 hours, the cytoplasm appears to thicken and 16 hours after invasion granules of the black pigment hematin, the end product of hemoglobin digestion, begin to appear. At this time receptors are expressed at the surface of the infected red blood cell that mediate adhesion to host ligands not only on venular endothelium but also on placenta, uninfected red blood cells, platelets and dendritic cells, and many of these interactions have been associated with pathology. These mature infected red blood cells or *trophozoites* are sequestered in tissue beds as they adhere to post-capillary venular endothelium. Nuclear division begins, at about 30 hours, to form *schizonts* containing up to 32 merozoites. At 48 hours the red blood cell is ruptured to release the

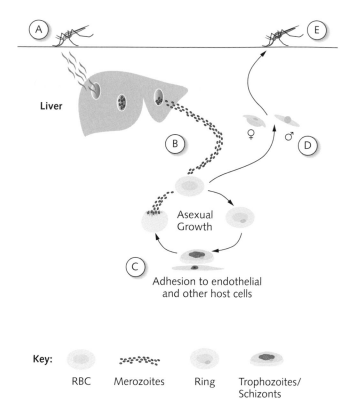

**Key:**

| RBC | Merozoites | Ring | Trophozoites/Schizonts |

**Fig. 16.2 Life cycle of *Plasmodium***
(A) The asexual life cycle begins when sporozoites from a female mosquito taking a blood meal enter the circulation and invade hepatocytes. (B) Up to 30 000 merozoites are formed. The hepatocyte becomes detached and migrates to the liver sinusoid where budding of parasite-filled vesicles or "merosomes" occurs. Following rupture of the merosome, infective merozoites are released and invade erythrocytes (RBC). (C) Within RBCs, the parasite develops through the stages of rings, trophozoites and schizonts. Mature schizonts burst to release erythrocytic merozoites which invade new RBCs. (D) A small proportion of merozoites in RBCs transform into male and female gametocytes, which are ingested by the mosquito. (E) The male and female gametes fuse and transform into an oocyst, which divides asexually into many sporozoites that migrate to the salivary gland from where they are released during the next blood meal.

merozoites into the circulation to continue further cycles of asexual multiplication.

The erythrocytic cycle of growth may yield a 10-fold increase in parasitemia *in vivo* and a patent or microscopically detectable infection 6 days after the liver stage is completed. After two or more cycles the infection becomes manifest by the paroxysms of fever that accompany the release of merozoites. Growth continues until parasite multiplication is reduced by chemotherapy, specific or non-specific defense mechanisms, or occasionally the demise of the host.

When fully grown, some merozoites become committed during the previous erythrocytic cycle to form male or female gametocytes, which are distinguished by dispersed pigment in a single nucleus. They are sequestered for the first 5 days of their development in the peripheral circulation but later appear as circulating, mature, crescent-shaped gametocytes. The sexual phase of the parasite life cycle begins after male and female gametocytes are ingested by a feeding female *Anopheles* mosquito. In the midgut of the mosquito the gametocytes shed the red blood cell membrane, which appears to be precipitated by a drop in ambient temperature. A female gametocyte forms a single macrogamete, but male gametocytes undergo several rounds of nuclear division to produced flagellated motile microgametes, which migrate to fertilize a macrogamete. The resulting zygote forms a mobile ookinete and migrates through the epithelial wall of the midgut to rest on the external surface. The oocyst divides repeatedly to form about 10 000 sporozoites, which enter the acinar cells of the salivary glands and are infective when injected into the host.

In *P. vivax* and *P. ovale* infections, some sporozoites entering the liver form dormant forms or *hypnozoites* which only begin to divide some months later to cause further relapses. In *P. malariae*, erythrocytic development takes 72 hours and thus causes quartan fever (i.e., on days 1 and 4).

## Invasion of red blood cells

The invasion of erythrocytes by malaria parasites is a complex process and requires many specific molecular interactions. These interactions are self-evidently required for the survival of the parasite and it would seem likely that the parasite proteins involved in these interactions would be promising candidates for malaria vaccines.

Erythrocyte invasion by malaria parasites is a multistep process. After initial binding with an erythrocyte, the merozoite reorients itself so that its apical end faces the erythrocyte. A junction forms between the apical surface of the merozoite and the erythrocyte, and several apical organelles such as the rhoptries, micronemes and dense granules discharge their contents to create an invagination in the erythrocyte surface. As the merozoite moves into this invagination, the junction at the apical end transforms into a circumferential ring that moves around the merozoite and pinches closed behind the merozoite when invasion is complete.

The receptors that mediate invasion of red blood cells are found in the rhoptries, micronemes and on the cell surface of merozoites. The intracellular location of many of these parasite receptors and a rapid invasion process may, at least in part, allow the parasite to evade protective immune responses.

## Use of host ligands during red blood cell invasion

*Plasmodium vivax*, and the simian (and occasionally human) malaria parasite *P. knowlesi*, are completely dependent on interaction with the Duffy blood group antigen for invasion of human red blood cells. Electron microscopy studies have shown that the interaction of *P. knowlesi*, and by analogy *P. vivax*, merozoites with the Duffy antigen as ligand is necessary for junction formation during invasion. This blood group antigen is a 38-kDa glycoprotein with seven putative transmembrane segments and 66 extracellular amino acids at the N-terminus (Figure 16.3). The Duffy antigen serves as a receptor for a family of proinflammatory cytokines that includes the chemokines interleukin (IL)-8, melanoma growth stimulating activity and monocyte chemotactic peptide 1. Indeed, IL-8 and melanoma growth stimulating activity inhibit invasion of Duffy-positive human erythrocytes by *P. knowlesi*, with 50% inhibition achieved at nanomolar concentrations *in vitro*, suggesting that it may be possible to block the critical step of junction formation during invasion. The binding site for *P. vivax* and *P. knowlesi* has been mapped to a 35-amino-acid segment of the extracellular region at the N-terminus of the Duffy antigen. Sulfation of tyrosine 41 within this region of the Duffy antigen is critical for recognition by *P. vivax* and *P. knowlesi*.

Unlike *P. vivax* and *P. knowlesi*, *P. falciparum* does not use the Duffy antigen as a ligand during invasion. Instead, studies have shown that sialic acid residues of glycophorin A are ligands for *P. falciparum* during invasion. A 175-kDa *P. falciparum* protein, also known as erythrocyte binding antigen (EBA)-175, binds sialic acid residues on glycophorin A during invasion. EBA-175 does not bind En(a$^-$) erythrocytes, which lack glycophorin A but retain glycophorin B and other sialoglycoproteins, suggesting that sialic acid residues and the peptides from glycophorin A are required for binding. A 63-amino-acid tryptic glycopeptide from the extracellular region of glycophorin A, which blocks binding of EBA-175 to human erythrocytes, serves as the binding site. It is possible that EBA-175 makes contact directly with the peptide backbone of glycophorin A or that the peptide backbone presents sialic acid residues in the correct conformation for binding.

While *P. vivax* is completely dependent on a single pathway for invasion, *P. falciparum* uses multiple invasion pathways and is not confined to using sialic acid residues of glycophorin A. Some *P. falciparum* laboratory strains use sialic acid residues on glycophorin B as ligands. Others invade neuraminidase-treated erythrocytes using sialic acid-independent ligands. Field or wild-type isolates collected from patients with malaria commonly use alternative

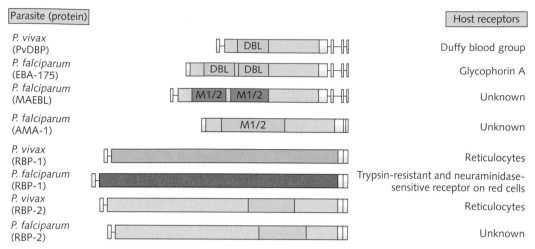

**Fig. 16.3 Apical protein families involved in erythrocyte invasion**

Bar diagrams represent the various protein families found in apical organelles of *Plasmodium* species merozoites that mediate erythrocyte invasion.

invasion pathways independent of sialic acid residues of glycophorin A. These multiple invasion pathways may provide *P. falciparum* with a survival advantage when faced with host immune responses or receptor heterogeneity in natural infections and pose a daunting challenge for vaccine design.

## Parasite receptors used during invasion

Parasite proteins that bind erythrocyte receptors during invasion belong to the erythrocyte-binding protein (EBP) family (Figure 16.3). The EBP family includes *P. vivax* and *P. knowlesi* Duffy binding proteins (PvDBP and PkDBP), *P. knowlesi* β and γ proteins, which bind Duffy-independent receptors on rhesus erythrocytes, and *P. falciparum* EBA-175.

The extracellular region of each EBP contains two conserved cysteine-rich domains, regions II and VI, which contain conserved cysteines and hydrophobic amino acid residues. *Plasmodium falciparum* EBA-175 contains a tandem duplication in region II of the N-terminal cysteine-rich region. The functional binding domain of each EBP maps to region II. Region II of PvDBP binds the human Duffy antigen, region II of PkDBP binds both human and rhesus Duffy antigens, *P. knowlesi* β region II binds sialic acid residues on rhesus erythrocytes, and *P. knowlesi* γ region II binds as yet unidentified Duffy-independent receptors on rhesus erythrocytes. In the case of *P. falciparum* EBA-175, region II binds sialic acid residues on human glycophorin A. Several EBA-175 paralogs have been identified and they may mediate sialic acid–glycophorin A-independent invasion pathways of *P. falciparum*.

## Structural basis for the interaction of EBPs with host receptors

Regions containing binding residues have been mapped to domains of PvDBP and *P. knowlesi* β protein, which contain approximately 350 amino acids with 12 conserved cysteines. Chimeric binding domains containing stretches of *P. vivax* region II fused to stretches of *P. knowlesi* β region II have been expressed and used to define binding residues for the Duffy antigen; these residues map to a 170-amino-acid stretch between the fourth and seventh cysteines of *P. vivax* region II and binding residues for sialic acid map to a 53-amino-acid stretch between the fourth and fifth cysteines of *P. knowlesi* β region II. EBPs are localized in micronemes, not on the surface of merozoites. Invasion studies using another Apicomplexan parasite, *Toxoplasma gondii*, have showed that discharge of microneme proteins such as MIC2 is regulated by cytoplasmic free calcium. It is possible that cytoplasmic calcium levels may serve as a second messenger to trigger release of EBPs to the merozoite surface from micronemes during invasion. The external signals that trigger microneme release in Apicomplexan parasites during host cell invasion are not yet known.

The relatively recent ability to transfect malaria parasites has allowed functional analysis of parasite proteins. Replacement of the EBA-175 gene with a mutant copy encoding a truncated EBA-175 protein without region VI and the transmembrane and cytoplasmic segments has no effect on localization of EBA-175 in micronemes. Disruption of the EBA-175 gene in the *P. falciparum* strain Dd2/NM, which uses sialic acid-independent invasion pathways, has no effect on invasion or growth rates. However, when the EBA-175 gene is disrupted in the *P. falciparum* strain W2Mef, which is dependent on sialic acid residues on glycophorin A, invasion is reduced. *Plasmodium falciparum* W2Mef transfectants expressing truncated EBA-175 use a sialic acid-independent invasion pathway, demonstrating that *P. falciparum* can switch to alternative invasion pathways. The ability to switch to alternative invasion pathways may allow *P. falciparum* to escape intervention strategies that target EBA-175.

Region II of EBA-175 and PvDBP have been expressed as secreted functional proteins that bind erythrocytes with the correct specificity. Antibodies directed against region II of PvDBP block the binding of PvDBP to erythrocytes, and antibodies to region II of EBA-175 inhibit the invasion of erythrocytes by *P. falciparum in vitro*, providing support for their development as malaria vaccines. Somewhat surprisingly, high-affinity antibodies to EBA-175 inhibit invasion by *P. falciparum* strains that use alternate sialic acid–glycophorin A-independent invasion pathways. Antibodies directed against EBA-175 region II may inhibit invasion via such other pathways by steric hindrance after binding to EBA-175 at the apical surface. Given the limited homology between region II of EBP homologs, it is unlikely that antibodies raised against EBA-175 will cross-react with its homologs to block receptor binding.

The crystal structures of PvDBP region II (PvRII) and region II (F1-F2) of EBA-175 (EBA175-RII), together with identification of binding residues, reveal interesting features of receptor recognition by these diverse DBL domains. While the three-dimensional structures of these domains are similar, EBA175-RII forms dimers whereas PvRII is monomeric. The receptor recognition site on PvRII is fully exposed, whereas four sialic acid-binding sites lie in channels at the dimer interface in the case of EBA175-RII. Significant conformational changes are predicted to be necessary for receptor engagement by EBA175-RII. Interestingly, the Duffy recognition site within PvRII is conserved. Regions of polymorphic clusters map to the face opposite the binding site, suggesting that the receptor recognition site is not under selective immune pressure upon natural infection. Indeed, in a field study conducted in children residing in a malaria endemic region of Papua New Guinea, high-titer binding inhibitory antibodies against PvRII were rare. However, once children developed anti-PvRII binding inhibitory antibodies, they were strain-transcending and protected against *P. vivax* infection. These observations support development of a vaccine for *P. vivax* malaria based on region II of *P. vivax* Duffy binding protein.

## MAEBL

Attempts to identify genes encoding EBP homologs from rodent malaria parasites led to the discovery of a related protein family called MAEBL from *P. yoelii* and *P. berghei* that infect rodents. MAEBL has a chimeric character in that it contains domains found in two different protein families (Figure 16.3). The carboxyl end of MAEBL contains a cysteine-rich domain homologous to region VI of EBPs, while the N-terminal end contains paired duplicated cysteine-rich domains, M1 and M2, that share homology with the *P. falciparum* apical merozoite antigen (AMA)-1. Domains M1 and M2 bind mouse erythrocytes. MAEBL can be detected in the rhoptries early in schizogeny. It is also seen evenly distributed on the surface of mature merozoites in late-stage schizonts. This pattern of localization and the fact that regions M1 and M2 of MAEBL bind erythrocytes suggest that MAEBL plays a role in invasion.

## Reticulocyte-binding proteins

*Plasmodium vivax* preferentially invades reticulocytes, which account for only about 1–4% of circulating red blood cells. Two *P. vivax* reticulocyte-binding proteins (PvRBP-1 and PvRBP-2) have been identified and are localized to the apical surface of *P. vivax* merozoites (Figure 16.3). They may therefore be responsible for recognition of reticulocytes by *P. vivax* during invasion. The Duffy antigen is expressed on the surface of mature erythrocytes as well as reticulocytes, but an irreversible junction forms only when the *P. vivax* merozoite encounters a reticulocyte. The interaction of PvRBP-1 and PvRBP-2 with erythrocyte receptors may thus be involved in junction formation during invasion. Sequencing of the *P. vivax* genome has revealed the presence of additional PvRBP homologs. Multiple *P. falciparum* PvRBP-2 orthologs, referred to as PfRH1, PfRH2a, PfRH3, PfRH4 and PfHR5, have also been identified (Figure 16.3). Like PvRBP-2, the *P. falciparum* orthologs are localized at the apical surface of merozoites and may bind erythrocyte receptors to mediate invasion. Erythrocyte binding has been established for PfRH1, PfRH2 and PfRH4 and the binding sites on PfRH1 and PfRH4 for sialic acid-dependent host ligands have now been identified.

A large family of closely related, high molecular weight (~235 kDa) rhoptry proteins from the murine malaria parasite *P. yoelii*, collectively known as the p235 family, share homology with PvRBP-2 (Figure 16.3). Each *P. yoelii* genome has as many as 50 copies of p235 rhoptry protein genes. Members of the p235 family bind mouse erythrocytes. Moreover, immunization with p235 and passive transfer of monoclonal antibodies directed against p235 limits *P. yoelii* infection to reticulocytes and protects mice from death on challenge with the lethal *P. yoelii* YM strain, suggesting a role for the p235 family of proteins in erythrocyte invasion. Individual merozoites isolated from a single schizont express different p235 proteins. This unique method of clonal phenotypic variation allows a schizont to produce a set of merozoites with distinct antigenic and adhesive phenotypes. This may allow the parasite to escape host immune responses or overcome heterogeneity of red blood cell surface ligands in host populations. Similar mechanisms for clonal phenotypic variation have not yet been found in either *P. falciparum* or *P. vivax*.

## Other invasion proteins

AMA-1 is a well-characterized rhoptry protein and a leading malaria vaccine candidate. Sequence analysis of AMA-1 from different primate and rodent malaria parasites reveals the presence of 16 conserved cysteine residues. The pattern of disulfide linkages formed by these cysteine residues in *P. falciparum* AMA-1 has been experimentally determined. Based on the pattern of disulfide linkages, AMA-1 can be divided into three domains (Figure 16.3). Regions M1 and M2 from the N-terminal cysteine-rich regions of MAEBL share homology with the first two domains of AMA-1. AMA-1 is detected in the rhoptries of mature merozoites in late-stage schizonts and is proteolytically processed at the time of schizont rupture, and is subsequently evenly distributed over the merozoite surface. Anti-AMA-1 antibodies inhibit erythrocyte invasion, and immunization with purified AMA-1 provides protection against parasite challenge. Furthermore, the gene for *P. falciparum* AMA-1 cannot be knocked out using gene-replacement methods. This evidence suggests that it plays a critical, non-redundant role in invasion, validating its inclusion in a blood-stage malaria vaccine.

Two other rhoptry-associated proteins from *P. falciparum*, referred to as RAP-1 and RAP-2, are involved in erythrocyte invasion and form a complex with a third protein, RAP-3. Antibodies directed against RAP-1 block erythrocyte invasion *in vitro*, and monkeys immunized with RAP-1 and RAP-2 are protected against parasite challenge, suggesting that these rhoptry proteins should be considered for malaria vaccine development. Gene-replacement methods can be used to disrupt the RAP-1 gene in *P. falciparum* and replace it with a mutant gene encoding truncated RAP-1. Although truncated RAP-1 targets to the rhoptries, it does not form a complex with RAP-2 and RAP-3. Moreover, RAP-2 does not localize to the rhoptries, indicating that it must complex with RAP-1 to correctly target to the rhoptries. *Plasmodium falciparum* transfectants expressing truncated RAP-1 have normal growth and invasion rates *in vitro*, indicating that full-length RAP-1 and the presence of the rhoptry complex containing RAP-1, RAP-2, and RAP-3 is not necessary for invasion. *Plasmodium falciparum* thus appears to have redundant mechanisms that mediate invasion in the absence of the rhoptry protein complex, raising questions about the use of RAP-1 and RAP-2 for malaria vaccine development.

### Merozoite surface protein 1 and invasion

Merozoite surface protein (MSP)-1 was the first merozoite surface protein to be identified and has been extensively investigated. Homologs of MSP-1 have been identified from a number of primate malaria parasites as well as several rodent malaria parasites. Sequence analysis shows that, within a species, MSP-1 contains conserved and more polymorphic regions. Interestingly, MSP-1 undergoes extensive proteolytic processing either during schizogeny or soon after merozoite release. Proteolysis results in four proteolytic fragments of 83 kDa (N-terminus), 30 kDa, 38 kDa, and 42 kDa (C-terminus). These polypeptides remain noncovalently associated at the merozoite surface. The C-terminal 42-kDa fragment is attached to the plasma membrane of the merozoite by a glycosylphosphatidylinositol (GPI) anchor. Final processing steps cleaves the 42-kDa fragment into a 33-kDa fragment and then into a 19-kDa fragment. Because MSP-1 is evenly distributed over the merozoite surface, it is suggested that MSP-1 may mediate the initial interaction with the erythrocyte. Full-length *P. falciparum* MSP-1 binds erythrocytes in a sialic acid-dependent manner.

Antibodies directed against MSP-1$_{19}$ block erythrocyte invasion, and immunization with recombinant MSP-1$_{19}$ protects mice as well as monkeys against parasite challenge, providing support for a blood-stage vaccine based on MSP-1. Invasion-inhibitory antibodies directed against *P. falciparum* MSP-1$_{19}$ block proteolytic processing of MSP-1. Following natural exposure to *P. falciparum* infections, individuals in endemic areas acquire antibodies that can block the binding of processing-inhibitory antibodies to MSP-1. It may be important to design a subunit vaccine based on MSP-1$_{19}$ that elicits processing-inhibitory antibodies without eliciting antibodies that block their binding to MSP-1.

It has not been possible to knock out the *P. falciparum* MSP-1 gene using gene targeting methods, indicating that MSP-1 is essential for invasion and survival. Moreover, *P. falciparum* MSP-1$_{19}$ has limited sequence diversity, possibly because of functional constraints, and this provides a further advantage for vaccine development. However, it has been shown that *P. chabaudi* MSP-1$_{19}$ can functionally replace the *P. falciparum* domain despite the fact that the two sequences are highly divergent, suggesting that the sequence of MSP-1$_{19}$ may not be tightly constrained by function. This observation raises the possibility that introduction of a vaccine based on MSP-1$_{19}$ may result in selection of *P. falciparum* parasites with mutant MSP-1$_{19}$ domains that are functional but antigenically divergent, allowing parasites to escape host immune responses.

Erythrocyte invasion by malaria parasites is a multistep process that is mediated by highly specific molecular interactions that once understood may help in the rational design of vaccines that attempt to block erythrocyte invasion and prevent malaria.

## Adhesion of infected red blood cells to host cells

*Plasmodium falciparum* is distinguished from the other human malarias by the adherence of a very high proportion of the more mature infected red blood cells, containing asexual parasites, and the first stages of gametocytes to post-capillary venular endothelium. The host ligands and parasite receptors that mediate the sequestration of ring-stage parasites have been widely studied as there is is considerable evidence that adhesion of infected red blood cells to some host ligands is associated with the development of severe clinical disease and evasion and indeed modulation of the immune system.

Sequestration of infected red blood cells begins with a similar sequence of events seen during adhesion of leukocytes. Using a flow cell chamber to mimic the shear forces believed to be present *in vivo*, infected red blood cells can be seen to roll across the substrate (indicating receptor–ligand interactions with very rapid on and off rates). Most host receptors are involved with tethering and rolling, but only two receptors, CD36 and chondroitin sulfate A (CSA), support adhesion of infected red blood cells under flow.

Electron microscopy of post-mortem tissues have shown that parasites are sequestered in various organs including heart, lung, brain, liver, kidney, subcutaneous tissues and placenta. Post-capillary venular endothelium and placental syncytiotrophoblasts in placenta express a variety of inducible and non-inducible receptors. Parasites isolated from natural infections or laboratory strains can bind in variable numbers to many different receptors. The total number of parasites, the specificity and degree of binding to host ligands, and the expression of these receptors are thought to determine the tissue and organ distribution of parasites and quite possibly the clinical syndromes observed in severe malaria.

Adhesion of falciparum-infected red blood cells to endothelium and other host receptors is mediated by a para-site protein expressed at the cell surface, the aptly named *P. falciparum* erythrocyte membrane protein 1 (PfEMP1). PfEMP1 is encoded by a large *var* gene family. As the name suggests, these proteins are highly variable, not only antigenically but also in their ability to bind host ligands. Each parasite cell contains 60 or so different *var* genes but only one is expressed at any one time and the cell can rapidly switch expression from one gene to another at a rate of 2–4% per cycle, a phenomenon known as *clonal antigenic variation*. Isolates of parasites from patients or laboratory lines therefore contain infected red blood cells that contain heterogeneous antigenic and adhesive phenotypes.

PfEMP1 has a complex domain structure (Figure 16.4). The extracellular region of PfEMP1 is composed of variable numbers of different DBL domains, named after their homology to the DBL domains involved in red blood cell invasion, and one or two cysteine-rich interdomain regions (CIDRs). DBL domains have been classified into five different classes and the binding domains for several host receptors have been mapped to various DBL and CIDR domains.

PfEMP1 is involved in many pathogenic processes (Plate 16.1). Almost all infected red blood cells can bind to thrombospondin and the platelet glycoprotein CD36, while a subset of infected cells expressing different members of the PfEMP1 family can bind to intercellular adhesion molecule (ICAM)-1, platelet endothelial cell adhesion molecule (PECAM)-1, P-selectin, $\alpha v \beta 3$ integrin, and vascular cell adhesion molecule (VCAM)-1. Adhesion of infected red blood cells or "rosetting" has been associated with severe disease, and in different strains may be mediated by CR1, ABO blood group antigens, glycosaminoglycans and/or IgM. Similarly, the ability of infected red blood cells to adhere to platelets and form large clumps has also been associated with severe disease and is mediated by adhesion of infected red blood cells to CD36 or to the complement receptor gC1qR. The exact relationship between these molecular adhesive phenotypes and disease is not entirely clear but it seems possible that the formation of multicellular aggregates and/or binding of infected cells to a ligand expressed on a particular endothelial bed could contribute to microvascular obstruction and tissue pathology and organ dysfunction (Plate 16.1).

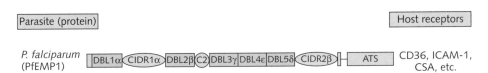

**Fig. 16.4 *Plasmodium falciparum* erythrocyte membrane protein (PfEMP)-1**
The extracellular region of PfEMP-1, which is expressed on the infected red blood cell surface, is composed of variable numbers of five possible DBL domains, named after their homology to the DBL domains involved in red blood cell invasion, and one or two cysteine-rich interdomain regions (CIDRs).

For example, sequestration of parasites in the brain may be related to cerebral malaria or coma and may involve adhesion of infected red blood cells to the ICAM-1 receptor, as vessels containing infected red blood cells are more likely to express ICAM-1 than vessels that do not contain infected red blood cells (Plate 16.1). Adhesion and accumulation of infected cells in the brain is likely to be the result of many different processes and pathways. Recent *in vitro* studies have demonstrated that platelets may act to bridge infected cells and endothelium and contribute to activation of endothelial cells. The relative contribution of these factors and phenotypes to cerebral malaria is not yet clear.

However, the closest linkage between tissue-specific adhesion and pathology is for malaria during pregnancy (Plate 16.1). Pregnant women are more susceptible to malaria and not only suffer severe acute malaria and chronic anemia but also experience premature delivery, low birthweights and increased neonatal mortality. Parasitized red blood cells are sequestered in the placenta in pregnant women and, unlike isolates from other groups of patients, are able to bind to CSA but not to CD36. This adhesive phenotype is linked to expression of a single PfEMP1 with a DBL domain that binds CSA and a non-CD36-binding CIDR1, while CD36-adherent parasites express a PfEMP1 with a CD36-binding CIDR1. The apparently restricted molecular structures associated with placental malaria suggest that the CSA-binding PfEMP1 may be a good candidate antigen to prevent malaria in pregnancy.

Immunity to malaria has a major role in controlling disease. Intriguingly, epidemiological evidence suggests that immunity to severe forms of malaria may be gained after one or two episodes of infection and experimentally this has been achieved in the absence of an antibody response. Even after many tens of exposures, people may develop immunity to disease but are not refractory to asymptomatic infection. Again, the immune responses that underlie this form of immunity are not clear. However, anti-PfEMP1 antibodies do play some role in protecting against pathogenic infections. Exposure to parasites that sequester in the placenta during pregnancy induces strain-transcending immunity that stops infected red blood cells adhering to CSA and may protect a multigravid mother and fetus from placental malaria. During the development of clinical immunity, particularly during early childhood, strain-specific antibodies to PfEMP1 are important in preventing infection with previously encountered isolates. It also appears that virulent isolates from children with severe malaria are not rare, but on the contrary are more commonly recognized by childrens' sera than isolates from cases with mild malaria. It remains possible that the functionally significant regions of PfEMP1 that mediate binding to CD36 or CSA have conserved epitopes that can be targeted for vaccine development.

The exact relationship between the adhesion of infected red blood cells and pathology is somewhat obscure but may involve obstruction of the microcirculation, initiation of a local inflammatory response and/or endothelial activation, damage or death. Understanding such processes may define possible routes for therapy of severe disease.

## Malarial anemia

In endemic areas the etiology of anemia is complex. In children, acute or chronic malaria infection is a major precipitating factor of severe anemia causing admission to hospital. Not infrequently, patients present with a hemoglobin level of less than 5 g/dL with or without respiratory distress secondary to metabolic acidosis. The sudden appearance of hemoglobin in the urine, indicating severe intravascular hemolysis leading to hemoglobinemia and hemoglobinuria (so-called blackwater fever), was described in early studies of anemia in expatriates living in endemic areas, but is rare in Africa and more common in Southeast Asia and Papua New Guinea, where some cases are associated with G6PD deficiency and treatment with a variety of drugs including quinine, mefloquine and artesunate.

The anemia of falciparum malaria is typically normocytic and normochromic, with a notable absence of reticulocytes. The anemia of malaria may be accompanied by modest leukocytosis, leukopenia, leukemoid reaction, monocytosis, lymphocytosis and thrombocytopenia but these changes are neither in themselves diagnostic nor do they help guide management. However, malarial pigment is often seen in neutrophils and monocytes and has been associated with severe disease and an unfavorable outcome.

Malaria provides ample reasons for both increased red cell destruction and reduced red cell production (see Plate 16.2 for overview). Destruction of red blood cells is inevitable as parasites complete their 48-hour growth cycle and lyse their temporary host cell. Some parasites may be removed from erythrocytes as immature ring forms by phagocytic cells, leaving the red blood cells with residual parasite antigens to continue to circulate, albeit with reduced survival. Infected erythrocytes may also be phagocytosed by macrophages following opsonization by immunoglobulins and/or complement components. Other signals for recognition of infected erythrocytes by macrophages include abnormally rigid membranes, exposure of phosphatidylserine and other altered host antigens.

Changes to uninfected red blood cells also contribute to their own enhanced clearance by phagocytes. The activity and number of macrophages are increased in malarial infection, and increased removal of uninfected cells may occur. Moreover, the signals for recognition of uninfected erythrocytes for removal by macrophages are enhanced. Uninfected erythrocytes bind increased amounts of immunoglobulin and/or complement as detected by the direct antiglobulin test (Coombs test). These antibodies do not have a particular specificity, but are more likely to represent immune complexes adsorbed onto the surface of red blood cells. More recent studies have shown that red cells from malaria patients were not only more susceptible to phagocytosis, but also showed increased surface IgG and deficiencies in CR1 and CD55 compared with controls. Uninfected red cells in children and adults with severe disease are less deformable and this is a significant predictor of the severity of anemia and indeed outcome, consistent with the notion that these cells are being removed by the spleen. Active erythrophagocytosis is a conspicuous feature within the bone marrow during *P. vivax* and *P. falciparum* malaria, and it is highly probable that this also occurs within the spleen. Children with acute *P. falciparum* malaria have high circulating levels of interferon (IFN)-γ and tumor necrosis factor (TNF)-α, a synergistic combination of cytokines that activates macrophages.

Parasite proteins may also contribute to the clearance of uninfected red blood cells. The ring surface protein (RSP)-2 is expressed shortly after merozoite invasion of red blood cells and is widely deposited on uninfected red blood cells by contact with merozoites in the circulation. Opsonization of these RSP-2-bearing uninfected red blood cells could contribute to erythrophagocytosis. Indeed, high levels of antibodies that could facilitate complement-mediated phagocytosis of cells expressing RSP-2 are found in sera from immune adults and children with severe anemia. The RSP-2 antigen is also present on the surface of erythroblasts in the bone marrow of *P. falciparum*-infected patients and it has been suggested that damage to developing erythroid cells by RSP-2 and anti-RSP-2 could also contribute to the development of anemia.

Thus, all the available evidence points to increased reticuloendothelial clearance in *P. falciparum* malaria, persisting long after recovery. These changes are presumably a host defense mechanism, maximizing the clearance of parasitized erythrocytes.

## Ineffective erythropoiesis in malaria

Reticulocytopenia has been confirmed in numerous clinical studies of malarial anemia. The histopathological study of the bone marrow of children with malarial anemia shows erythroid hyperplasia with increased numbers of erythroid precursors. However, maturation is abnormal by light and electron microscopy. Abdalla and Weatherall described the hallmark characteristics of such abnormal maturation, namely cytoplasmic and nuclear bridging and irregular nuclear outline. They later confirmed that the distribution of the erythroid progenitors through the cell cycle is abnormal in malarial anemia, with an increased proportion of cells in $G_2$ phase compared with normal controls. Ineffective erythropoiesis also contributes to anemia in animal models of malaria. A recent study has shown that vaccinated *Aotus* monkeys, after a challenge infection, may develop moderate to severe anemia following rapid clearance of uninfected erythrocytes but with low reticulocyte counts, indicating bone marrow dysfunction.

Given the importance of EPO to erythropoiesis, attention has focused on the levels of this crucial cytokine in malarial infection. Serum EPO was appropriately raised in a single study of African children suffering from malarial anemia. However, other studies in adults from Thailand and Sudan have suggested that EPO concentration, although raised, was inappropriate for the degree of anemia. The most recent studies of EPO in African children have shown a supraphysiological rise in EPO levels compared with age-matched community controls with non-malarial anemia, and there appears to be a defective response to EPO in malaria at least in these children.

The prime candidates for the host factors mediating dyserythropoiesis are imbalances in TNF-α, IFN-γ and IL-10. The concentrations of TNF-α and IFN-γ have been correlated with the severity of the disease. While low concentrations of TNF-α (<1 ng/mL) stimulate erythropoiesis, higher levels of TNF-α have been shown to suppress erythropoiesis. Furthermore, it is possible that high levels of these inflammatory cytokines may contribute to reduced and abnormal production of erythrocytes, and also to increased erythrophagocytosis. Recent evidence has also suggested that the release of macrophage inhibitory factor (MIF) inhibits the growth of early erythroid and myeloid progenitors during murine malaria infection and that MIF$^{-/-}$ mice are protected from anemia during experimental malaria infection. However, the role of MIF in human malaria infection has not been established.

High levels of the Th2 cytokine IL-10 might prevent the development of severe malarial anemia. Low levels of IL-10 have been described in African children with severe malarial anemia. It has been suggested that IL-10 may induce heme oxygenase and so reduce oxidative damage to red blood cells and/or developing erythroid cells. Similarly, IL-12 may be associated with a protective innate immune response to malaria and low IL-12 levels have been associated with severe malaria in African children.

There is also substantial evidence that the lysate of infected erythrocytes may directly modulate the function of host cells. During its blood stage, the malaria parasite proteolyzes host hemoglobin in an acidic vacuole to obtain amino acids, releasing heme as a byproduct, which is autoxidized to potentially toxic hematin [aquaferriprotoporphyrin IX or $H_2O$-Fe(III)PPIX]. β-Hematin forms as a crystalline cyclic dimer of Fe(III)PPIX and is complexed with protein and lipid products as malarial pigment or hemozoin. Arese and colleagues showed that the function of monocytes and of monocyte-derived macrophages is severely inhibited after ingestion of malaria pigment or hemozoin. These cells are unable to repeat phagocytosis and to generate oxidative burst when appropriately stimulated. Furthermore, after phagocytosis of hemozoin, myeloid cells are unable to kill ingested fungi, bacteria and tumor cells and to respond to IFN-γ stimulation, but instead respond by increased release of IL-1β, TNF-α and macrophage inflammatory protein (MIP)-1α and MIP-1β.

The hemozoin polymer of heme moieties may be complexed with biologically active compounds. The oxidation of membrane lipids catalyzed by ferric heme produces lipoperoxides. There is accumulating evidence that 4-hydroxynonenal and other lipoperoxides including 15-hydroxy-arachidonic acid (15-HETE) may play a role in the pathophysiology of malaria. Endoperoxides produced in pigment-containing monocytes or macrophages may impair erythroid growth. Hemozoin may also directly inhibit erythroid development *in vitro* and increased levels of plasma hemozoin and pigment in monocytes have been associated with anemia.

A further class of parasite products that may contribute to malarial anemia are the GPI anchors of merozoite proteins, such as MSP-1, MSP-2 and MSP-4, which are found in plasma during infections. GPIs are likely to contribute to anemia since their injection into mice results in a transient decrease in the number of circulating red blood cells, probably through induction of TNF-α from macrophages. More recently, it has been demonstrated that the proinflammatory response from human monocytes is through interaction of GPIs with TLR2 and, to a lesser extent, TLR4. Antibodies specific to GPIs were present in sera of adults from endemic regions in Kenya, but the level of these antibodies was less in younger children who in general have more severe disease and malarial anemia.

Many possible molecular mechanisms of red blood cell clearance have been described in a variety of experimental and clinical systems. The challenge now is to determine the relative contribution of these mechanisms to anemia in children with malaria and to seek ways to prevent anemia without increasing susceptibility to disease.

## Future prospects

Molecular methods and the application of modern proteomic and genomic biology are likely to transform our approach to the diagnosis, treatment and prevention of malaria. The diagnosis of malaria is based on the identification of circulating blood-stage parasites in thick and thin films. In endemic areas, laboratory staff are skilled at the examination of thick films and are routinely able to detect 1 parasite in 100 high-power fields of a thick film, which corresponds to a sensitivity of approximately 5–50 parasites/μL. Nevertheless, the diagnosis of malaria by microscopy in non-endemic countries has proven problematic. Routine laboratories may only achieve sensitivities of the order of 500 parasites/μL using thick films. Detection of circulating malarial antigens is another potentially attractive, but ultimately limited, alternative to the laborious method of screening blood films. The widely available tests detect *Plasmodium* histidine-rich protein 2 and *Plasmodium*-specific lactate dehydrogenase by immunochromatography. The formulation of the tests using dipstick antigens allows rapid testing to be performed by laboratory staff. However, the sensitivity is 100–1000 parasites/μL and this is comparable to the sensitivity achieved by inexperienced microscopists. The current recommendations for malaria diagnosis in the UK emphasize clearly that these tests only have a place when experienced staff are not available. Amplification of circulating parasite DNA using the repeated rRNA genes is an extremely sensitive method of malaria diagnosis. The sensitivity may be as low as 0.005 parasites/μL or 5 parasites/mL. This approach may be developed as a future method for routine diagnostic use.

Malaria requires urgent effective chemotherapy to prevent progression of disease and may be the most crucial public health intervention to reduce global mortality from malaria. Resistance to the first-line treatment of chloroquine and to dihydrofolate reductase inhibitors has led to artemisinin-based combination treatments. This group of drugs has a remarkable history and represents a novel class of chemical compounds known as the artemisinins. Chinese scientists rediscovered the activity of extracts of the plant *Artemisia annua* from careful re-reading of medieval pharmacopeias. The active substance was crystallized and identified as artemisinin in 1973, and derivatives dihydroartemisinin (DHA), artemether, artesunate and arteether were first prepared in China in the 1970s. The mechanism of action of these drugs was proposed to be within the "food vacuole," where the drug could inhibit digestion of hemoglobin. However, artemisinins act very early in the parasite life cycle, killing ring-stage parasites, and other studies have indicated that artemisinins could also inhibit the function of the mitochondrion or the translationally controlled tumor protein (TCTP) and PfATP6, a parasite-encoded sarcoplasmic reticulum calcium-ATPase. Understanding the mechanism of action and the routes by which drug resistance can be developed will be of crucial importance given the central role artemisinin-based combination therapy has for controlling malaria (http://www.rbm.who.int/gmap).

The search for a malaria vaccine could almost be a case study in the triumph of hope over experience. However, there have been some recent trials showing significant efficacy. The RTS, S vaccine was developed by Joe Cohen at GlaxoSmithKline and uses a recombinant *P. falciparum* circumsprozoite protein, which is naturally expressed in high levels on the surface of the infective forms injected by mosquitoes, fused to the hepatitis B surface protein. A series of trials have shown a reduction in episodes of severe malaria by 50% and further Phase III studies are planned. There are over 40 subunit vaccines in different stages of development, many of which are based on the antigens described above (see http://www.malariavaccine.org).

This chapter has described the essential features of the epidemiology, clinical presentations and life cycle of the parasite and the main features of our present molecular understanding of key features of invasion of red blood cells, adhesion of infected erythrocytes to host ligands and how these and other host–parasite interactions lead to cerebral and placental malaria and anemia. The data revealed by sequencing the parasite, human and mosquito genomes are just beginning to be applied, increasing our understanding not only of the pathogenesis of disease, for example by large-scale genetic association studies of single-nucleotide poly-morphisms associated with protection from malaria, but also of the biology of the parasite. The genomic approach to unraveling parasite biology has been boosted by the availability of sequences from many wild isolates and laboratory strains of *P. falciparum* and all the major human, simian and rodent malaria species. It is to be hoped that the "new biology" will lead to novel methods for diagnosing, treating and preventing malaria to complement the huge efforts in public health now targeted at rolling back and perhaps one day eradicating malaria.

## Further reading

Cowman AF, Crabb BS. (2006) Invasion of red blood cells by malaria parasites. *Cell*, **124**, 755–766.

Kwiatkowski DP. (2005) How malaria has affected the human genome and what human genetics can teach us about malaria. *American Journal of Human Genetics*, **77**, 171–192.

Miller LH, Baruch DI, Marsh K, Doumbo OK. (2002) The pathogenic basis of malaria. *Nature*, **415**, 673–679.

Snow RW, Guerra CA, Noor AM, Myint HY, Hay SI. (2005) The global distribution of clinical episodes of *Plasmodium falciparum* malaria. *Nature*, **434**, 214–217.

White NJ. (2008) Qinghaosu (artemisinin): the price of success. *Science*, **320**, 330–334.

Winzler EA. (2008) Malaria research in the post-genomic era. *Nature*, **455**, 751–756.

# Chapter 17 Molecular coagulation and thrombophilia

## Björn Dahlbäck & Andreas Hillarp

*Department of Laboratory Medicine, Section of Clinical Chemistry, Lund University, University Hospital, Malmö, Sweden*

## Introduction

Venous thrombosis is a major medical problem affecting millions of individuals worldwide each year. It is a typical multifactorial disease, the pathogenesis involving both environmental and genetic risk factors. A mutation in the factor V (FV) gene (Arg506Gln or FV Leiden) is the most common genetic risk factor known to date. Activated protein C (APC) regulates the activity of FVa by cleaving several sites in FVa, and Arg506 is one of them. APC resistance, which is the consequence of the FV mutation, results in a lifelong hypercoagulable state. A point mutation in the prothrombin gene is another relatively common risk factor, whereas deficiencies of the anticoagulant proteins antithrombin, protein C or protein S are less common. Owing to the high prevalence of the FV and prothrombin mutations, combinations of genetic defects are relatively common in the general population. Such individuals have highly increased risk of thrombosis.

## Blood coagulation

At sites of vascular damage, circulating platelets adhere to subendothelial structures and undergo a series of reactions that lead to primary hemostasis due to the formation of a platelet plug. Concomitant to these events, the subendothelial membrane protein tissue factor (TF) is exposed to blood. A small amount of activated factor VII (FVIIa) present in circulating blood binds to TF and triggers a series of proteolytic reactions that culminate in the formation of thrombin and the conversion of fibrinogen to insoluble fibrin.

FVIIa bound to TF specifically cleaves and activates the two vitamin K-dependent plasma proteins, factor IX (FIX) and factor X (FX) (Plate 17.1). Activated FX (FXa) activates prothrombin to thrombin, whereas activated FIX (FIXa) activates FX. Both FIXa and FXa are poor enzymes that require protein cofactors, calcium ions and negatively charged phospholipid surfaces for expression of full biological activity. The protein cofactors for FIXa and FXa are the activated forms of factor VIII (FVIIIa) and factor V (FVa), respectively (Plate 17.2). As a result of multiple protein–protein and protein–phospholipid interactions, enzymatically highly efficient complexes are assembled on the phospholipid surface.

The initiation of blood coagulation by TF is usually referred to as the *extrinsic pathway* or the TF pathway. In association with injury, this is the physiologically most important mechanism of blood coagulation. However, coagulation can also be activated through the *intrinsic pathway*, triggered by activation of the contact phase proteins (FXII, FXI, prekallikrein and high-molecular-weight kininogen) that follows exposure of blood to certain negatively charged surfaces. The intrinsic pathway does not appear to be physiologically important for injury-related coagulation *in vivo*, illustrated by the lack of bleeding problems in individuals with deficiency of FXII.

Thrombin generated at sites of vascular injury expresses a number of procoagulant properties. It amplifies the coagulation process by activating FXI and in addition it activates platelets and converts fibrinogen to fibrin. Moreover, in a positive feedback reaction, thrombin converts the procofactors FV and FVIII into their biologically active counterparts (FVa and FVIIIa).

*Molecular Hematology*, 3rd edition. Edited by Drew Provan and John Gribben.
© 2010 Blackwell Publishing.

# Regulation of blood coagulation

The efficient reactions of the coagulation system have considerable biological potential and strict regulation is required. For this purpose, several plasma proteins and protein–cell interactions are involved in constant monitoring of the circulation. At each level of the coagulation pathway, membrane-bound molecules expressed on the surface of intact endothelial cells, circulating inhibitors and negative feedback mechanisms provide efficient control.

Antithrombin (AT) is the most important serine protease inhibitor (serpin) involved in the regulation of blood coagulation. AT inhibits thrombin as well as FXIa, FIXa and FXa and, under certain conditions, also FVIIa. AT forms a highly stable complex with the protease and, as a consequence, the protease is trapped and eliminated from the circulation. The activity of AT is stimulated by heparin, which accelerates the rate of formation of the AT–protease complexes. Under normal physiological conditions, heparan sulfate proteoglycans present on the endothelial cell surface stimulate the activity of AT, whereas heparin injections are used in clinical situations. During inhibition of thrombin, an important role of heparin is to function as a bridge between thrombin and AT. In addition, heparin induces conformational changes in AT that are associated with the generation of a more efficient inhibitor. In the inhibition of FXa, the conformational change appears to be more important than the bridging mechanism.

The tissue factor pathway inhibitor (TFPI) regulates the TF pathway. TFPI is composed of three protease inhibitory domains belonging to the Kunitz type of inhibitors. TFPI has the unique capacity to inhibit the FVIIa–TF–FXa complex and is therefore highly efficient in turning off the TF pathway. The inhibition mediated by TFPI occurs in two steps: the first involves inhibition of FXa by the middle Kunitz domain; the first Kunitz domain then binds and inhibits FVIIa. The majority of TFPI is bound to glucosaminoglycans on endothelial cells (approximately 80%) and only a minor fraction of TFPI is present in plasma, where it is mainly associated with low-density lipoprotein.

The highly efficient procoagulant reactions of thrombin are physiologically adequate at sites of vascular injury and are instrumental in efficient hemostasis. However, the same reactions pose a threat to the organism as uncontrolled coagulation leads to thrombus formation. Nature has solved this dilemma in intricate and fascinating ways, one of which is the transformation of thrombin into an efficient initiator of a natural anticoagulant pathway, the protein C system. The conversion of thrombin from a procoagulant into an anticoagulant enzyme depends on the presence of intact endothelium. Thus, thrombin generated at sites of intact vasculature binds to the endothelial membrane protein thrombomodulin, which is a potent modulator of thrombin activity and a cofactor to thrombin in the activation of protein C (Plate 17.3). A recently discovered receptor for protein C, the endothelial protein C receptor (EPCR), has been shown to stimulate the activation of protein C by the thrombin–thrombomodulin complex. APC inactivates membrane-bound FVa and FVIIIa by limited proteolysis in reactions that are potentiated by a cofactor protein designated protein S and, in the case of FVIIIa degradation, also by the non-activated form of FV (Plate 17.4).

Under physiological conditions, procoagulant and anticoagulant mechanisms are balanced in favor of anticoagulation, whereas the anticoagulant system is downregulated and procoagulant forces prevail at sites of vascular damage. Defects in this ingenious system are associated with increased thrombin generation and a hypercoagulable state, leading to an increased risk of thrombosis.

## Protein C anticoagulant system

Protein C is a vitamin K-dependent plasma protein that is synthesized mainly in the liver. It is homologous to FVII, FIX and FX and shares with them a common modular organization. From the N-terminus, these proteins contain a vitamin K-dependent $\gamma$-carboxyglutamic acid (Gla)-rich module, two epidermal growth factor (EGF)-like modules and a serine protease module. The Gla domains bind calcium ions and provide the vitamin K-dependent clotting proteins with phospholipid-binding properties. Upon activation by the thrombin–thrombomodulin complex, the serine protease module is converted to an active enzyme. APC is highly specific in its proteolytic activity, cleaving a limited number of peptide bonds in FVa and FVIIIa.

Intact FV is a high-molecular-weight protein and shares with the homologous FVIII molecule the modular arrangement A1, A2, B, A3, C1 and C2 (Figure 17.1). On activation of FV by thrombin or FXa, peptide bonds surrounding the B-module (positions 709 and 1545) are cleaved, releasing the B-module, which is thus not part of FVa. FVIII is activated by thrombin in a similar fashion, leading to release of the B-module. In circulation, FVIII is bound to von Willebrand factor (VWF) and the thrombin-mediated activation of FVIII results in the release of FVIIIa from VWF. APC cleaves three peptide bonds in FVa at Arg306, Arg506 and Arg679, whereas FVIIIa is cleaved at Arg336 and Arg526. As a consequence of the APC-mediated cleavages, FVa and FVIIIa lose their procoagulant properties.

APC alone has poor anticoagulant activity and it is only in the presence of its cofactors protein S and FV that efficient anticoagulant function is expressed. This was demonstrated in an experimental system based on the degradation of

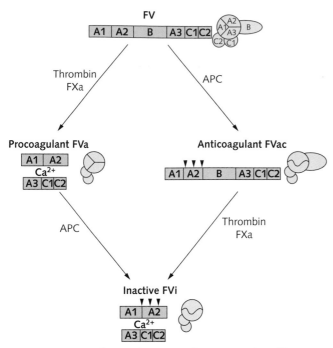

**Fig. 17.1 Procoagulant and anticoagulant properties of factor V**
Proteolytic modification of single-chain FV results in the expression of either procoagulant or anticoagulant properties. Thrombin and FXa cleaves peptide bonds in and surrounding the B domain (positions 709, 1018, 1545) and thus activates FV to procoagulant FVa, which functions as a cofactor to FXa in the activation of prothrombin. Intact FV is sensitive to cleavage by APC (at positions 306, 506, and 679), which recruits FV into an anticoagulant path. FV modified by APC (FVac) functions as a synergistic APC cofactor with protein S in the degradation of FVIIIa. The anticoagulant properties of FV are lost on further proteolysis by thrombin or FXa. Likewise, the procoagulant effects of FVa are lost as a result of cleavage by APC. Thus, FV plays a crucial and central role, balancing procoagulant and anticoagulant forces. Arrowheads denote the three APC-cleavage sites at position 306, 506 and 679.

FVIIIa. In this system, it was found that full anticoagulant activity of APC was obtained in the presence of the combination of FV and protein S. The synergistic APC cofactor activity of FV requires APC-mediated proteolysis of at least the Arg506 cleavage site (Figure 17.1). Thus the Arg506 → Gln mutation is important for understanding the mechanism of APC resistance (FV Leiden; *see below*). The APC cofactor activity of FV appears specific for the degradation of FVIIIa, whereas the FVa degradation is unaffected by this FV activity. FV loses its APC cofactor activity upon proteolysis by thrombin, but it gains procoagulant properties as a cofactor to FXa. Thus, FV is similar to thrombin in being able to

express both procoagulant and anticoagulant effects. However, whereas the anticoagulant effects of thrombin depend on its binding to thrombomodulin, the anticoagulant properties of FV are dependent on APC-mediated proteolysis of the non-activated form of FV. The detailed mechanisms by which FV functions as an APC cofactor remain to be elucidated.

Protein S is also a vitamin K-dependent plasma protein, but unlike the other vitamin K-dependent coagulation proteins it is not a serine protease. It is a multimodular protein containing a Gla module, a thrombin-sensitive module, four EGF-like modules and a large module homologous to sex hormone-binding globulin (SHBG) (*see Figure 17.4*). Protein S also has functions outside the protein C system and 60–70% of protein S in plasma circulates bound to C4b-binding protein (C4BP), a regulator of the complement system. The Gla module of protein S provides both free protein S and the protein S–C4BP complex with phospholipid-binding ability. This is important for the localization of coagulation and complement regulatory activities to certain cell membranes, for example to the phosphatidylserine that is exposed on apoptotic cells. Protein S binding to such cells has been shown to be involved in stimulation of phagocytosis of these cells.

During the degradation of free FVa (i.e., not bound to FXa) by APC, the cleavage at Arg506 is faster than that at Arg306. The cleavage at Arg506 leads only to partial loss of FVa activity, whereas the cleavage at Arg306 leads to efficient inactivation of FVa. Protein S serves as cofactor for the cleavage at Arg306 but has minor effects on the Arg506 cleavage. This, together with a specific protection of the Arg506 site exerted by FXa, indicates that the Arg306 site is the most important site for regulation of FVa activity in the prothrombinase complex. On the other hand, FVa that is not part of a prothrombinase complex is first cleaved at the Arg506 site, because the kinetics of this cleavage are more favorable than those for the cleavage site at Arg306. In experiments *in vitro*, protein S has been shown to express an anticoagulant activity that is independent of the presence of APC. The exact mechanism is still unclear despite considerable research. Recently, it has been suggested that the direct anticoagulant effect of protein S is due to interaction with TFPI and direct stimulation of the TFPI activity. Other proposals suggest that protein S inhibits prothrombin activation through direct interactions of protein S with FVa, FXa and the phospholipid membrane. The *in vivo* physiological significance of this APC-independent anticoagulant activity is unclear. Regardless of its mode of action, protein S is an important anticoagulant protein *in vivo* as demonstrated by animal studies and by the association between protein S deficiency and venous thrombosis.

# Molecular genetics of venous thromboembolism

The annual incidence of venous thrombosis in Western societies is approximately 1–2 per 1000. Thrombotic episodes tend to occur in conjunction with surgery, fractures, pregnancy, the use of oral contraceptives, and immobilization. In addition, genetic defects are frequently involved and many patients report positive family histories. Genetic defects known to predispose to thrombosis include inherited APC resistance due to FV Leiden, a point mutation in the prothrombin gene (G20210A) and deficiencies of anticoagulant protein C, protein S or AT. These inherited causes of thrombophilia are autosomal dominant disorders and the prothrombotic mutations result in a lifelong increased risk of thrombosis. However, the penetrance of the disease may be variable and the individual risk profile is still difficult to predict.

## Factor V gene mutation (FV Leiden) causing APC resistance

In 1993, APC resistance was described as a cause of inherited thrombophilia and it was soon demonstrated to be highly prevalent (20–60%) among thrombosis patients. In APC resistance, APC does not give a normal prolongation of the clotting time. In more than 95% of cases the molecular defect associated with APC resistance is a single point mutation in the FV gene, *F5* (GeneID 2153, OMIM ID 227400). The mutation is a G → A substitution at nucleotide position 1691 in the FV gene, which predicts replacement of Arg506 with a Gln (Figure 17.1). The mutant FV is known as FVR506Q, FV Leiden or FV:Q506 (R and Q are one-letter codes for Arg and Gln, respectively).

The FV Leiden allele is found only in Caucasians, and its prevalence varies considerably in the general population of Western societies. High prevalence (up to 15%) is found in southern Sweden, Germany, Greece, Arab countries and Israel. In the Netherlands, the UK and the USA, around 3–5% of the population carry the mutant allele. Lower prevalence (around 2%) is found in Hispanics. The high prevalence of the FV Leiden allele in certain populations suggests a possible survival advantage, and there is a reduced risk of bleeding after delivery in women carrying the mutation. In the history of humankind, the slightly increased risk of thrombosis associated with the FV Leiden allele has presumably not been a negative survival factor because thrombosis develops relatively late in life and does not influence fertility. In addition, many of the circumstantial risk factors for thrombosis, such as a sedentary lifestyle, surgery and the use of oral contraceptives, did not affect our ancestors.

The high prevalence of the FV Leiden allele in Western societies is the result of a founder effect. It has been estimated that the mutation event occurred around 21 000 years ago, after the "Out of Africa Exodus" that took place 100 000 years ago and also after the separation of Asians from Europeans. This explains why the mutant FV allele is common among European populations but is not present among Japanese, Chinese or in the original populations of Africa, Australia or America.

A large number of studies have demonstrated a relationship between the presence of APC resistance (FV Leiden) and an increased risk of venous thrombosis. Differences in selection criteria of patients and in the prevalence of the mutant allele in the general population explain the wide variation in results obtained from different studies. However, the general consensus is that the FV Leiden allele is the most common genetic risk factor for venous thrombosis in Western societies. The odds ratio, describing the increased risk of thrombosis in affected individuals, has been calculated to be sixfold to eightfold for those carrying the defect in a heterozygous form, whereas homozygous individuals are at 30–140-fold increased risk of thrombosis. The FV Leiden allele does not appear to be a strong risk factor for arterial thrombosis, such as myocardial infarction. Two different mutations affecting the Arg306 site have recently been found in thrombosis cases, FV Cambridge and FV Hong Kong, but such mutations appear to be rare. They do not result in APC resistance and are not major risk factors for thrombosis.

The FV Leiden allele is associated with a hypercoagulable state, which is reflected by increased levels of prothrombin activation fragments in plasma of individuals with inherited APC resistance. Two molecular mechanisms are involved (Figure 17.1 and Plate 17.4). One is that an APC cleavage site in FVa is lost, which impairs the normal degradation of FVa by APC. The other surprising observation is that FV Leiden is a poor APC cofactor in the degradation of FVIIIa because the cleavage at Arg506 is required for expression of APC cofactor activity of FV.

In the degradation of normal FVa, the APC cleavage at Arg506 has favorable kinetics compared with cleavages at other sites. The Arg506 cleavage is approximately 10-fold faster than the cleavage at Arg306 and the activity of FVa:Q506 (FVa Leiden) is therefore inhibited at an approximately 10-fold lower rate than FVa:R506. Generated FVa Leiden persists longer than normal FVa and can form active prothrombinase complexes with FXa. However, degradation of free FVa (i.e., FVa not bound to FXa) is different from that of FVa which is part of the prothrombinase complex. In the prothrombinase complex, the Arg506 site is protected from degradation by APC by both FXa and prothrombin. In addition, protein S functions as an APC cofactor primarily for the Arg306 cleavage. As a consequence, APC-mediated degradation of FVa, which is part of the prothrombinase complex, follows a different pathway compared with that of free FVa. Therefore, when FVa:R506 and FVa:Q506 are part of assembled prothrombinase complexes, the rates of their degradation by APC plus protein S are similar.

Laboratory investigation of inherited APC resistance due to the FV Leiden allele can be done using both a functional APC-resistance test and molecular biology assays. A modified APC-resistance test involving dilution of the patient's plasma in FV-deficient plasma is highly sensitive and specific for the presence of the FV Leiden allele. The most commonly used molecular biology assay for FV Leiden involves polymerase chain reaction (PCR) amplification of genomic DNA and subsequent allele-specific mutation analysis.

## Deficiency of antithrombin

Subjects with inherited AT deficiency are, with few exceptions, heterozygotes. It is caused by mutations in the AT gene, *SERPINC1* (GeneID 462, OMIM ID 107300), which is located at chromosome 1q23–q25. Heterozygous AT deficiency is found in 0.02–0.05% of the general population and in 1–2% of thrombosis patients, suggesting that the genetic defect to be associated with a 10- to 20-fold increased risk

of thrombosis – somewhat higher than estimated for APC resistance. AT deficiency may be of either type I or type II. Type I deficiency is characterized by low levels of both immunological and functional AT, whereas type II denotes functional defects. Type II cases can be further divided into three subtypes: RS (reactive site mutants), HBS (heparin-binding site mutants) or PE (mutants giving pleiotropic effects). A large number of AT deficiencies are caused by missense mutations, which alter key amino acid residues in the primary structure of the protein (Figure 17.2).

According to the AT deficiency database maintained at Imperial College in London (www1.imperial.ac.uk/medicine/about/divisions/is/haemo/coag/antithrombin), there are at least 127 distinct mutations causing a deficiency phenotype. In a majority of cases, the genetic defect is a point mutation leading to missense, nonsense or splice-site mutations. Other mutations involve small deletions or insertions, which result in frameshift alterations that are often deleterious. Partial or whole gene deletions are relatively uncommon causes of AT deficiency (<10% of the reported mutations). Type II RS variants are defective in protease inactivation and mutations in the vicinity of the reactive site have been found. The type II HBS deficiency carries mutations in the heparin-binding site, and type II PE variants are caused by a limited number of mutations between amino acids 402 and 429.

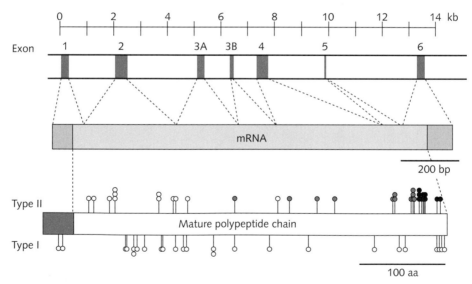

**Fig. 17.2 Structure of the human antithrombin gene and location of detrimental missense mutations in the antithrombin molecule**
The gene for antithrombin (*SERPINC1*) is localized to chromosome 1q23–q25 and spans 13.4 kb of DNA (upper part). It comprises seven exons and results in an mRNA of 1.7 kb (middle part). The antithrombin molecule (lower part) is synthesized as a single polypeptide chain comprising a mature protein of 432 amino acid residues and a signal peptide (shaded) of 32 amino acid residues. Many mutations of different types causing antithrombin deficiency have been described. Shown here are only missense mutations leading to amino acid substitutions associated with type I deficiency (indicated by open circles below the polypeptide chain) or type II deficiency (open, shaded and filled circles denote type II HBS, type II RS and type II PE variants, respectively).

## Protein C deficiency

Protein C deficiency is caused by mutations in the protein C gene, *PROC* (GeneID 5624, OMIM ID 176860), which is located on chromosome 2q13–q21. Clinically, there are two types of protein C deficiency. Type I is characterized by a parallel reduction in protein C antigen and functional activity. Type II is characterized by a functional defect in the protein, and its plasma concentration may be normal. The majority of reported cases of protein C deficiency are of type I. However, plasma assays can sometimes have limited discriminative power between the different types. There is also an overlap between plasma concentrations at the low end of the normal distribution and at the upper end of protein C deficiency, which can complicate correct phenotyping.

Heterozygous deficiency of protein C is identified in 2–5% of thrombosis patients. The prevalence of protein C deficiency in the population is estimated to be approximately 0.3%. The 10-fold higher prevalence of protein C deficiency in thrombosis cohorts suggests that carriership is associated with a 10-fold increased risk of venous thrombosis, essen-tially similar to the risk associated with APC resistance. Protein C deficiency is not a risk factor for arterial thrombosis, although there are studies claiming that protein C deficiency may have an impact on the onset of arterial occlusive diseases. Homozygous or compound heterozygous protein C deficiency is a rare condition (1 in 200 000 to 1 in 400 000) that often leads to severe and fatal thrombosis in the neonatal period. The clinical picture is that of purpura fulminans and the symptoms include necrotic skin lesions due to microvascular thrombosis. Other major symptoms are thrombosis in the brain and disseminated intravascular coagulation. Several cases have been successfully treated with fresh frozen plasma or with protein C concentrates.

Genetic analysis has been performed in a large number of cases with protein C deficiency and there are more than 200 mutations in the Human Gene Mutation Database (www.hgmd.cf.ac.uk/ac) associated with protein C deficiency. Most genetic defects are missense mutations, which lead to single amino acid substitutions, or nonsense mutations located within the coding region of the gene. The locations of reported missense mutations are indicated in Figure 17.3.

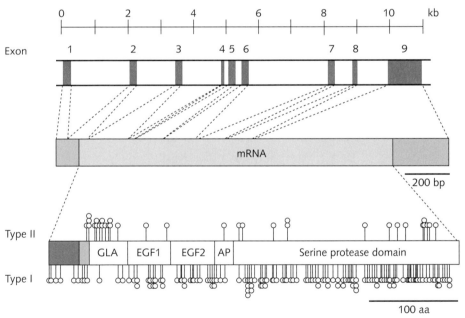

**Fig. 17.3 Structure of the human protein C gene and location of detrimental missense mutations in the protein C molecule**
Human protein C is encoded by the *PROC* gene, localized to chromosome 2q13–q14, which spans approximately 11 kb of DNA (upper part). The gene comprises nine exons which yield about a 1.8-kb mRNA transcript (middle part). The protein C mRNA encodes a pre-pro-protein C sequence of 461 amino acid residues (lower part). The pre-sequence (dark shading) serves as a signal peptide and the pro-sequence (light shading) functions as a signal for proper γ-carboxylation of the protein. The mature protein consists of 419 residues and can be divided into a γ-carboxyglutamic acid (GLA) domain, two epidermal growth factor (EGF) domains and a serine protease domain. During processing of the protein, an internal dipeptide is removed from the protein and the mature protein circulates as a covalently linked two-chain molecule. Between the second EGF domain and the protease part of the molecule is an activation peptide (AP) region, which is released on protein C activation. The open circles indicate the location of known missense mutations, leading to amino acid substitutions associated with type I deficiency (indicated below the polypeptide chain) or type II deficiency (above the polypeptide chain).

Missense mutations causing type I deficiency are scattered over the entire polypeptide chain. Mutations leading to type II deficiency are less common but have also been found in almost all the modules of protein C, including the propeptide, the Gla module, EGF1, the activation peptide, and the serine protease domain. Mutations in the promoter region of the gene, which affect the plasma protein concentration, and mutations affecting RNA splicing have also been found.

## Protein S deficiency

Protein S deficiency is linked to the protein S gene, *PROS1* (GeneID 5627, OMIM ID 176880). The *PROS1* gene is located close to the centromere at chromosome 3p11.1–q11.2. A homologous pseudogene (*PROSP*, GeneID 5628) is located in close vicinity and shares more than 95% similarity with *PROS1* exon and intron sequences, which must be taken into consideration when designing genetic investigations of *PROS1*.

Phenotyping for protein S deficiency is dependent on the correct measurement of protein S plasma concentration in the laboratory. This is not a simple task to perform and will be further complicated by the presence of pools of free and C4BP-bound protein S. However, the level of free protein S discriminates better between those with and without protein S deficiency than the level of total protein S. This is because the concentrations of protein S and C4BPβ⁺, which is the protein S-binding isoform of C4BP, are equimolar in protein S-deficient individuals and most of the protein S is bound to C4BPβ⁺. Protein S deficiency with low levels of both free and total protein S is called type I, whereas protein S deficiency with low free protein S and normal total protein S has been believed to constitute a separate genetic type (type III). However, coexistence of the two types in many protein S-deficient families demonstrates that they represent different phenotypic variants of the same genetic disease. Mutations that cause functional defective protein S are referred to as type II deficiency. To date, very few type II deficiencies have been found, presumably related to the poor diagnostic performance of available functional protein S assays.

Heterozygous protein S deficiency is present in 1–10% of thrombosis patients; the wide variety may be explained by several factors such as different inclusion and exclusion criteria and geographical/ethnic differences between studies. The prevalence of protein S deficiency in the general population has been estimated to be 0.03–0.13% in European populations but higher figures have been reported from Japanese and Thai populations. Family studies suggest that heterozygous carriers have a fivefold to tenfold increased risk of thrombosis compared with their healthy relatives, which is similar to the rates in protein C deficiency and APC resistance. Homozygous protein S deficiency is extremely rare but appears to give a similar picture to homozygous protein C deficiency, with purpura fulminans in the neonatal period.

The *PROS1* database, published by the International Society on Thrombosis and Haemostasis in 2000, contained more than 200 entries, in which 131 different mutations were considered to be detrimental. In the Human Gene Mutation Database there are 178 different *PROS1* mutations that may be associated with a protein S deficiency phenotype. Most of the gene defects are missense or nonsense mutations, and mutations affecting splicing or small insertion/deletion defects are less common (Figure 17.4). Due to the large size of the protein S gene and the presence of a closely linked and highly similar pseudogene, identification of mutations is not easy. Furthermore, in many families with phenotypically established protein S deficiency, *PROS1* gene mutations are not found although linkage between the *PROS1* locus and protein S deficiency has been established. The reason for the difficulties in identifying protein S gene mutations in some families may be explained by the fact that common genetic screening techniques may miss large deletions as a cause for quantitative protein S deficiency. This was also shown to be the case by extensive segregation analysis using a dense set of genetic single-nucleotide polymorphism (SNP) and microsatellite markers in families where mutations in the *PROS1* gene have not been found. By this approach, three of eight investigated families could be explained by large and unique deletions. If this finding, of an unusually high frequency of large deletions, is reproduced in other family materials, then such mutations must be considered a major explanatory factor for protein S deficiency.

## Prothrombin mutation

A point mutation in the prothrombin gene, *F2* (GeneID 2147, OMIM ID 176930), has been identified as the second most common independent risk factor for venous thrombosis. The mutation involves a G → A base substitution at nucleotide position 20210, which is located in the 3′ untranslated regions of the *F2* gene (Figure 17.5). Thus the point mutation does not lead to protein structure alterations. Instead, the mutation is associated with increased plasma levels of prothrombin through a gain-of-function phenotype that has been explained by increased efficiency of the *F2* gene mRNA. The prevalence of the mutation in the general population is 1–2% and the mutation is associated with an approximately threefold increased risk of thrombosis. Similar to the FV Leiden mutation, the *F2* 20210A variant originated from a single mutational event and the allele is only found in Caucasian populations.

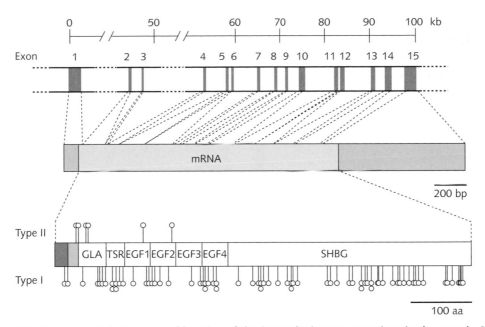

**Fig. 17.4 Structure of the human protein S gene and location of detrimental missense mutations in the protein S molecule**
The gene for human protein S (*PROS1*) comprises 15 exons (upper part) and spans 100 kb of DNA and is localized to chromosome 3p11.1–q11.2. Exons are denoted by open bars and introns by lines. Introns denoted by dashed lines between exons indicate gaps and are not drawn to scale. The *PROS1* mRNA is approximately 3.5 kb in size (middle part). The mRNA is translated into a pre-pro-protein S of 676 amino acid residues (lower part). The polypeptide chain can be divided into a signal peptide (dark shading), a pro-peptide (light shading), a thrombin-sensitive region (TSR), a γ-carboxyglutamic acid (GLA) domain, four epidermal growth factor (EGF)-like domains, and a large carboxy-terminal domain homologous to sex hormone-binding globulin (SHBG). The circles indicate the location of known missense mutations, leading to amino acid substitutions associated with type I deficiency (indicated below the polypeptide chain) or type II deficiency (above the polypeptide chain).

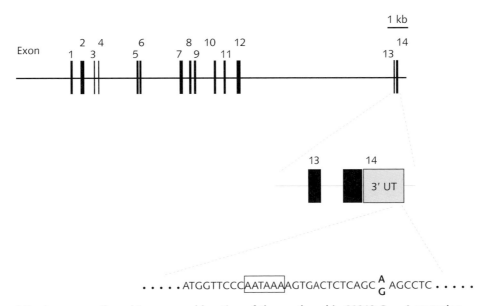

**Fig. 17.5 Structure of the human prothrombin gene and location of the prothrombin 20210 G → A mutation**
The human gene for prothrombin (*F2*) comprises 14 exons and spans approximately 20 kb of DNA on chromosome 11p11–q12. The nucleotide sequence flanking the G → A transition at nucleotide 20210 (indicated in bold) in the 3′ untranslated region of the *F2* gene is shown below. The putative polyadenylation signal is boxed. The 20210A allele represents a gain-of-function mutation associated with elevated levels of plasma prothrombin and an increased risk of venous thrombosis.

## Severe thrombophilia is a multigenic disease

Venous thrombosis is a typical multifactorial disease involving one or more environmental and/or genetic risk factors. In Western societies, many individuals carry more than one genetic risk factor because the FV Leiden allele is so common. In contrast, in countries where the FV Leiden allele is rare, few individuals carry more than one genetic defect. This may explain the difference in incidence of thromboembolic disease between Japan and China on the one hand and Europe and the USA on the other. The frequency of individuals carrying two or more genetic defects can be calculated on the basis of the prevalence of the individual genetic defects in the general population. In a country where the prevalence of FV Leiden is 10%, combinations of protein C deficiency and FV Leiden are expected to be present in between 1 in 3000 and 1 in 10 000 individuals. A similar calculation for the combination of the prothrombin mutation and FV Leiden allele suggests the prevalence of combined defects to be 1–2 per 1000 individuals. Thus, a large number of people carry more than one genetic defect and such individuals have considerably increased risk of thrombosis. The FV Leiden allele is thus found to be an additional genetic risk factor in certain thrombophilic individuals with deficiency of protein C, protein S or AT as well as in cases with the prothrombin mutation (Figure 17.6).

The thrombotic tendency in individuals with inherited genetic defects is highly variable and some individuals never develop thrombosis, whereas others develop recurrent severe thrombotic events at an early age. This depends on the particular genotype, the coexistence of other genetic defects, and the presence of environmental risk factors such as oral contraceptives, trauma, surgery and pregnancy. Thus, women with heterozygosity for the FV Leiden allele who also use oral contraceptives have been estimated to have a 35- to 50-fold increased risk of thrombosis, whereas those with homozygosity have a several hundred-fold increased risk.

## Management of thrombophilia

Decisions about medical intervention due to the presence of one or more genetic defects should be based on careful consideration of the clinical picture, including the patient's family history. The impact of the medical history on the use of oral anticoagulants is perhaps even more important in individuals with APC resistance (FV Leiden) or the prothrombin mutation than in those with the more rare deficiencies of protein C, protein S or AT. The risk of bleeding complications due to anticoagulant therapy must always be weighed against the benefits of anticoagulation, especially if an oral anticoagulant is used for periods exceeding 3–6 months when the risk of thrombotic recurrence probably declines. New clinical data are continually emerging and no general consensus regarding screening, prophylaxis and the treatment of symptomatic patients has yet been established.

When the FV Leiden allele is present in homozygous form, or heterozygosity is combined with a second genetic defect, prophylactic treatment with heparin or oral antico-

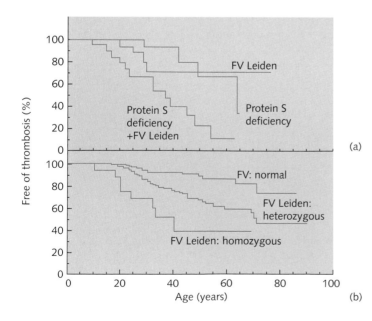

(a)

(b)

**Fig. 17.6 Thrombosis-free survival curves for individuals with different FV genotypes and co-inherited protein S deficiency**

(a) The increased risk of thrombosis with combined defects is illustrated with thrombosis-free survival curves for 21 individuals with single defects, FV Leiden or protein S deficiency, and 18 individuals with both defects. There was no significant difference between those with single defects, whereas differences between individuals with the FV Leiden allele or protein S deficiency and those with combined defects were significant. (b) Probability of being free of thrombotic events at a certain age for 146 normal individuals, 144 heterozygotes and 18 homozygotes for the FV Leiden allele (Kaplan–Meier analysis). Highly significant differences were observed between normals and heterozygotes and between heterozygotes and homozygotes.

agulants is recommended in situations known to be associated with a high risk of thromboembolic complications, such as surgery or pregnancy, even if the patient has never experienced any thrombosis or has no family history of such complications. For heterozygous asymptomatic carriers lacking a family history of thrombosis, short-term prophylaxis has been recommended in high-risk situations, but it remains to be established whether prophylaxis should be given in all situations associated with a risk of thrombosis.

Symptomatic heterozygous patients should be managed in the same way as any other patient with thrombotic events until more specific recommendations are established. It is not known whether the presence of a genetic defect is associated with an increased risk of recurrence, even though most studies on APC resistance tend to suggest that this is indeed the case. Patients with combined defects, and probably also patients with single gene defects, may be at increased risk of recurrence and should accordingly be given long-term anticoagulation therapy beyond 6 months, even after an isolated thromboembolic event. However, more data are needed before these recommendations can be considered generally applicable.

The potential benefits of general screening for APC resistance and/or the FV Leiden allele prior to thrombotic events or in the presence of such circumstantial factors as oral contraceptive use, pregnancy and surgery are obvious, but more prospective data are needed, not least in terms of cost–benefit ratios before any general recommendations can be made.

## Conclusions

Inherited APC resistance, caused by the Arg506Gln mutation in the FV gene (FV Leiden), is the most common genetic risk factor for thrombosis identified to date. The mutated FV has normal procoagulant properties, but the loss of the APC cleavage site at position 506 in FV results in impaired regulation of coagulation and a hypercoagulable state. The prevalence of FV Leiden in Caucasian populations varies between 2 and 15%. A genetic variant in the prothrombin gene (G20210A) is another common prothrombotic risk factor, with a prevalence of approximately 2% in the general population. Other less common independent genetic risk factors include abnormalities in the genes for AT, protein C and protein S. Families with thrombophilia present with variable penetrance of thrombosis explained by different combinations of genetic defects and environmental risk factors. Patients with combined genetic defects are at higher risk of thrombosis than those with single gene defects. Thus, evaluation of patients with thrombosis must be performed in order to fully estimate the risk for thrombosis in each case.

## Further reading

### Blood coagulation: introduction and regulation

Dahlbäck B. (2005) Blood coagulation and its regulation by anticoagulant pathways: genetic pathogenesis of bleeding and thrombotic diseases. *Journal of Internal Medicine*, **257**, 209–223.

Dahlbäck B, Villoutreix BO. (2005) Regulation of blood coagulation by the protein C anticoagulant pathway: novel insights into structure–function relationships and molecular recognition. *Arteriosclerosis, Thrombosis, and Vascular Biology*, **25**, 1311–1320.

Furie B, Furie BC. (2005) Thrombus formation in vivo. *Journal of Clinical Investigation*, **115**, 3355–3362.

Mann KG, Brummel-Ziedins K, Orfeo T, Butenas S. (2006) Models of blood coagulation. *Blood Cells, Molecules and Diseases*, **36**, 108–117.

Rapaport SI, Rao LVM. (1995) The tissue factor pathway: how it has become a "prima ballerina". *Thrombosis and Haemostasis*, **74**, 7–17.

Rau JC, Beaulieu LM, Huntington JA, Church FC. (2007) Serpins in thrombosis, hemostasis and fibrinolysis. *Journal of Thrombosis and Haemostasis*, **5** (Suppl 1), 102–115.

van Boven HH, Lane DA. (1997) Antithrombin and its inherited deficiency states. *Seminars in Hematology*, **34**, 188–204.

### Molecular genetics of venous thromboembolism, APC resistance and FV Leiden

Bertina RM, Koeleman BP, Koster T et al. (1994) Mutation in blood coagulation factor V associated with resistance to activated protein C. *Nature*, **369**, 64–67.

Bezemer ID, Bare LA, Doggen CJM et al. (2008) Gene variants associated with deep venous thrombosis. *Journal of the American Medical Association*, **299**, 1306–1314.

Dahlbäck B, Carlsson M, Svensson PJ. (1993) Familial thrombophilia due to a previously unrecognized mechanism characterized by poor anticoagulant response to activated protein C: prediction of a cofactor to activated protein C. *Proceedings of the National Academy of Sciences of the United States of America*, **90**, 1004–1008.

Greengard JS, Sun X, Xu X et al. (1994) Activated protein C resistance caused by Arg506Gln mutation in factor Va. *Lancet*, **343**, 1361–1362.

Griffin JH, Evatt B, Wideman C, Fernandez JA. (1993) Anticoagulant protein C pathway defective in majority of thrombophilic patients. *Blood*, **82**, 1989–1993.

Heit JA. (2008) The epidemiology of venous thromboembolism in the community. *Arteriosclerosis, Thrombosis, and Vascular Biology*, **28**, 370–372.

Koster T, Rosendaal FR, de Ronde H et al. (1993) Venous thrombosis due to poor anticoagulant response to activated protein C: Leiden Thrombophilia Study. *Lancet*, **342**, 1503–1506.

Lindqvist PG, Svensson PJ, Dahlbäck B, Marsal K. (1998) Factor V R506Q mutation (activated protein C resistance) associated with reduced intrapartum blood loss: a possible evolutionary selection mechanism. *Thrombosis and Haemostasis,* **79**, 69–73.

Moll S. (2008) A clinical perspective of venous thromboembolism. *Arteriosclerosis, Thrombosis, and Vascular Biology,* **28**, 373–379.

Moll S, Mackman N. (2008) Venous thromboembolism: a need for more public awareness and research into mechanisms. *Arteriosclerosis, Thrombosis, and Vascular Biology,* **28**, 367–369.

Rosendaal FR. (1997) Risk factors for venous thrombosis: prevalence, risk, and interaction. *Seminars in Hematology,* **34**, 171–187.

Svensson PJ, Dahlbäck B. (1994) Resistance to activated protein C as a basis for venous thrombosis. *New England Journal of Medicine,* **330**, 517–522.

Vandenbroucke JP, Koster T, Briet E *et al.* (1994) Increased risk of venous thrombosis in oral-contraceptive users who are carriers of factor V Leiden mutation. *Lancet,* **344**, 1453–1457.

Voorberg J, Roelse J, Koopman R *et al.* (1994) Association of idiopathic venous thromboembolism with single point-mutation at Arg506 of factor V. *Lancet,* **343**, 1535–1536.

Wakefield TW, Myers DD, Henke PK. (2008) Mechanisms of venous thrombosis and resolution. *Arteriosclerosis, Thrombosis, and Vascular Biology,* **28**, 387–391.

## Antithrombin deficiency

Lane DA, Bayston T, Olds RJ *et al.* (1997) Antithrombin mutation database: 2nd (1997) update. *Thrombosis and Haemostasis,* **77**, 197–211.

Perry DJ, Carrell RW. (1996) Molecular genetics of antithrombin deficiency. *Human Mutation,* **7**, 7–22.

Picard V, Nowak-Göttl U, Biron-Andreani C *et al.* (2006) Molecular bases of antithrombin deficiency: twenty-two novel mutations in the antithrombin gene. *Human Mutation,* **27**, 600. [Erratum in *Human Mutation* 2006, **27**, 1160.]

Van Boven HH, Vandenbroucke JP, Briet E, Rosendaal FR. (1999) Gene–gene and gene–environment interactions determine the risk of thrombosis in families with inherited antithrombin deficiency. *Blood,* **94**, 2590–2594.

## Protein C system and protein C deficiency

Alhenc-Gelas M, Gandrille S, Aubry M-L, Aiach M. (2000) Thirty-three novel mutations in the protein C gene. *Thrombosis and Haemostasis,* **83**, 86–92.

Dahlbäck B, Villoutreix BO. (2005) Regulation of blood coagulation by the protein C anticoagulant pathway: novel insights into structure–function relationships and molecular recognition. *Arteriosclerosis, Thrombosis and Vascular Biology,* **25**, 1311–1320.

Esmon CT. (2003) The protein C pathway. *Chest,* **124**, 26S–32S.

Mosnier LO, Zlokovic BV, Griffin JH. (2007) The cytoprotective protein C pathway. *Blood,* **109**, 3161–3172.

Reitsma PH, Bernardi F, Doig RG *et al.* (1995) Protein C deficiency: a database of mutations, 1995 update. *Thrombosis and Haemostasis,* **73**, 876–889.

Segers K, Dahlbäck B, Nicolaes GA. (2007) Coagulation factor V and thrombophilia: background and mechanisms. *Thrombosis and Haemostasis,* **98**, 530–542.

## Protein S deficiency

Dahlbäck B. (2007) The tale of protein S and C4b-binding protein, a story of affection. *Thrombosis and Haemostasis,* **98**, 90–96.

Gandrille S, Borgel D, Sala N *et al.* (2000) Protein S deficiency: a database of mutations. Summary of the first update. *Thrombosis and Haemostasis,* **84**, 918–934.

Garcia de Frutos G, Fuentes-Prior P, Hurtado B, Sala N. (2007) Molecular basis of protein S deficiency. *Thrombosis and Haemostasis,* **98**, 543–556.

Johansson AM, Hillarp A, Säll T, Zöller B, Dahlbäck B, Halldén C. (2005) Large deletions of the PROS1 gene in a large fraction of mutation negative patients with protein S deficiency. *Thrombosis and Haemostasis,* **94**, 951–957.

Persson KE, Dahlbäck B, Hillarp A. (2003) Diagnosing protein S deficiency: analytical considerations. *Clinical Laboratory,* **49**, 103–110.

## Prothrombin gene mutation

Danckwardt S, Hartmann K, Gehring NH, Hentze MW, Kulozik AE. (2006) 3′ End processing of the prothrombin mRNA in thrombophilia. *Acta Haematologica,* **115**, 192–197.

Gehring NH, Frede U, Neu-Yilik G *et al.* (2001) Increased efficiency of mRNA 3′ end formation: a new genetic mechanism contributing to hereditary thrombophilia. *Nature Genetics,* **28**, 389–392.

Poort SR, Rosendaal FR, Reitsma PH, Bertina RM. (1996) A common genetic variation in the 3′-untranslated region of the prothrombin gene is associated with elevated plasma prothrombin levels and an increase in venous thrombosis. *Blood,* **88**, 3698–3703.

# Chapter 18 The molecular basis of hemophilia

## Paul LF Giangrande

*Oxford Haemophilia and Thrombosis Centre, Churchill Hospital, Oxford, UK*

## Introduction: clinical features of hemophilia

The clinical severity (phenotype) is critically determined by the concentration of circulating factor VIII (or IX) in the blood, and severe hemophilia is defined by a clotting factor concentration below 1 IU/dL (Table 18.1). The hallmark of severe hemophilia is recurrent and spontaneous hemarthrosis. Typically, hinge joints such as the knees, elbows and ankles are affected but bleeds may also occur in the wrist or shoulder. Bleeding into the hip joint is unusual. The affected joint is swollen and warm, and held in a position of flexion (Figure 18.1), with no external discoloration or bruising around the joint. It is unusual for an infant to suffer spontaneous hemarthroses in the first few months of life, and the first joint to be affected tends to be the ankle as the child learns to crawl. The first sign of a hemarthrosis in an infant will often be obvious discomfort and distress, accompanied by limping or reluctance to use a limb. Recurrent bleeds into a joint lead to synovitis and joint damage resulting in crippling arthritis (Figure 18.2). Bleeding into muscles is also a feature of hemophilia, but this is usually a consequence of direct injury, albeit often minor (Figure 18.3). Bleeds into certain areas are particularly dangerous because of the risk of compression of neighboring structures. Patients with inhibitory antibodies are particularly at risk in this regard, as bleeds may be more difficult to control. Bleeds in the tongue can obstruct the airway, and retroperitoneal bleeding within the iliopsoas muscle may result in femoral nerve compression, causing weakness and wasting of leg muscles (Figure 18.3). Bleeding from the gastrointestinal tract (melena) and bleeding into the urinary tract (hematuria) may also occur. There is also a significant risk of intracranial hemorrhage in severe hemophilia, which in the past was a significant cause of mortality when treatment was not so readily available. Higher levels of factor VIII (or IX) above 5 IU/dL are associated with a milder form of the disease, with no spontaneous joint bleeds but a definite risk of bleeding after even relatively minor injury.

Treatment of bleeding episodes involves the intravenous injection of coagulation factor concentrates; the total dose and frequency of treatment will also be determined by the severity and site of bleeding. The great majority of joint bleeds will resolve with a single infusion, if the bleed is recognized early and treated promptly. There is an increasing move to prophylactic therapy, in which patients inject coagulation factor concentrate two or three times a week to prevent bleeds rather than just treating on demand when bleeds occur. Patients on prophylactic therapy experience few or even no spontaneous bleeds, and thus progressive joint damage and arthritis can be avoided. The quality of life of patients on prophylaxis may be greatly enhanced, allowing them to lead much more independent lives.

Approximately 15% of patients with severe hemophilia A can be expected to develop inhibitory antibodies to factor VIII at some stage. In contrast, inhibitor development in hemophilia B is very rare and encountered in less than 1% of patients. The development of such antibodies poses considerable problems in treatment as these immunoglobulins (IgG) are capable of rapidly inactivating infused factor VIII, and furthermore the antibody titer may rise dramatically after a course of factor VIII. Very occasionally, acquired hemophilia may arise in a previously normal individual due to the formation of autoantibodies directed against factor VIII, and both males and females may be affected. Hemarthrosis is unusual in acquired hemophilia, and the principal manifestations are usually extensive superficial

*Molecular Hematology*, 3rd edition. Edited by Drew Provan and John Gribben.
© 2010 Blackwell Publishing.

**Table 18.1** The relation of blood levels of factor VIII (or IX) to the severity of hemorrhagic manifestations.

| Level (IU/dL) | Hemorrhagic manifestations |
| --- | --- |
| 50–100 | Normal level, no bleeding problems |
| 25–50 | No problems in day-to-day life. Tendency to bleed after major surgery |
| 5–25 | Mild hemophilia. Bleeding typically occurs only after significant injuries |
| 2–5 | Moderately severe hemophilia: occasionally apparently spontaneous bleeds. Most bleeds associated with injury, albeit often relatively minor |
| <1 | Severe hemophilia with spontaneous and recurrent bleeding into muscles and joints |

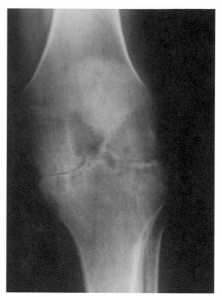

**Fig. 18.2 Radiograph of the knee of a patient with severe hemophilic arthropathy**
Joint replacement surgery was subsequently carried out in this case.

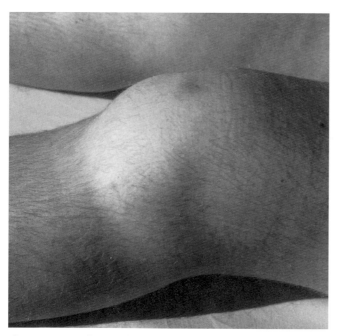

**Fig. 18.1 Acute hemarthrosis in severe hemophilia**
This usually arises in the absence of injury. The joints most frequently involved are the knees, elbows and ankles. The joint is swollen, warm and tender but there is no external bruising or discoloration.

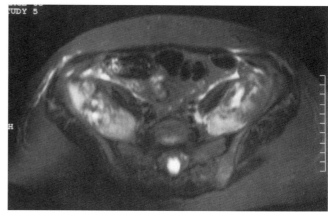

**Fig. 18.3 Magnetic resonance imaging (MRI) scan showing bilateral iliopsoas hemorrhage**
This bleed was associated with a complete but transient paralysis in both legs, as the femoral nerve is located on the anterior surface of the muscle and may be compressed in such cases.

purpura and muscle bleeds. Acquired hemophilia arises most often in the elderly, and there is an association with underlying malignant or autoimmune diseases.

## Inheritance of hemophilia

The genes for factors VIII and IX are both located at the telomeric end of the X chromosome and thus hemophilia is

inherited as an X-linked recessive condition (Figure 18.4). The daughters of affected males are obligate carriers but the sons are normal. The phenotype remains constant within a family, so the daughter of a man with only mild hemophilia may be reassured that she will not pass on a severe form of the condition. However, approximately one-third of all cases of hemophilia arise in the absence of a previous family history and are due to a new mutation. The most famous example is that of Queen Victoria, who had a hemophilic

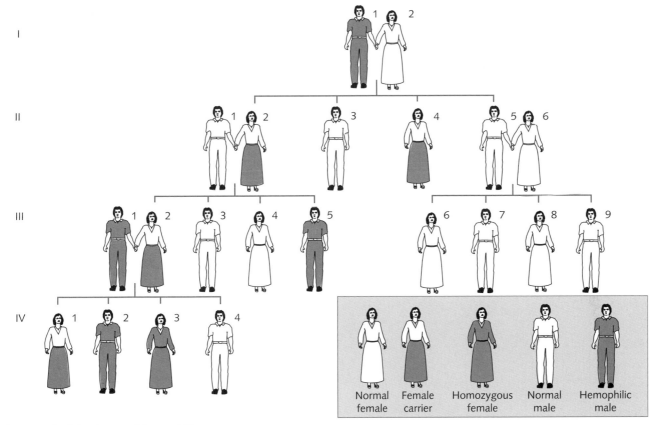

**Fig. 18.4 The inheritance of hemophilia**

The gene for factors VIII and IX are both encoded on the X chromosome, and inheritance is thus sex-linked. The daughter of a man with hemophilia is an obligate carrier, but the son of a hemophiliac will not be affected. Hemophilia may thus be transmitted to a grandson via a carrier daughter. Color blindness and Duchenne muscular dystrophy are other examples of conditions which are X-linked disorders.

son (Leopold) and two daughters (Alice and Beatrice) who turned out to be carriers. There are instances of hemophilia affecting females due to inheritance of the defective gene from both parents, and there are also case reports of hemophilia in females with Turner syndrome (XO karyotype) and androgen insensitivity syndrome (XY karyotype).

## Molecular basis of hemophilia A

Factor VIII is an essential cofactor for the activation of factor X by activated factor IX (*see Chapter 17*). Factor VIII must itself undergo proteolytic cleavage at two distinct sites through the action of thrombin before it becomes physiologically active. It circulates in plasma as a large glycoprotein bound non-covalently to the larger protein, von Willebrand factor (VWF). The factor VIII gene (*F8*) was first cloned in 1984. It is 186 kb in length and is situated on the long arm of the X chromosome at Xq28 (Figure 18.5). The factor VIII gene consists of 26 exons, which range in size from 69 bp

(exon 5) to 3.1 kb (exon 14). The factor VIII message is nearly 9 kb in size and encodes a mature protein of 2332 amino acids. Approximately half of all cases of severe hemophilia and all cases of mild and moderate hemophilia result from heterogeneous mutations that occur throughout the factor VIII gene.

By far the commonest single genetic defect causing severe hemophilia is an inversion in intron 22, which is encountered in as many as 45% of people with severe hemophilia in all ethnic groups (Figure 18.6). The inversion mechanism involves an intronless gene of unknown function, designated *F8A*. Two copies of this gene are located near the tip of the X chromosome and there is another copy within intron 22 of the factor VIII gene itself. During meiosis, either of the two telomeric copies may cross over with the intronic copy, resulting in a division of the gene into two halves facing in opposite directions and separated by approximately 500 kb. Crossover with the distal copy is much more common than crossover with the proximal copy, and accounts for approximately 80% of all inversions. It is now recognized that

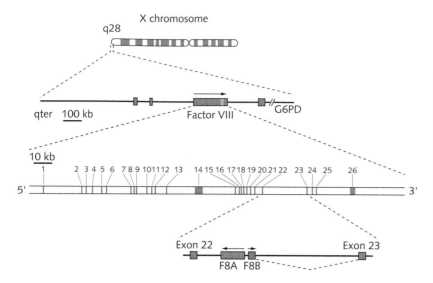

**Fig. 18.5 The factor VIII gene**
The factor VIII gene was cloned in 1984 and is located toward the telomeric end of the long arm of the X chromosome (Xq28). It maps distal to the gene encoding glucose 6-phosphate dehydrogenase (G6PD), about 1 Mb from the Xq telomere. The gene is composed of 26 exons, of which exon 14 is the largest. The large intron 22 contains a nested intronless gene termed *F8A* (the function of the gene and its transcript are unknown). There are two further copies of *F8A* located about 400 kb telomeric to the factor VIII gene. The spliced factor VIII mRNA is ~9 kb in length and the mature factor VIII molecule is composed of 2332 amino acids.

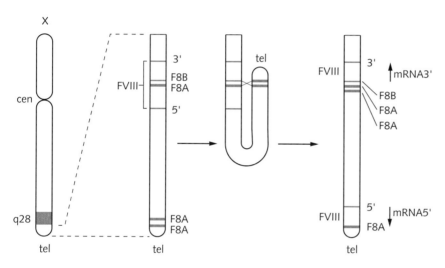

**Fig. 18.6 "Flip tip inversion"**
This unique inversion of the tip of the X chromosome is now recognized to be responsible for about half of all cases of severe hemophilia in all ethnic groups. Crossover occurs between a copy of *F8A* within the factor VIII gene and one of the two telomeric copies. Crossover with the distal copy is more common, occurring in approximately 80% of cases where an inversion is identified.

inversion almost always forms during a male meiosis. It is believed that the presence of a large region of non-homology between the X and Y chromosomes during meiotic pairing may favor a misalignment and the presence of a second X chromosome with a complementary region may act as a stabilizing factor. An important clinical consequence of this observation is that when an apparently new and spontaneous case of hemophilia is diagnosed in which the gene inversion is identified, it is likely that the defect arose in the maternal grandfather's allele and thus the mother can generally be assumed to be a carrier and at risk of having another affected male child. The resulting truncated protein product is presumably unstable, resulting in severe hemophilia. The inversion is not found in individuals with mild forms of hemophilia. The inversion is easily detected and the identi-

fication of this defect as the commonest cause of severe hemophilia has simplified both screening for carriers and antenatal diagnosis of hemophilia. The inversion may be identified with Southern blotting, although many laboratories now use either inverse polymerase chain reaction (PCR) or long-range PCR for identification of this inversion. More recently, inversions in intron 1 of the factor VIII gene have been identified as a cause of severe hemophilia and this abnormality appears to be responsible for approximately 5% of all cases of severe hemophilia. Since approximately half of all cases of severe hemophilia are associated with these two inversions, it is usual practice to screen samples from new cases for these two abnormalities first.

Developments in molecular biology have permitted more rapid identification of defects in hemophilia. Southern blotting has been superseded by methods involving PCR amplification of either patient DNA or material derived from the reverse transcription of mRNA (RT-PCR). Although automated sequence analyzers have been developed, gene sequencing of the entire factor VIII gene is both expensive and labor-intensive. Methods have been developed to identify restricted areas of abnormal DNA in patients with hemophilia, which may then be targeted for specific attention. These methods include amplification and mismatch detection (AMD), conformation-sensitive gel electrophoresis (CSGE), denaturing gradient gel electrophoresis (DGGE), high-resolution melting analysis (HRM), and pyrosequencing. Approximately 4% of cases of hemophilia are the consequence of gene deletions, which have been reported throughout the gene and which are very variable in size. As with the intron 22 inversion, most deletions are associated with a severe clinical phenotype. To date, around 650 different single base substitutions have been described, of which approximately 75% predict a single amino acid change from the wild-type sequence (missense). Such mutations affect RNA processing, mRNA translation or the fine structure of factor VIII itself. A further 100 lead to creation of preliminary peptide chain termination or Stop codons and the production of truncated factor VIII molecules devoid of any functional activity. Frameshift mutations resulting from insertions or small deletions have also been identified as a cause of severe hemophilia. Duplications within one or more exons of the factor VIII gene have recently been identified in a small minority of patients with hemophilia A using multiplex ligation-dependent probe amplification (MLPA). A full list of mutations described in association with hemophilia is outside the scope of this chapter, but additional information is provided in the Further reading section.

Approximately 40% of all missense mutations arise at CG dinucleotide sites, resulting in a change to TG or CA sequences. It is generally believed that CG nucleotides represent genomic hotspots. Cytosine is predominantly methylated in human DNA, but this is relatively unstable and 5-methylcytosine is prone to spontaneous deamination to yield a GT mismatch that is inefficiently repaired. It is also of interest that a missense mutation may be associated with varying degrees of clinical severity. Thus a C → T mutation at nucleotide 1689 within exon 14 resulting in replacement of arginine by cysteine has been reported in association with both severe and mild clinical phenotypes.

## Molecular basis of hemophilia B

The factor IX gene (*F9*) is also located on the long arm of the X chromosome at band Xq27, and is encoded by a stretch of DNA spanning 33.5 kb that contains eight exons (Figure 18.7). The basic structure of the gene is similar in organization to that of protein C and coagulation factors VII and X, and it is likely that they all originated in the distant past from a common ancestral gene by duplication. Factor IX mRNA comprises 2.8 kb and encodes a mature protein of 415 amino acids. This is made up of a glutamic acid-rich sequence (Gla domain) and two epidermal growth factor (EGF)-like domains separated from the serine protease domain by an activation region. The 12 glutamic acid residues in the Gla domain undergo post-translational γ-carboxylation, which is necessary for binding of calcium, and exon 2 encodes a recognition site for the carboxylase. Exon 1 encodes the signal peptide necessary for transport into the endoplasmic reticulum. Exon 6 encodes the

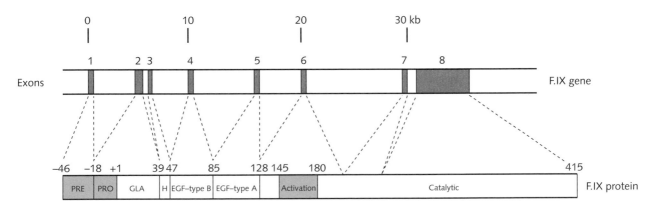

**Fig. 18.7 The factor IX gene**
The factor IX gene was first cloned in 1982. It is located on the long arm of the X chromosome at band Xq27. The gene spans 34 kb and encodes eight exons (exons are shown as colored boxes, and dotted lines between the gene and protein indicate protein domains encoded by each exon). The signal peptide and propeptide sequences are cleaved during processing and activation of factor IX. GLA, γ-carboxyglutamic acid domain; EGF, epidermal growth factor domains.

activation peptide that is cleaved off during the activation of factor IX by either factor XI or a complex of tissue factor and factor VII. Exons 7 and 8 encode the catalytic regions of factor IX, which are responsible for subsequent activation of factor X in the coagulation cascade. The gene is controlled by a promoter.

The gene for factor IX, which was cloned in 1982, is considerably smaller than that of factor VIII, and patients with hemophilia B have been studied more extensively than those with hemophilia A. The first defects identified in hemophilia B were gross deletions, detected by Southern blotting. However, it is now recognized that gene deletions account for only approximately 3% of all cases of hemophilia B. No equivalent of the factor VIII gene inversion has been encountered in hemophilia B and it is now clear that point mutations account for the vast majority of cases of hemophilia B; over 500 have been described from families around the world. The great majority involve single base changes, which have been identified in all domains of the protein. The unusually high frequency of mutations at CG dinucleotide sites in hemophilia B probably reflects the high number of CG dinucleotides at critical sites in the factor IX gene. Exon 8 is the largest at 1.9 kb in length and half of all mutations are found in this exon. However, about 20–30% of cases of mild hemophilia B are due to a small number of founder mutations. The original case of Christmas disease has been identified as a G → C mutation at nucleotide 31170, resulting in substitution of cysteine by serine within exon 8.

Mutations in the promoter region of the factor IX gene (e.g., T → A at −20 and G → A at −6) are relatively rare and account for around 2% of all cases. However, they are of particular interest as they can give rise to the unique hemophilia B Leyden phenotype, where the factor IX level rises significantly after puberty with loss of the bleeding tendency. Most of these mutations have been shown to be located in regions that contain binding sequences for liver-enriched transcription factors, which are presumably influenced by androgenic steroids.

Full details of the many genetic abnormalities associated with hemophilia B can be found at the websites listed at the end of this chapter.

## Inhibitor formation: etiology and clinical implications

A minority of patients with hemophilia will develop immunoglobulins directed against infused factor VIII (or IX) after exposure to these blood products for treatment of bleeding episodes. This is potentially very serious, as patients are generally refractory to conventional doses of coagulation factor concentrates and bleeding can be very difficult to control.

Inhibitory antibodies interfere with the normal function of factor VIII in a number of different ways. The most frequent site of inhibitor binding occurs within the A2 and C2 domains. Inhibitors may thereby block the ability of activated factor VIIIa to bind and activate factors IXa and X, or inhibit the binding of factor VIII to VWF or negatively charged phospholipid surfaces. Inhibitors may also hinder the activation of factor VIII by thrombin, or the subsequent release of factor VIII from VWF. Proteolysis of factor VIII has recently been identified as a novel additional mechanism of inactivation in some cases.

Activated prothrombin complex concentrates (e.g., FEIBA) and recombinant activated factor VIIa (NovoSeven) are valuable therapeutic materials in controlling bleeding in those patients with inhibitory antibodies. Recombinant porcine factor VIII has also been developed for this indication and is under evaluation in clinical trials. The rationale is that the porcine molecule is sufficient similar to human factor VIII to exert a hemostatic effect but at the same time sufficiently different to avoid rapid neutralization by antibodies. Another important strategy in the management of these patients who develop inhibitory antibodies is immune tolerance, which involves the daily administration of coagulation factor concentrate over a period of some months. This usually results in the eventual disappearance of the antibody, as the body becomes tolerant of the protein and inhibitor formation is suppressed.

Following the elimination of the risk of transmission of viruses by coagulation factor concentrates, the risk of inhibitor development is perhaps the principal danger faced by people with hemophilia nowadays. Data from the UK registry suggest that approximately 15% of all patients with severe hemophilia A will develop antibodies at some time, but it is quite likely that this figure underestimates the true prevalence as transient and low-titer inhibitors may not be detected. As a general rule, if an individual is susceptible to inhibitor development, they will become apparent at a fairly young age. Data from prospective studies involving recombinant factor VIII products suggests a median of approximately 10 exposure days for inhibitor development if this is to occur.

It is now clear that the major factor which determines the predisposition to inhibitor development is the underlying molecular defect. Certain types of gene defects in hemophilia are undoubtedly associated with a significantly increased risk of inhibitor development (Figure 18.8). The risk of inhibitor development in patients with severe molecular defects, such as large deletions, nonsense mutations and the intron-22 inversion, is seven to ten times higher than in patients with other defects such as missense mutations, small deletions and splice-site mutations. The overall risk of inhibitor development in patients with the common intron-22 inversion is approximately 30%.

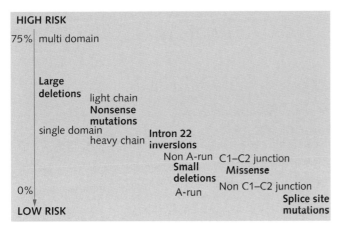

**Fig. 18.8 Mutation types and risk of inhibitor development**

However, there is also additional evidence from family and twin studies that other subtle genetic factors play a role, although no associations with specific human leukocyte antigens (HLA) or other linkages have been conclusively identified. Race may also influence the risk of inhibitor development, and several studies have shown that people of Afro-Caribbean origin are more susceptible to inhibitor formation. Major histocompatibility complex (MHC) molecules on cell surfaces play a pivotal role in such reactions but to date no strong association between any one particular MHC molecule and an increased risk of inhibitor development has been shown. Links between structural variants (polymorphisms) in the genes of two important proteins involved in inflammatory and immunological responses, interleukin (IL)-10 and tumor necrosis factor (TNF)-$\alpha$, have been reported. Such variants might have an impact on inhibitor development by increasing the production and secretion of chemicals that ultimately enhance the production of antibodies directed against factor VIII. In the case of IL-10, one particular polymorphism (134-bp variant of a CA repeat microsatellite in the promoter region of the *IL10* gene) was found to be associated with a 4.4-fold increased risk of inhibitor development. This same polymorphism has already been shown to influence the level of antibody production in such diverse diseases as myasthenia gravis, multiple myeloma and systemic lupus erythematosus. More recently, the same group reported that a particular polymorphism (C/T at −318) in the cytotoxic T-lymphocyte-associated protein-4 receptor of certain immune cells actually confers protection against inhibitor development. It is to be hoped that increasing knowledge about the role of molecular genetics in inhibitor development will lead to new strategies to prevent and treat patients with inhibitors or even prevent their development in the first place.

Inhibitor development in hemophilia B is a rare event, occurring in probably less than 1% of patients, and these patients often have an underlying large gene deletion. In contrast with the immunoglobulin inhibitors in patients with hemophilia A, inhibitory antibodies in patients with hemophilia B are often capable of fixing complement proteins. The administration of coagulation factor concentrate in such cases may therefore trigger severe, often anaphylactic, allergic reactions. The development of nephrotic syndrome has also been reported in patients with hemophilia B and inhibitors undergoing immune tolerance induction treatment with factor IX concentrates.

## Therapeutic applications of molecular biology to patient care

### Carrier testing

Ideally, carriers of hemophilia should be identified before a pregnancy, and offered counseling. The inheritance of hemophilia is sex-linked, as with other disorders such as color blindness and Duchenne muscular dystrophy. The daughters of men with hemophilia are thus obligate carriers of the condition, with a 50:50 chance of passing on the condition to a son, and there is a similar chance that a daughter of a carrier will also herself be a carrier of the condition. No special genetic tests are therefore required to determine the carrier status of daughters of men with hemophilia, although the results of DNA-based studies are likely to be useful for subsequent antenatal diagnostic procedures. The phenotype of hemophilia remains constant within a family, so that the daughter of a man with only mild hemophilia may be reassured that she can only transmit a similarly mild form of the condition. However, a more common problem is to be confronted with a woman with only a vague history of a bleeding disorder in a distant relative. National patient registers can be very helpful in establishing the type and severity of bleeding disorder of an affected relative as a first step in determining which tests need to be carried out. It may seem logical to initiate carrier testing to determine carrier status as soon as possible in girls with a family history of the condition, as this would facilitate management in the case of an early and possibly unexpected pregnancy. There are significant differences in legislation as well as clinical practice among healthcare professionals in various countries with regard to the timing of testing of children for genetic disorders. Some take the view that it is unethical to test very young children in order to determine carrier status for inherited disorders for conditions which have no immediate implications for their own health. In the UK, most hematologists would generally be prepared to offer carrier testing to girls in their early teens, with the proviso that the issues must be discussed with the family and the children deemed able to understand the implications of such testing.

It is important to emphasize that the plasma level of factor VIII (or IX) alone should not be used to determine whether a female is a carrier of hemophilia and that only DNA-based tests should be used. Indirect testing of carrier status using the tracking of restriction fragment length polymorphisms (RFLPs) has now been superseded by direct identification of the underlying causative genetic abnormality such as mutation or inversion. Once the molecular defect has been identified in an individual with either hemophilia A or B, direct screening for that defect could be applied in subsequent generations for both carrier testing and also antenatal diagnosis. It is recommended that hemophilia centers collate information on the family pedigree ("family tree") to identify potential carriers and facilitate screening.

RFLP analysis may still be employed in the few cases where, for example, a mutation has not been identified or verified in a potential carrier. This technique is also still widely used in countries around the world which do not yet have access to more sophisticated technology. The method is based on the fact that there are some genetic polymorphisms that represent natural variations of the genome sequence, without any adverse impact on the function of the molecule. The polymorphisms are detected by cleavage of patient DNA with restriction enzymes, which generate fragments of varying size according to the presence or absence of the polymorphism. Only intragenic markers should be used because the small possibility of recombination may result in erroneous diagnoses when extragenic probes are used. The most widely intragenic markers used are dinucleotide repeats in introns 13 and 22; *Xba*I dimorphism in intron 22; and digestion products using *Bcl*I in intron 18. The limitations of this approach include the fact that samples have to be taken from several members to permit the tracking of the mutant gene responsible for hemophilia in the family. Blood from an affected family member will be required, and this may not be possible in some cases. It should also be appreciated that there is ethnic variation of the allelic frequencies of the various polymorphisms, more so with factor IX than factor VIII, and this may influence the choice of probes used in some family studies. Furthermore, non-paternity may confound attempts to track the gene in families.

Germline and somatic mosaicism may complicate the picture. This needs particular consideration in cases of sporadic hemophilia where the mother of a child with hemophilia does not appear to carry the mutation in her own leukocyte DNA. This has been reported to be a particular problem when the apparently *de novo* mutation is a point mutation. For this reason, it is recommended not to state that the mother of a child with hemophilia is not a carrier, even when the mutation is not identified in her somatic DNA.

## Antenatal diagnosis of hemophilia

As a general rule, it is the practice in the UK to perform antenatal procedures to determine whether or not a fetus has hemophilia *only* where a termination is being contemplated. The general experience in the UK has been that only a minority of women subsequently take up the offer of antenatal diagnosis with a view to termination if an affected fetus is identified. This may well reflect the fact that many women with affected relatives appreciate that major advances in treatment in recent years, such as the introduction of recombinant products for children and the wider adoption of prophylaxis, offer the prospect of an essentially normal life for the younger generation of people with hemophilia.

Amniocentesis was the first technique employed for antenatal diagnosis of hemophilia and other X-linked disorders such as muscular dystrophy. Whilst amniocentesis is both technically simple and safe, an important limitation is the fact that it may only be employed in the second trimester of pregnancy, after approximately 15 weeks' gestation. Chorionic villus sampling (CVS) was first applied to antenatal diagnosis of a number of genetic disorders in the early 1980s, but is now the principal method used for antenatal diagnosis of hemophilia and several other single gene disorders. The main advantage is that the method may be applied for antenatal diagnosis during the first trimester, so that if termination of the pregnancy is required this is easier to carry out. Furthermore, the results of the test are often available within only a few days of the procedure as (in contrast to amniocentesis) there is no need to culture cells before genetic analysis. A sample is obtained by either a transabdominal or transvaginal route, under ultrasound guidance (Figure 18.9). CVS should not be undertaken before 11 weeks of pregnancy in order to minimize the risk of inducing congenital limb abnormalities. A recent development has been the determination of fetal sex early in pregnancy through flow cytometric analysis of maternal blood at around 8 weeks. The advantage of this non-invasive technique, which is now widely available, is that identification of a female fetus obviates the need for CVS. It is likely that in the not too distant future this technique will be developed to allow full antenatal diagnosis of hemophilia (and other genetic disorders) based on isolation of fetal cells such as normoblasts from the maternal circulation.

Direct fetal blood sampling may also be used for antenatal diagnosis of hemophilia but this method is usually only offered as a last resort, either because it was not possible to carry out DNA-based family studies in time or because

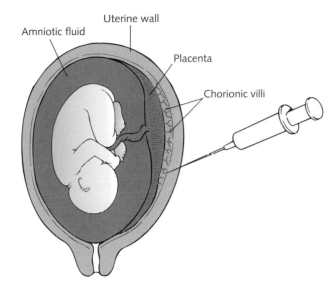

**Fig. 18.9 Chorionic villus sampling (CVS)**
A sample of trophoblastic tissue from the placental area is aspirated with a fine needle under general anesthesia. The procedure is usually carried out after 11 weeks' gestation. DNA isolated from the fetal tissue can then be analyzed to determine fetal sex and status with regard to hemophilia.

such studies were carried out but did not yield results. In this technique, fetal blood is taken from fetal umbilical vessels under ultrasound guidance. The procedure requires considerable expertise and will thus not be available in all hospitals. It is usually carried out at a minimum of 18 weeks' gestation. The levels of factor VIII and IX in a normal fetus at around 19 weeks' gestation are significantly lower than those in an adult, approximately 40 IU/dL and 10 IU/dL, respectively.

The need to abort an implanted fetus is a formidable ethical concern for many female carriers of hemophilia. Preimplantation diagnosis is another technique that has been developed, and this may prove to be particularly attractive to women who would not be prepared to undergo conventional termination of a well-established pregnancy. The female partner must undergo an *in vitro* fertilization cycle and the fertilized ova are then biopsied. Embryos shown to be unaffected by hemophilia can then be transferred to the uterus. The initial approach was to offer determination of embryonic sex alone using dual fluorescence *in situ* hybridization of blastomere cells with labeled probes specific for the sex chromosomes. More recently, specific mutation analysis has become possible, although it must be emphasized that this has only been performed in a very limited number of cases and is still far from being a service that is available on a routine basis even in major hospitals. Sperm sorting has been developed as a cheaper and easier method for preim-

plantation sex determination, using flow cytometry to sort spermatozoa labeled with a fluorescent dye that binds to DNA. The resulting higher fluorescence of X chromosomes, which contain more DNA than Y chromosomes, facilitates separation.

## Recombinant blood products

The development of plasma-derived coagulation factor concentrates in the early 1970s dramatically improved both the longevity and quality of life of patients with hemophilia, and the demand for factor VIII and IX has risen steadily. The burgeoning global demand for factor VIII can no longer be met by products derived from volunteer blood donors. The manufacture of recombinant coagulation factor proteins offers the promise of unlimited supplies, albeit at increased cost. However, the most important advantage of recombinant products is safety with regard to transmission of human pathogens. Many patients with hemophilia were infected with HIV and/or hepatitis C before the introduction of physical methods of viral inactivation of plasma-derived coagulation factor concentrates in 1985. More recently, there has been concern about the possibility of transmission of variant Creutzfeldt–Jakob disease (vCJD) via blood products, as the prions believed to be the cause of this neurological disorder are extremely resistant to the usual viral inactivation procedures such as heat treatment and exposure to a solvent/detergent mixture. Many clinicians now regard recombinant products as the treatment of choice for all patients with hemophilia as they offer the best possible protection from transmission of blood-borne pathogens. However, the increased cost with regard to conventional plasma-derived products has limited the availability of these products in many parts of the world.

Recombinant coagulation factor concentrates are manufactured by insertion of the human gene into mammalian cell lines (such as Chinese hamster ovary cells or baby hamster kidney cells), which are then grown in culture on an industrial scale. Factor VIII (or IX) is then secreted into the growth medium, from which it is subsequently extracted by monoclonal or other immunoaffinity chromatography (Figure 18.10). The original recombinant factor VIII products all contained added human albumin as a stabilizer. However, third- and fourth-generation products are now available in which alternative stabilizers are used. Human albumin and all bovine proteins have also been eliminated from the culture media of these modern products and the incorporation of specific viral elimination/inactivation steps further increases the margin of safety. Recombinant factor VIII has an essentially identical structure and glycosylation profile to natural plasma factor VIII (although one brand has no B domain).

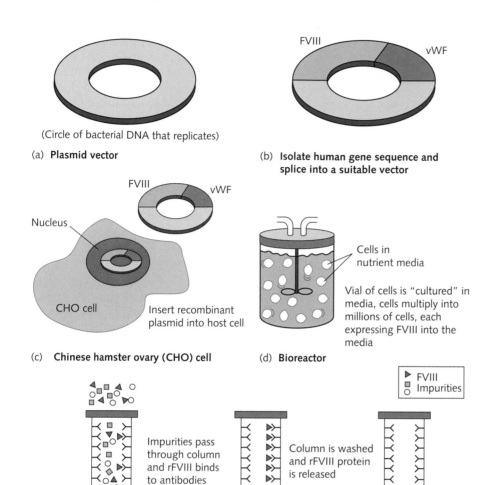

(a) **Plasmid vector**

(Circle of bacterial DNA that replicates)

(b) **Isolate human gene sequence and splice into a suitable vector**

FVIII  vWF

Nucleus

CHO cell  Insert recombinant plasmid into host cell

(c) **Chinese hamster ovary (CHO) cell**

Cells in nutrient media

Vial of cells is "cultured" in media, cells multiply into millions of cells, each expressing FVIII into the media

(d) **Bioreactor**

FVIII
Impurities

Impurities pass through column and rFVIII binds to antibodies

Column is washed and rFVIII protein is released

Impurities

rFVIII Protein

(e) **FVIII is purified from media using a monoclonal Ab column and ion-exchange columns**

**Fig. 18.10 Manufacture of recombinant factor VIII**

The gene for human factor VIII is incorporated into a bacterial vector (a, b). Inclusion of the von Willebrand factor gene also enhances production of factor VIII. The vector is then inserted into a mammalian host cell (c). The cells grow and multiply in a nutrient medium, and then secrete factor VIII (d). Factor VIII can be extracted and purified by immunoaffinity chromatography (e). The final product also contains no von Willebrand factor.

The pharmacokinetic profiles and post-infusion recoveries are also essentially identical to those observed for plasma-derived concentrates. Initial concerns about a potential increase in the incidence of inhibitors among people with hemophilia receiving recombinant products have proved unfounded. Although randomized and controlled trials comparing the incidence of inhibitor development in previously untreated patients receiving recombinant and plasma-derived products have never been conducted, it would be fair to say that the consensus is that the incidence of inhibitor development is similar for both types of product.

Recombinant factor IX is also available. Recombinant factor IX is identical in amino acid sequence to the Ala148 (as opposed to the less common Thr148) human polymorphic variant. Plasma factor IX is synthesized in the liver and undergoes post-translational glycosylation of a number of glutamic acid residues. Vitamin K is a vital cofactor in this process, which is essential for its activity, but recombinant factor IX is not as effectively carboxylated. The post-infusion recovery does appear to be reduced when compared with plasma-derived products, although the plasma half-life is identical. It is a smaller molecule than factor VIII and requires no albumin, or other material, to be added to the final product as a stabilizer. The cell line is grown in media that contain no animal or human-derived proteins but the product is subjected to nanofiltration to enhance its safety profile. There is no suggestion of an increased risk of inhibitor development associated with the use of recombinant factor IX.

Another useful recombinant product is recombinant activated factor VII (NovoSeven; Novo Nordisk). It is now recognized that factor VII plays a key role in initiation of the coagulation cascade through contact with tissue factor released from damaged tissues, to form activated factor VII (*see also Chapter 17*). Recombinant activated factor VII is very useful in the clinical management of patients with either hemophilia A or B and inhibitory antibodies, as well as those with acquired hemophilia.

Looking to the future, it is likely that the direction of future research in genetic engineering will increasingly be applied to production of modified molecules with more favorable properties. For example, it would obviously be useful to produce factor VIII molecules with a longer plasma half-life or reduced propensity to stimulate inhibitor development. A number of companies are developing pegylated coagulation factor molecules (including both factors VIII and IX as well as VWF) for clinical trials. The stability and thus duration of action of factor VIII can be enhanced by structural modifications, for example cross-linking of the A2 and A3 domains by covalent disulfide bonding. Circulating factor VIII is cleared from the bloodstream by binding to lipoprotein receptor-related protein (LRP), a hepatic receptor with broad ligand specificity. Pharmacological blockade of these catabolic receptors represents another potential target for prolonging the plasma-half life of infused factor VIII in patients with hemophilia. Hybrid factor VIII molecules have been developed in which epitopes within the A2 and C2 domains have been replaced by porcine equivalents. Since almost 90% of inhibitory antibodies bind to these two domains of the human factor VIII molecule, it is hoped that these new constructs may be of clinical use in the treatment of people with inhibitory antibodies. A further development has been the generation of transgenic livestock, such as sheep, pigs and goats, for production of human coagulation proteins. Transgenic animals that secrete antithrombin, factor VIII or factor IX into their milk have been produced, and this approach is being explored with a view to production of relatively cheap and unlimited supplies of biologically active products free of the risk of transmission of human pathogens (Figure 18.11). More recently, this work has been extended by successful cloning of sheep. Production of transgenic animals by nuclear transfer may permit the establishment of large breeding colonies of livestock more quickly and efficiently than would be possible through production of individual transgenic sheep by pronuclear microinjection.

## Gene therapy for hemophilia (*see also Chapter 25*)

Gene therapy offers the prospect of a cure for hemophilia in the long term, but it must be emphasized that there is no prospect of widescale application for some years. Gene therapy poses a number of ethical problems, particularly since effective and safe treatment with recombinant coagulation factors is already available for patients with both hemophilia A and B. The use of viral vectors introduces risks such as oncogenesis and infection, or even modification of patient germlines.

There are two basic approaches to gene delivery into cells. The first technique involves the direct injection of transducing vector into the bloodstream or target tissue, with subsequent *in vivo* transformation of the cells which take up the gene. Alternatively, target cells may be modified by removal of cells from a patient, with subsequent modification *ex vivo* of these cells followed by reinfusion. Retroviruses and adenoviruses have been used extensively as vectors. The principal advantage of using retroviruses as vectors is that the genetic material is actually integrated into the genome of the target cell, so expression of the transfected gene is permanent. However, integration is random, introducing the potential for oncogenesis through disruption of oncogenes. A further problem with the use of retroviruses as vectors is that there is a physical size limit of approximately 8 kb in the size of cassette that can be accommodated within the virus. The factor IX gene may be accommodated, but the full-length factor VIII gene cannot. Lentiviruses have the advantage that they transduce non-dividing cells. Adenoviruses permit transfer of larger genes and can transfect non-dividing cells but transferred DNA does not integrate permanently, so expression of the transfected gene is only transient. A further limitation is that immune response to adenoviral proteins, commonly encountered in everyday life, may limit efficiency of transfer. It is likely that gene therapy for hemophilia B will be achieved earlier than gene therapy for classical hemophilia A since the smaller size of the factor IX gene compared with the factor VIII gene permits the use of retroviral vectors; furthermore, factor IX (in contrast to factor VIII) may be absorbed from subcutaneous tissues after local injection. Although the liver is the site of synthesis of factor IX, a number of other cells can produce factor IX very effectively after transfection with the human factor IX gene, even in the absence of vitamin K. Both human fibroblasts and keratinocytes can produce factor IX, but keratinocytes are particularly attractive cells for gene therapy as they are very accessible, grow well in culture and can be grafted with ease.

A total of six small clinical trials have been conducted in humans so far. The results have yielded encouraging results, with expression of low levels of coagulation factor in the blood for up to 3 months and apparent reduction in bleeding tendency.

## Conclusions

Hemophilia is an inherited disorder of coagulation, associated with congenital deficiency of factor VIII (or IX). It is

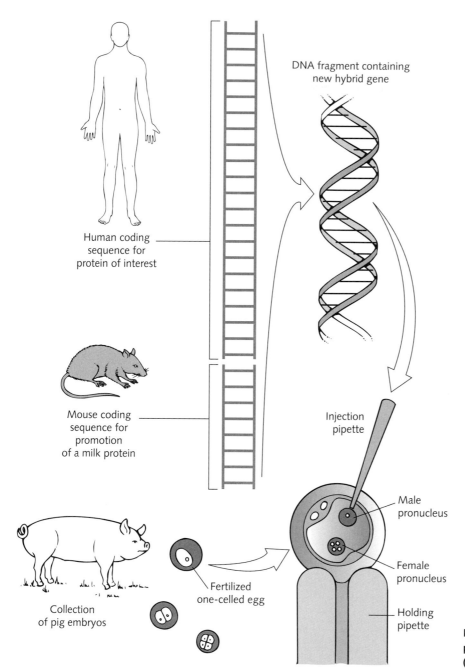

DNA fragment containing
new hybrid gene

Human coding
sequence for
protein of interest

Mouse coding
sequence for
promotion
of a milk protein

Injection
pipette

Male
pronucleus

Female
pronucleus

Holding
pipette

Collection
of pig embryos

Fertilized
one-celled egg

**Fig. 18.11 Production of recombinant proteins using transgenic livestock ("pharming")**

inherited in a sex-linked fashion, so that only males are affected. Approximately one-third of cases arise in families with no previous family history, and represent new mutations. The typical features of severe hemophilia include spontaneous bleeding into joints, but in the absence of treatment more serious complications (such as intracranial hemorrhage) will lead to early death.

The first products used for the treatment of hemophilia were derived from human plasma, but unfortunately the use of pooled plasma products before 1985 resulted in the trans-

mission of serious viral infections such as HIV and hepatitis to many patients. In recent years, the development of recombinant blood products has eliminated the risk of transmission of these infections, and also offers the prospect of unlimited supplies. The life expectancy of the younger generation of hemophiliacs now approaches that of the normal population.

The commonest molecular defect in severe hemophilia A is an inversion in intron 22 of the factor VIII gene on the X chromosome, which accounts for approximately half of all cases. Genetic testing is now readily available in many centers to document the genetic defect in each family, and identify carriers within families. Antenatal diagnosis is now readily available, facilitating early termination of the pregnancy if hemophilia is identified. Recent trials of gene therapy for hemophilia have yielded encouraging results.

## Hemophilia resources on the internet

Factor VIII (and VII) HAMSTeRS (Haemophilia A Mutation, Structure, Test and Resource Site) database. Available at europium.csc.mrc.ac.uk

Factor IX mutation database. Available at www.kcl.ac.uk/ip/petergreen/haemBdatabase.html

World Federation of Haemophilia. Available at www.wfh.org

United Kingdom Haemophilia Centre Doctors' Organisation (UKHCD). Available at www.ukhcdo.org

European Association for Haemophilia and Allied Disorders (EAHAD). Available at www.eahad.org

## Further reading

### Introduction

Key NS, Negrier C. (2007) Coagulation factor concentrates: past, present and future. *Lancet*, **370**, 439–448.

Mannucci PM. (2008) Back to the future: a recent history of haemophilia treatment. *Haemophilia*, **14** (Suppl 3), 10–18.

Lee CA, Berntorp E, Hoots WK (eds) (2005) *Textbook of Hemophilia*. Oxford: Blackwell Publishing.

Darby SC, Kan SW, Spooner RJ *et al.* (2007) Mortality rates, life expectancy, and causes of death in people with hemophilia A or B in the United Kingdom who were not infected with HIV. *Blood*, **110**, 815–825.

Zeepvat C. (1998) *Prince Leopold: the Untold Story of Queen Victoria's Youngest Son*. Stroud, UK: Sutton Publishing.

### Hemophilia A

Antonarakis SE, Rossiter JP, Young M *et al.* (1995) Factor VIII gene inversions in severe hemophilia A: results of an international consortium study. *Blood*, **86**, 2206–2212.

Bagnall RD, Waseem N, Green PM, Giannelli F. (2002) Recurrent inversion breaking intron 1 of the factor VIII gene is a frequent cause of severe hemophilia A. *Blood*, **99**, 168–174.

Keeney S, Mitchell M, Goodeve A. (2005) The molecular analysis of haemophilia A: a guideline from the UK haemophilia centre doctors' organization haemophilia genetics laboratory network. *Haemophilia*, **11**, 387–397.

Leuer M, Oldenburg J, Lavergne JM *et al.* (2001) Somatic mosaicism in hemophilia A: a fairly common event. *American Journal of Human Genetics*, **69**, 75–87.

Rost S, Löffler S, Pavlova A, Müller CR, Oldenburg J. (2008) Detection of large duplications within the factor VIII gene by MLPA. *Journal of Thrombosis and Haemostasis*, **6**, 1996–1999.

### Hemophilia B

Giangrande PLF. (2005) Haemophilia B: Christmas disease. *Expert Opinion in Pharmacotherapy*, **6**, 1517–1524.

Mitchell M, Keeney S, Goodeve A. (2005) The molecular analysis of haemophilia B: a guideline from the UK haemophilia centre doctors' organization haemophilia genetics laboratory network. *Haemophilia*, **11**, 398–404.

Reijnen MJ, Peerlinck K, Maasdam D, Bertina RM, Reitsma PH. (1993) Hemophilia B Leyden: substitution of thymine for guanine at position −21 results in a disruption of a hepatocyte nuclear factor 4 binding site in the factor IX promoter. *Blood*, **82**, 151–158.

Yoshitake S, Schach B, Foster DC, Davie EW, Kurachi K. (1985) Nucleotide sequencing of the gene for human factor IX (antihemophilic factor B). *Biochemistry*, **24**, 3736–3750.

### Inhibitors

Astermark J, Oldenburg J, Escobar M, White GC, Berntorp E. (2005) The Malmö International Brother Study (MIBS). Genetic defects and inhibitor development in siblings with severe hemophilia A. *Haematologica*, **90**, 924–931.

Astermark J, Oldenburg J, Pavlova A, Berntorp E, Lefvert AK. (2006) Polymorphisms in the IL10 but not in the IL1beta and IL4 genes are associated with inhibitor development in patients with hemophilia A. *Blood*, **107**, 3167–3172.

Hay CR, Brown SA, Collins PW, Keeling DM, Liesner R. (2006) The diagnosis and management of factor VIII and IX inhibitors: a guideline from the United Kingdom Haemophilia Centre Doctors' Organisation (UKHCDO). *British Journal of Haematology*, **133**, 591–605.

Huth-Kühne A, Baudo F, Collins P *et al.* (2009) International recommendations on the diagnosis and treatment of patients with acquired hemophilia A. *Haematologica*, **94**, 566–575.

Oldenburg J, Pavlova A. (2006) Genetic risk factors for inhibitors to factor VIII and IX. *Haemophilia*, **12** (Suppl 6), 15–22.

Saint Remy JM. (2008) How to get rid of inhibitors. *Haemophilia*, **14** (Suppl 3), 33–35.

Saint Remy JM, Lacroix-Desmazes S Oldenburg J. (2004) Inhibitors in haemophilia: pathophysiology. *Haemophilia*, **10** (Suppl 4), 146–151.

**Verbruggen B. (2009) Diagnosis and quantification of factor VIII inhibitors. *Haemophilia* [Epub ahead of print].

### Carrier testing and antenatal diagnosis

Dunn NF, Miller R, Griffioen A, Lee CA. (2008) Carrier testing in haemophilia A and B: adult carriers' and their partners' experiences and their views on the testing of young females. *Haemophilia*, **14**, 584–592.

Finning KM, Chitty LS. (2008) Non-invasive fetal sex determination: impact on clinical practice. *Seminars in Fetal and Neonatal Medicine*, **13**, 69–75.

Lavery S. (2009) Preimplantation genetic diagnosis of haemophilia. *British Journal of Haematology*, **144**, 303–307.

Ludlam CA, Pasi KJ, Bolton-Maggs P *et al.* (2005) A framework for genetic service provision for haemophilia and other inherited bleeding disorders. *Haemophilia*, **11**, 145–163.

Street AM, Ljung R, Lavery S. (2008) Management of carriers and babies with haemophilia. *Haemophilia*, **14** (Suppl 3), 181–187.

## Recombinant blood products

Pipe SW. (2008) Recombinant clotting factors. *Thrombosis and Haemostasis*, **99**, 840–850.

Van Cott KE, Monahan PE, Nichols TC, Velander WH. (2004) Haemophilic factors produced by transgenic livestock: abundance that can enable alternative therapies worldwide. *Haemophilia*, **10** (Suppl 4), 70–76.

## Gene therapy

Murphy SL, High KA. (2008) Gene therapy for haemophilia. *British Journal of Haematology*, **140**, 479–487.

Pipe SW, High KA, Ohashi K, Ural AU, Lillicrap D. (2008) Progress in the molecular biology of inherited bleeding disorders. *Haemophilia*, **14** (Suppl 3), 130–137.

Viiala NO, Larsen SR, Rasko JEJ. (2009) Gene therapy for hemophilia: clinical trials and technical tribulations. *Seminars in Thrombosis and Haemostasis*, **35**, 81–92.

# Chapter 19 The molecular basis of von Willebrand disease

## Luciano Baronciani and Pier Mannuccio Mannucci

*Angelo Bianchi Bonomi Hemophilia and Thrombosis Center, University of Milan and IRCCS Maggiore Hospital, Mangiagalli and Regina Elena Foundation, Milan, Italy*

## Introduction

Von Willebrand disease (VWD) is a common inherited bleeding disorder. Precise data regarding its prevalence are not available due to the extreme variability in clinical symptoms of mild VWD. However, population-based studies give an estimate of clinically significant VWD, with a prevalence of at least 100 per million. VWD is caused by the deficiency or dysfunction of a multimeric plasma glycoprotein, von Willebrand factor (VWF). Because of its ability to bind to a number of ligands, VWF is involved in hemostasis via a number of mechanisms but can be considered as having two main roles: in primary hemostasis and in intrinsic blood coagulation. VWF is directly involved in platelet binding to the subendothelium and in platelet–platelet interactions, and also acts as the carrier of procoagulant factor VIII (FVIII). Mutations at the *VWF* locus can affect VWF synthesis, its complex biosynthetic assembly, stability in the circulation, and its binding interactions with specific ligands.

## Function of von Willebrand factor in primary hemostasis

At the time of a hemostatic challenge, VWF acts as a bridge between platelets and the subendothelium of blood vessels, and is involved in the formation of the platelet plug. The role of platelets in hemostasis is to become irreversibly attached

at sites of injury. The primary physical factor that affects platelet binding to the vessel wall is the rate of blood flow in the vessel, which is faster at the center and slower close to the wall. These variations in velocity create a shearing effect, or shear stress, between layers of fluid. Disruption of the vascular endothelial surface leads to exposure of the subendothelium and results in an alteration of the rate of blood flow and an increase in shear stress. Plasma VWF binds rapidly and tightly to subendothelial collagen. VWF does not constitutively bind platelets, but in high blood flow conditions is capable of tethering platelets and to expose thrombogenic surfaces through the interaction of its A1 domain with the platelet receptor glycoprotein (GP)Ib. However, the VWF–GPIb interaction does not provide irreversible platelet adhesion because of the fast dissociation rate, and platelets tethered to the vessel wall still move constantly in the direction of the flow, but at a much slower rate. A second molecule on the platelet surface is required to obtain firm platelet adhesion: the integrin GPIIb-IIIa ($\alpha$IIb$\beta$3). This molecule is responsible for platelet–platelet interaction, which is mediated by VWF and, under slow-flow conditions, by fibrinogen. $\alpha$IIb$\beta$3 does not appear to be involved in the first events of platelet adhesion, probably because its rate of binding to VWF is too slow to mediate the initial platelet attachment to the vessel wall under high-flow conditions. However, when platelets become activated as a consequence of the VWF–GPIb interaction, $\alpha$IIb$\beta$3 increases its affinity for its ligand VWF. This event, together with the slow motion of platelets due to the VWF–GPIb interaction, allows $\alpha$IIb$\beta$3 to bind platelets irreversibly to the vessel wall (Figure 19.1). In all vessels with a high shear rate, VWF is the primary mediator of platelet binding to the vessel wall and of platelet aggregation.

*Molecular Hematology*, 3rd edition. Edited by Drew Provan and John Gribben.
© 2010 Blackwell Publishing.

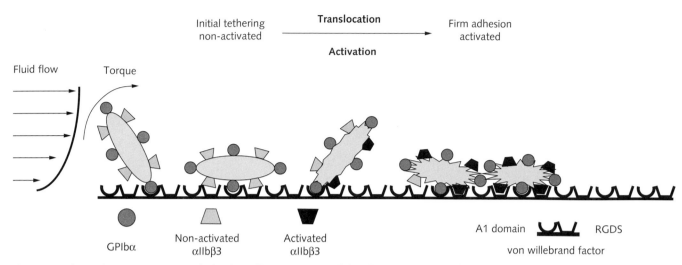

**Fig. 19.1 Schematic representation of platelet adhesion to immobilized von Willebrand factor (VWF)**
At first, platelets are tethered to the subendothelium through the interaction of their GPIbα with VWF (A1 domain), and the inactivated αIIbβ3 does not bind to the RGDS sequence of VWF. Because of the torque imposed by the flowing fluid, platelets begin to roll. New bonds are formed as different regions of the membrane of the rolling platelets come into contact with the surface and the translocation continues until αIIbβ3 becomes activated and binds firmly to the RGDS of VWF. Adapted from Ruggeri ZM. (1997) von Willebrand factor. *Journal of Clinical Investigation*, 99, 559–564, with permission.

## Function of von Willebrand factor in blood coagulation

Von Willebrand factor circulates in plasma as a complex associated with FVIII. The binding of VWF to FVIII is required to stabilize FVIII in the circulation, preventing cleavage by activated protein C (APC) or factor Xa. This interaction with VWF is crucial in prolonging the half-life of FVIII and concentrating FVIII at the point of bleeding. When patients with severe VWD (type 3) are treated with purified FVIII, this is cleared with a half-life of less then 2 hours, whereas the VWF–FVIII complex infused in the same patient has a half-life of about 12–14 hours. VWF binds to FVIII via regions within the first 272 residues of the mature polypeptide, in the D' and D3 domains of VWF.

## Gene organization, synthesis and multimeric structure of von Willebrand factor

The gene encoding VWF has been mapped on chromosome 12, has a length of approximately 178 kb with 52 exons, and transcribes an mRNA of about 8.2 kb. Analysis of the *VWF* gene is complicated by the existence of a partial unprocessed pseudogene on chromosome 22. The pseudogene extends from exon 23 to exon 34 and shares a high degree of homology with the gene (97%). VWF is synthesized in megakaryocytes and endothelial cells as a precursor of 2813 amino acids, the prepro-VWF. It is composed of a 22-residue signal peptide, a 741-residue propeptide and a 2050-residue mature subunit. More than 95% of the sequence accounts for structural domains that are arranged in the following order: D1-D2-D'-D3-A1-A2-A3-D4-B1-B2-B3-C1-C2-CK (Figure 19.2). The biosynthesis of VWF is a complex process, involving post-translational processing of the protein prior to storage or release into the circulation. The initial dimerization occurs by disulfide bonding between cysteine residues in the cysteine knot (CK) carboxyl-terminal region of the monomer (tail-to-tail dimerization). The signal peptide is cleaved before it enters the Golgi apparatus. The tail-to-tail glycosylated dimers are then transported to the Golgi apparatus where multimerization and further glycosylation occur. The propeptide of VWF mediates the assembly of VWF multimers. This process requires the presence of the D1 and D2 domains (propeptide) and the D' and D3 domains of the mature polypeptide. This is followed by cleavage of the propeptide sequence (Figure 19.3) and secretion of both the mature polypeptide and the propeptide into the circulation, or storage within the Weibel–Palade bodies of endothelial cells or the α-granules of platelets. The molecular mass of the mature subunit is 220 kDa but circulates as multimers of up to 20 000 kDa.

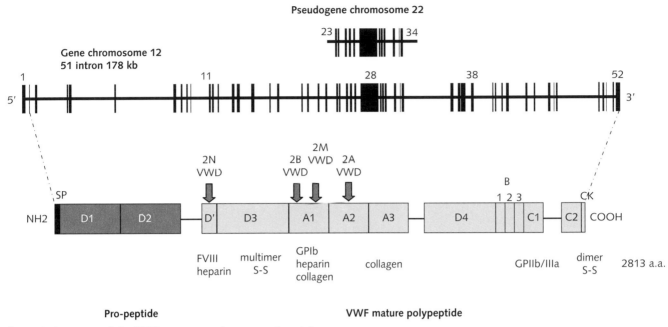

Fig. 19.2 **Structure of the VWF gene, pseudogene and protein**
The schematic structure of the prepro-VWF is shown, along with the homologous repeated domain. Also shown are the locations of intersubunit disulfide bonds involved in dimerization and multimerization, and the binding sites for several ligands.

## Von Willebrand disease and its classification

The most common symptoms of mild VWD are mucosal bleeding (epistaxis, gingival bleeding, menorrhagia) and prolonged bleeding after surgical procedures and dental extractions. Hemarthroses and soft-tissue hematomas are rare, but they occur in severely affected individuals (type 3). The diagnosis of VWD is suspected in individuals with these symptoms and a family history of bleeding. Several VWF assays are used in the diagnosis of VWD and its subtypes, such as those that measure the plasma levels of VWF antigen (VWF:Ag), VWF binding to type I or type III collagen (collagen binding activity, VWF:CB), the ability of VWF to bind FVIII (VWF:FVIIIB), and VWF interactions with the antibiotic ristocetin and platelet GPIb (VWF ristocetin cofactor activity, VWF:RCo; and ristocetin-induced platelet aggregation, RIPA, in platelet-rich plasma). This large number of measurements reflects the fact that none is by itself sensitive and specific enough for a diagnosis of VWD.

VWD is a highly heterogeneous disease in which there are quantitative and qualitative abnormalities of VWF, caused by mutations at the *VWF* locus. The classification identifies three basic types (Table 19.1). Type 1 is characterized by partial quantitative deficiency of VWF. Type 2 is character-

ized by qualitative abnormalities of VWF and is further categorized into subgroups (2A, 2B, 2M and 2N) depending on the nature of the qualitative defect (*see below*). Type 3 is the most severe form of the disease and is characterized by the complete absence of VWF in plasma and platelets. Transmission of type 1 VWD is usually dominant, type 2 is dominant in the majority of cases, whereas transmission of type 3 is recessive (Figure 19.4). The severity of the disease due to the same mutation can be variable, even within the same family.

In the last decades, many molecular defects of the *VWF* gene have been identified in VWD patients. At first, most of the mutations were identified in patients with the functional variants (types 2A, 2B and 2N), then in the more rare type 3 and, quite recently, in the most common type 1. The unique phenotypes of the type 2 variants made it possible to restrict the genetic analysis to the exons encoding for specific structural domains, such as the A1 domain for the variants 2B and 2M, A2 domain for the variant 2A, and D'–D3 domains for the variant 2N. On the other hand, characterization of molecular defects in types 1 and 3 VWD requires extensive screening, since mutations are not restricted to specific regions and are usually scattered throughout the *VWF* gene. In addition, whereas the identification of a nonsense mutation or a small deletion, more common in type 3 VWD, can undoubtedly be considered the cause of the

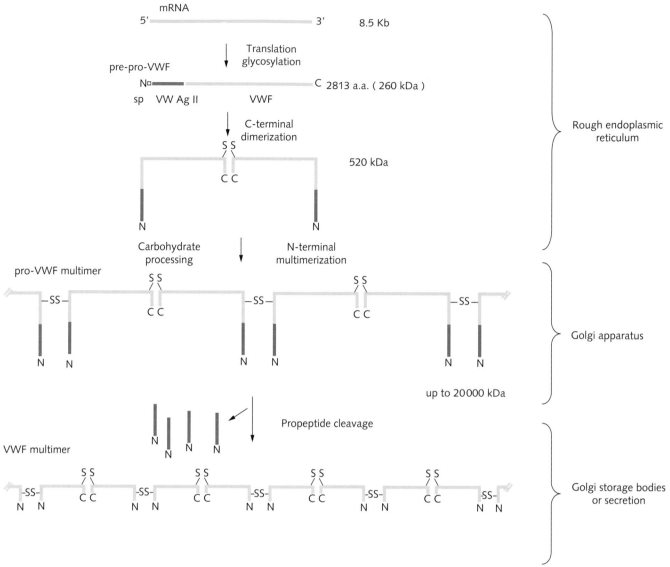

**Fig. 19.3 Processing steps of VWF multimer synthesis and subcellular localization of the post-translational modification events**
The propeptide is shown as a dark tint, the mature subunit as a light tint. The N and C prefixes represent, respectively, the amino- and carboxyl-terminal ends of the protein. Monomers are linked together at the C-termini by disulfide bonds to form dimers (endoplasmic reticulum), which further multimerize in the Golgi apparatus. The cleavage of the propeptide occurs prior to secretion.

**Table 19.1** Current classification of von Willebrand disease.

| | |
|---|---|
| Type 1 | Partial quantitative deficiency of VWF |
| Type 2 | Qualitative deficiency of VWF |
| 2A | Decreased platelet-dependent VWF function, with lack of high-molecular-weight multimers (HMWM) |
| 2B | Increased VWF platelet-dependent VWF function, with lack of HMWM |
| 2M | Decreased platelet-dependent VWF function, with normal multimeric structure |
| 2N | Decreased VWF affinity for FVIII |
| Type 3 | Complete deficiency of VWF |

disease, the identification of missense mutations, more common in type 1 VWD, requires supplementary studies in order to confirm their relationship with the disease, causing further complexity in the molecular characterization of the most common variant. In most type 2 cases the mutations consist of amino acid substitutions (missense mutations), although small in-frame deletions or insertions have been reported. In type 3 VWD the majority of molecular defects identified are responsible for null alleles (nonsense mutations, splice-site mutations, small deletions, small insertions and, more rarely, large gene deletions). Nevertheless, several missense mutations have been identified. In type 1, the

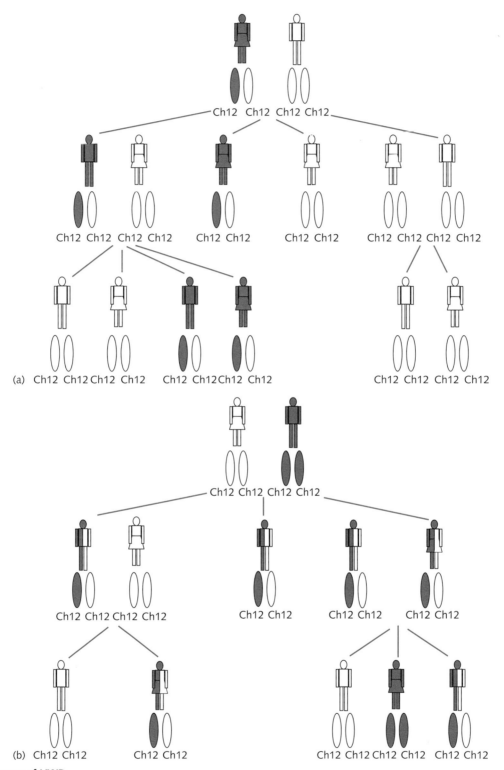

**Fig. 19.4 Inheritance of VWD**
(a) A family pedigree with autosomal dominant segregation as found in VWD types 1, 2A, 2B and 2M. (b) A family pedigree with autosomal recessive segregation as found in VWD types 2N and 3.

opposite seems to be the case, with a majority of missense mutations and a minority of splice-site mutations, small deletions and insertions (sometimes in-frame) and more rarely nonsense mutations.

## Genetic defects in von Willebrand disease

### Type 1 VWD

This is the most common form, comprising approximately 70% of all cases of VWD. Patients have mild to moderate bleeding symptoms, a normal or variably prolonged bleeding time, decreased levels of VWF in plasma, and a normal multimeric structure of VWF, although some cases show a slightly decreased level of high-molecular-weight multimers. Type 1 VWD may be difficult to diagnose due to natural variations in circulating VWF levels related to the influence of environmental factors, such as exercise, thyroid hormone, estrogens and ABO blood type. VWF levels are lower by as much as 30% in individuals with blood group O compared with individuals with other blood groups.

Quite recently, a number of studies have significantly advanced our knowledge of type 1 VWD, in particular the genetic basis of the disorder. Linkage analysis has showed complete cosegregation of the *VWF* gene and VWD in just over 50% of the families investigated. Direct sequencing analysis of the whole coding region and exon/intron boundaries has allowed the identification of mutations in about 67% of patients with type 1 VWD. Most of these are missense mutations (75%), with the remainder being splice-site mutations (7%), small insertions and deletions (5%; one-quarter in-frame), nonsense mutations (2%), and promoter changes (11%). Only 15% of the mutations cause null alleles. Further studies are currently investigating the causative role of mutations such as missense, splice-site and promoter changes. At variance with that found in type 2 VWD, the missense mutations are found throughout the entire *VWF* gene, even though approximately one-third of them are in exon 28. Patients with type 1 VWD could be divided roughly into three groups: (i) patients with a fully penetrant dominant mutation with low VWF levels; (ii) patients with an incomplete penetrant mutation, where not all the family members with the mutation have low VWF levels; and (iii) patients with no apparent mutations in the *VWF* gene.

The first group is characterized by penetrant missense mutations like C1130F or C1149R. An *in vitro* study has clarified the molecular mechanism of these dominant-negative mutations found in the D3 domain. In a random dimerization process occurring in the endoplasmic reticulum, mutant and wild-type pro-VWF subunits form both

homodimers and heterodimers. Retention of all mutant subunits in the endoplasmic reticulum reduces the transport of wild-type subunits to the Golgi apparatus by about 50%, whereas subunits reaching the Golgi assemble into large multimers and are normally secreted (25% of the total VWF subunits). In this group also, accelerated clearance can cause dominant type 1 VWD, similar to the effects of the mutation S2179F which produces a VWF with a reduced half-life after desmopressin treatment.

In the second group, incomplete penetrant mutations, such as Y1584C, have been identified. In the heterozygous state this mutation does not always results in low VWF levels and bleeding symptoms. Apparently, only the co-inheritance of blood group O, which has been linked with increased VWF proteolysis, results in type 1 VWD in individuals with the mutation Y1584C. The third group of patients, with no identified mutations, remains to be clarified. These are usually patients with low borderline VWF levels, who should perhaps not be classified as type 1 VWD. In this group of patients there is the highest percentage of subjects with blood group O. However, it cannot be excluded that mutations in genes other than *VWF* engaged in VWF biosynthesis and processing could be the cause of reduced plasma levels of VWF. The classification of VWD has recently changed and is not now restricted to *VWF* gene mutations.

### Type 2 VWD

Type 2 VWD accounts for approximately 20% of all VWD cases, is caused by a variety of mechanisms, and is associated with a variety of specific defects, reflecting the multifunctional role of VWF and the complicated post-translational processing of this moiety.

#### Type 2A

This is characterized by decreased platelet-dependent function due to the reduction or absence of high- and intermediate-molecular-weight multimers (Figure 19.5). The bleeding diathesis is caused by the lack of the most biologically active high-molecular-weight multimers. At least two mechanisms are known to produce type 2A VWD, subclassified as group 1 and group 2. Group 1 mutations lead to a VWF subunit that is improperly folded, retained in the endoplasmic reticulum by the cell quality control machinery, and subsequently degraded. Multimers formed by the interactions between normal and mutant subunits are retained in the cell. The largest multimers, as a result of a greater content of the mutant subunit, are more efficiently retained, accounting for the characteristic type 2A multimer pattern and autosomal dominant inheritance. The defect of group 2 does not interfere with biosynthesis and secretion,

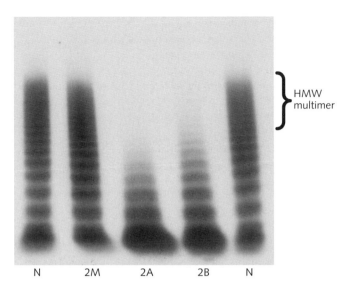

**Fig. 19.5 Comparison of multimeric structure of plasma VWF from VWD patients and normal subjects**
Lane 3 (VWD type 2A) and lane 4 (VWD type 2B) show the lack of high-molecular-weight multimers. Lane 2 (VWD type 2M) shows a normal multimeric pattern. Lanes 1 and 5 show a normal multimeric structure from a normal control.

but instead renders the mutant subunit more susceptible to proteolytic cleavage (between amino acids Y1605 and M1606 of the A2 domain) by the plasma metalloproteinase ADAMTS-13. This enhanced plasma proteolysis results in the selective loss of the largest VWF multimers, similar to that seen in group 1. More recently, computer modeling suggests that mutations of both groups impaired the folding of the VWF A2 domain, exposing the proteolytic site and causing increased degradation by ADAMTS-13. Group 1 mutations appears to have a more disruptive effect on A2 domain structure, which may account for their additional effect on multimer assembly. At least 50 distinct mutations have been reported, responsible for both groups, and 30 of these are in the A2 VWF structural domain, the most frequent being R1597W and I1628T.

## Type 2B

This uncommon subtype accounts for approximately 5% of all VWD cases. The 2B variant VWF shows increased affinity for platelet GPIb and is usually associated with the absence of high-molecular-weight multimers in circulating plasma but not in platelets (Figure 19.5). Therefore, type 2B mutations do not impair the assembly of large VWF multimers, but after secretion the multimers bind spontaneously to platelets leading to low plasma levels. The variable thrombocytopenia, which may be present in these patients, is believed

to be secondary to the formation of platelet–VWF aggregates. Type 2B is inherited as a dominant trait. Mutations responsible for this subtype are nearly all contained within the A1 domain, which binds to the GPIb receptor. With a few exceptions, all mutations result in amino acid substitutions, and a few of them (R1306W, R1308W, V1316M and R1341Q) account for 80–90% of reported cases. Type 2B VWD is sometimes misdiagnosed and treated as autoimmune thrombocytopenia. Thrombocytopenia and the absence of the larger multimers are not constantly present in type 2B VWD. For instance, mutation P1266L causes increased GPIb binding with no apparent loss of large multimers and absence of thrombocytopenia before and after desmopressin, leading to earlier classification among type 1 variants (type 1 New York or type 1 Malmo). Patients carrying this mutation usually have mild bleeding symptoms and in some cases may have none.

## Type 2M

Type 2M VWD refers to qualitative variants with decreased platelet-dependent function not caused by the absence of the largest VWF multimers (Figure 19.5). With a pattern of VWF laboratory measurements similar to that of type 2A, type 2M shows a normal multimer distribution (hence M for multimer) or may even show the presence of ultra-large multimers (2M Vicenza). Type 2M is inherited as a dominant trait. The molecular defects are identified in the A1 domain, but in a region different from that of the 2B mutations. These defects, which in most cases are missense mutations (G1324S, R1374H, R1374C and R1379C), seem to downregulate the binding of the A1 domain to its platelet receptor. An important exception is the 2M Vicenza variant, the candidate mutation being in the D3 domain (R1205H). It is characterized by low levels of VWF:Ag, normal platelet VWF and ultra-large plasma VWF multimers. Compared with healthy controls, the half-life of VWF Vicenza is reduced 4.4-fold after desmopressin, suggesting that rapid clearance accounts for the moderately severe VWF deficiency. In addition, rapid clearance decreases the time during which large circulating VWF multimers can be cleaved by ADAMTS-13, resulting in partial preservation of ultra-large multimers. The classification of this variant has been controversial; recently, on the basis of the proportionately low level of VWF:Ag and VWF:RCo, it was classified under type 1 VWD.

## Type 2N

Type 2N VWD refers to all the qualitative variants characterized by decreased affinity for FVIII. The first description of this type of variant was that of a patient from Normandy (hence the N). This subtype is characterized by low levels of

FVIII; however, VWF levels are usually normal and have an intact VWF multimeric pattern. It is difficult to distinguish type 2N from mild hemophilia A. Hemophilia is an X-linked disease, whereas type 2N VWD is an autosomal recessive disease. A definitive diagnosis can be made by demonstrating the reduced binding of FVIII to VWF with assays exploring this VWF property. Since the majority of mutations are located in the N-terminus of the mature VWF subunit (D′–D3), diagnosis can be confirmed by screening for mutations in exons 18, 19 and 20. Three mutations (T791M, R816W and R854Q) account for 90% of the type 2N mutations.

## Type 3 VWD

Type 3 VWD is an autosomal recessive, clinically severe disorder characterized by the complete or nearly complete absence of VWF. As in type 2N VWD, there is a secondary deficiency of FVIII and the patients therefore present a double defect of primary hemostasis and intrinsic coagulation. Type 3 VWD is rare and accounts for 1–2% of all VWD cases, with a prevalence in the general population of 0.5–1 per million. The parents of type 3 patients are obligatory heterozygotes and in most cases are asymptomatic, but a minority of them have mild bleeding symptoms. Because of the large size of the gene, the presence of the pseudogene, the low prevalence of the disease and the absence of a specific location for the mutations, the characterization of the molecular defects in type 3 has been relatively slow. Southern blot analysis first allowed the identifications of large gene deletions, found in the majority of the patients who had developed alloantibodies to VWF after transfusion. However, the use of more specific and sensitive screening methods, such as single-stranded conformational polymorphisms, chemical cleavage mismatch analysis, conformation-sensitive gel electrophoresis and others, allowed the identification of most of the mutations in these patients. The most common mutations in type 3 VWD are nonsense mutations, small deletions, small insertions and splice-site mutations. Among the nonsense mutations, a few hotspot mutations at the arginine codons (R365X, R1659X, R1853X and R2535X) have been found repeatedly in different populations. A single cytosine deletion, in a stretch of six cytosines in exon 18 appears to be particularly common in patients from Sweden and Germany. Although most of the mutations cause null alleles, a few in-frame deletions and several missense mutations have been identified. Patients with type 3 VWD may develop alloantibodies to VWF, which render replacement therapy ineffective. This complication is strongly associated with the presence of homozygous large gene deletions, although a few cases have been reported due to nonsense mutations.

## Treatment of von Willebrand disease

While the treatment of patients with hemophilia A and B is facilitated by the close relationships between the content of FVIII or factor IX in the replacement material, the plasma levels attained after infusion and clinical efficacy, this model cannot be easily translated into the evaluation of products for treatment of VWD, because it is still unclear which FVIII or VWF measurement in therapeutic products or in patient plasma better correlates with the severity of clinical bleeding and the efficacy of treatment. The situation is further complicated by the fact that VWD subtypes may respond differently to treatment. Two main therapeutic agents are currently used to stop spontaneous bleeding and to prevent bleeding at the time of surgical procedures: the non-transfusional agent desmopressin and blood products that contain FVIII and VWF concentrated from plasma. Ancillary forms of treatment include platelet concentrates, synthetic fibrinolysis inhibitors, and combined estrogen/progestogen preparations, which in some clinical situations are adjunctive or sometime alternative to the two main treatments.

### Desmopressin

Desmopressin (1-deamino-8-D-arginine vasopressin, DDAVP) is a synthetic analog of the antidiuretic hormone vasopressin that, when administered to healthy volunteers or patients with mild hemophilia and VWD, transiently increases FVIII and VWF by releasing these moieties from storage sites into plasma. Endothelial cell Weibel–Palade bodies appear to be the source of VWF, but the source of FVIII has not been determined as yet. Desmopressin induces VWF release into plasma by binding to the vasopressin $V_2$ receptor and thereby activating cyclic AMP-mediated signaling in vascular endothelial cells.

The advantage of this compound is that it is relatively inexpensive and carries no risk of transmitting blood-borne infectious agents. When infused intravenously over 30 min at a dose of 0.2–0.3 μg/kg, desmopressin is expected to increase plasma FVIII and VWF twofold to fourfold above basal levels. In general, high FVIII/VWF concentrations last in plasma for at least 8–10 hours. Patients with baseline plasma levels of FVIII/VWF in the range of 10–20 IU/dL or more are those who are more likely to reach post-desmopressin levels sufficient to attain hemostasis, taking into account variables such as the type and severity of the bleeding episode and the levels of FVIII/VWF that must be attained and maintained to secure hemostasis. Even though most patients with mild hemophilia A treated repeatedly with desmopressin become less responsive to therapy, this problem is less frequent and prominent in patients with type 1 VWD. The drug is also available in concentrated forms for subcutaneous and intranasal administration (at doses of 0.3 µg/kg and 150–300 µg, respectively), which can be convenient for home treatment.

Side effects of desmopressin usually include mild tachycardia, headache and facial flushing. Hyponatremia and volume overload due to the antidiuretic effect of desmopressin are relative rare if fluid intake is not excessive during treatment. Even though no thrombotic episodes have been reported in VWD patients treated with desmopressin, this compound should be used with caution in elderly patients with cardiovascular disease, because a few cases of myocardial infarction and stroke have occurred in treated patients with hemophilia and uremia. Desmopressin has little or no oxytocic activity and has been used without mishap during the early period of pregnancy in 31 women with low FVIII levels (including carriers of hemophilia A and VWD patients) in order to prevent bleeding at the time of invasive diagnostic procedures such as chronic villus sampling and amniocentesis.

Desmopressin is particularly effective in patients with type 1 VWD. In these patients, FVIII, VWF and the bleeding time are usually corrected to normal values by desmopressin. In other VWD subtypes, responsiveness is less certain (Table 19.2). In type 2A, FVIII levels are usually increased by desmopressin but the bleeding time is shortened in only a minority of cases. Desmopressin is contraindicated in type 2B, because of the transient appearance of thrombocytopenia. There is little experience in type 2M, but a poor response is predicted because VWF is dysfunctional in this subtype. In type 2N, FVIII coagulant activity (FVIII:C) levels increase following desmopressin, but released FVIII circulates for a relatively short time in patients' plasma because the stabilizing effect of VWF on FVIII is impaired. Therefore, plasma concentrates containing FVIII and VWF are usually preferable. Patients with type 3 VWD are unresponsive to desmopressin, because they lack releasable stores of VWF.

**Table 19.2** Indications for desmopressin in different types of von Willebrand disease.

| Type | Response |
| --- | --- |
| 1 | Usually effective |
| 2A | Usually ineffective |
| 2B | May be contraindicated |
| 2M | Predicted to be ineffective |
| 2N | Rarely effective |
| 3 | Ineffective |

## Transfusional therapies

Transfusional therapy with plasma products containing both FVIII and VWF is the treatment of choice when bleeding occurs or must be prevented and the predicted response to desmopressin is considered suboptimal for hemostasis. FVIII and VWF may be infused as fresh frozen plasma but the large volumes required severely limit its use. Cryoprecipitate contains five to ten times more FVIII and VWF than fresh frozen plasma (each bag contains approximately 80–100 IU). Early studies indicated that cryoprecipitate administered every 12–24 hours normalized plasma FVIII levels and stopped or prevented bleeding in VWD. On the basis of these observations, cryoprecipitate has been the mainstay of treatment for many years. However, virucidal methods cannot be applied to cryoprecipitate as produced by blood banks, so that this product carries a small risk of transmitting blood-borne infectious agents. Therefore, virus-inactivated FVIII/VWF concentrates, originally developed for the treatment of hemophilia A, are currently perceived as safer and are preferred in the management of VWD patients unresponsive to desmopressin or unsuitable for treatment with this drug.

Two commercially available concentrates have been evaluated in prospective clinical studies and these have demonstrated their efficacy in preventing or stopping bleeding. One, licensed in the USA and in several European countries for the treatment of VWD, contains relatively larger amounts of VWF (measured as VWF:RCo) than of FVIII (approximately two to three times more in terms of IU). The virucidal method adopted is pasteurization. The other, licensed in Europe and in the USA, differs because it contains similar relative amounts of FVIII and VWF:RCo. Two virucidal methods, solvent/detergent and heating at high temperatures, are included in the manufacturing step, with the goal of inactivating both enveloped and non-enveloped virus. Other virally inactivated FVIII/VWF concentrates have been employed in VWD patients, but clinical experience is much more limited. Recently, a chromatography-purified concentrate particularly rich in VWF but with a very low FVIII content has also been produced. As many as three viral inactivation methods are used in the production of this concentrate (solvent/detergent, heating and nanofiltration). The concentrate was clinically efficacious when tested in a large number of European patients with clinically severe forms of VWD at the time of spontaneous bleeding episodes and surgical procedures.

The dosages recommended for the control or prevention of bleeding are summarized in Table 19.3. Dosages are expressed in IU/kg of FVIII because the majority of the available concentrates, being originally manufactured for treatment of patients with hemophilia A, are labeled in terms of FVIII content only. Since FVIII has a longer half-life in

**Table 19.3** Dosages of FVIII coagulant activity (FVIII:C) recommended in patients with von Willebrand disease treated with FVIII/VWF concentrates.*

| Type of bleeding | Dose (IU/kg) | Number of infusions | Target |
|---|---|---|---|
| Major surgery | 40–60 | Once a day | Maintain plasma FVIII:C >50 IU/dL until healing is complete depending on the type of surgery |
| Minor surgery | 30–50 | Once a day or every other day | FVIII:C >30 IU/dL until healing is complete depending on the type of surgery |
| Dental extractions | 20–30 | Single | FVIII:C >30 IU/dL for at least 12 hours |
| Spontaneous bleeding episodes | 20–30 | Single | FVIII:C >30 IU/dL |

* For concentrates labeled in terms of VWF:RCo, the recommended doses for adults, the number of infusions and the target plasma levels are the same as those for FVIII:C.

**Table 19.4** Summary of management of different types and subtypes of von Willebrand disease.

| | Treatment of choice | Alternative or adjunctive therapy |
|---|---|---|
| Type 1 | Desmopressin | Antifibrinolytic amino acids |
| Type 2A | Factor VIII/VWF concentrates | Antifibrinolytic amino acids |
| Type 2B | Factor VIII/VWF concentrates | Antifibrinolytic amino acids |
| Type 2M | Factor VIII/VWF concentrates | Antifibrinolytic amino acids |
| Type 2N | Factor VIII/VWF concentrates | Desmopressin |
| Type 3 | Factor VIII/VWF concentrates | Antifibrinolytic amino acids, platelet concentrates |
| Type 3 complicated by alloantibodies | Recombinant factor VIII | Recombinant activated factor VII |

VWD patients than in patients with hemophilia A (20–24 vs. 12–14 hours), the infusion of one daily dose is sufficient to reach and maintain adequate plasma levels for the treatment of spontaneous bleeding episodes and to prevent excessive bleeding. Since in the USA the Food and Drug Administration (FDA) requires that plasma products licensed for treatment of VWD patients are labeled in terms of the actual defective protein to be replaced, most concentrates are now also labeled in terms of VWF:RCo content. The doses of this concentrate recommended for their demonstrated efficacy in large prospective clinical trials are 40–60 IU/kg of VWF:RCo (50–75 IU/kg in children because of the lower *in vivo* recovery), which usually results in VWF:RCo plasma levels of 80–120 IU/dL or higher. Even though the plasma half-life of VWF:RCo is much shorter than that of FVIII:C (8–10 vs. 20–24 hours), usually these doses do not need to be repeated more often than every 24 hours, although sometimes treatment intervals must be tailored to the clinical situation.

It is usually not necessary to carry out laboratory tests to monitor replacement therapy in patients with spontaneous bleeding episodes. For surgical procedures, we recommend measuring FVIII every 12 hours on the operation day and then every 24 hours. Those who use concentrates labeled in terms of VWF:RCo content may choose to monitor the plasma levels of this moiety, although this is more complex

to measure in the clinical setting and less standardized than the FVIII level. It remains to be demonstrated whether laboratory measurements such as the collagen binding assay will be simpler and more predictive of outcome.

Monitoring the bleeding time is usually not necessary. The prolonged bleeding time is frequently not normalized nor even shortened in patients treated with FVIII/VWF concentrates. Despite no or partial correction of the bleeding time, major surgical procedures are successfully carried out and spontaneous bleeding episodes controlled following the infusion of FVIII/VWF concentrates. In the relatively rare instances when bleeding is not controlled and the bleeding time remains prolonged, platelet concentrates (given immediately after FVIII/VWF-containing preparations, at doses of $4$–$5 \times 10^{11}$ platelets) are effective, particularly in patients with type 3 VWD, both in terms of bleeding time correction and control of hemorrhage. Platelets from type 3 VWD patients lack VWF completely and there is no uptake of the protein from plasma after infusion of concentrates. The hemostatic effectiveness of the transfusion of normal platelets is likely to be due to the fact that these cells transport and localize VWF at sites of vascular injury. From a practical standpoint, it must be emphasized that in one of the largest prospective studies carried out so far in VWD patients, platelet concentrates became necessary to prevent or stop bleeding in one case only.

In conclusion, the different options currently available for the management of VWD are summarized in Table 19.4. Treatment of spontaneous bleeding episodes and their prevention at the time of invasive procedures is relatively simple and can certainly be tackled by the average clinical hematologist with access to a minimum of laboratory testing (FVIII assays). However, patients need to be well characterized phenotypically, because the choice of treatment must be tailored to the different types and subtypes of the disease. Such characterization is not simple, so that in the majority of clinical centers it is probably not worthwhile setting up relatively complicated tests such as multimer analysis and VWF:RCo assays when samples can be sent for analysis to more expert laboratories that have become proficient during the study of large series of patients. Genotyping is not necessary for treatment but one should be cognizant that patients with type 3 disease due to large homozygous deletions are more likely to develop anti-VWF alloantibodies and often severe anaphylactic reactions.

## Von Willebrand disease resources on the internet

International Society for Thrombosis and Haemostasis Scientific and Standardization Subcommittee VWF Online Database. Available at http://www.vwf.group.shef.ac.uk/index.html

Human Gene Mutation Database, Cardiff. Available at http://www.hgmd.cf.ac.uk/ac/index.php

Online Mendelian Inheritance in Man. http://www.ncbi.nlm.nih.gov/entrez/dispomim.cgi?cmd=entry&id=193400

GeneCards™ is a database of human genes. Available at http://www.genecards.org/cgi-bin/carddisp.pl?gene=VWF

## Further reading

### General

Sadler JE, Mannucci PM, Berntorp E *et al.* (2000) Impact, diagnosis and treatment of von Willebrand disease. *Thrombosis and Haemostasis*, **84**, 160–174.

Michiels JJ (ed.) (2001) Von Willebrand factor and von Willebrand disease. *Best Practice and Research. Clinical Haematology*, **14**, 235–462.

### Von Willebrand factor

Bonthron DT, Orr EC, Mitsock LM, Ginsburg D, Handin RI, Orkin SH. (1986) Nucleotide sequence of pre-pro-von Willebrand factor cDNA. *Nucleic Acids Research*, **14**, 7125–7127.

Dong Z, Thoma RS, Crimmins DL, McCourt DW, Tuley EA, Sadler JE. (1994) Disulfide bonds required to assemble functional von Willebrand factor multimers. *Journal of Biological Chemistry*, **269**, 6753–6758.

Foster PA, Fulcher CA, Marti T, Titani K, Zimmerman TS. (1987) A major factor VIII binding domain resides within the amino-terminal 272 amino acid residues of von Willebrand factor. *Journal of Biological Chemistry*, **262**, 8443–8446.

Ginsburg D, Handin RI, Bonthron DT *et al.* (1985) Human von Willebrand factor (vWF): isolation of complementary DNA (cDNA) clones and chromosomal localization. *Science*, **228**, 1401–1406.

Jaffe EA, Hoyer LW, Nachman RL. (1974) Synthesis of von Willebrand factor by cultured human endothelial cells. *Proceedings of the National Academy of Sciences of the United States of America*, **71**, 1906–1909.

Kroll MH, Hellums JD, McIntire LV, Schafer AI, Moake JL. (1996) Platelets and shear stress. *Blood*, **88**, 1525–1541.

Mancuso DJ, Tuley EA, Westfield LA *et al.* (1989) Structure of the gene for human von Willebrand factor. *Journal of Biological Chemistry*, **264**, 19514–19527.

Mancuso DJ, Tuley EA, Westfield LA *et al.* (1991) Human von Willebrand factor gene and pseudogene: structural analysis and differentiation by polymerase chain reaction. *Biochemistry*, **30**, 253–269.

Shelton-Inloes BB, Titani K, Sadler JE. (1986) cDNA sequences for human von Willebrand factor reveal five types of repeated domains and five possible protein sequence polymorphisms. *Biochemistry*, **25**, 3164–3171.

Wagner DD, Marder VJ. (1984) Biosynthesis of von Willebrand protein by human endothelial cells: processing steps and their intracellular localization. *Journal of Cell Biology*, **99**, 2123–2130.

Weiss HJ, Sussman II, Hoyer LW. (1977) Stabilization of factor VIII in plasma by the von Willebrand factor. Studies on posttransfusion and dissociated factor VIII and in patients with von Willebrand's disease. *Journal of Clinical Investigation*, **60**, 390–404.

### Genetic defects in von Willebrand disease

Baronciani L, Cozzi G, Canciani MT *et al.* (2003) Molecular defects in type 3 von Willebrand disease: updated results from 40 multiethnic patients. *Blood Cells, Molecules and Diseases*, **30**, 264–270.

Bodo I, Katsumi A, Tuley EA, Eikenboom JC, Dong Z, Sadler JE. (2001) Type 1 von Willebrand disease mutation Cys1149Arg causes intracellular retention and degradation of heterodimers: a possible general mechanism for dominant mutations of oligomeric proteins. *Blood*, **98**, 2973–2979.

Bowen DJ, Collins PW. (2006) Insights into von Willebrand factor proteolysis: clinical implications. *British Journal of Haematology*, **133**, 457–467.

Cumming A, Grundy P, Keeney S *et al.* (2006) An investigation of the von Willebrand factor genotype in UK patients diagnosed to have type 1 von Willebrand disease. *Thrombosis and Haemostasis*, **96**, 630–641.

Eikenboom JCJ, Matsushita T, Reitsma PH *et al.* (1996) Dominant type I von Willebrand disease caused by mutated cysteine residues in the D3 domain of von Willebrand factor. *Blood*, **88**, 2433–2441.

Federici AB. (1998) Diagnosis of von Willebrand disease. *Haemophilia*, **4**, 654–660.

Gill JC, Endres-Brooks J, Bauer PJ, Marks WJ Jr, Montgomery RR. (1987) The effect of ABO blood group on the diagnosis of von Willebrand disease. *Blood*, **69**, 1691–1695.

Ginsburg D. (1999) Molecular genetics of von Willebrand disease. *Thrombosis and Haemostasis*, **82**, 585–591.

Goodeve A, Eikenboom JCJ, Castaman G *et al.* (2007) Phenotype and genotype of a cohort of families historically diagnosed with type 1 von Willebrand disease in the European study. Molecular and Clinical Markers for the Diagnosis and Management of Type 1 von Willebrand disease (MCMDM-1VWD). *Blood*, **109**, 112–121.

Haberichter SL, Balistreri M, Christopherson P *et al.* (2006) Assay of the von Willebrand factor (VWF) propeptide to identify patients with type 1 von Willebrand disease with decreased VWF survival. *Blood*, **108**, 3344–3351.

Holmberg L, Dent JA, Schneppenheim R, Budde U, Ware J, Ruggeri ZM. (1993) von Willebrand factor mutation enhancing interaction with platelets in patients with normal multimeric structure. *Journal of Clinical Investigation*, **91**, 2169–2177.

James PD, Notley C, Hegadom C *et al.* (2007) The mutational spectrum of type 1 von Willebrand disease: results from a Canadian cohort study. *Blood*, **109**, 145–154.

Jenkins PV, Pasi KJ, Perkins SJ. (1998) Molecular modeling of ligand and mutation sites of the type A domains of human von Willebrand factor and their relevance to von Willebrand's disease. *Blood*, **91**, 2032–2044.

Lyons SE, Bruck ME, Bowie EJW, Ginsburg D. (1992) Impaired intracellular transport produced by a subset of type IIA von Willebrand disease mutations. *Journal of Biological Chemistry*, **267**, 4424–4430.

Mancuso DJ, Tuley EA, Castillo R, de Bosch N, Mannucci PM, Sadler JE. (1994) Characterization of partial gene deletions in type III von Willebrand disease with alloantibody inhibitors. *Thrombosis and Haemostasis*, **72**, 180–185.

Mannucci PM, Federici AB. (1995) Antibodies to von Willebrand factor in von Willebrand disease. In: Aledort LM, Hoyer LW, Reisner HM, White II GC (eds). *Inhibitors to Coagulation Factors*. New York: Plenum Press, pp. 87–92.

Mannucci PM, Bloom AL, Larrieu MJ, Nilsson IM, West RR. (1984) Atherosclerosis and von Willebrand factor. I. Prevalence of severe von Willebrand's disease in western Europe and Israel. *British Journal of Haematology*, **57**, 163–169.

Mannucci PM, Lombardi R, Castaman G *et al.* (1988) von Willebrand disease "Vicenza" with larger-than-normal (supranormal) von Willebrand factor multimers. *Blood*, **71**, 65–70.

Mazurier C, Meyer D. (1996) Factor VIII binding assay of von Willebrand factor and the diagnosis of type 2N von Willebrand disease: results of an international survey. *Thrombosis and Haemostasis*, **76**, 270–274.

Meyer D, Fressinaud E, Gaucher C *et al.* (1997) Gene defects in 150 unrelated french cases with Type 2 von Willebrand disease: from patient to the gene. *Thrombosis and Haemostasis*, **78**, 451–456.

Miller CH, Graham JB, Goldin LR, Elston RC. (1979) Genetics of classic von Willebrand's disease. I. Phenotypic variation within families. *Blood*, **54**, 117–136.

Sadler JE, Budde U, Eikenboom JCJ *et al.* (2006) Update on the pathophysiology and classification of von Willebrand disease: a report of the Subcommittee on von Willebrand Factor. *Journal of Thrombosis and Haemostasis*, **4**, 1–12.

Schneppenheim R, Krey S, Bergmann F *et al.* (1994) Genetic heterogeneity of severe von Willebrand disease type III in the German population. *Human Genetics*, **94**, 640–652.

Schneppenheim R, Federici AB, Budde U *et al.* (2000) von Willebrand disease type 2M "Vicenza" in Italian and German patients: identification of the first candidate mutation (G3864A; R1205H) in 8 families. *Thrombosis and Haemostasis*, **83**, 136–140.

Shelton-Inloes BB, Chehab FF, Mannucci PM, Federici AB, Sadler JE. (1987) Gene deletions correlate with the development of alloantibodies in von Willebrand disease. *Journal of Clinical Investigation*, **79**, 1459–1465.

Sutherland JJ, O'Brien LA, Lillicrap D, Weaver DF. (2004) Molecular modeling of the von Willebrand factor A2 domain and the effects of associated type 2A von Willebrand disease mutations. *Journal of Molecular Modeling*, **10**, 259–270.

Zhang ZP, Blombäck M, Egberg N, Falk G, Anvret M. (1994) Characterization of the von Willebrand factor gene (vWF) in von Willebrand disease type III patients from 24 families of Swedish and Finnish origin. *Genomics*, **21**, 188–193.

## Treatment of von Willebrand disease

Bond L, Bevan D. (1988) Myocardial infarction in a patient with hemophilia treated with DDAVP [Letter]. *New England Journal of Medicine*, **318**, 121.

Borel-Derlon A, Federici AB, Roussel-Robert V *et al.* (2007) Treatment of severe von Willebrand disease with a high-purity von Willebrand factor concentrate (Wilfactin): a prospective study of 50 patients. *Journal of Thrombosis and Haemostasis*, **5**, 1115–1124.

Byrnes JJ, Larcada A, Moake JL. (1988) Thrombosis following desmopressin for uremic bleeding. *American Journal of Hematology*, **28**, 63–65.

Castillo R, Escolar G, Monteagudo J, Aznar-Salatti J, Reverter JC, Ordinas A. (1987) Hemostasis in patients with severe von Willebrand disease improves after normal platelet transfusion and normalizes with further correction of the plasma defect. *Transfusion*, **37**, 785–790.

Castillo R, Monteagudo J, Escolar G, Ordinas A, Magallon M, Villar JM. (1991) Hemostatic effect of normal platelet transfusion in severe von Willebrand disease patients. *Blood*, **77**, 1901–1905.

Chang AC, Rick ME, Ross PL, Weinstein MJ. (1998) Summary of a workshop on potency and dosage of von Willebrand factor concentrates. *Haemophilia*, **4** (Suppl 3), 1–6.

Dobrkovska A, Krzensk U, Chediak JR. (1998) Pharmacokinetics, efficacy and safety of Humate-P in von Willebrand disease. *Haemophilia*, **4** (Suppl 3), 33–39.

Favaloro EJ, Dean M, Grispo L, Exner T, Koutts J. (1994) von Willebrand's disease: use of collagen binding assay provides potential improvement to laboratory monitoring of desmopressin (DDAVP) therapy. *American Journal of Hematology*, **45**, 205–211.

Hanna WT, Bona RD, Zimmerman CE, Carta CA, Hebert GZ, Rickles FR. (1994) The use of intermediate and high purity factor VIII products in the treatment of von Willebrand disease. *Thrombosis and Haemostasis*, **71**, 173–179.

Holmberg L, Nilsson IM, Borge L, Gunnarsson M, Sjorin E. (1983) Platelet aggregation induced by 1-desamino-8-D-arginine vasopressin (DDAVP) in type IIB von Willebrand's disease. *New England Journal of Medicine*, **309**, 816–821.

Kaufmann JE, Oksche A, Wollheim CB, Gunther G, Rosenthal W, Vischer UM. (2000) Vasopressin-induced von Willebrand factor secretion from endothelial cells involves V2 receptors and cAMP. *Journal of Clinical Investigation*, **106**, 107–116.

Kohler M, Hellstern P, Wenzel E. (1985) The use of heat-treated Factor VIII-concentrates in von Willebrand's disease. *Blut*, **50**, 25–27.

Kumar RA, Moake JL, Nolasco L *et al.* (2006) Enhanced platelet adhesion and aggregation by endothelial cell-derived unusually large multimers of von Willebrand factor. *Biorheology*, **43**, 681–691.

Lethagen S, Berntorp E, Nilsson IM. (1992) Pharmacokinetics and hemostatic effect of different factor VIII/von Willebrand factor concentrates in vo Willebrand's disease type III. *Annals of Hematology*, **65**, 253–259.

Mannucci PM. (1997) Desmopressin (DDAVP) in the treatment of bleeding disorders: the first 20 years. *Blood*, **90**, 2515–2521.

Mannucci PM. (2005) Use of desmopressin (DDAVP) during early pregnancy in factor VIII-deficient women. *Blood*, **105**, 3382.

Mannucci PM, Ruggeri ZM, Pareti FI, Capitanio A. (1977) 1-Deamino-8-D-Arginine vasopressin: a new pharmacological approach to the management of haemophilia and von Willebrand disease. *Lancet*, **i**, 869–872.

Mannucci PM, Canciani MT, Rota L, Donovan BS. (1981) Response of factor VIII/von Willebrand factor to DDAVP in healthy subjects and patients with haemophilia A and von Willebrand's disease. *British Journal of Haematology*, **47**, 283–293.

Mannucci PM, Bettega D, Cattaneo M. (1992) Consistency of responses to repeated DDAVP infusions in patients with severe vWD and alloantibodies to vWF. *European Journal of Haematology*, **82**, 87–93.

Mannucci PM, Tenconi PM, Castaman G, Rodeghiero F. (1992) Comparison of four virus-inactivated plasma concentrates for treatment of severe von Willebrand disease: a cross-over randomized trial. *Blood*, **79**, 3130–3137.

Mannucci PM, Lattuada A, Ruggeri ZM. (1994) Proteolysis of von Willebrand factor in therapeutic plasma concentrates. *Blood*, **83**, 3018–3027.

Mannucci PM, Chediak J, Hanna W *et al.* (2002) Treatment of von Willebrand disease with a high-purity factor VIII/von Willebrand factor concentrate: a prospective, multicenter study. *Blood*, **99**, 450–456.

Mazurier C, De Romeuf C, Parquet-Gernez A, Goudemand M. (1989) In vitro and in vivo characterization of a high-purity, solvent/detergent-treated factor VIII concentrate: evidence for its therapeutic efficacy in von Willebrand's disease. *European Journal of Haematology*, **43**, 7–14.

Mazurier C, Gaucher C, Jorieux S, Goudeman MatCG. (1994) Biological effect of demopressin in eight patients with type 2N ("Normandy") von Willebrand disease. *British Journal of Haematology*, **88**, 849–854.

Menache D, Aronson DL, Darr F *et al.* (1996) Pharmacokinetics of von Willebrand factor and factor VIIIC in patients with severe von Willebrand disease (type 3 VWD): estimation of the rate of factor VIIIC synthesis. *British Journal of Haematology*, **94**, 740–745.

Pasi KJ, Williams MD, Enayat MS, Hill FGH. (1990) Clinical and laboratory evaluation of the treatment of von Willebrand's disease patients with heat-treated factor VIII concentrate (BPL8Y). *British Journal of Haematology*, **75**, 228–233.

Perkins HA. (1967) Correction of the hemostatic defects in von Willebrand disease. *Blood*, **30**, 375–380.

Rodeghiero F, Castaman G, Meyer D, Mannucci PM. (1992) Replacement therapy with virus-inactivated plasma concentrates in von Willebrand disease. *Vox Sanguinis*, **62**, 193–199.

Siekmann J, Turecek PL, Schwarz HP. (1998) The determination of von Willebrand factor activity by collagen binding assay. *Haemophilia*, **4**, 15–24.

Smith TJ, Gill JC, Ambroso DR, Hathaway WE. (1989) Hyponatremia and seizures in young children given DDAVP. *American Journal of Hematology*, **31**, 199–202.

# Chapter 20 Platelet disorders

## Kenneth J Clemetson

*University of Berne, Theodor Kocher Institute, Berne, Switzerland*

## Introduction

Over the past few decades a large number of disorders caused by genetic mutations in platelet components have been diagnosed at a molecular level. These include defects in platelet receptors, signaling pathways and cytoskeletal proteins. Generally, these were originally detected in bleeding disorders, varying from severe through moderate to mild. Platelets have a major role in hemostasis, particularly primary hemostasis, where platelets adhere to sites of vascular damage, become activated and bind further platelets by aggregation to form a thrombus. The platelet plug formed is then stabilized by secondary hemostasis, which involves coagulation factors that assemble on the surface of the activated platelets, becoming activated in turn and leading to formation of thrombin and cleavage of fibrinogen to form fibrin. Many components have active roles in the overall process, from first platelet contact to stable platelet plug. Most large hospitals see over 100 patients annually with mild to moderate bleeding disorders that are not caused by coagulation factor problems and which can be ascribed to uncharacterized congenital platelet defects. While major defects in known receptors may lead to severe bleeding and are relatively easy to diagnose, others are often very difficult to diagnose at a molecular level and each represents a challenging research project; most remain effectively undiagnosed. However, new methods are beginning to become available, which could make such diagnoses more straightforward. This chapter deals with genetic defects in platelet components that cause human disease. Although these are mostly bleeding disorders, genetic differences leading to an enhanced tendency to thrombosis are increasingly suspected.

## Normal platelet function

Following damage to the endothelium that protects the vascular system, which may simply be caused by loss of "old" endothelial cells due to the high shear stress in the arterial system, platelets adhere to the subendothelium via glycoprotein (GP)Ib on the platelet and von Willebrand factor (VWF) attached to extracellular matrix proteins, particularly collagen (Plate 20.1). This interaction alone is sufficient to start platelet activation, but following initial platelet adhesion other receptors such as the collagen receptor GPVI are recruited. GPVI comes into contact with collagen and signals via its Fcγ subunit to enhance platelet activation and recruit integrins, which increase the binding of adherent platelets and provide attachment for further aggregating platelets. Activation of αIIbβ3 allows platelet–platelet aggregation via ligands such as fibrinogen. Activated platelets release ADP, ATP, serotonin and $Ca^{2+}$ from dense granules and a wide range of proteins from α-granules that contribute to platelet activation and aggregation, including fibrinogen, high-multimer VWF and thrombospondin, as well as growth factors and chemokines that affect endothelial cells and leukocytes involved in wound repair. The major collagen adhesive receptor α2β1 is also activated, increasing platelet adhesion to the exposed collagen of the subendothelium. Both these integrins use disulfide bond reshuffling mechanisms via thiol isomerase to change disulfide bond patterns in the β subunits to control the resting or active state.

Activated platelets also show surface changes, with exposure of negatively charged phospholipids that act, together with surface receptors such as GPIb, to assemble and activate

*Molecular Hematology*, 3rd edition. Edited by Drew Provan and John Gribben.
© 2010 Blackwell Publishing.

coagulation factors, leading to conversion of prothrombin to thrombin. The major effect of thrombin is to convert fibrinogen to fibrin, stabilizing and solidifying the thrombus. However, thrombin also feeds back to platelets via receptors including GPIb and the seven-transmembrane PAR1 and PAR4, activating them further.

# Diagnosis of platelet defects in bleeding disorders

Most patients with clinically relevant platelet defects seek medical assistance because of bleeding problems, ranging from easy or excessive bruising, epistaxis, gingival bleeding, menorrhagia to excessive bleeding following tooth extraction or other surgery. Such patients are normally screened for coagulation defects; if none are detected, examination for platelet problems is the next logical step. Normally, a complete blood count is done to exclude thrombocytopenia and a peripheral blood smear is examined to check platelet morphology. A number of whole-blood techniques are now available to check platelet function including PFA-100 and Impact technologies. These should indicate the presence of a platelet defect and its likely origin. Platelet aggregation tests with a battery of agonists, including ADP, collagen, TRAP (thrombin receptor activation peptide), arachidonic acid, epinephrine and ristocetin, should also help to narrow down which responses are defective. Flow cytometry or Western blotting with specific monoclonal antibodies may be used to check for the absence of receptors or to determine the amounts present. Flow cytometry may also be used to examine the expression of P-selectin or the activation of αIIbβ3 or the exposure of negatively charged phospholipids in response to the classic agonists. All these techniques can provide valuable information in leading to a molecular diagnosis. If a defect can be ascribed to a given platelet molecule, coding regions can be amplified from genomic DNA and sequenced. In rare cases it may also be necessary to sequence non-coding regions to establish a genetic reason for a particular platelet protein deficiency. Regardless of whether a disorder is homozygous or compound heterozygous in recessive disease, or present in only one allele in dominant disease, it is extremely useful to establish the familial inheritance by analyzing DNA from other family members.

# Platelet adhesion disorders

## Bernard–Soulier syndrome

Bernard–Soulier syndrome (BSS) is a rare bleeding disorder caused by defective expression or function of the GPIb–V–IX receptor complex (Figure 20.1). With a few still unclear exceptions, it is inherited in an autosomal recessive way and homozygous cases are often associated with consanguinity. BSS is characterized by thrombocytopenia, giant platelets (up to 20 μm diameter), decreased platelet adhesion, reduced platelet survival, and abnormal prothrombin consumption. BSS platelets do not aggregate in response to ristocetin or botrocetin and show weaker and slower responses to thrombin due to the lack/deficiency of GPIb as thrombin receptor that accelerates responses. As well as interacting with VWF and thrombin, GPIb is a receptor for a wide range of ligands with various physiological roles, including P-selectin, thrombospondin 1, factors XI and XII, αMβ2 and high-molecular-weight kininogen; its absence in BSS may therefore contribute to other aspects of this disorder. Four separate genes, *GPIBA* (chromosome 17), *GPIBB* (chromosome 22), *GP5* and *GP9* (chromosome 3), code for the subunits of the GPIb complex, which are expressed relatively late in megakaryocyte maturation. All four subunits belong to the leucine-rich repeat (LRR) family of proteins, with eight, two, 16 and two repeats present, respectively. GPIbα and GPIbβ are linked covalently via disulfide bonds, probably in a 1:2 ratio, while GPIX and GPV associate non-covalently with GPIb, probably in 1:1 and 2:1 ratios, respectively (Plate 20.2). While GPIbβ and GPIX are certainly critical for the function of the complex, with structural and signaling roles, the function of GPV remains controversial; it has been suggested that it has a role in the thrombin response (it contains a thrombin-binding and cleavage site) as well as in platelet collagen binding.

Mutations and other genetic defects causing BSS have now been collected on a website (http://www.bernardsoulier.org) and will therefore not be listed in detail here. Many of the mutations found to cause BSS lie in the LRR domains and appear to destabilize their folding. The subunits also contain typical disulfide bridge patterns and thus mutation of the constituent cysteines or of other amino acids close to cysteine have deleterious effects on folding, leading to lack of expression of the affected subunit and hence decrease in expression of the rest of the complex.

No cases of BSS due to defects in GPV have been described and mice lacking GPV express GPIb–IX normally. On the other hand, expression of GPIb–IX appears to be essential for stable expression of GPV on platelets, possibly by protecting it from proteolysis. Most mutations in GPIbα either cause folding problems or are nonsense mutations leading to premature termination. Rare BSS variants have been described as having dominant inheritance and lead to expression of non-functional GPIb, although only one allele is affected. The molecular mechanism involved is not understood, although it has been suggested that the defective GPIbα molecule prevents the normal one from functioning. This class of mutation includes Leu57Phe, Leu129Pro,

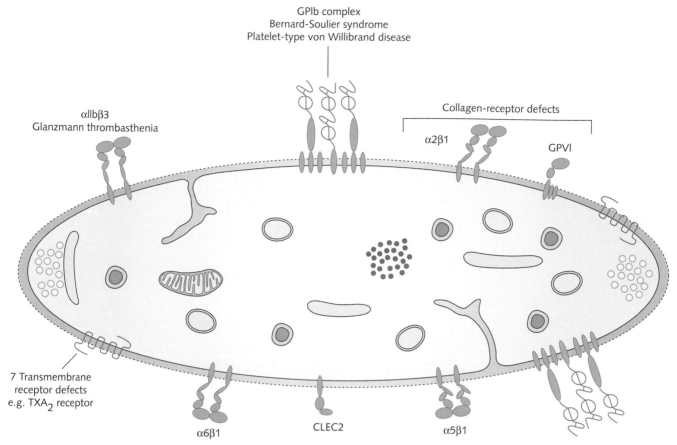

**Fig. 20.1 Diagram of a resting platelet indicating the major receptors implicated in inherited bleeding disorders**

Ala156Val (known as BSS Bolzano) and Leu179del (known as BSS Nancy). Mutations in GPIbβ generally have the same effect as those in GPIbα concerning expression. Mutations in GPIX, while causing many of the classic symptoms of BSS, generally do not produce such a severe phenotype because trace amounts (up to 10%) of functional GPIb are often still expressed, enough to support basic levels of hemostasis if other aspects, such as coagulation factors, are normal. The Asn45Ser mutation in GPIX is the commonest cause of BSS among northern Europeans, accounting for the majority of cases among these populations. Because this mutation generally does not cause such a marked phenotype as many of the GPIbα and GPIbβ mutations, patients have not been easily detected and diagnosis is only now catching up. This mutation has also been found in patients of Turkish origin.

Mice models of BSS have been produced through targeted knockout of GPIbα or GPIbβ but so far not GPIX. The phenotype is essentially the same as in humans. Research on megakaryocytes from these mice indicates that pro-platelet formation and microtubule coil assembly are defective. As noted above, GPV knockout mice do not show

major differences in phenotype using the present selection criteria and, in particular, do not have characteristics of BSS.

## Platelet-type von Willebrand disease

Platelet-type von Willebrand disease (VWD) is an inherited dominant bleeding disorder resembling VWD type IIB but caused by mutations in GPIbα rather than in the A1 domain of VWF (see Figure 20.1 and Plate 20.2). Unlike BSS, platelet-type VWD shows a gain of function, with spontaneous binding of VWF to platelets. In platelet-type VWD, platelets are often enlarged like those in BSS, although the reasons for this are not yet clear. It may be due to enhanced binding of VWF to GPIb, which blocks other GPIb functions. The platelet-type VWD mutations that have been described include Gly233Val/Ser and Met239Val, and a 27-bp deletion in the region of the gene coding for the macroglycopeptide domain of GPIbα has been reported to produce a similar effect. Studies on mutant proteins suggest that similar mutations in other amino acids of the flexible β-loop structure of GPIbα can also produce this phenotype.

## Collagen receptor defects

### α2β1 integrin

A few patients have been reported with bleeding problems related to an α2β1 integrin deficiency, showing defective platelet adhesion to collagen while responses to other agonists were normal. Both patients were female and became normal following the menopause, suggesting a hormonal role in the disorder. Neither α2$^{-/-}$ nor β1$^{-/-}$ mice have major hemostatic problems but defects were reported in aggregation to fibrillar collagen and adhesion to soluble collagen. Differences in occlusion times in thrombosis models in α2$^{-/-}$ or β1$^{-/-}$ mice seem to be dependent on the model used and remain controversial.

### GPVI

Several patients have been described with mild bleeding disorders related to low levels or deficiency of GPVI (Plate 20.3). Most of the defects have not been diagnosed on a molecular level. There are two recent reports of bleeding disorders caused by compound heterozygous mutations in GPVI. One patient with a lifelong history of bleeding problems had structurally normal platelets but a functional platelet defect. Platelet aggregation was normal except for an absent response to collagen, convulxin and the collagen-related peptide. ATP dense granule secretion was normal with ADP but defective with collagen. Thrombus formation on a collagen surface in flowing blood was reduced but more single platelets are attached. PFA-100 analysis showed a shortened collagen/ADP closure time. Flow cytometry showed absence of GPVI expression while immunoblotting showed strongly reduced levels of GPVI. The patient is compound heterozygous for an out-of-frame 16-bp deletion and a missense mutation S175N in a highly conserved residue of the second immunoglobulin-like GPVI domain. The parents, who do not have clinical bleeding problems, are heterozygous carriers. The mother carries the S175N mutation and has a mild platelet functional defect. *In vitro* studies showed reduced membrane expression and convulxin binding in the S175N mutant compared with the wild-type GPVI receptor.

The other patient, a 10-year-old girl, had a tendency to bruising since infancy, a prolonged bleeding time despite a normal platelet count and no antiplatelet antibodies. Collagen-induced platelet activation was null, although there was an incomplete deficiency of GPVI detected by flow cytometry. Immunoblotting showed abnormal residual GPVI, and no FcγR defect. DNA sequencing revealed an R38C mutation in exon 3 of one allele of GPVI and an

insertion of five nucleotides in exon 4 of the other allele, leading to a premature nonsense codon and absence of the corresponding mRNA. Expression of the R38C mutation gave an abnormal protein migration and loss of collagen binding. This composite genetic GPVI defect leads to absence of platelet responses to collagen and a mild bleeding phenotype.

Platelets from GPVI$^{-/-}$ mice do not adhere to collagen under static conditions, probably because the α2β1 integrin is not activated. GPVI is probably important for platelet activation on subendothelium under low-shear conditions. Under high-shear conditions in GPVI$^{-/-}$ mice, α2β1 is probably activated via GPIb/VWF interactions, with VWF bound to collagen. Stable adhesion and spreading are strongly affected in GPVI$^{-/-}$ platelets, indicating that GPVI has an important role in downstream signaling to molecules critical for thrombus formation. Tail bleeding times in GPVI$^{-/-}$ mice are only slightly prolonged compared with wild type. Thrombosis models using both GPVI$^{-/-}$ and Fcγ$^{-/-}$ (the GPVI signaling subunit) mice are controversial because the type of vascular wall damage involved is variable. Thus, laser-induced injuries did not implicate GPVI as a major factor in thrombosis, whereas FeCl$_3$-induced injuries suggested a more substantial role. Other research pointed to thrombin production as a major factor in overcoming GPVI/Fcγ deficiencies in mice thrombosis models. There is a clear need for research involving mouse thrombosis models that are more closely related to human pathology, such as in the presence of fragile vascular plaque, before any definitive conclusions can be reached about collagen receptors in human thrombosis.

## Platelet aggregation defects

### Glanzmann thrombasthenia

Glanzmann thrombasthenia (GT) is an autosomal recessive bleeding disorder caused by defects in the αIIbβ3 integrin or its signaling (see Figure 20.1 and Plate 20.4). If this receptor is absent or defective, it is unable to interact with its ligands, including fibrinogen and VWF but also fibronectin and vitronectin. Thus, platelet aggregates are not formed or are limited in extent, preventing efficient recruitment of platelets to a damaged vessel site. In addition, αIIbβ3–fibrinogen binding has an important role in clot retraction, the process by which wound edges are drawn together to help seal the wound. Thus, GT patients form more scar tissue than normal because wounds tend to reopen. Patients with platelets lacking, or with a severe deficiency (<5% of normal) in, αIIbβ3 are traditionally designated as type I, those with a moderate deficiency (10–50% of normal) as type II, and others as variants. The latter includes patients who express non-functional αIIbβ3 on their platelets. There is a very wide range of molecular defects in αIIb or β3 and as a consequence the clinical symptoms are highly variable. However, even the same defect may show some variability in symptoms in different patients depending on other factors such as levels of coagulation factors. Typical symptoms include purpura, epistaxis, gum bleeding and menorrhagia, but gastrointestinal and interjoint bleeding and hematuria are rare. Problems generally follow trauma and are rarely spontaneous. Diagnostic criteria are prolonged bleeding time and defective clot retraction. Platelet aggregation to all agonists except ristocetin is absent or defective. Molecular diagnosis of GT includes flow cytometry and/or Western blotting to establish whether both subunits are absent or present in reduced amounts.

Mutations and other genetic defects causing GT have now been collected on a database (http://sinaicentral.mssm.edu/intranet/research/glanzmann) and are therefore not listed in detail here. GT can be caused by mutations in either subunit αIIb or β3 and may show some distinct differences. Since fibrinogen is not synthesized in the megakaryocyte but in the liver and transported to the α-granules from the plasma by αIIbβ3-dependent endocytosis, GT patients often lack or are deficient in platelet α-granule fibrinogen, a contributory factor to their poor hemostatic function. In patients lacking β3, who as a consequence lack the vitronectin receptor αvβ3 as well as αIIbβ3, the platelet α-granules, in addition to fibrinogen deficiency, also contain up to five times normal amounts of vitronectin. Vitronectin is synthesized in megakaryocytes so these results suggest a possible role for αvβ3 in transporting vitronectin from α-granules out of platelets. Both αIIb and β3 have a complex gene structure, with the αIIb gene (*ITGA2B*) composed of 30 exons and spanning 17 kb, while the β3 gene (*ITGB3*) consists of 15 exons and spans 46 kb. Both are located on chromosome 17q21–23. Genetic defects are distributed over the entire region.

Mutations/deletions may prevent subunit biosynthesis or transport of precursors from the endoplasmic reticulum to the Golgi or plasma membrane. When mutations do not affect folding too seriously, expression of lower levels of the complex may occur with some functions retained. Several GT mutations lead to expressed dysfunctional receptor. Thus, an Asp119Tyr mutation in β3 affects the key RGD binding site, while Ser752Pro removes a key phosphorylation site involved in outside-in signaling. A stop codon truncating β3 (Arg724tTer), so that only eight of the normal 47 amino acids of the cytoplasmic domain are present, removes binding sites for the cytoskeletal proteins talin and kindlin-2. Cys560Arg and Cys598Tyr mutations in β3 produces

platelets that spontaneously bind fibrinogen because the β3 in their αIIbβ3 has its disulfide bridges blocked in the activated pattern and because the disulfide isomerase activity that normally switches between resting and activated and vice versa is unable to do so. A heterozygous cytoplasmic domain mutation in the αIIb subunit Arg995Gln within the critical GFFKR sequence reduces expression of the complex and produces mild "thrombasthenia-like" symptoms. There is some evidence for cases of GT caused by replacement of DNA segments lying outside coding regions and affecting mRNA stability. A more general syndrome affecting inside-out activation of several classes of integrins present in platelets, neutrophils and lymphocytes has been shown to be due to mutations in the *CalDAG-GEFI* gene, preventing signaling to the small GTPase Rap1.

# Agonist receptor defects

## ADP and ATP receptor defects

Platelets interact with ADP via the purinergic seven-transmembrane receptors P2Y$_1$ and P2Y$_{12}$. P2Y$_1$ signals to release Ca$^{2+}$ from the dense tubular system and cytoskeletal changes leading to shape change. P2Y$_{12}$ signals to αIIbβ3 leading to platelet aggregation. Thus, platelet defects in P2Y$_{12}$ were first thought to be GT variants. Platelets from rare patients in both France and Italy showed decreased and reversible platelet aggregation to ADP but normal shape change and calcium mobilization. This was due to an autosomal recessive hereditary disease affecting one allele of the P2Y$_{12}$ gene. No patients with P2Y$_1$ defects have been described so far but knockout mice lacking this receptor have been prepared. P2X$_1$ is the platelet receptor for ATP. Three molecules form a calcium channel that is regulated when platelets are activated, to control intracellular calcium levels. One case of a young girl with a bleeding syndrome caused by deletion of a single amino acid in P2X$_1$ has been described. That this is a dominant inherited disease is presumably due to the defective molecule preventing the active calcium channel from forming.

## Other primary agonist receptor defects

Rare examples of an Arg60Leu mutation in the thromboxane (TX)A$_2$ receptor have been reported in some Japanese families that result in defective signaling. Mutations in other agonist receptors have been reported but it is not clear that these affect platelet function. In particular, there have been no reports of bleeding disorders linked to defects in the PAR1 and PAR4 thrombin receptors.

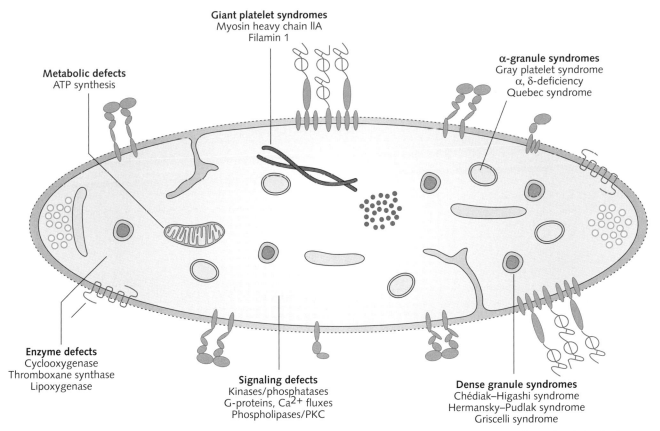

**Giant platelet syndromes**
Myosin heavy chain IIA
Filamin 1

**Metabolic defects**
ATP synthesis

**α-granule syndromes**
Gray platelet syndrome
α, δ-deficiency
Quebec syndrome

**Enzyme defects**
Cyclooxygenase
Thromboxane synthase
Lipoxygenase

**Signaling defects**
Kinases/phosphatases
G-proteins, Ca$^{2+}$ fluxes
Phospholipases/PKC

**Dense granule syndromes**
Chédiak–Higashi syndrome
Hermansky–Pudlak syndrome
Griscelli syndrome

**Fig. 20.2 Diagram of a resting platelet indicating the major internal organelles and other structures implicated in inherited bleeding disorders**

# Defects in intracellular signaling pathways

A wide range of defects in signaling molecules are known, often affecting other cells as well as platelets (Figure 20.2). These include defects in phospholipase C (PLC) activation, calcium mobilization and plekstrin phosphorylation. Studies in one of these patients with impaired PLC activation indicated a decrease only in PLC-β2 while other isoforms were normal. Coding sequence was normal but mRNA for PLC-β2 was decreased, suggesting sequence changes in the gene outside the coding region affecting mRNA stability. Eight patients were described with bleeding problems and abnormal aggregation and secretion in response to several different agonists. Receptor-mediated calcium mobilization and/or plekstrin phosphorylation were abnormal in seven of these patients. Several patients have been reported with platelet cyclooxygenase deficiency, a milder bleeding disorder and impaired platelet aggregation responses. Thromboxane synthase deficiency has been described in two patients. In other patients a deficiency of the PLC-γ2

isoform or a specific decrease in platelet $G_{\alpha q}$ have been reported.

Defects in signaling molecules probably account for many of the undiagnosed patients with mild to moderate bleeding problems. Techniques to diagnose these on a molecular basis are only starting to be developed and even proteomics by itself cannot be expected to detect all of these. There is still a large unmet need here.

# Platelet secretion defects (storage pool disease)

This is a large and heterogeneous group of inherited disorders caused by intracellular defects of platelets (Figure 20.2). Since secretion is a function of many cell types, it is clear that the phenotype may extend beyond hemostasis depending on which molecule is affected.

## Defects of α-granules

Proteins in α-granules are either synthesized in megakaryocytes or endocytosed from plasma. Membranes of α-granules also contains specific receptors, such as P-selectin and CD63, synthesized in megakaryocytes that translocate to the plasma membrane during platelet activation and secretion and are good markers for these processes. Inherited deficiencies of plasma proteins that are taken up into α-granules will be reflected in their content.

### Gray platelet syndrome

Gray platelet syndrome is characterized by the absence of platelet contents and has a mostly autosomal recessive inheritance. Packaging or storage of proteins during platelet production in megakaryocytes is defective and the proteins are directly released from the megakaryocytes. The platelets are often larger than normal and the patients are somewhat thrombocytopenic. Platelet aggregation responses are variously affected and differ between patients. Tissue inhibitors of metalloproteinases (TIMPs) are still present in gray platelet syndrome and may account for some of this variability. The genetic defect underlying gray platelet syndrome has not yet been convincingly described.

### Quebec platelet disorder

As the name implies, this autosomal dominant bleeding disorder was described in this region of Canada. Many α-granule proteins are degraded proteolytically, including membrane receptors such as P-selectin. Defective platelet aggregation is particularly strong with epinephrine as agonist. The problem is caused by overexpression of urokinase plasminogen activator, a protease normally stored in α-granules and released on platelet activation.

## Dense (δ) granule defects

Platelet dense granules are storage sites for a number of small molecules including ADP, ATP, serotonin and calcium. Defects in these granules therefore affect platelet aggregation responses (Figure 20.2). Granule deficiencies are variable and disorders are known in which α-granules are also affected, in which common pathway molecules are defective (αδ-storage pool deficiency). Since similar types of organelles exist in other cells, these are often disorders that affect pigmentation of the skin and hair, such as Hermansky–Pudlak, Chédiak–Higashi and Griscelli syndromes. Mouse models exist for several of these.

### Hermansky–Pudlak syndrome

Hermansky–Pudlak syndrome manifests as albinism and absence of ceroid-lipofuscin storage in the reticuloendothelial system. The syndrome is common in Puerto Rico and is caused by a frameshift due to a 16-bp duplication in exon 15 of the *HPS-1* gene, which normally encodes a 79-kDa protein with two membrane-spanning domains. Defects in at least eight genes cause distinct subtypes of Hermansky–Pudlak syndrome in humans.

### Chédiak–Higashi syndrome

Severe immunological defects and progressive neurological dysfunction accompany bleeding problems. The major diagnostic criterion is the presence of giant inclusion bodies in a variety of cells with granules, including platelets. The gene responsible (*LYST*) has been cloned and a series of frameshift and nonsense mutations identified that produce a truncated LYST protein. A milder form of the disease is thought to be due to rare missense mutations. LYST protein is large and complex with domains suggesting that it regulates organelle protein trafficking and membrane–membrane interactions.

### Griscelli syndrome

Patients with Griscelli syndrome are partially albino with silver hair. Neurological defects and/or immunodeficiency are linked to lymphocyte cytotoxicity defects. Clinical manifestations include fatal complications caused by lymphoid cell activation and cytokine release. Griscelli syndrome is associated with mutations in the genes for myosin Va, Rab27a (a small GTPase) or melanophilin. A mouse model for this disease has recently been characterized with a mutation in Rab27a, a variant of the ashen mouse with a phenotype resembling Hermansky–Pudlak syndrome. Rab27a deficiency in humans was identified in a young patient with psychomotor retardation. The patient's platelets lacked dense granules but had normal α-granules; epinephrine-induced aggregation was defective.

## Wiskott–Aldrich syndrome

Platelets in Wiskott–Aldrich syndrome (WAS) aggregate poorly and have few granules. This is an X-linked recessive disease characterized by thrombocytopenia, small platelets, eczema, immunodeficiency and increased autoimmunity and malignancy problems. Hereditary X-linked thrombocytopenia is a milder form lacking the immune problems. T lymphocytes are the other major blood cells affected. The 502-amino-acid WAS protein is encoded by the large *WAS* gene, which consists of 12 exons. Mutations in exons 1 and 2 mostly lead to the mild form. WAS protein regulates actin polymerization in hematopoietic cells and its deficiency leads to premature proplatelet formation in the bone marrow.

## Procoagulant regulation defects

### Scott syndrome

Scott syndrome is a very rare disorder found in a few humans and some dogs. So far there is no mouse model. When normal platelets are activated, one of the changes produced is the exposure of negatively charged phospholipids on the surface, critical for procoagulant activity. This is absent in Scott syndrome platelets and as a consequence less thrombin and fibrin are formed in the platelet plug, leading to bleeding complications. This defect also affects membrane vesiculation, suggesting a common mechanism. Under *in vitro* conditions, this phenomenon requires platelet activation by thrombin and collagen (or a GPVI agonist such as convulxin or collagen-related peptide). Despite much research on platelet scramblases, a convincing molecular defect in Scott syndrome has not yet been demonstrated.

### Stormorken syndrome

Stormorken syndrome is an even rarer disorder confined so far to one family, implying a dominant inheritance. Unlike Scott syndrome, the platelets are constitutively activated with surface exposure of negatively charged phospholipids and raised levels of microvesicles even under resting conditions. As with Scott syndrome the molecular basis remains unknown.

## Giant platelet syndromes and cytoskeletal defects

Although this group is diverse, many of the patients have mutations or other defects in the *MYH9* gene coding for non-muscle myosin heavy chain IIA (see Plate 20.2 and Figure 20.2). Since this is expressed in a variety of cells, not only platelets are affected. Macrothrombocytopenia (variable, up to leukocyte size) is accompanied by variable phenotypes in other cells/tissues. Döhle bodies in leukocytes with distinctive distribution of myosin IIA detected by immunofluorescence is a major diagnostic criterion. Hearing loss caused by defective cilia, nephritis and cataracts are all possible symptoms in later life. Characteristic mutation zones in the protein seem linked to particular symptoms: mutations in the head reagion can affect folding of the entire molecule and can yield more serious symptoms, whereas mutations toward the C-terminus have less dramatic effects possibly because function is partly maintained and there is less tendency to form denatured protein clusters. While non-muscle myosin has an important role in many cells/

tissues, the presence of the IIB and IIC forms may compensate in some of these.

Giant platelets have also been reported in patients with mutations in the *FLNA* gene coding for filamin A. As well as platelets, neuronal migration was abnormal in these patients. In platelets, filamin A is a major attachment site for the GPIb complex, stabilizing the connection between the membrane and the cytoskeleton, and anchoring GPIb in platelets when they attach during adhesion under high shear. Myosin IIA may play a role in this process as well providing a rationale for the giant platelets in these disorders as well as BSS. It is important to distinguish these large platelet syndromes (including BSS), particularly when accompanied by thrombocytopenia, from idiopathic thrombocytopenic purpura and to avoid treatments such as splenectomy, which are not useful in these disorders.

## Transcription factor defects

Autosomal dominant Paris–Trousseau syndrome is a typical example of this class of disorder, with decreased platelet production and a mild bleeding tendency associated with a deletion at 11q23. Platelets are often larger than normal with giant α-granules. The defect leads to a hemizygous loss of the *FLI1* gene coding for Fli1 transcription factor. A subpopulation of megakaryocyte precursors fails to mature adequately to produce platelets. Other disorders including thrombocytopenia are caused by mutations in the *GATA-1* gene. Platelets may be larger than normal with poor response to collagen. The phenotype depends on whether the mutations affect GATA-1 interactions with DNA or FOG-1. GATA-1-dependent platelet molecules include members of the GPIb complex and α-granule components. Defects in RUNX1 lead to platelets with a deficiency in protein kinase C-θ and lack of phosphorylation of its downstream targets but also an increased tendency to develop leukemia.

## Platelet protein polymorphisms and tendency to thrombosis

Platelet activation responses vary widely in the population but are reproducible for individuals and show a strong genetic component. Following the demonstration of major polymorphisms in coagulation factors affecting thrombotic tendencies, there has been a major effort to identify polymorphisms in platelet proteins such as receptors that could explain the interindividual variation. There is also considerable interest in polymorphisms that affect patient responses to antithrombotic treatments because this could be an important way to improve treatment and reduce mortality.

Common polymorphisms in αIIbβ3 were among the first targets for statistical investigation. Each of the subunits contains a common amino acid dimorphism: β3 has two isoforms, Leu33/Pro33, that lead to conformational differences in the proteins; the Ile843/Ser843 dimorphism in αIIb has also been intensively investigated. Most of the studies were controversial, with only minor effects detected.

The situation in GPIbα is more complicated, with two major polymorphic systems present: (i) a Thr145/Met145 dimorphism and (ii) several versions of a tandem repeat structure of 13 amino acids within the macroglycopeptide domain; these have the nomenclature VLTR-A, -B, -C and -D with four, three, two and one copies, respectively, of the tandem repeat. The incidence varies widely depending on ethnic origins between Europe and East Asia. Again there has been no consensus reached about a role in thrombosis susceptibility and many studies have given contradictory results. Polymorphisms in collagen receptors α2β1 and GPVI have also been implicated in thrombosis susceptibility but these studies still remain controversial.

Perhaps if one considers that many individual genetic differences may contribute to the overall thrombosis susceptibility, it is not so surprising that these single differences do not have more pronounced effects. However, several newly discovered polymorphisms, particularly in signaling molecules, are still under investigation.

One area which is less controversial is the effect of cytochrome P450 polymorphisms on activation of clopidogrel and therefore on its ability to inhibit the ADP receptor P2Y$_{12}$. Among persons treated with clopidogrel, carriers of a reduced-function *CYP2C19* allele had significantly lower levels of the active metabolite of clopidogrel, diminished platelet inhibition, and a higher rate of major adverse cardiovascular events, including stent thrombosis, than did non-carriers.

## Further reading

### Overview of platelet function

Clemetson KJ. (2007) A short history of platelet glycoprotein Ib complex. *Thrombosis and Haemostasis*, **98**, 63–68.

Clemetson KJ, Clemetson JM. (2001) Platelet collagen receptors. *Thrombosis and Haemostasis*, **86**, 189–197.

Coller BS, Shattil SJ. (2008) The GPIIb/IIIa (integrin alphaIIbbeta3) odyssey: a technology-driven saga of a receptor with twists, turns, and even a bend. *Blood*, **112**, 3011–3025.

Farndale RW, Slatter DA, Siljander PR, Jarvis GE. (2007) Platelet receptor recognition and cross-talk in collagen-induced activation of platelets. *Journal of Thrombosis and Haemostasis*, **5**, 220–229.

Hartwig JH, Italiano JE Jr. (2006) Cytoskeletal mechanisms for platelet production. *Blood Cells, Molecules and Diseases*, **36**, 99–103.

Jackson SP. (2007) The growing complexity of platelet aggregation. *Blood*, **109**, 5087–5095.

Lau TL, Kim C, Ginsberg MH, Ulmer TS. (2009) The structure of the integrin αIIbβ3 transmembrane complex explains integrin transmembrane signalling. *EMBO Journal*, **28**, 1351–1361.

Ozaki Y, Asazuma N, Suzuki-Inoue K, Berndt MC. (2005) Platelet GPIb-IX-V-dependent signaling. *Journal of Thrombosis and Haemostasis*, **3**, 1745–1751.

Plow EF, Qin J, Byzova T. (2009) Kindling the flame of integrin activation and function with kindlins. *Current Opinion in Hematology*, **16**, 323–328.

Prevost N, Woulfe D, Tognolini M, Brass LF. (2003) Contact-dependent signaling during the late events of platelet activation. *Journal of Thrombosis and Haemostasis*, **1**, 1613–1627.

Ren Q, Ye S, Whiteheart SW. (2008) The platelet release reaction: just when you thought platelet secretion was simple. *Current Opinion in Hematology*, **15**, 537–541.

Rivera J, Lozano ML, Navarro-Nunez L, Vicente V. (2009) Platelet receptors and signaling in the dynamics of thrombus formation. *Haematologica*, **94**, 700–711.

Ruggeri ZM, Mendolicchio GL. (2007) Adhesion mechanisms in platelet function. *Circulation Research*, **100**, 1673–1685.

### Laboratory assessment of platelet disorders

Harrison P. (2009) Assessment of platelet function in the laboratory. *Hamostaseologie*, **29**, 25–31.

Hayward CP, Favaloro EJ. (2009) Diagnostic evaluation of platelet disorders: the past, the present, and the future. *Seminars in Thrombosis and Hemostasis*, **35**, 127–130.

### Overview of inherited platelet disorders

Lanza F. (2007) [Murine models of platelet diseases.] *Transfusion Clinique et Biologique*, **14**, 35–40.

Nurden P, Nurden AT. (2008) Congenital disorders associated with platelet dysfunctions. *Thrombosis and Haemostasis*, **99**, 253–263.

Rao AK, Jalagadugula G, Sun L. (2004) Inherited defects in platelet signaling mechanisms. *Seminars in Thrombosis and Hemostasis*, **30**, 525–535.

Salles II, Feys HB, Iserbyt BF, De Meyer SF, Vanhoorelbeke K, Deckmyn H. (2008) Inherited traits affecting platelet function. *Blood Reviews*, **22**, 155–172.

### Bernard–Soulier syndrome

#### Overview

Dumas JJ, Kumar R, McDonagh T *et al.* (2004) Crystal structure of the wild-type von Willebrand factor A1–glycoprotein Ibα complex reveals conformation differences with a complex bearing von Willebrand disease mutations. *Journal of Biological Chemistry*, **279**, 23327–23334.

Lanza F. (2006) Bernard–Soulier syndrome (hemorrhagiparous thrombocytic dystrophy). *Orphanet Journal of Rare Diseases*, **1**, 46.

Pham A, Wang J. (2007) Bernard–Soulier syndrome: an inherited platelet disorder. *Archives of Pathology and Laboratory Medicine*, **131**, 1834–1836.

Uff S, Clemetson JM, Harrison T, Clemetson KJ, Emsley J. (2002) Crystal structure of the platelet glycoprotein Ibα N-terminal domain reveals an unmasking mechanism for receptor activation. *Journal of Biological Chemistry*, **277**, 35657–35663.

### New GPIbα mutations

Imai C, Kunishima S, Takachi T *et al.* (2009) A novel homozygous 8-base pair deletion mutation in the glycoprotein Ibα gene in a patient with Bernard–Soulier syndrome. *Blood Coagulation and Fibrinolysis*, **20**, 470–474.

Rosenberg N, Lalezari S, Landau M, Shenkman B, Seligsohn U, Izraeli S. (2007) Trp207Gly in platelet glycoprotein Ibα is a novel mutation that disrupts the connection between the leucine-rich repeat domain and the disulfide loop structure and causes Bernard–Soulier syndrome. *Journal of Thrombosis and Haemostasis*, **5**, 378–386.

Vettore S, Scandellari R, Moro S *et al.* (2008) Novel point mutation in a leucine-rich repeat of the GPIbα chain of the platelet von Willebrand factor receptor, GPIb/IX/V, resulting in an inherited dominant form of Bernard–Soulier syndrome affecting two unrelated families: the N41H variant. *Haematologica*, **93**, 1743–1747.

### New GPIbβ mutations

Hadjkacem B, Elleuch H, Gargouri J, Gargouri A. (2009) Bernard–Soulier syndrome: novel nonsense mutation in GPIbα gene affecting GPIb–IX complex expression. *Annals of Hematology*, **88**, 465–472.

### Velocardiofacial syndrome

Liang HP, Morel-Kopp MC, Curtin J *et al.* (2007) Heterozygous loss of platelet glycoprotein (GP)Ib-V-IX variably affects platelet function in velocardiofacial syndrome (VCFS) patients. *Thrombosis and Haemostasis*, **98**, 1298–1308.

### New GPIX mutations

Kunishima S, Yamada T, Hamaguchi M, Saito H. (2006) Bernard–Soulier syndrome due to GPIX W127X mutation in Japan is frequently misdiagnosed as idiopathic thrombocytopenic purpura. *International Journal of Hematology*, **83**, 366–367.

### Variant forms

Balduini A, Malara A, Pecci A *et al.* (2009) Proplatelet formation in heterozygous Bernard–Soulier syndrome type Bolzano. *Journal of Thrombosis and Haemostasis*, **7**, 478–484.

Vettore S, Scandellari R, Scapin M *et al.* (2008) A case of Bernard–Soulier syndrome due to a homozygous four bases deletion (TGAG) of GPIbα gene: lack of GPIbα but absence of bleeding. *Platelets*, **19**, 388–391.

## Platelet-type von Willebrand disease

Matsubara Y, Murata M, Sugita K, Ikeda Y. (2003) Identification of a novel point mutation in platelet glycoprotein Ibα Gly to Ser at residue 233, in a Japanese family with platelet-type von Willebrand disease. *Journal of Thrombosis and Haemostasis*, **1**, 2198–2205.

Nurden P, Lanza F, Bonnafous-Faurie C, Nurden A. (2007) A second report of platelet-type von Willebrand disease with a Gly233Ser mutation in the GPIBA gene. *Thrombosis and Haemostasis*, **97**, 319–321.

Othman M, Notley C, Lavender FL *et al.* (2005) Identification and functional characterization of a novel 27-bp deletion in the macro-glycopeptide-coding region of the GPIBA gene resulting in platelet-type von Willebrand disease. *Blood*, **105**, 4330–4336.

Suva LJ, Hartman E, Dilley JD *et al.* (2008) Platelet dysfunction and a high bone mass phenotype in a murine model of platelet-type von Willebrand disease. *American Journal of Pathology*, **172**, 430–439.

## Collagen receptor defects

### α2β1 integrin

Joutsi-Korhonen L, Smethurst PA, Rankin A *et al.* (2003) The low-frequency allele of the platelet collagen signaling receptor glycoprotein VI is associated with reduced functional responses and expression. *Blood*, **101**, 4372–4379.

Sarratt KL, Chen H, Zutter MM, Santoro SA, Hammer DA, Kahn ML. (2005) GPVI and α2β1 play independent critical roles during platelet adhesion and aggregate formation to collagen under flow. *Blood*, **106**, 1268–1277.

### GPVI

Arthur JF, Dunkley S, Andrews RK. (2007) Platelet glycoprotein VI-related clinical defects. *British Journal of Haematology*, **139**, 363–372.

Dumont B, Lasne D, Rothschild C *et al.* (2009) Absence of collagen-induced platelet activation caused by compound heterozygous GPVI mutations. *Blood*, **114**, 1900–1903.

Hermans C, Wittevrongel C, Thys C, Smethurst PA, Van Geet C, Freson K. (2009) A compound heterozygous mutation in glycoprotein VI in a patient with a bleeding disorder. *Journal of Thrombosis and Haemostasis*, **7**, 1356–1363.

Hughan SC, Senis Y, Best D *et al.* (2005) Selective impairment of platelet activation to collagen in the absence of GATA1. *Blood*, **105**, 4369–4376.

## Glanzmann thrombasthenia

### Overview

Fang J, Hodivala-Dilke K, Johnson BD *et al.* (2005) Therapeutic expression of the platelet-specific integrin, αIIbβ3, in a murine model for Glanzmann thrombasthenia. *Blood*, **106**, 2671–2679.

French DL. (1998) The molecular genetics of Glanzmann's thrombasthenia. *Platelets*, **9**, 5–20.

Jayandharan G, Nelson EJ, Baidya S, Chandy M, Srivastava A. (2007) A new multiplex PCR and conformation-sensitive gel electrophoresis strategy for mutation detection in the platelet glycoprotein αIIb and β3 genes. *Journal of Thrombosis and Haemostasis*, **5**, 206–209.

Manickam N, Sun X, Li M, Gazitt Y, Essex DW. (2008) Protein disulphide isomerase in platelet function. *British Journal of Haematology*, **140**, 223–229.

### αIIb defects

Losonczy G, Rosenberg N, Boda Z *et al.* (2007) Three novel mutations in the glycoprotein IIb gene in a patient with type II Glanzmann thrombasthenia. *Haematologica*, **92**, 698–701.

Vijapurkar M, Ghosh K, Shetty S. (2009) Novel mutations in GPIIb gene in Glanzmann's thrombasthenia from India. *Platelets*, **20**, 35–40.

### β3 defects

Chen P, Melchior C, Brons NH, Schlegel N, Caen J, Kieffer N. (2001) Probing conformational changes in the I-like domain and the cysteine-rich repeat of human α3 integrins following disulfide bond disruption by cysteine mutations: identification of cysteine 598 involved in αIIbβ3 activation. *Journal of Biological Chemistry*, **276**, 38628–38635.

D'Andrea G, Bafunno V, Del Vecchio L *et al.* (2008) A α3 Asp217αVal substitution in a patient with variant Glanzmann thrombasthenia severely affects integrin αIIbβ3 functions. *Blood Coagulation and Fibrinolysis*, **19**, 657–662.

Gonzalez-Manchon C, Butta N, Larrucea S *et al.* (2004) A variant thrombasthenic phenotype associated with compound heterozygosity of integrin α3-subunit: (Met124Val)α3 alters the subunit dimerization rendering a decreased number of constitutive active αIIbβ3 receptors. *Thrombosis and Haemostasis*, **92**, 1377–1386.

Liu J, Jackson CW, Gruppo RA, Jennings LK, Gartner TK. (2005) The α3 subunit of the integrin αIIbβ3 regulates αIIb-mediated outside-in signaling. *Blood*, **105**, 4345–4352.

Mor-Cohen R, Rosenberg N, Peretz H *et al.* (2007) Disulfide bond disruption by a α3-Cys549Arg mutation in six Jordanian families with Glanzmann thrombasthenia causes diminished production of constitutively active αIIbβ3. *Thrombosis and Haemostasis*, **98**, 1257–1265.

Nurden P, Poujol C, Winckler J, Combrie R, Caen JP, Nurden AT. (2002) A Ser752βPro substitution in the cytoplasmic domain of α3 in a Glanzmann thrombasthenia variant fails to prevent interactions between the αIIbβ3 integrin and the platelet granule pool of fibrinogen. *British Journal of Haematology*, **118**, 1143–1151.

Ruiz C, Liu CY, Sun QH *et al.* (2001) A point mutation in the cysteine-rich domain of glycoprotein (GP) IIIa results in the expression of a GPIIb-IIIa (αIIbβ3) integrin receptor locked in a high-affinity state and a Glanzmann thrombasthenia-like phenotype. *Blood*, **98**, 2432–2441.

Wang R, Shattil SJ, Ambruso DR, Newman PJ. (1997) Truncation of the cytoplasmic domain of α3 in a variant form of Glanzmann thrombasthenia abrogates signaling through the integrin αIIbβ3 complex. *Journal of Clinical Investigation*, **100**, 2393–2403.

### Other

Pasvolsky R, Feigelson SW, Kilic SS *et al.* (2007) A LAD-III syndrome is associated with defective expression of the Rap-1 activator CalDAG-GEFI in lymphocytes, neutrophils, and platelets. *Journal of Experimental Medicine*, **204**, 1571–1582.

### ADP and ATP receptor defects

Cattaneo M. (2006) Disorders of platelet function. Abnormalities of the platelet P2 receptors. *Pathophysiology of Haemostasis and Thrombosis*, **35**, 10–14.

Daly ME, Dawood BB, Lester WA *et al.* (2009) Identification and characterization of a novel P2Y$_{12}$ variant in a patient diagnosed with type 1 von Willebrand disease in the European MCMDM-1VWD study. *Blood*, **113**, 4110–4113.

Leon C, Hechler B, Freund M *et al.* (1999) Defective platelet aggregation and increased resistance to thrombosis in purinergic P2Y$_1$ receptor-null mice. *Journal of Clinical Investigation*, **104**, 1731–1737.

Oury C, Toth-Zamboki E, Vermylen J, Hoylaerts MF. (2002) Does the P2X$_1$del variant lacking 17 amino acids in its extracellular domain represent a relevant functional ion channel in platelets? *Blood*, **99**, 2275–2277.

Oury C, Toth-Zamboki E, Vermylen J, Hoylaerts MF. (2006) The platelet ATP and ADP receptors. *Current Pharmaceutical Design*, **12**, 859–875.

Remijn JA, Ijsseldijk MJ, Strunk AL *et al.* (2007) Novel molecular defect in the platelet ADP receptor P2Y$_{12}$ of a patient with haemorrhagic diathesis. *Clinical Chemistry and Laboratory Medicine*, **45**, 187–189.

### Other primary agonist receptor defects

Hirata T, Kakizuka A, Ushikubi F, Fuse I, Okuma M, Narumiya S. (1994) Arg$^{60}$ to Leu mutation of the human thromboxane A$_2$ receptor in a dominantly inherited bleeding disorder. *Journal of Clinical Investigation*, **94**, 1662–1667.

### Intracellular signaling pathway defects

Bellucci S, Huisse MG, Boval B *et al.* (2005) Defective collagen-induced platelet activation in two patients with malignant haemopathies is related to a defect in the GPVI-coupled signalling pathway. *Thrombosis and Haemostasis*, **93**, 130–138.

Dunkley S, Arthur JF, Evans S, Gardiner EE, Shen Y, Andrews RK. (2007) A familial platelet function disorder associated with abnormal signalling through the glycoprotein VI pathway. *British Journal of Haematology*, **137**, 569–577.

Mao GF, Vaidyula VR, Kunapuli SP, Rao AK. (2002) Lineage-specific defect in gene expression in human platelet phospholipase C-α2 deficiency. *Blood*, **99**, 905–911.

Patel YM, Patel K, Rahman S *et al.* (2003) Evidence for a role for Gαi1 in mediating weak agonist-induced platelet aggregation in human platelets: reduced Gαi1 expression and defective Gi signaling in the platelets of a patient with a chronic bleeding disorder. *Blood*, **101**, 4828–4835.

### Platelet secretion defects (storage pool disease)

#### Gray platelet syndrome

Drouin A, Favier R, Masse JM *et al.* (2001) Newly recognized cellular abnormalities in the gray platelet syndrome. *Blood*, **98**, 1382–1391.

Nurden AT, Nurden P. (2007) The gray platelet syndrome: clinical spectrum of the disease. *Blood Reviews*, **21**, 21–36.

Nurden P, Jandrot-Perrus M, Combrie R *et al.* (2004) Severe deficiency of glycoprotein VI in a patient with gray platelet syndrome. *Blood*, **104**, 107–114.

## Quebec platelet disorder

Diamandis M, Veljkovic DK, Maurer-Spurej E, Rivard GE, Hayward CP. (2008) Quebec platelet disorder: features, pathogenesis and treatment. *Blood Coagulation and Fibrinolysis*, **19**, 109–119.

Veljkovic DK, Rivard GE, Diamandis M, Blavignac J, Cramer-Borde EM, Hayward CP. (2009) Increased expression of urokinase plasminogen activator in Quebec platelet disorder is linked to megakaryocyte differentiation. *Blood*, **113**, 1535–1542.

## Hermansky–Pudlak syndrome

Gautam R, Novak EK, Tan J, Wakamatsu K, Ito S, Swank RT. (2006) Interaction of Hermansky–Pudlak syndrome genes in the regulation of lysosome-related organelles. *Traffic*, **7**, 779–792.

Huizing M, Parkes JM, Helip-Wooley A, White JG, Gahl WA. (2007) Platelet α-granules in BLOC-2 and BLOC-3 subtypes of Hermansky–Pudlak syndrome. *Platelets*, **18**, 150–157.

Spritz RA. (1998) Molecular genetics of the Hermansky–Pudlak and Chediak–Higashi syndromes. *Platelets*, **9**, 21–29.

Walker M, Payne J, Wagner B, Vora A. (2007) Hermansky–Pudlak syndrome. *British Journal of Haematology*, **138**, 671.

## Chédiak–Higashi syndrome

Kaplan J, De Domenico I, Ward DM. (2008) Chediak–Higashi syndrome. *Current Opinion in Hematology*, **15**, 22–29.

Nagle DL, Karim MA, Woolf EA *et al.* (1996) Identification and mutation analysis of the complete gene for Chediak–Higashi syndrome. *Nature Genetics*, **14**, 307–311.

Westbroek W, Adams D, Huizing M *et al.* (2007) Cellular defects in Chediak–Higashi syndrome correlate with the molecular genotype and clinical phenotype. *Journal of Investigative Dermatology*, **127**, 2674–2677.

## Griscelli syndrome

Barral DC, Ramalho JS, Anders R *et al.* (2002) Functional redundancy of Rab27 proteins and the pathogenesis of Griscelli syndrome. *Journal of Clinical Investigation*, **110**, 247–257.

Novak EK, Gautam R, Reddington M *et al.* (2002) The regulation of platelet-dense granules by Rab27a in the ashen mouse, a model of Hermansky–Pudlak and Griscelli syndromes, is granule-specific and dependent on genetic background. *Blood*, **100**, 128–135.

## Wiskott–Aldrich syndrome

Imai K, Nonoyama S, Ochs HD. (2003) WASP (Wiskott–Aldrich syndrome protein) gene mutations and phenotype. *Current Opinion in Allergy and Clinical Immunology*, **3**, 427–436.

Lutskiy MI, Shcherbina A, Bachli ET, Cooley J, Remold-O'Donnell E. (2007) WASP localizes to the membrane skeleton of platelets. *British Journal of Haematology*, **139**, 98–105.

Ochs HD, Filipovich AH, Veys P, Cowan MJ, Kapoor N. (2008) Wiskott–Aldrich syndrome: diagnosis, clinical and laboratory manifestations, and treatment. *Biology of Blood and Marrow Transplantation*, **15** (1 Suppl), 84–90.

Sabri S, Foudi A, Boukour S *et al.* (2006) Deficiency in the Wiskott–Aldrich protein induces premature proplatelet formation and platelet production in the bone marrow compartment. *Blood*, **108**, 134–140.

## Procoagulant regulation defects

Solum NO. (1999) Procoagulant expression in platelets and defects leading to clinical disorders. *Arteriosclerosis, Thrombosis and Vascular Biology*, **19**, 2841–2846.

Weiss HJ. (2009) Impaired platelet procoagulant mechanisms in patients with bleeding disorders. *Seminars in Thrombosis and Hemostasis*, **35**, 233–241.

## Scott syndrome

Bettache N, Gaffet P, Allegre N *et al.* (1998) Impaired redistribution of aminophospholipids with distinctive cell shape change during $Ca^{2+}$-induced activation of platelets from a patient with Scott syndrome. *British Journal of Haematology*, **101**, 50–58.

Zwaal RF, Comfurius P, Bevers EM. (2004) Scott syndrome, a bleeding disorder caused by defective scrambling of membrane phospholipids. *Biochimica Biophysica Acta*, **1636**, 119–128.

## Stormorken syndrome

Stormorken H, Holmsen H, Sund R *et al.* (1995) Studies on the haemostatic defect in a complicated syndrome. An inverse Scott syndrome platelet membrane abnormality? *Thrombosis and Haemostasis*, **74**, 1244–1251.

## Giant platelet syndromes and cytoskeletal defects

Althaus K, Greinacher A. (2009) MYH9-related platelet disorders. *Seminars in Thrombosis and Hemostasis*, **35**, 189–203.

Chen Z, Shivdasani RA. (2009) Regulation of platelet biogenesis: insights from the May-Hegglin anomaly and other MYH9-related disorders. *Journal of Thrombosis and Haemostasis*, **7**, 272–276.

Leon C, Eckly A, Hechler B *et al.* (2007) Megakaryocyte-restricted MYH9 inactivation dramatically affects hemostasis while preserving platelet aggregation and secretion. *Blood*, **110**, 3183–3191.

Nurden AT, Federici AB, Nurden P. (2009) Altered megakaryocytopoiesis in von Willebrand type 2B disease. *Journal of Thrombosis and Haemostasis*, **7**, 277–281.

Provaznikova D, Geierova V, Kumstyrova T *et al.* (2009) Clinical manifestation and molecular genetic characterization of MYH9 disorders. *Platelets*, **26**, 1–8.

Saito H, Matsushita T, Yamamoto K, Kojima T, Kunishima S. (2005) Giant platelet syndrome. *Hematology*, **10**, 41–46.

Toren A, Rozenfeld-Granot G, Heath KE *et al.* (2003) MYH9 spectrum of autosomal-dominant giant platelet syndromes: unexpected association with fibulin-1 variant-D inactivation. *American Journal of Hematology*, **74**, 254–262.

White JG. (2007) Platelet pathology in carriers of the X-linked GATA-1 macrothrombocytopenia. *Platelets*, **18**, 620–627.

## Transcription factor defects

Breton-Gorius J, Favier R, Guichard J *et al.* (1995) A new congenital dysmegakaryopoietic thrombocytopenia (Paris–Trousseau) associated with giant platelet α-granules and chromosome 11 deletion at 11q23. *Blood*, **85**, 1805–1814.

Escher R, Wilson P, Carmichael C *et al.* (2007) A pedigree with autosomal dominant thrombocytopenia, red cell macrocytosis, and an occurrence of t(12:21) positive pre-B acute lymphoblastic leukemia. *Blood Cells, Molecules and Diseases*, **39**, 107–114.

Freson K, Devriendt K, Matthijs G *et al.* (2001) Platelet characteristics in patients with X-linked macrothrombocytopenia because of a novel GATA1 mutation. *Blood*, **98**, 85–92.

Sun L, Gorospe JR, Hoffman EP, Rao AK. (2007) Decreased platelet expression of myosin regulatory light chain polypeptide (MYL9) and other genes with platelet dysfunction and CBFA2/RUNX1 mutation: insights from platelet expression profiling. *Journal of Thrombosis and Haemostasis*, **5**, 146–154.

White JG. (2007) Platelet pathology in carriers of the X-linked GATA-1 macrothrombocytopenia. *Platelets*, **18**, 620–627.

## Platelet protein polymorphisms and tendency to thrombosis

Jones CI, Bray S, Garner SF *et al.* (2009) A functional genomics approach reveals novel quantitative trait loci associated with platelet signalling pathways. *Blood*, **114**, 1405–1416.

Martini CH, Doggen CJ, Cavallini C, Rosendaal FR, Mannucci PM. (2005) No effect of polymorphisms in prothrombotic genes on the risk of myocardial infarction in young adults without cardiovascular risk factors. *Journal of Thrombosis and Haemostasis*, **3**, 177–179.

Mega JL, Close SL, Wiviott SD *et al.* (2009) Cytochrome P-450 polymorphisms and response to clopidogrel. *New England Journal of Medicine*, **360**, 354–362.

Meisel C, Lopez JA, Stangl K. (2004) Role of platelet glycoprotein polymorphisms in cardiovascular diseases. *Naunyn Schmiedebergs Archives of Pharmacology*, **369**, 38–54.

Ouwehand WH. (2007) Platelet genomics and the risk of atherothrombosis. *Journal of Thrombosis and Haemostasis*, **5**, 188–195.

Ouwehand WH. (2009) The discovery of genes implicated in myocardial infarction. *Journal of Thrombosis and Haemostasis*, **7**, 305–307.

# Chapter 21 The molecular basis of blood cell alloantigens

## Willem H Ouwehand[1] & Cristina Navarrete[2]

[1] Department of Haematology, University of Cambridge, Cambridge, UK
[2] NHS Blood and Transplant, London; and Department of Immunology and Molecular Pathology, University College London, London, UK

## Introduction

The transfusion of blood and fetal–maternal hemorrhage during pregnancy have provided unique models for studying the immune response against a plethora of polymorphic blood cell surface markers, including the alloantigens of the human leukocyte antigen (HLA) system. Many blood cell membrane determinants show allelic variation, which can elicit the formation of alloantibodies. In nearly all transfusion situations and pregnancies, the recipient's immune system is challenged by blood cells mismatched for multiple alloantigen systems. As the difference between self and non-self is limited, alloantibodies are only formed by a subset of recipients. Red cell alloantibodies are detected in 1–1.5% of pregnant women and in 2–3% of transfused individuals, and can increase significantly in multitransfused patients. The HLA alloantigens are more immunogenic than those of the red cells, and 15–25% of multiparous women and 30–40% of patients on long-term prophylactic platelet transfusions are positive for HLA class I antibodies.

Alloantigens were initially defined as polymorphic membrane determinants identified by polyclonal alloantibodies in serum samples from alloimmunized patients or pregnant women, but the molecular basis of most alloantigens has now been resolved and it is possible to use DNA-based techniques to further characterize their polymorphism. Alloantigens can be categorized as those shared by all blood cells, for example HLA class I and those unique to one blood cell type, such as Rh on red cells and human platelet antigen (HPA) on platelets (Table 21.1). When expression is limited

to one type of blood cell, destruction of cells in the newborn by maternal blood cell alloantibodies may lead to the development of immune-mediated anemia, thrombocytopenia or neutropenia of the newborn. In contrast, HLA class I alloantibodies do not cause cytopenias in the newborn but may compromise the effectiveness of platelet transfusions, complicate organ transplantation, cause febrile non-hemolytic transfusion reactions or, on rare occasions, precipitate transfusion-related acute lung injury and occasionally delay engraftment in hemopoietic stem cell transplantation.

The formation of alloantibodies after an incompatible challenge in the form of blood transfusion is more the exception than the rule. In contrast to our detailed understanding of the molecular basis of blood cell alloantigens, we remain relatively ignorant about the mechanism of non-responsiveness. We have learned from animal experiments that restriction in the ability to mount an immune response is largely controlled by genes of the major histocompatibility complex (MHC) or HLA. However, the reason why, for example, some 25% of RhD-negative individuals fail to mount an anti-D response on repeated challenge with RhD-positive red cells remains elusive. An exception to this is our detailed understanding of the immune response against the HPA-1a alloantigen on platelets. There is a near-complete restriction on the ability to form HPA-1a antibodies by the HLA class II allele DRB3*0101. However, except for this example, our ability to identify the genes controlling the risk of alloimmunization remains limited and further research is needed to identify the genetic basis of this variability in responsiveness.

This chapter reviews the recent developments in the molecular aspects of blood cell alloantigens and highlights their impact on clinical management. Recognizing the wide variety of clinical conditions in which the HLA alloantigens play a role, we have placed the main emphasis on:

*Molecular Hematology*, 3rd edition. Edited by Drew Provan and John Gribben.
© 2010 Blackwell Publishing.

**Table 21.1** Antigen expression on peripheral blood cells.

| Antigens | Erythrocytes | Platelets | Neutrophils | B lymphocytes | T lymphocytes | Monocytes |
|---|---|---|---|---|---|---|
| A, B, H | + + + | + + /(+) | – | – | – | – |
| I | + + + | + + | + + | – | – | – |
| Rh* | + + + | – | – | – | – | – |
| K | + + + | – | – | – | – | – |
| HLA class I | –/(+) | + + + | + + + | + + + | +++ | +++ |
| HLA class II | – | – | –/+ + +† | + + + | –/+++† | +++ |
| GPIIb/IIIa | – | + + + | (+ )‡ | – | – | – |
| GPIa/IIa | – | + + + | – | – | – | – |
| GPIb/IX/V | – | + + + | – | – | – | – |
| FcγRIIIB | – | – | + + + | – | – | –/+++§ |

\* Non-glycosylated.
† When activated.
‡ Inconclusive.
§ When differentiated to macrophages expressing FcγRIIIA.

• antibody-mediated cytopenias in the newborn by maternal blood cell-specific alloantibodies;
• the complication of HLA class I alloimmunization in patients receiving prophylactic platelet transfusions.
The HLA antigens have also been used to introduce the molecular techniques currently used to identify alleles of genes.

## Identification of HLA gene polymorphism

The impact of molecular biological techniques on our ability to scan and identify allelic variation of human genes is best exemplified by the HLA system. For decades the enormous diversity of the alloantigens of the HLA system has been a challenge in both the technical and the clinical sense. It is now obvious that the use of molecular techniques, including sequencing-based high-resolution typing, is contributing to improved outcome in transplant patients. Improved matching allows graft maintenance at lower levels of immunosuppression, which is of great importance with the emerging evidence that long-term use of potent immunosuppressive drugs is not without side effects. The following sections review a number of current molecular techniques used to define alleles of the HLA genes. The same techniques may be used to define allelic variation in genes encoding other blood cell alloantigens.

### Molecular typing techniques

Initially, the definition and characterization of the HLA molecules and polymorphisms was carried out using serological and cellular techniques. With the development of gene cloning and DNA-based molecular techniques, it is now possible to perform a detailed analysis of these molecules at the single-nucleotide level. The result of this analysis has shown the existence of shared nucleotide sequences between alleles of the same and/or different loci. Similarly, it has been shown that there are certain locus-specific nucleotide sequences in both the coding regions (exons) and the noncoding regions (introns) of the various genes.

DNA sequencing of a number of alleles at various MHC loci has demonstrated that most of the nucleotide substitutions are located in exons 2 and 3 of HLA class I and exon 2 of HLA class II molecules. These exons code for the distal membrane domains of the molecules, which form the peptide-binding groove (Figure 21.1). On the basis of this information, a number of techniques have been developed to identify this polymorphism using the polymerase chain reaction (PCR) to amplify specific genes or regions to be analyzed. These include PCR-SSOP (sequence-specific oligonucleotide probing), PCR-SSP (sequence-specific priming) and sequencing-based typing (SBT).

### PCR-SSOP

In this technique the gene of interest is amplified by PCR using generic primers complementary to highly conserved gene segments. The PCR products are then immobilized onto support membranes (e.g., nylon membranes) and analyzed by probing the membranes with labeled oligonucleotides designed to anneal with polymorphic sequences present in the various alleles. By scoring the probes that bind to specific regions, it is possible to assign an HLA type. A

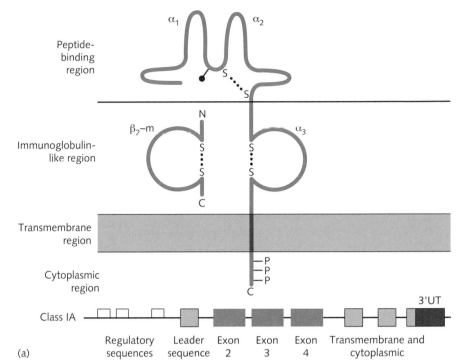

**Fig. 21.1 a Schematic presentation of HLA class I**

The non-covalent association between the HLA class I protein (with three immunoglobulin-like domains, $\alpha_1$, $\alpha_2$ and $\alpha_3$) and $\beta_2$-microglobulin ($\beta_2$-m) is shown. The three $\alpha$ domains are encoded by three exons of the HLA class IA gene on chromosome 6.

(a)

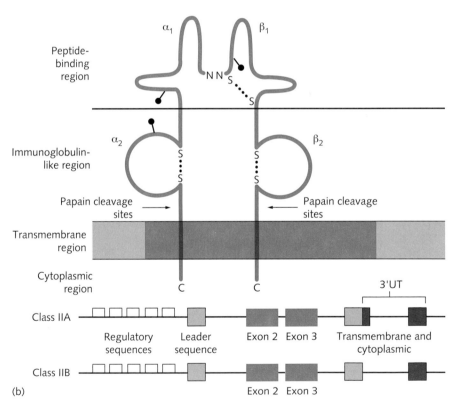

**Fig. 21.1 b Schematic presentation of HLA class II**

The $\alpha$ and $\beta$ chains of the HLA class II protein (each with two distinct immunoglobulin-like domains, $\alpha_1$ and $\alpha_2$, and $\beta_1$ and $\beta_2$) are non-covalently associated. Both domains of each chain are encoded by their respective exons of the $\alpha$ and $\beta$ class II genes on chromosome 6.

(b)

recent modification includes the addition of PCR-amplified product to labeled probes immobilized on membranes or plates. This technique, which has been called reverse SSOP, is particularly useful when testing large number of samples, such as those required for bone marrow donor registries.

A modification of the reverse SSOP technique has recently been described whereby the relevant PCR product is labeled with biotin and, following denaturation and neutralization steps, the product is hybridized with oligonucleotide-specific probes coupled to color beads. Following the addition of R-phycoerythrin-conjugated streptavidin (SAPE) to the reaction, the fluorescence is then measured using a flow cytometer-based instrument, the Luminex LABtype. Currently, there are two commercial kits to perform this test, Tepnel LIFECODES and One Lambda LABType. There are a number of advantages and disadvantages of these two kits but the main difference is that in the Tepnel LIFECODES kit there is asymmetric amplification of double-stranded and single-stranded products and therefore there no need for denaturation prior to the hybridization step (Plate 21.1).

### PCR-SSP

This technique involves the use of allele-specific primers in the PCR. The amplified DNA is detected by gel electrophoresis and this allows the rapid identification of the HLA alleles in individual samples, since the read-out of this method is the presence or absence of an amplicon for which a specific primer was used. PCR-SSP was first developed to define the various HLA-DRB3 alleles (Figure 21.2). Although this is a rapid technique, many PCR reactions have to be set up for each sample, for example 24 reactions for low-resolution DR typing. An obvious advantage of PCR-SSP is that, as two sequences are detected in *cis*, ambiguities which may arise from PCR-SSOP typing can be resolved. For PCR-SSP typing, however, the target sequence of the alleles must be known, and novel unknown sequences may not always be detected. PCR-SSP is also the technique of choice for HPA typing (*see section The molecular basis of platelet-specific antigens or HPA*). Using the PCR-SSP technique, it is possible to determine whether the detected sequences are in *cis* or in *trans*.

### Sequencing-based typing

The principle of DNA sequencing is relatively straightforward. It involves the denaturation of the DNA to be analyzed to provide a single-strand template; a sequencing primer is then added and the extension is performed by the addition of polymerase in the presence of excess nucleotides. The sequencing mixture is divided into four tubes, each of which contains a specific dideoxyribonucleoside triphosphate

(ddATP). When this is incorporated into the DNA strand, elongation is interrupted, leading to chain termination. In each reaction there is random incorporation of the chain terminators and therefore products of all sizes are generated. The products of the four reactions are then analyzed by electrophoresis in parallel lanes of a polyacrylamide–urea gel and the sequence is read by combining the results of each lane using an automated DNA sequencer.

## HLA antigens

These are a group of highly polymorphic cell surface molecules that play a central role in the induction and regulation of immune responses, and as such they are involved in self/non-self recognition, tolerance, rejection of allografts and graft-versus-host disease. The genes coding for these molecules form part of a complex genetic system called the MHC, located on the short arm of chromosome 6. This region spans a distance of approximately 4000 kb and is divided into HLA class I, class II and class III genes. Class III includes a group of non-MHC genes coding for proteins with various immunological functions, such as the complement factor 4 and tumor necrosis factor (TNF)-$\alpha$.

The development of recombinant DNA technology has led to increased understanding of the genetic complexity, structure and function of the HLA genes and molecules.

### HLA class I genes

The HLA class I genes have been classified according to their structure and function as classical and non-classical, or class Ib genes. The classic HLA class I genes, HLA-A, HLA-B and HLA-Cw, code for heterodimers formed by a heavy ($\alpha$) chain of approximately 43 kDa, non-covalently linked to the $\beta_2$-microglobulin light chain of 12 kDa. The latter is coded for by a gene located outside the HLA region on chromosome 15. The extracellular portion of the $\alpha$ chain has three domains ($\alpha_1$, $\alpha_2$ and $\alpha_3$) encoded by exons 2, 3 and 4, respectively. Each domain is approximately 90 amino acids in length. The transmembrane and cytoplasmic domains are encoded by exons 5, 6 and 7, respectively. The $\beta_2$-microglobulin, which confers stability on the molecule, is non-covalently linked to the $\alpha_3$ domain (see Figure 21.1a).

The $\alpha_1$ and $\alpha_2$ domains are the most polymorphic regions of these molecules and form a groove consisting of two $\alpha$ helices, with an antiparallel-running $\beta$-pleated sheet forming the floor of the groove. This groove, which is approximately 2.5 nm long and 1 nm wide, can accommodate a variety of antigen-derived peptides of about eight to ten amino acids to be presented to T cells.

Allele-specific PCR (PCR–SSP)

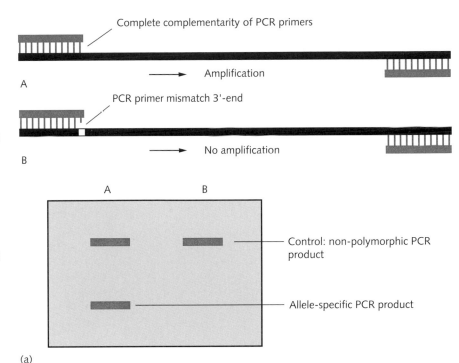

**Fig. 21.2 a PCR-SSP**
With allele-specific PCR, specificity is obtained during the PCR. A single nucleotide mismatch at the 3′-end of the allele-specific primer (B primer in the figure) will prevent the polymerase from commencing DNA amplification. Therefore, no amplification of template DNA will occur with the B allele primer, whereas with the A allele primer a product is obtained. Ethidium bromide is used to reveal amplified DNA with ultraviolet light after DNA gel electrophoresis. Allele-specific DNA is obtained in the A reaction (lower band) but not in the B reaction. In both reactions a control PCR product is generated by amplification of a segment of the growth hormone gene (upper two bands).

**Fig. 21.2 b PCR-SSP for DR and DQ alleles**
Results of PCR-SSP with template DNA from a single donor. Each lane represents the result of gel electrophoresis of a single PCR reaction with one of the allele-specific DR or DQ primers. From the pattern of positive results, a DR (upper panel) and DQ (lower panel) type can be concluded, in this case DR1, DR13, DRB3 and DQ5, DQ6.

In addition to the classical HLA class I genes, the non-classical HLA class I genes are also located in this region. They include HLA-E, HLA-F and HLA-G and their exon/intron organization is similar to that of the classical class I genes, but they have a more restricted polymorphism. The HLA class I genes are expressed on most tissues and blood cells, including T and B lymphocytes and platelets (Table 21.1). The non-classical class I genes HLA-E and HLA-F are expressed on most tissues tested so far, whereas HLA-G has so far only been detected on trophoblasts and monocytes.

More recently, two MHC class I chain-related genes (MIC-A and MIC-B), located centromeric to HLA-B, have been described. Unlike the classical and non-classical HLA class I, MIC genes do not require binding to the $\beta_2$-microglobulin or peptide in order to be expressed on the cell surface. So far, MIC expression has been detected on freshly isolated endothelial cells, fibroblasts, keratinocytes and monocytes. They have also been found to be expressed on intestinal epithelial cells as a result of stress, and on a variety of tumors of epithelial origin.

HFE is another non-classical class I gene, located 4 Mb telomeric of HLA-A. This gene has been found to be responsible for the development of hereditary hemochromatosis (HH). A single point mutation, 845A, replacing cysteine with tyrosine at position 282 (C282Y) is found in over 90% of HH patients in the UK. The other two mutations, replacing histidine by aspartate at amino acid position 63 (H63D) and serine by cysteine at amino acid 65 (S65C), appear to be associated with milder forms of HH. This gene does not have a direct immune function as it has lost the ability to bind antigenic peptides due to closure of the antigen-binding groove. However, since HFE can bind to the transferrin receptor, and in this way regulate iron uptake and availability, it is possible that HFE may indirectly be involved in the regulation of immune responses.

## HLA class II genes

The HLA class II genes DR, DQ and DP are all located within the HLA class II region. There is one non-polymorphic DRA and nine highly polymorphic DRB genes, of which DRB2, B6 and B9 are pseudogenes. These genes code for heterodimers formed by an α and a β chain both encoded by genes within the MHC. The extracellular portion of these molecules has two domains ($\alpha_1$ and $\alpha_2$ and $\beta_1$ and $\beta_2$) encoded by exon 2 and 3 of each gene respectively. The $\alpha_1$ and $\beta_1$ domains form the peptide-binding groove (see Figure 21.1b).

The number of DRB genes expressed in each haplotype varies depending on the DRB1 allele expressed; for example, HLA DR1, DR103, DR8 and DR10 haplotypes only express the DRB1 gene. DR15 and DR16 haplotypes additionally express the DRB5 gene, which codes for the DR51 product. The HLA DR17, DR18, DR11, DR12, DR13 and DR14 haplotypes also express the DRB3 genes, which code for the DR52 specificity, while the HLA DR4, DR7 and DR9 alleles also express the DRB4 gene, which encodes the DR53 product. There are a few exceptions to this gene distribution; for example, a DRB5 gene has been found linked to a DR1 haplotype, and null DRB5 and DRB4 genes have been identified.

In contrast, there are two DQA and three DQB genes; of these, only A1 and B1 are expressed and both are polymorphic. Similarly, there are two DPA and two DPB genes of which only DPA1 and DPB1 are expressed and are polymorphic. There are more x number of alleles identified so far (http://web17110.vs.netbenefit.co.uk?HIG/data.html).

Other HLA-related genes located within the MHC class II region include LMP2, LMP7, TAP1 and TAP2, which are involved in the transport and processing of peptides presented by class I molecules, and the HLA DMA, DMB, DOA and DOB genes, which participate in the loading of peptides in the HLA class II molecules.

The HLA class II genes (DR, DQ and DP) are constitutively expressed on B lymphocytes, monocytes and dendritic cells, and on activated T lymphocytes and granulocytes (Table 21.1). HLA class II expression can also be induced on non-hematopoietic cells such as fibroblasts and endothelial cells, as the result of activation or by the effect of certain inflammatory cytokines, such as interferon (IFN)-γ and TNF-α.

## Function

The HLA molecules play a pivotal role in the induction and regulation of the immune response. Both the phenomenon of MHC restriction and the development of tolerance, learnt as T cells pass through the thymus, result in the selection of a T-cell repertoire that will form the basis of an individual's capacity to respond to antigens. HLA class I molecules are primarily but not exclusively involved in the presentation of endogenous antigens to CD8$^+$ cytotoxic T cells, whereas HLA class II molecules present primarily, but not exclusively, exogenous antigenic peptides to CD4$^+$ helper T cells. These cells, once activated, can initiate and regulate a variety of processes leading to the maturation and differentiation of cellular and humoral effector cells, including the secretion of cytokines. The presentation of antigenic peptides is a highly regulated process and requires fine interaction between the antigenic peptide, the antigen-binding groove of the HLA molecules, and the T-cell receptor. Allelic variation of the HLA molecules can profoundly affect the ability to present certain peptides because of the presence or absence of critical contact residues in the peptide-binding groove.

HLA molecules on donor cells loaded with donor-derived peptides can also be recognized directly by T cells of the host by a mechanism called allorecognition. Two pathways of allorecognition, direct and indirect, have been identified, both of which lead to the strong alloimmunization seen in patients receiving blood transfusions or a solid organ or bone marrow/stem cell transplantation.

More recently, it has been shown that both classical and non-classical HLA class I molecules interact with two functionally distinct types of receptors, inhibitory and activating, present on natural killer (NK) cells. These receptors belong to two families, the immunoglobulin superfamily, also called killer immunoglobulin receptors (KIRs), and the C-type lectin superfamily CD94, which can covalently assemble with several members of the NKG2 family. The KIRs interact with products of the HLA-A, -B, -Cw and -G loci, whereas CD94-NKG2 recognize the non-classical HLA-E molecule presenting peptides derived from several HLA class I, A, B or C alleles and from HLA-G. MIC-A and MIC-B gene products are recognized by receptors present on both NK and γδ T cells.

Thus, HLA molecules have become increasingly relevant in a variety of clinical situations, such as susceptibility to certain autoimmune and infectious diseases and in solid organ and stem cell transplantation and blood cell alloimmunization. With regard to the latter, two examples will be discussed: refractoriness for prophylactic platelet transfusion by HLA alloimmunization and HLA class II restriction of the formation of anti-HPA-1a antibodies.

## Prophylactic and therapeutic platelet transfusions

Prophylactic platelet transfusions are essential for preventing bleeding during intensive chemotherapy or other myeloablative therapies. Increments in the platelet count after the infusion of an adult dose of donor platelets ($>250 \times 10^9$/L) are frequently disappointing. Non-immune factors, such as splenomegaly, bleeding, sepsis, fever and certain drugs (e.g., amphotericin), can compromise the beneficial effect of donor platelet infusions. In 10–20% of patients the problem of poor increments is further compounded by antibody-mediated destruction of donor platelets. Despite this, the clinical definition of refractoriness remains much disputed; clinically, the picture of an increased frequency of platelet transfusions to maintain satisfactory platelet counts and effective hemostasis requires further laboratory investigations for HLA class I and for HPA alloantibodies, platelet autoantibodies or high-titer anti-A or anti-B antibodies.

The ability to type donors and patients for HLA class I A and B and HPA by molecular techniques using genomic DNA (*see sections Molecular typing techniques, p. 260, and The molecular basis of platelet-specific antigens or HPA, p. 270*) has resulted in more accurate matching of donors with patients, with improved platelet recovery. The algorithm currently used for the management of the alloimmunized patient with poor increments is shown in Figure 21.3.

Traditionally, HLA matching for the provision of compatible platelets for patients who have become immunologically refractory to random platelet transfusion has been based on the serological definition of these antigens at the specificity level. More recently, a new approach based on the identifica-

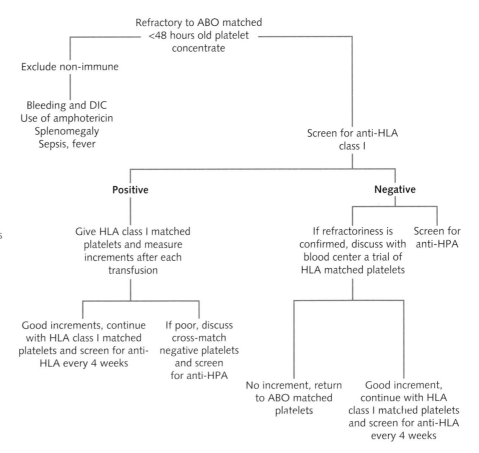

**Fig. 21.3 Platelet transfusions in alloimmunized patients**
An algorithm outlining the decision process for the management of alloimmunized patients refractory for random donor platelets. After confirmation of refractoriness for random donor platelets, patients are screened for HLA class I alloantibodies and, if positive, HLA class I-matched platelets are transfused. In 20–30% of patients, increments with HLA class I-matched platelets are poor and screening for HPA antibodies should follow. Also, the possible presence of potent anti-A or anti-B should be excluded since platelets do carry ABO blood group antigens. If there are no detectable HLA class I antibodies, a trial of HLA-matched platelets and screening for HPA antibodies should be considered (right arm of algorithm).

**Table 21.2** Amino acid sequence of the RhD and RhCE proteins.

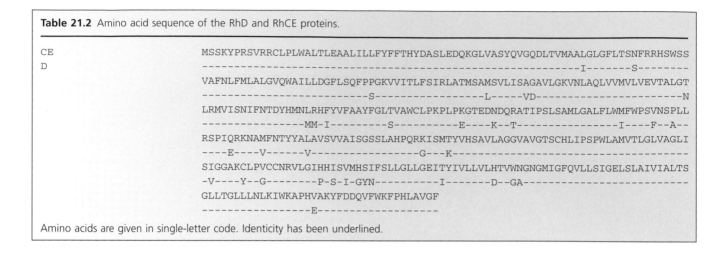

```
CE        MSSKYPRSVRRCLPLWALTLEAALILLFYFFTHYDASLEDQKGLVASYQVGQDLTVMAALGLGFLTSNFRRHSWSS
D         ----------------------------------------------------------------I-------S--------
          VAFNLFMLALGVQWAILLDGFLSQFPPGKVVITLFSIRLATMSAMSVLISAGAVLGKVNLAQLVVMVLVEVTALGT
          -----------------------S-----------------L-----VD----------------------N
          LRMVISNIFNTDYHMNLRHFYVFAAYFGLTVAWCLPKPLPKGTEDNDQRATIPSLSAMLGALFLWMFWPSVNSPLL
          ---------------MM-I---------S----------E----K--T---------------I----F--A--
          RSPIQRKNAMFNTYYALAVSVVAISGSSLAHPQRKISMTYVHSAVLAGGVAVGTSCHLIPSPWLAMVTLGLVAGLI
          ----E----V------V----------------G---K----------------------------
          SIGGAKCLPVCCNRVLGIHHISVMHSIFSLLGLLGEITYIVLLVLHTVWNGNGMIGFQVLLSIGELSLAIVIALTS
          -V----Y--G--------P-S-I-GYN----------I-------D--GA------------------
          GLLTGLLLNLKIWKAPHVAKYFDDQVFWKFPHLAVGF
          ----------------E------------------
```

Amino acids are given in single-letter code. Identity has been underlined.

tion of conformational epitopes present in each HLA allele has been described. According to this strategy, each HLA antigen is converted into a string of potentially immunogenic epitopes, which are represented by amino acid triplets (called eplets) on exposed parts of the HLA chains accessible to alloantibodies. These eplet epitopes are amino acid residues located within small clusters (with diameters of about 0.3–0.35 nm) around a non-self residue and are formed by amino acids in linear sequences as described in the triplet model but also include amino acids from discontinuouss regions of the sequence brought together by the folding of the molecule. This is therefore considered to be a more accurate representation of the epitope than that derived from the triplet HLAMatchmaker model developed by Duquesnoy. Consequently, it is possible to determine the number of triplets (eplets) which are either shared or different between the donor and the recipient The algorithm also performs intra- and inter-locus comparisons of polymorphic eplets in amino acid sequence positions in order to determine the spectrum of non-shared eplets between HLA antigens of the donor and the patient.

## Hemolytic disease of the newborn

### Rh system

The Rh system is the most immunogenic red cell blood group system after the ABO system. While the antigens of the latter have a carbohydrate nature, the Rh antigens are non-glycosylated proteins. Two-dimensional gel electrophoresis of trypsin digests of Rh proteins, which could be performed once human monoclonal antibodies specific for Rh alloantigens became available, provided evidence of a high level of homology between the proteins carrying the RhD and the RhC/c and RhE/e alloantigens.

### Rh genes

Cloning of the *RhD* and *RhCE* genes (carrying the RhD antigen and the RhC/c and RhE/e antigens, respectively) revealed a high level of sequence homology (Table 21.2), confirming the observation made by gel electrophoresis. These molecular studies suggested that the C/c and E/e antigens are localized on a single protein, the RhCE protein encoded by the *RhCE* gene and its allelic variants. The recent expression of the *RhD* and *RhCE* genes in K562 cell lines by retroviral transfection provided the ultimate proof that the RhD alloantigen and the RhC/c and E/e alloantigens are localized on two distinct proteins encoded by these two genes and their respective allelic variants.

The 75-kb *RhD* gene, with 10 exons, encodes a 30-kDa non-glycosylated protein of 417 amino acids of unknown function which traverses the red cell membrane 12 times (Figure 21.4). The gene is deleted in RhD-negative individuals (15% of the Caucasian population). The RhC/c and E/e alloantigens are carried on the highly homologous 30-kDa RhC/cE/e protein, which differs by only 36 of the 417 amino acids from RhD (Table 21.2). The difference between RhC and Rhc is associated with six nucleotide substitutions, of which four result in a replacement. One of these, residue 103, is exofacial and seems to be the most critical one of the C/c polymorphism. The difference between RhE and Rhe is defined by a single Pro226Ala replacement in the fourth extracellular loop of the RhCE protein (Figure 21.4).

### Immunogenicity of RhD and prevention of immunization

The absence of the RhD protein in RhD-negative individuals is the most plausible explanation of its relatively high immunogenicity, as the immune system has not been tolerized by a lookalike RhD protein encoded by an allele of the *RhD* gene. Until the late 1960s, the formation of anti-D in RhD-

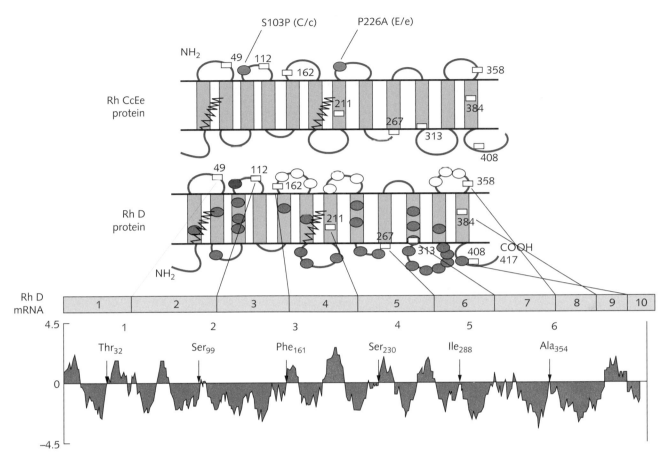

**Fig. 21.4 RhD and RhCE proteins**
Schematic representation of the topography of the RhCE (upper figure) and RhD (lower figure) proteins. Both 30-kDa non-glycosylated proteins traverse the red cell membrane 12 times. The difference between RhD and RhCE is defined by 36 of the 417 amino acids (colored circles indicate RhD-specific residues; shaded circles indicate C/c and E/e polymorphisms). The rectangular boxes (1–10) indicate the positions of exon–exon boundaries in the RhD mRNA, and a hydropathy plot of the RhD protein is shown at the bottom.

negative pregnant women had a high incidence and was associated with significant neonatal morbidity and mortality because of hydrops fetalis and kernicterus. The discovery that the formation of anti-D could be prevented by the administration of passive IgG anti-D, combined with a much reduced family size, has led to a steep decline in mortality associated with hemolytic disease of the newborn (HDN). It is estimated that, per annum in the UK, approximately 150–200 cases of severe RhD immunization require intrauterine treatment. The officially reported annual mortality for RhD HDN is nine cases, but estimates from screening laboratories suggest that the figure is closer to 50.

Knowledge of the structure of the *RhD* gene now makes it possible to give better support to RhD-immunized women, as the fetal *RhD* genotype can be determined in the first trimester from amniocyte DNA or from maternal serum. The former is now routinely used in cases of severe RhD immunization with an *RhD* (*D/d*) heterozygous partner,

whereas the latter technique, which is non-invasive, will need further validation before routine application in genetic counseling. The immunogenicity of RhE in RhE-negative individuals is low and the change in severe HDN because of anti-E is infinitely small when compared with anti-D. Its poor immunogenicity is best explained by the relatively small difference between self and non-self. The greater sequence difference between RhC and Rhc is reflected in a greater risk of potent alloantibody formation during pregnancy, although severe HDN by anti-C and anti-c antibodies is relatively uncommon.

## Kell system

The K antigen of the Kell system is, after RhD, the second most immunogenic protein blood group alloantigen system on the red cell membrane. The Kell alloantigens K and k are carried on a 93-kDa, type II transmembrane protein of 732 amino acids. The *KEL* gene spans about 21.5 kb, with 19 exons, and has sequence homology with genes of the protein family of zinc-binding endopeptidases, like the CALLA (CD10) antigen and human common acute lymphoblastic leukemia antigen. The difference between K and k is a single base change in exon 6, causing a Met193Thr replacement. It is of interest to note that despite this minor difference between the two forms, K is one of the most immunogenic blood group substances. This is possibly explained, although not proven, by the absence of an *N*-glycosylation site in the k protein at residue 191.

### Immunogenicity of K and the mechanism of fetal anemia

Transfusion frequently triggers the formation of anti-K. As anti-K antibodies can cause severe HDN, it is recommended that K-negative blood should be transfused to all girls and women of childbearing age. In K alloimmunization, fetal anemia seems to be mainly caused by antibody-mediated inhibition of erythroid maturation. The question of why anti-K downregulates erythropoiesis has not been answered, but it points to a possible regulatory role of the K-carrying endopeptidase in erythroid differentiation and maturation. Owing to the aplastic nature of the anemia, the degree of fetal anemia cannot be assessed by measurement of bilirubin levels in the amniotic fluid, but should be based on the obstetric history, maternal anti-K level, and paternal K status. If there is a high-risk scenario, with a K-positive partner, the fetal K type should be determined by PCR on amniocyte DNA. If the fetus is K-positive, fetal anemia should be assessed and treated by periumbilical blood sampling (PUBS).

## Red cell alloantigens other than Rh and K

As is the case for the Rh and K systems, the molecular structure of most other blood group alloantigens has been resolved over the last two decades. Detailed discussion of these systems is beyond the scope of this chapter, but PCR-based typing can now be performed for most clinically relevant blood group systems (e.g., Duffy, Jk, M/N and S/s). This knowledge is of use when blood group alloantibodies are associated with severe HDN. These users include patients with thalassemia, in whom blood transfusion has been given before a complete red cell phenotype is established.

The high level of sequence homology between the *RhD* and *RhCE* genes and the occurrence of crossover events, which are often associated with reduced expression of the Rh antigens, requires ample expertise in the use of PCR for prenatal diagnosis. Therefore, such tests should be performed in laboratories with a scientific interest in blood group genetics.

## Frequency

Of all pregnant women, 1–1.5% screen positive for red cell alloantibodies. In roughly half of them, the antibodies are of possible clinical significance, and antibody potency needs monitoring during pregnancy to determine the risk of significant hemolysis requiring therapy. Severe disease with intrauterine intravascular transfusion therapy occurs in approximately 1 in 5000 pregnancies and is mainly due to anti-D or anti-K.

## Pathology

Maternal alloantibodies can be formed against a blood group alloantigen present on the fetal red cells but absent from the maternal ones. RhD, K, Rhc and RhC are the main culprits with respect to HDN. Red cell alloantibodies of the IgG class can cross the placenta, bind to the fetal red cells and shorten their survival. In K immunization, hyperbilirubinemia is a less reliable parameter for the prediction of the severity of fetal anemia, and these pregnancies can be complicated by early fetal loss.

## Treatment of HDN

An increased concentration of unconjugated bilirubin in the neonate poses the risk of kernicterus. Treatment of severe hemolytic anemia and hyperbilirubinemia in the post-delivery setting is by exchange transfusion with compatible donor red cells. When a pregnancy is preceded by one with a history of severe HDN, intrauterine intravascular transfusion of compatible donor red cells by PUBS is the treatment of choice and has a good outcome in 90% of cases. Genetic counseling of couples with a heterozygous partner has been greatly helped by the discovery of the *Rh* and *K* genes (*see above*).

## Prevention of HDN

Before the introduction of anti-D prophylaxis, most HDN cases were caused by RhD immunization. The routine RhD testing of all pregnant women, combined with anti-D prophylaxis for RhD-negative individuals carrying an RhD-positive infant, has been extremely successful in lowering HDN-associated morbidity and mortality. Screening for clinically significant red cell alloantibodies in pregnant women is the standard of care in most European countries and cases of possible severe disease should be identified early in pregnancy to allow the prevention of morbidity or mortality.

# Neonatal alloimmune thrombocytopenia

## Platelet-specific or HPA alloantigen systems

Besides the alloantigens shared with other blood cells (e.g., HLA class I A and B alloantigens), platelets also express alloantigens which are carried on proteins uniquely expressed on platelets but not on other blood cells (see Table 21.1). Alloimmunization against platelet-specific antigens or HPA is associated with three clinical syndromes:

1 neonatal/fetal alloimmune thrombocytopenia (NAITP);
2 post-transfusion purpura;
3 refractoriness for platelet transfusions.

NAITP was first described by van Loghem in 1959 and was initially thought to be a rare disorder. Prospective screening studies in pregnant (Caucasian) women have shown that 1 in 1100 neonates have severe thrombocytopenia ($<50 \times 10^9$/L) due to maternal anti-HPA-1a, confirming the notion that the most frequent cause of severe thrombocytopenia in the term newborn is maternal alloantibodies against a fetal HPA alloantigen.

This serious clinical condition is caused by the destruction of fetal/neonatal platelets by maternal HPA alloantibodies of the IgG class. Cerebral bleeds in the perinatal period are the most concerning complication, which either occur *in utero* or during delivery. In cases of severe thrombocytopenia ($<20 \times 10^9$/L), there remains a small but definite risk of this serious complication in the first days of life, warranting treatment. For proper clinical management, the cause of

**Table 21.3** Platelet-specific alloantigen systems.

| System | Antigen | Alternative names | Glycoprotein | Nucleotide change | Amino acid change |
|---|---|---|---|---|---|
| HPA-1 | 1a | Zw$^a$, Pl$^{A1}$ | GPIIIa | T196 | Leucine33 |
| | 1b | Zw$^b$, Pl$^{A2}$ | | C196 | Proline33 |
| HPA-2 | 2a | Ko$^b$ | GPIb$\alpha$ | C524 | Threonine145 |
| | 2b | Ko$^a$, Sib$^a$ | | T524 | Methionine145 |
| HPA-3 | 3a | Bak$^a$, Lek$^a$ | GPIIb | T2622 | Isoleucine843 |
| | 3b | Bak$^b$ | | G2622 | Serine843 |
| HPA-4 | 4a | Yuk$^b$, Pen$^a$ | GPIIIa | G526 | Arginine143 |
| | 4b | Yuk$^a$, Pen$^b$ | | A526 | Glutamine143 |
| HPA-5 | 5a | Br$^b$, Zav$^b$ | GPIa | G1648 | Glutamic acid505 |
| | 5b | Br$^a$, Zav$^a$, Hc$^a$ | | A1648 | Lysine505 |
| HPA-6w | | | GPIIIa | G1564 | Arginine489 |
| | 6bw | Ca$^a$, Tu$^a$ | | A1564 | Glutamine489 |
| HPA-7w | | | GPIIIa | C1267 | Proline407 |
| | 7bw | Mo | | G1267 | Alanine407 |
| HPA-8w | | | GPIIIa | T2004 | Arginine636 |
| | 8bw | Sr$^a$ | | C2004 | Cysteine636 |
| HPA-9w | | | GPIIb | G2603 | Valine837 |
| | 9bw | Max$^a$ | | A2603 | Methionine837 |
| HPA- | | | GPIIIa | G281 | Arginine62 |
| 10w | 10bw | La$^a$ | | A281 | Glutamine62 |
| | | | GPIIIa | G1946 | Arginine633 |
| | | Gro$^a$ | | A1946 | Histidine633 |
| | | Iy$^a$ | GPIb$\beta$ | G141 | Glycine15 |
| | | | | A141 | Glutamic acid15 |
| | | Oe$^a$ | GPIIIa | | |
| | | Va$^a$ | GPIIb/IIIa | | |
| | | Gov$^a$ | CD109 | | |
| | | Gov$^b$ | | | |
| | | Pl$^T$ | GPV | | |
| | | Vis | GPIV | | |
| | | Pe$^a$ | GPIb$\alpha$ | | |
| | | Sit$^a$ | GPIa | | |

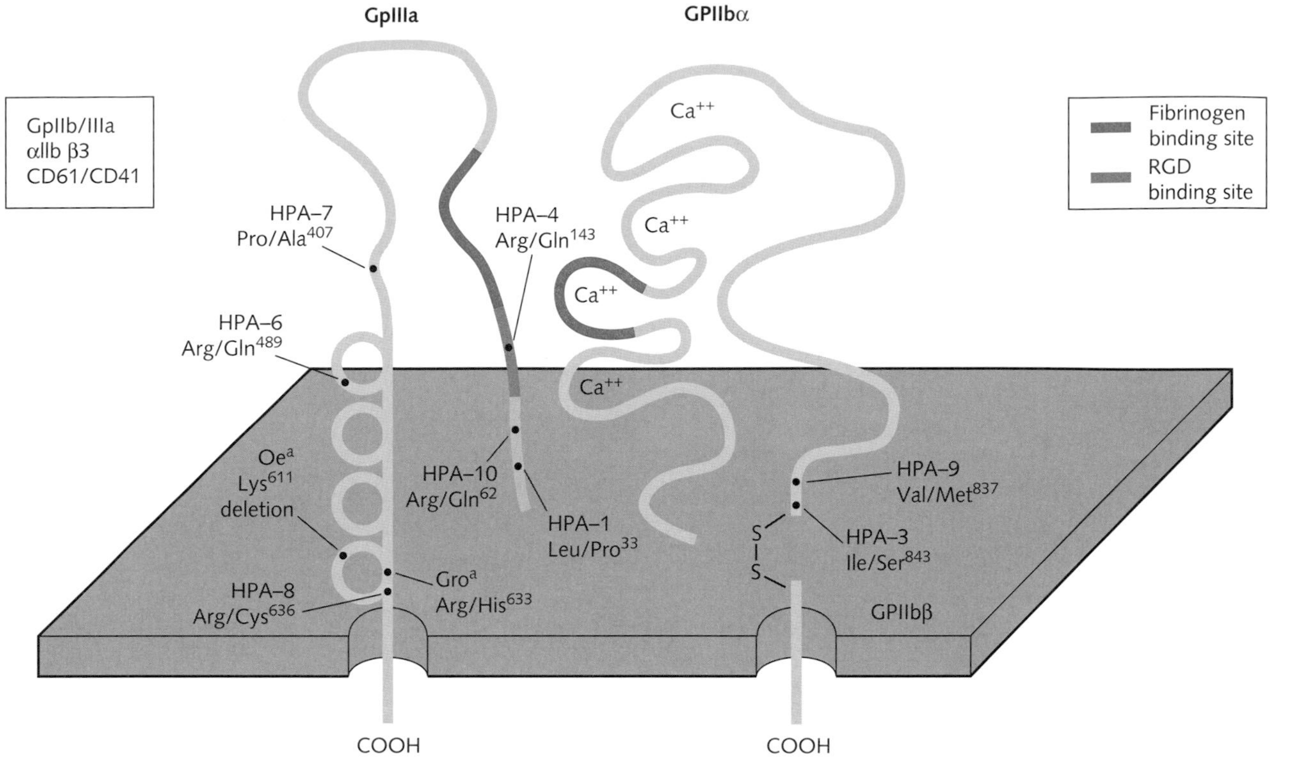

GpIIIa                 GPIIbα

GpIIb/IIIa
αIIb β3
CD61/CD41

Ca⁺⁺

Ca⁺⁺

Ca⁺⁺

Ca⁺⁺

Fibrinogen
binding site

RGD
binding site

HPA–7
Pro/Ala⁴⁰⁷

HPA–4
Arg/Gln¹⁴³

HPA–6
Arg/Gln⁴⁸⁹

Oeᵃ
Lys⁶¹¹
deletion

HPA–10
Arg/Gln⁶²

HPA–9
Val/Met⁸³⁷

HPA–3
Ile/Ser⁸⁴³

HPA–1
Leu/Pro³³

HPA–8
Arg/Cys⁶³⁶

Groᵃ
Arg/His⁶³³

GPIIbβ

COOH                 COOH

**Fig. 21.5 Schematic presentation of GPIIb/IIIa**

Schematic presentation of platelet GPIIb/IIIa or the αIIbβ3 integrin. GPIIIa is recognized by murine monoclonal antibodies of the CD61 cluster and the heterodimer by antibodies of the CD41 cluster. The amino acid substitutions arising from allelic variation of the GPIIb and GPIIIa genes are depicted by black dots and the name of the HPA system is noted. Amino acids are given as three-letter acronyms. The fibrinogen-binding site is indicated in color and the Arg-Gly-Asp (RGD)-binding site in dark gray. The RGD peptide is the minimal fibrinogen-derived peptide that binds GPIIb/IIIa.

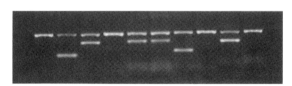

**Fig. 21.6 PCR-SSP for HPA alleles**

Results of agarose gel electrophoresis of PCR products obtained by amplification of segments of the GPIIIa, GPIbα, GPIIb and GPIa genes using allele-specific primers for the "a" and "b" alleles of the HPA-1, HPA-2, HPA-3, HPA-4 and HPA-5 systems. The results for this donor are HPA-1b1b, 2a2a, 3a3b, 4a4a and 5a5a. Products of the allele-specific amplification are the lower bands. In all reactions a set of control primers has been included to produce an amplicon (upper band) derived from the growth hormone gene.

severe thrombocytopenia in an otherwise healthy term neonate should be determined with urgency and correction of a count less than 20 × 10⁹/L by platelet transfusion is of utmost importance. This should precede the outcome of platelet antibody investigation, as this can be time-consuming.

## The molecular basis of platelet-specific antigens or HPA

So far, 19 platelet-specific alloantigen systems have been described. All are biallelic and have been mapped to certain membrane proteins. Of the 19 alloantigen systems, 11 are on the integrin heterodimer αIIbβ3 or glycoprotein (GP)IIb/IIIa (Table 21.3 and Figure 21.5); of the remaining eight, three are on GPIb–IX–V, two on the integrin α2β1 or GPIa/IIa and one each on GPIV, GPV and CD109. With the advent of PCR, the molecular basis of all but five of the systems has been resolved in the last decade. With the exception of one system, the difference between the two alleles is a single-nucleotide substitution in the gene encoding the relevant glycoprotein (Table 21.3). Amplification of genomic DNA by PCR-SSP (Figure 21.6) and SBT can be used to type donors and patients, even when the latter are thrombocytopenic. High-throughput donor HPA typing can also be performed using the 5'-nuclease (TaqMan) assay.

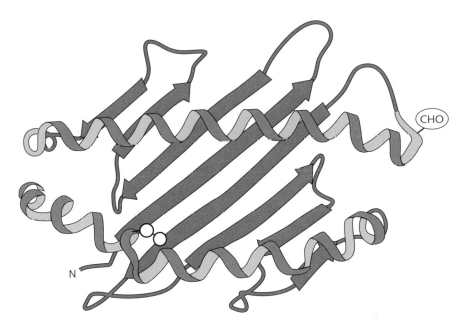

**Fig. 21.7 Structure of HLA DRB3*0101 molecule**
A view of the peptide-binding site of the HLA class II DRB3*0101 molecule as seen by the T-cell receptor of a T lymphocyte. Two α helices (see Figure 21.1b) are resting on a base of antiparallel-running β-pleated sheets. The antigen-derived peptide is not shown, but in our example of immune response restriction an oligopeptide derived from fetal GPIIIa-Leu33 will be juxtaposed between the two helices. The presence of this peptide defines the difference between self and non-self and triggers the proliferation of GPIIIa-Leu33 (HPA-1a) alloantigen-specific helper T cells.

## Immunogenicity and immune response restriction

As the difference between self and non-self is defined by a single amino acid substitution, the immunogenicity of the HPA alloantigens is relatively poor when compared with that of some of the other blood cell alloantigens (e.g., RhD and HLA class I). The two most clinically relevant HPA antigens are HPA-1a and HPA-5b on the β3 and α2 integrins, namely those on platelet glycoproteins GPIIIa and GPIa, respectively. Alloantibodies against other HPA alloantigens are observed infrequently in pregnancy but do occur, albeit at a low frequency, in hemato-oncological and other patients on long-term prophylactic platelet transfusion.

The HPA-1a and -1b alloantigens are based on a C → G mutation in the GPIIIa gene, resulting in a Leu33Pro mutation. Why the immunogenicity of HPA-1a (Leu33) is magnitudes higher than that of its antithetical antigen HPA-1b (Pro33) was initially not well understood. In the early 1980s, it was discovered that the formation of anti-HPA-1a in pregnancy was positively associated with the HLA haplotype A1, B8, DR3. Further study revealed that nearly all antibody formers were positive for the 0101 allele of the DRB3 gene (DRB3*0101 or DR52a; *see section HLA class II genes, p.* ••) (Figure 21.7). A prospective study in 25 000 pregnant women showed that this class II marker has an odds ratio of 140, which makes it one of the most reliable HLA associations reported to date, with negative predictive power equal to that of HLA B27 in ankylosing spondylitis. A difference in

the efficiency of presentation of the GPIIIa-Leu33 (HPA-1a)-derived oligopeptide between DRB3*0101-positive and -negative antigen-presenting cells to CD4+ T cells is the most likely explanation of this restriction in alloimmunization. The frequency of the HLA DRB3*0101 allele in Caucasians is 33%, and this marker therefore has a high negative predictive value but a low positive one for anti-HPA-1a formation.

## Allele frequencies

In Caucasians, the allele frequency for most HPA systems is skewed toward the "a" allele. The allele frequencies vary between populations; for example, GPIIIa-Pro33 (HPA-1b) is extremely rare or absent in the Far East, while the opposite is the case for the GPIIIa-Gln143 form (HPA-4b).

## Incidence of NAITP

Alloantibodies against the HPA-1a (Pl$^{A1}$, Zw$^a$) alloantigen occur in 1 in 365 pregnancies and cause severe thrombocytopenia, with a neonatal platelet count of less than $50 \times 10^9$/L in 1 in 1100 term neonates.

## Pathology

Maternal IgG alloantibodies against a fetal HPA alloantigen can cross the placenta and bind to the fetal platelets, thus reducing platelet survival. HPA-1a and HPA-5b are the two clinically most relevant alloantigens.

## Characteristics

Neonatal alloimmune thrombocytopenia presents in the otherwise healthy newborn as petechiae or ecchymoses, or is found coincidentally by a whole blood count. Severe cases can present with neurological symptoms because of cerebral bleeds or with hydrops fetalis or cerebral cysts. Diagnosis is based on the detection of HPA alloantibodies in the maternal serum combined with a parental HPA incompatibility, as determined by PCR-SSP.

## Inheritance

All systems described to date are biallelic with codominant expression of both alleles. Homozygous women can produce alloantibodies against a paternally inherited platelet alloantigen present on the fetal platelets but absent from the maternal ones. In cases where the partner is homozygous for the relevant alloantigen, there is a 100% chance that his future offspring will be at risk, whereas in the case of heterozygosity 50% will be affected.

## Treatment

A neonatal platelet count below $20 \times 10^9$/L should be corrected immediately, preferably with HPA-1a- and HPA-5b-negative donor platelets, as these will be compatible with the maternal HPA alloantibody in over 95% of cases. In cases of absence of HPA-compatible platelets, initial transfusion of random ABO/RhD-compatible platelets should be considered, followed by the transfusion of compatible ones if the platelet count dips again. In a typical case the platelet count should recover to normal within a week, although a more protracted recovery can occur.

In a subsequent pregnancy a decision needs to be taken on whether treatment of the fetus, the mother or both is indicated, or whether conservative management is acceptable. When conservative management is acceptable, the pregnancy should be closely monitored and the mother should be advised to avoid any non-steroidal anti-inflammatory drugs and aspirin. The delivery needs careful planning between obstetric and pediatric teams in close consultation with the consultant hematologist. Treatment during pregnancy should be reserved for cases in which the estimated risk of severe fetal/neonatal thrombocytopenia is considerable, and the treatment should be in collaboration with a fetal medicine unit. The available treatments for the mother during pregnancy are (i) intrauterine intravascular transfusion of compatible platelets by PUBS at weekly intervals or just before delivery, (ii) intravenous IgG or corticosteroids or (iii) a combination of both. As no randomized trials have been performed on either therapy, firm evidence of efficacy is lacking. However, weekly platelet transfusion by PUBS, although invasive and technically demanding, has shown good outcome in families with previously severely affected children. Repeated infusion of intravenous IgG to the mother remains highly controversial, as the initial report of its possible effectiveness made use of a historical control group. The costs are high and there remains a small but definite risk of transmission of infectious agents by a protein concentrate obtained from large plasma pools. The precise mechanism of action, if any, of corticosteroids administered to the mother on the severity of fetal disease is poorly understood.

## Counseling

Counseling of couples with an index case about the risks of severe fetal/neonatal thrombocytopenia in a subsequent pregnancy needs to be based on the severity of disease in the index case and the outcome of immunological investigations. The following should be taken into account.
• Thrombocytopenia in subsequent cases is as severe or generally more severe.
• Antibody specificity and titer have some correlation with severity; for example, HPA-5b antibodies generally cause mild thrombocytopenia, which rarely results in a cerebral bleed. The latter is generally associated with HPA-1a antibodies.
• A high-titer HPA antibody is more likely to be associated with severe thrombocytopenia, but cerebral bleeds also occur with low titers.

# Neonatal alloimmune neutropenia

Maternal alloimmunization against neutrophil-specific alloantigens on fetal/neonatal neutrophils is rare, although there are no precise prevalence figures. Clinical presentation is one of mainly bacterial infection with a selective neutropenia on a whole blood cell count. The number of well-characterized neutrophil-specific alloantigen systems is limited.

## HNA system

Neutrophils, like all other cells present in blood, express polymorphic molecules that are able to induce strong antibodies when transfused or transplanted or during pregnancy. These antigens are now called human neutrophil antigens (HNA). On the other hand, HNA-specific antibodies have been implicated in the development of neonatal alloimmune neutropenia, transfusion-related acute lung injury (TRALI), and other alloimmune or autoimmune neutropenias. So far five HNA antigenic systems have been described (HNA-1 to HNA-5), all of them with a limited degree of polymorphism.

• HNA-1 is located on a glycosylphosphatidylinositol (GPI)-anchored glycoprotein that forms the low-affinity Fcγ receptor. HNA-1 is encoded by the FcγRIIIB (*FCGR3B*) gene located on chromosome 1 and mediates IgG-induced phagocytosis. Three HNA-1 alleles have been described, HNA-1a, HNA-1b and HNA-1c (previously known as NA1, NA2 and SH respectively). Four amino acid substitutions at positions 36, 65, 82 and 106 determine the a and b alleles whereas the c allele is determined by a single substitution at position 78 of the b allele (Plate 21.2). In individuals expressing the HNA-3c allele, a third *FCGR3B* gene has been identified. Some individuals who do not express the *FCGR3B* gene and carry a null phenotype can develop isoantibody of known clinical significance in cases of NAITP. The FcγRIIIB null phenotype is rare and is based on a double deletion of the *FCGR3B* gene, and is in some cases associated with a deletion of the FcγRIIC (*FCGR2C*) gene. Deficiency for the most abundant Fc receptor on neutrophils does not seem to be associated with an obvious clinical phenotype. This is in contrast with a mutation in the FcγRIIIA (*FCGR3A*) gene, which encodes a Leu48His substitution in the first extracellular domain of the NA cell FcγRIIIA which, although only described in one infant, was associated with recurrent and serious respiratory tract viral infection from birth. The FcγRIIIB null phenotype can cause immune neutropenia in the newborn due to maternal anti-FcγRIIIB isoantibodies. PCR techniques can be used to determine the NA, SH and FcγRIIIB null genotypes, and transfectants expressing the FcγRIIIB NA allotypes are useful probes for alloantibody detection. HNA-1 alloantibodies have also been implicated in cases of autoimmune and alloimmune neutropenia, including neonatal alloimmune neutropenia and TRALI.

• HNA-2 (previously known as NB1) is expressed on a 58–64 kDa glycoprotein (CD177) found on the plasma membrane and secondary granules of neutrophils. This glycoprotein is linked to the plasma membrane by a GPI anchor and is coded for by a gene located on chromosome 19. HNA-2 is expressed in approximately 50% of the total neutrophils by 95% of individuals. Some individuals do not express HNA-2 due to a CD177 transcription defect. The gene encoding the NB protein has not been cloned and NB alloantigen typing is based on the use of human immune antisera and immunofluorescence. The clinical relevance of HNA-2 antibodies is not yet clear but they have been found in patients with alloimmune and autoimmune neutropenia.

• HNA-3 (previously known as 5b) is located on a 70–90 kDa glycoprotein and so far only one allele has been identified serologically, HNA-3a. HNA-3 antibodies are rare but they are known to be implicated in TRALI reactions.

• HNA-4 (previously known as Mart^a) is located on the αM chain (CD11b) of the β2 integrin MAC-1. This system has one antigen, the result of a single amino acid substitution at position 61.

• HNA-5 (previously known as Ond^a) is located on the αL integrin unit of the leucocyte function-associated antigen (LFA)-1, also known as CD11b. The antigen is determined by a single amino acid substitution at position 766. The clinical significance of both HNA-4 and HNA-5 antibodies is not yet certain (Table 21.4).

Some HNA antigens are uniquely expressed on neutrophils (HNA-1 and HNA-2), whereas others are also present on other cells or tissues (HNA-3, HNA-4 and HNA-5). The detection of these antigens was for many years limited by the lack of specific and reliable alloantisera, and by the difficulties in preserving viable cells to perform these tests. With the development of monoclonal antibodies and the cloning of some of the genes coding for these molecules, it is now possible to detect most of the polymorphism present on HNA using the monoclonal antibody immobilization of granulocyte antigens (MAIGA) or DNA-based

**Table 21.4** Human neutrophil antigens (HNA).

| Antigen system | Antigen | Former name | Alleles/genes | Location | CD |
|---|---|---|---|---|---|
| HNA-1 | HNA-1a | NA1 | *FCGR3B*1* | FcγRIIIB | CD16 |
| | HNA-1b | NA2 | *FCGR3B*2* | FcγRIIIB | CD16 |
| | HNA-1c | SH | *FCGR3B*3* | FcγRIIIB | CD16 |
| HNA-2* | HNA-2a | NB1 | | 58–64 kDa glycoprotein | CD177 |
| HNA-3 | HNA-3a | 5b | Not defined | 70–95 kDa glycoprotein | Not known |
| HNA-4 | HNA-4a | Mart | *ITGAM*01* (230G) | MAC-1; CR3; αMβ2 integrin | CD11b |
| HNA-5 | HNA-5a | Ond | *ITGAL*01* (2372G) | LFA-1; αLβ2 integrin | CD11a |

* HNA-2 is defined by isoantibodies.

techniques including PCR-amplified DNA and PCR-SSP, PCR-SSOP, a combination of PCR-SSP and restriction fragment length polymorphism (RFLP), or direct DNA sequencing. However, the detection of HNA-specific antibodies is still difficult, unreliable and time-consuming and involves use of the granulocyte agglutination test, granulocyte immunofluorescence test, chemiluminescence test, and MAIGA. Indeed, the majority of these techniques (with the exception of MAIGA) are not able to distinguish specific HNA from HLA antibodies. There is a need to develop a new generation of techniques for the detection and characterization of HNA-specific antibodies. Once these are available, it may be possible to reassess the clinical significance of these antibodies.

In addition to neonatal neutropenia, neutrophil-specific antibodies are implicated in non-hemolytic febrile transfusion reactions, TRALI and autoimmune neutropenia. Severe but reversible neutropenia in the newborn might require treatment with antibiotics to control bacterial infection. So far, there is minimal or no evidence that the mutations in the FcγRIIIB protein have any functional consequences, exemplified by the recently described FcγRIIIB null phenotype, which is not linked with an obvious pathological phenotype. In sharp contrast, the single amino acid mutation in the NK cell *FCGR3A* gene, which might be rare, may be associated with a more grave clinical condition.

## Conclusions

The molecular basis of most blood cell alloantigens, including those of the HLA system, has been discovered over the last two decades. The use of molecular techniques allows their reliable definition at high resolution, replacing previous less reliable techniques that were based on the use of polyclonal antibody reagents. This new body of knowledge has already made a significant contribution to current clinical management. On the one hand, first-trimester fetal typing for blood cell-specific alloantigens can now be used in cases of severe maternal alloimmunization to prevent fetal and neonatal morbidity, and improved selection of HLA- and HPA-matched donor platelets aids the management of hemato-oncological patients. On the other hand, it is envisaged that in the near future bone marrow and solid organ transplants across apparent mismatches can progress because of the identification of so-called permissive mismatches, and better HLA matching will allow accommodation of the graft at lower levels of immune suppression. Finally, more complete understanding of the molecular rules defining a subject's immune response status should lead to the identification of high responders, in order to target these for more specific manipulation of their immune system with the aim of establishing alloantigen-specific non-responsiveness.

## Further reading

Bennett PR, Le Van Kim C, Colin Y *et al.* (1993) Prenatal determination of fetal RhD type by DNA amplification. *New England Journal of Medicine*, **329**, 607–610.

Bux J. (2008) Human neutrophil alloantigens. *Vox Sanguinis*, **94**, 277–285.

Deo YM, Graziano RF, Repp R *et al.* (1997) Clinical significance of IgG Fc receptors and Fc gamma R-directed immunotherapies. *Immunology Today*, **18**, 127–135.

Duquesnoy R. (2006) A structurally based approach to determine HLA compatibility at the humoral immune level. *Human Immunology*, **67**, 847–862.

Gruen JR, Weissman SM. (1997) Evolving views of the major histocompatibility complex. *Blood*, **90**, 4252–4265.

Howell WM, Navarrete C. (1996) The HLA system: an update and relevance to patient–donor matching strategies in clinical transplantation. *Vox Sanguinis*, **71**, 6–12.

Huizinga TW, Roos D, von dem Borne AE. (1990) Neutrophil Fc-gamma receptors: a two-way bridge in the immune system. *Blood*, **75**, 1211–1214.

Kuijpers RW, von dem Borne AE, Kiefel V *et al.* (1992) Leucine33–proline33 substitution in human platelet glycoprotein IIIa determines HLA-DRw52a (Dw24) association of the immune response against HPA-1a (Zwa/PIA1) and HPA-1b (Zwb/PIA2). *Human Immunology*, **34**, 253–256.

Le van Kim C, Mouro I, Cherif Zahar B *et al.* (1992) Molecular cloning and primary structure of the human blood group RhD polypeptide. *Proceedings of the National Academy of Sciences of the United States of America*, **89**, 10925–10929.

Madrigal JA, Arguello R, Scott I *et al.* (1997) Molecular histocompatibility typing in unrelated donor bone marrow transplantation. *Blood Reviews*, **11**, 105–117.

Maslanka K, Yassai M, Gorski J. (1996) Molecular identification of T cells that respond in a primary bulk culture to a peptide derived from a platelet glycoprotein implicated in neonatal alloimmune thrombocytopenia. *Journal of Clinical Investigation*, **98**, 1802–1808.

Mouro I, Colin Y, Cherif Zahar B *et al.* (1993) Molecular genetic basis of the human Rhesus blood group system. *Nature Genetics*, **5**, 62–65.

Newman PJ, Valentin N. (1995) Human platelet alloantigens: recent findings, new perspectives. *Thrombosis and Haemostasis*, **74**, 234–239.

Smythe JS, Avent ND, Judson PA *et al.* (1996) Expression of RhD and RhCE gene products using retroviral transduction of K562 cells establishes the molecular basis of Rh blood group antigens. *Blood*, **87**, 2968–2973.

van Loghem JJ, Dorfmeyer H, van de Hart M *et al.* (1959) Serological and genetical studies on the platelet antigen (zw). *Vox Sanguinis*, **4**, 161–169.

Vaughan JI, Manning M, Warwick RM *et al.* (1998) Inhibition of erythroid progenitor cells by anti-Kell antibodies in fetal alloimmune anemia. *New England Journal of Medicine*, **338**, 798–803.

von dem Borne AE, Ouwehand WH. (1989) Immunology of platelet disorders. *Baillière's Clinical Haematology*, **2**, 749–781.

von dem Borne AE, de Haas M, Roos D *et al.* (1995) Neutrophil antigens, from bench to bedside. *Immunological Investigation*, **24**, 245–272.

Warkentin TE, Smith JW. (1997) The alloimmune thrombocytopenic syndromes. *Transfusion Medicine Reviews*, **11**, 296–307.

Williamson LM, Hackett G, Rennie J. (1998) The natural history of fetomaternal alloimmunization to the platelet-specific antigen HPA-1a (PlA1, Zwa) as determined by antenatal screening. *Blood*, **92**, 2280–2287.

# Chapter 22 Functions of blood group antigens

## Jonathan S Stamler[1] & Marilyn J Telen[2]

[1] *Department of Medicine, Division of Cardiovascular Medicine and Pulmonary Medicine, Duke University Medical Center, Durham, NC, USA*
[2] *Department of Medicine, Division of Hematology, Duke University Medical Center, Durham, NC, USA*

## Introduction

Erythrocyte blood group antigens are, by definition, polymorphic epitopes of red cell surface structures that are recognizable by antibodies. These epitopes generally represent relatively small changes, such as the substitution of one amino acid, in molecules that are largely the same from one individual to another. After the initial discovery of ABO blood groups at the beginning of the 20th century, red cell serologists went on to discover hundreds of such polymorphic epitopes and gradually succeeded in organizing them into blood groups, antigens that arise from polymorphisms of a single parent molecule. During the late 20th century, most of these blood groups were localized to carrier structures (proteins or polysaccharides). Discovery of the biochemical and genetic basis for blood group antigens has now led to exploration of the function of these proteins beyond their importance in transfusion medicine.

This chapter reviews current knowledge about erythrocyte membrane proteins that bear blood group antigens and whose functional importance has been characterized. Primary attention is paid to two of the most interesting of these proteins: the anion exchanger protein, which bears antigens of the Diego blood group system, and the Rh proteins. Functional information about other proteins is summarized briefly.

## Anion-exchanger protein 1 (band 3 protein)

Anion-exchanger protein 1 (AE1) is the most prevalent integral protein of the red blood cell (RBC) membrane

*Molecular Hematology*, 3rd edition. Edited by Drew Provan and John Gribben.
© 2010 Blackwell Publishing.

(~1 million copies/cell), constituting 25–30% of the protein mass. Previously referred to as band 3 protein, on the basis of its original electrophoretic migration profile, AE1 is a 95–102 kDa variably glycosylated protein constructed of 911 amino acids, yielding three distinct structural and functional domains: the N-terminal 45-kDa cytoplasmic domain, the 55-kDa C-terminal hydrophobic transmembrane domain, and a small 28-amino-acid acidic cytoplasmic C-terminus (Figure 22.1). Extracellular domains of AE1 express the Diego blood group system, composed of two sets of antithetical antigens, Diego (Di$^a$/Di$^b$) and Wright (Wr$^a$/Wr$^b$). AE1 also expresses ABH and Ii antigens on a single multibranched N-linked oligosaccharide attached to the fourth extracellular domain.

## Transmembrane domain

The transmembrane segment of AE1 (amino acids 404–882) is responsible for the electroneutral cotransport of $HCO_3^-$ for $Cl^-$, accommodating the tide of $HCO_3^-$ generated by the activity of erythrocytic carbonic anhydrase on $CO_2$ entering the RBC, thus increasing the capacity of the blood to carry $CO_2$ from the tissues to the lungs. In the peripheral tissues, $CO_2$ taken up by RBCs is converted to $H^+$ and $HCO_3^-$ by the action of carbonic anhydrase. The transmembrane domain of AE1 exports $HCO_3^-$ in exchange for $Cl^-$ to maintain physiological pH in the plasma, while $H^+$ binds to hemoglobin (Hb), right-shifting its oxygen affinity to facilitate $O_2$ unloading. The reverse occurs in the lungs. The anion exchange domain is not specific for $HCO_3^-/Cl^-$ and can also transport other anions ( $SO_4^{2-}$, $H_2PO_4^-$), anionic phospholipids, and even divalent cations. Of particular interest, AE1 also transports $NO_2^-$, $NO_3^-$ and $OONO^-$, all products of nitric oxide (NO) metabolism (*see below*). An N-terminal truncated form of AE1 is expressed by the basolateral membrane of the

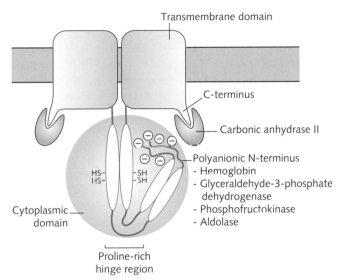

**Fig. 22.1 Schematic representation of an anion-exchanger 1 protein dimer**

The cytoplasmic domains (CDAE1) are enclosed by the tinted circle. CDAE1 cysteine thiols are indicated by –SH, and $\ominus$ indicates the negative charges of acidic amino acids in the N-terminus. Proteins known to bind specifically to the N-terminus are also listed.

α-intercalated cells in the renal collecting ducts and mediates acid secretion.

## C-terminal cytoplasmic domain

The C-terminus of the transmembrane domain of AE1 concludes in a 33-residue cytoplasmic protrusion consisting predominantly of acidic amino acids and has been shown to possess a binding site for the carbonic anhydrase II isoform. Using glutathione S-transferase (GST) fusion proteins with normal and mutated constructs, Vince and colleagues demonstrated that the critical binding site for carbonic anhydrase II is the acidic residue 887–890 region of AE1. A GST fusion protein containing the C-terminal 33 amino acids of AE2 could also bind carbonic anhydrase II, suggesting that this tethering of carbonic anhydrase II to anion exchangers is a general mechanism promoting bicarbonate transport across membranes. AE2 is the most widely expressed form of AE, located in the basolateral membrane of nearly all epithelial cells.

## N-terminal cytoplasmic domain

The primary function of the N-terminal cytoplasmic domain (amino acids 1–403) of AE1 (CDAE1) is to maintain erythrocyte integrity and stability by bracing the cytoskeleton to the plasma membrane. This large hydrophilic domain

projects into the RBC cytoplasm with a spatial orientation that is strongly pH-dependent. Under alkaline conditions (pH 10) the appendage is fully extended, whereas a slightly acidic milieu (pH 6.5) induces flexion such that the N-terminus is brought close to the cell membrane. Flexibility in this part of AE1 is conferred by a proline-rich hinge region between amino acids 175 and 190. The actual orientation of CDAE1 is likely to be a semi-flexed state because the internal pH of RBCs is closer to 7.0–7.2. However, given that carbonic anhydrase II binds to the C-terminus of AE1 in a juxtamembrane location and that each AE1 channel can export 2000–3000 molecules of $HCO_3^-$ per second, the micromilieu immediately adjacent to CDAE1 may experience much lower pH values under certain conditions, inducing greater degrees of CDAE1 flexion. These regions were once thought to be discrete operational units, but it is now clear that remote alterations in membrane domain structure can influence cytoplasmic domain activity, suggesting that these regions are functionally linked.

CDAE1 contains high-affinity binding sites for three peripheral membrane proteins that link AE1 to the underlying cytoskeletal meshwork. Ankyrin is a 206-kDa pyramidal protein that interacts with several sites throughout the length of CDAE1, hinting that ankyrin binds to a flexed conformation of CDAE1 in vivo. Ankyrin also possesses three structural–functional domains: an N-terminal AE1 and tubulin-binding domain, a middle spectrin-binding domain, and a C-terminal domain containing sequences that regulate ankyrin binding to AE1 and spectrin. CDAE1 also binds protein 4.2, or pallidin, a 77-kDa protein that binds to ankyrin as well, acting to reinforce the AE1–ankyrin interaction. Pallidin shows striking homology to transglutaminases but lacks enzymatic activity owing to loss of a necessary conserved active site residue. Finally, CDAE1 interacts (at least in vitro) with protein 4.1, a 66-kDa moiety that firmly binds spectrin near the actin-binding site, thus intensifying the spectrin–actin interaction. The spectrin-binding activity of protein 4.1 is concurrently regulated by phosphorylation/dephosphorylation, $Ca^{2+}$–calmodulin association, and phosphatidylinositol pathways.

The N-terminus of CDAE1 also includes specific high-affinity binding sites for the glycolytic enzymes glyceraldehyde 3-phosphate dehydrogenase (GAPDH), phosphofructokinase (PFK), and aldolase. Binding to CDAE1 results in a decrease in enzymatic activity (90% for aldolase and 100% for GAPDH), while at the same time enzyme substrates, products and cofactors displace the bound enzyme, suggesting that specific CDAE1–enzyme interactions take place at the catalytic site or a linked allosteric site. Aldolase and PFK mutually inhibit each other from binding CDAE1, but neither enzyme can displace bound GAPDH, indicative of a unique binding site for GAPDH.

Phosphorylation of tyrosine 8 of AE1 also regulates glyco-lytic enzyme binding, and thus activity. Binding affinities of the glycolytic enzymes for CDAE1 are strongly dependent on $H^+$ and salt concentration, decreasing dramatically as the pH and ionic strength are raised into the physiological range, calling into question the extent of binding *in vivo*. However, several studies support the notion of significant enzyme–CDAE1 binding in the intact erythrocyte.

## Nitric oxide export

The role of NO as a critical third gas in the human respiratory cycle (in addition to $O_2$ and $CO_2$) is gaining rapid acceptance. Vascular NO is generated chiefly by endothelial NO synthase and is a principal vasodilator and inhibitor of platelet activation. A portion of vascular NO penetrates circulating RBCs, where it interacts with Hb at the heme prosthetic groups or with β-chain cysteine thiols (Cysβ93) to form biologically active *S*-nitrosohemoglobin (SNO-Hb). Under low oxygen tension or oxidative conditions, SNO-Hb can release NO to effect vasodilation (and potentially inhibit platelet activation) (Figure 22.2). However, effective NO export from the RBC requires that the reactive NO species be shielded from the scavenging activities of the heme groups. Erythrocytes protect bioactive NO by complexing it with cysteine thiols (SNO). These "SNO-RBCs" elicit relaxation of vascular tissue *in vitro* at physiological tissue $Po_2$ (5–30 mmHg), while contracting smooth muscle under normoxic arterial conditions (>60 mmHg). RBCs can therefore sense ambient $O_2$ levels through an Hb-$O_2$ binding function and adjust NO bioavailability. In turn, RBCs can cause microvessels to dilate or constrict using SNO-Hb as a vasoactive intermediate. To the extent that tissue $Po_2$ is determined principally by blood flow, impairment in RBC-SNO func-tion would be expected to lower tissue $Po_2$. The implications for disorders of RBCs such as sickle cell disease are considered below.

Compartmentalization of SNO in the erythrocyte membrane by SNO-Hb requires close interaction between the hemoprotein and the inner membrane surface. Hemoglobin binds to the cytoplasmic face of the RBC membrane via both non-specific binding and specific protein–protein interactions. The predominant site of specific interaction between Hb and the RBC membrane is through high-affinity binding to the N-terminal cytoplasmic domain of AE1. More specifically, the site of Hb binding within CDAE1 has been localized to the polyanionic extreme N-terminus, which contains 18 acidic amino acids, thus forming an anionic milieu at physiological pH. Analysis of co-crystals of Hb and a CDAE1 N-terminal peptide has shown that this stretch of acidic residues inserts deeply into the 2,3-diphosphoglycerate-binding pocket formed between β-globin subunits of tetrameric Hb. CDAE1 thus binds with higher affinity to deoxyHb than to oxyHb (in which the β-cleft is occluded), and consistent with the requirements of thermodynamic linkage, the oxygen affinity of Hb is reduced in the presence of isolated CDAE1. Interestingly, the AE1 of kidney intercalated cells is a truncated isoform, lacking the N-terminal 65 residues of the CDAE1, and does not bind Hb, suggesting that these residues perform an AE1-related function specific to the RBC. Binding of Hb to CDAE1 is non-cooperative but causes a rightward shift in the oxygen dissociation curve. Simply stated, binding of Hb to CDAE1 stabilizes the "T" or deoxy conformation of Hb. CDAE1 also binds oxidized $Fe^{3+}$ or metHb more avidly than oxyHb. Because AE1 is present in insufficient quantity to bind a significant fraction of the total Hb in an RBC, the influence of AE1 on overall Hb oxygen delivery is probably negligible. This raises the possibility that AE1 may select a subpopulation of Hb molecules (e.g., SNO-Hb) to interact with, subserving an alternate function sufficiently executed by a small fraction of total Hb molecules. Specifically, SNO-Hb binding to AE1 would promote the T structure and enhance NO group release. Thus, the CDAE1/SNO-Hb interaction would appear designed to accelerate NO release from SNO-Hb (Figure 22.3). In support of this assertion, sequestration of SNO in RBC membranes following treatment with NO is markedly reduced by prior treatment with AE1 inhibitors such as DIDS (4,4′-diisothiocyanostilbene-2,2′-disulfonic acid), phenylglyoxal and niflumic acid. Further, SNO-Hb can trans-nitrosylate inside-out vesicles (IOVs) of RBC membranes, an effect blocked in IOVs purified from RBCs treated with AE1 inhibitors. CDAE1 contains two cysteine residues (Cys201 and Cys317) with reactive thiols that are clustered at the subunit interface of dimeric AE1. These thiols are removed by chymotrypsin (which cleaves CDAE1 from the

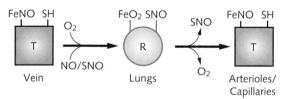

**Fig. 22.2 Simplified allosteric model of NO–hemoglobin interactions**
Nitric oxide (NO) binds to the heme groups of deoxygenated or T-state hemoglobin (Hb). On oxygenation, Hb assumes the R conformation and NO is transferred to the cysteine thiol in position 93 of the β-chain (Cysβ93) to form S-nitrosohemoglobin (SNO-Hb). During transit through the physiological oxygen gradient, Po2 falls, SNO-Hb converts to the T state, and NO is released from Cysβ93 to evoke vasodilation (thus regulating blood flow) or to inhibit platelet activation.

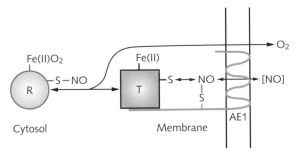

**Fig. 22.3 Interaction between S-nitrosohemoglobin (SNO-Hb) and the cytoplasmic domain of erythrocyte anion-exchanger 1 (CDAE1)**

Binding to CDAE1 stabilizes the T state of SNO-Hb and reduces NO affinity. SNO-Hb transfers NO to vicinal thiols in CDAE1, which can then release NO bioequivalents to effect vasodilation or inhibit platelet activation.

transmembrane domain) and are surrounded by amino acids that fit an *S*-nitrosylation motif. Accordingly, transnitrosylation of RBC IOVs by SNO-Hb is blocked by thiol-alkylating agents or enzymatic digestion of the IOVs with chymotrypsin. In cross-linking studies, Hb forms a disulfide bond (−S−S−) between its Cysβ93 thiols and the cytoplasmic domain cysteines of AE1, suggesting close spatial interplay in this region. Hemichromes, which are native Hb molecules with altered conformation near the heme, have a very high affinity for CDAE1. Moreover, hemichromes formed by the covalent modification of the Cysβ93 thiol (an SNO-Hb mimetic) bind preferentially to AE1. Therefore, transnitrosylation of a vicinal thiol within the cytoplasmic domain of AE1 is a strong candidate mechanism for transfer of the NO group from Cysβ93 of SNO-Hb to the RBC membrane (Figure 22.3). In fact, like Hb, SNO-Hb forms disulfide links with AE1 under oxidative conditions, confirming the proximity of SNO-Hb and CDAE1 thiols. Further, *S*-nitrosylated AE1 can be immunoprecipitated from the membranes of RBCs and from IOVs treated with SNO-Hb. Thus, a role for the anion exchange function of AE1 in transmembrane movement of NO bioactivity is enticing. It is important to note in this regard that RBCs can release small *S*-nitrosothiols, but AE1-mediated transport of an NO congener has not been shown. AE1-liganded (S)NO may directly exchange NO groups with receptors on the vascular wall.

SNO-Hb in RBCs is distributed equally between the cytosol and plasma membrane. However, only the plasma membrane fraction is bioactive. Deficiency of plasma membrane SNO can result from defects in either SNO-Hb synthesis or its transfer of NO groups into the membrane. In either case, RBC vasoactivity is compromised. Vasodilation by RBCs is impaired in several diseases, including sickle cell disease, which is characterized by a triune defect in SNO processing: SNO-Hb synthesis is reduced (an intrinsic property of Hb S); the interaction between Hb S and AE1 is disrupted; and the transfer of NO into the membrane is impaired. Most notably, Cys residues of AE1 that would otherwise accept the NO groups are oxidized in sickle RBCs. Membrane SNO is therefore greatly diminished. Impaired vasodilation in sickle patients corresponds with clinical symptoms (painful crises and organ damage) and may therefore represent a molecular corollary of vaso-occlusive disorders. A deficiency in plasma membrane SNO-AE1 has also been found in banked blood, which likewise exhibits impaired vasodilation.

## Deficiencies and mutations of AE1

Clinical conditions resulting from mutations or deficiencies in AE1 range from asymptomatic to severe, with manifestations predictably reflecting perturbation of one or both of the two primary functions of AE1, $HCO_3^-/Cl^-$ exchange and cytoskeletal membrane stability. A significant segment of the population (5–20%) are heterozygous for an AE1 polymorphism called "band 3 Memphis," involving a lysine to glutamic acid substitution in codon 56 resulting in a functionally normal AE1.

Southeast Asian ovalocytosis (SAO), characterized genotypically as a deletion of amino acids 400–408 in AE1, results in oval RBCs with increased rigidity, decreased osmotic fragility, and reduced expression of certain red cell antigens. Natural selection dramatically increases the prevalence of SAO in areas with endemic malarial infection, given that this defect confers reduced parasitemia and disease severity. However, homozygosity for the SAO mutation appears to be incompatible with life, as homozygotes have never been observed (even in areas with 40% prevalence), and the incidence of miscarriage in heterozygous parents is twice that for normals (20% vs. 9.8%).

Over 40 mutations of the AE1 protein have been found to be associated with a subset of individuals with dominant hereditary spherocytosis, a condition characterized by loss of erythrocyte surface area and a mild to severe hemolysis almost invariably improved by splenectomy. Despite being scattered throughout the entire protein, many mutations in the membrane-spanning domain involve substitutions of highly conserved arginine residues thought to be important in maintaining proper membrane orientation. Other mutations causing hereditary spherocytosis, including those in the cytoplasmic domain, lead to decreased binding affinities for the cytoskeletal bridging proteins ankyrin and pallidin.

Complete AE1 deletion in a murine model results in a deadly hypercoagulable state in which only 5–10% of AE1 null mice survive the neonatal period. Almost uniformly, animals were found at necropsy to have large thrombotic lesions of the heart, subcapsular liver necrosis suggesting arteriolar ischemia, and large vein thrombi. Inaba and colleagues similarly described a total deficiency of AE1 in Japanese black cattle homozygous for a nonsense mutation (CGA→TGA) in codon 646 causing an early stop signal. These animals exhibit moderate uncompensated anemias, spherocytosis, and mild acidosis at rest that is exacerbated by exercise. The only reported human case of total absence of AE1 occurred in a Portuguese female delivered by cesarean section at 36 weeks of gestation. The neonate was hydropic and severely anemic and had massive hepatosplenomegaly. Polymerase chain reaction (PCR) demonstrated homozygosity for the Coimbra mutation (V488M), complete absence of AE1 and protein 4.2, and reduction of spectrin and ankyrin by 43 and 57%, respectively. Spherocytes and erythroblasts dominated the peripheral blood morphology, while hyperchloremic acidosis was identified by age 3 months. The patient is being treated with an intensive transfusion regimen, chelator therapy, and oral base replacement to counteract the acidosis. Other than slightly delayed psychomotor development and stable nephrocalcinosis, her condition remains stable.

In addition, hereditary renal tubular acidosis can result from mutations in the genes encoding AE1, carbonic anhydrase II, or different subunits of the $H^+$-ATPase. Mutations of AE1 may account for up to 70% of cases in some areas of the world. These mutations, which affect the renal isoform of AE1, cause defects in urinary acidification and also lead to hypokalemia.

# Rh protein

The rhesus (Rh) blood group antigens constitute the most polymorphic family of human erythrocyte antigens and are also the most frequent inducers of transfusion- and parturition-related alloantibodies. Three separate proteins make up the Rh family of proteins, including RhD and RhCE, which are unglycosylated proteins of 417 amino acids with 97% homology, and Rh-associated glycoprotein (RhAG), which shows about 40% homology to RhD/CE. While scores of individual Rh antigens are recognized, only five epitopes (D, C, c, E and e) carried on the RhD or CE proteins are routinely identified; RhAG is thought to carry only the high-frequency Duclos antigen. RhCE expresses the antithetical Cc/Ee antigens, while no antithetical antigen exists for D. However, the presence (Rh-positive) and absence (Rh-negative) of the D antigen have sometimes been designated as D and d, respectively. Thus, the eight most common haplotypes associated with the Rh system are DCe, DcE, Dce,

dce, DCE, dcE, dCe, and dCE. The D antigen is a collection of conformation-dependent epitopes along the entire RhD protein. Deletion of the *RHD* gene characterizes most D-negative Caucasians, while in other populations (mainly Japanese and African blacks) the D-negative phenotype appears to arise from a variety of missense and nonsense mutations in otherwise intact *RHD* genes. In addition, there are multiple "weak D," "D category" and other variant D phenotypes. These are cataloged by several websites, including RhesusBase (www.uni-ulm.de/~fwagner/RH/RB/). RhAG is a glycosylated 409-amino-acid 50-kDa protein that appears to serve as a chaperone for RhD and RhCE to the RBC membrane; Rh antigens are only expressed if RhAG is also present.

Using known amino acid sequences, studies using both topology prediction and immunochemical analysis suggest that Rh proteins span the erythrocyte membrane 12 times, with both termini in the cytoplasm. Many multi-spanning membrane proteins have a transporter function. Thus, its structure, as well as its partial homology to a family of ammonium transport proteins, led to investigation of a possible transport function for Rh proteins. Interestingly, RhAG and the related proteins RhBG and RhCG found in non-erythroid tissues share a molecular architecture much more similar to the *Escherichia coli* AmtB channel than do RhD and RhCE. Marini and colleagues, having found sequence similarity between RhAG, and to a lesser extent RhCE, and the $NH_4^+$ transporters Mep1 protein in yeast and the Amt1 protein in the plant *Arabidopsis thaliana*, explored this possible function of Rh proteins. They showed that RhAG expressed in a yeast mutant with deletions in the three endogenous ammonium transporters (*mep1Δ mep2Δ mep3Δ*) could restore growth defects elicited by low-ammonium medium. However, this study has been criticized because the expressed RhAG was not glycosylated and the authors failed to show actual $NH_4^+$ uptake. Westhoff and colleagues showed that *Xenopus* oocytes expressing solely human RhAG protein were able to specifically transport $NH_4^+$ in a saturable, non-electrogenic, and pH-dependent manner, suggesting that the RhAG transport mechanism involves exchange of $NH_4^+$ for $H^+$, resulting in the net transport of $NH_3$ into the cell. More recent work has suggested that erythroid RhAG may serve to sequester ammonia in red cells, since it has been noted that blood plasma $NH_3$ and $NH_4^+$ levels are three times lower than the levels found in erythrocytes. Furthermore, in non-erythroid tissues, RhBG and RhCG are located at specific cellular surfaces where there is a disparate concentration of ammonia, such as at the luminal surface in the kidney.

Others have argued that Amt proteins act as gas channels handling $NH_3$, rather than as transporters of $NH_4^+$ cations, and that both erythrocytic and non-mammalian Rh proteins represent $CO_2$ transporters. Supporting this assertion, Soupene and colleagues found that Rh protein expression in the green alga *Chlamydomonas reinhardtii* was significantly higher under elevated $CO_2$ conditions (air + 3% $CO_2$ for 3 hours) than in air alone (0.035% $CO_2$). Further, Rh mRNA and protein expression remained low under conditions in which methylammonium uptake was high (nitrogen-limiting, with arginine as the sole nitrogen source instead of $NH_4Cl$). The same group went on to show that mutant algae without RH1 mRNA or protein grow slowly at high $CO_2$. Other evidence suggests that such algae fail to equilibrate this gas normally, and that gene regulation downstream of the effect of $CO_2$ is also abnormal. At this point, further studies in mammalian systems will be needed to confirm the function(s) of Rh and RhAG proteins.

$Rh_{null}$ disease is characterized by the complete absence of Rh proteins in the RBCs of affected subjects. The resulting erythrocytes exhibit stomatocytic and spherocytic changes, increased osmotic fragility, and deviations in ionic fluxes and cell volume. Two variations of $Rh_{null}$ disease have been identified, historically termed "amorph" and "regulator," based on the underlying molecular defect from which they arise. The amorph variety involves a genetic change in the *RhCE* gene coupled with deletion or inactivation of *RHD*, while the regulator phenotype results from two mutant *RHAG* genes (homozygote or compound heterozygote). These null phenotypes also display marked reductions in Rh-associated membrane proteins, including the LW glycoprotein (ICAM-4), integrin-associated protein (IAP) and glycophorin B (a type I membrane glycoprotein that bears the Ss antigens and may serve to couple Rh with larger complexes containing AE1 and GPA).

## Glycophorins C and D

Glycophorins C and D (GPC/GPD) are 32- and 23-kDa membrane glycoproteins arising from the same four-exon gene (2q14–q21) via alternative in-frame mRNA translation initiation sites, giving rise to the Gerbich erythrocyte antigens, Ge:2 and Ge:3. GPC and GPD are identical except that GPD has been truncated by 21 amino acids at the N-terminus. There are two or three copies per cell of GPC for each copy of GPD. While being infrequent targets of alloantibodies, GPC/GPD appear to be vital membrane-stabilizing components serving as high-affinity binding sites for the peripheral membrane protein 4.1, which acts to affix actin and spectrin elements. In addition to AE1–ankyrin–spectrin, the GPC/GPD–protein 4.1–spectrin/actin bridge is believed to constitute the other major connection site between the erythrocyte membrane and its spectrin skeleton. Evidence

for the importance of GPC/GPD in membrane/cytoskeletal stability originally arose from observations in cells containing natural defects in one or more members of this bridge. For instance, complete absence of erythrocyte GPC/GPD (termed the Leach phenotype) results in a rare form of hereditary elliptocytosis characterized by impaired red cell mechanical properties. However, these same GPC/GPD-deficient elliptocytic cells were also found to contain reduced amounts of protein 4.1. In addition, GPC interacts with p55, a member of the membrane-associated guanylate kinase family. The C-terminal region of GPC and GPD interacts with the PDZ domain in p55 as part of the ternary complex.

GPC/GPD deficiency is relatively common in Southeast Asia. One particular variant, the Melanesian Gerbich negativity phenotype, has been shown to reach a high frequency (46.5%) in coastal areas of Papua New Guinea, where *Plasmodium falciparum* malaria is hyperendemic, suggesting that it may confer protection against erythrocyte invasion by the parasite. This polymorphism is characterized genotypically by deletion of exon 3 (thus *GPCΔex3*) and phenotypically by ovalocytic RBCs. The *P. falciparum* erythrocyte-binding antigen EBA-140 appears to bind with high affinity to GPC, and this interaction mediates a principal invasion pathway into human erythrocytes. EBA-140 does not bind to GPC in Ge-negative erythrocytes from Papua residents homozygous for *GPCΔex3*, nor can *P. falciparum* infect such cells using this invasion pathway.

Interestingly, while the invasion of *GPCΔex3* erythrocytes by *P. falciparum* parasites is less efficient *in vitro*, no differences in infection rates for either *P. falciparum* or *P. vivax* in Ge-negative subjects have been observed to date. However, subjects with other RBC polymorphisms that are found in high frequencies in endemic malaria regions, notably sickle cell hemoglobin (Hb S), also demonstrate infectivity rates similar to those of subjects lacking the sickle trait phenotype. Nevertheless, individuals with Hb S trait show reduced parasite density and experience fewer cases of cerebral or severe malaria. Thus, it may be that the *GPCΔex3* phenotype is selected for by reducing erythrocyte invasion rates by malaria parasites, thus lessening disease severity. Studies to determine whether there has been natural selection of the *GPCΔex3* allele as a safeguard against severe malaria remain to be conducted.

## Blood group antigen proteins that function as adhesion molecules

A number of erythrocyte membrane proteins have been identified as adhesion molecules. As shown in Table 22.1, these include the proteins that bear the Lutheran, LW and Indian blood group antigens.

CD44 bears the Indian antigens and was first described on erythrocytes as *In(Lu)*-related p80, because expression on erythrocytes is downregulated by the *In(Lu)* gene. CD44 was the first erythrocyte membrane protein to be characterized as an adhesion molecule and bears homology to the cartilage link and proteoglycan core proteins, which are known to interact with hyaluronan. This similarity led to the demon-

**Table 22.1** Adhesion molecules of erythrocytes.

| Blood group antigen | Alternative name(s) | Ligand/adhesive function |
| --- | --- | --- |
| In$^a$/In$^b$ | CD44, *In(Lu)*-related p80 | Hyaluronan, possibly also fibronectin |
| JMH | CD108, semaphorin K1 (SEMA7A) | Possible role in adhesion of activated lymphocytes |
| Lutheran | B-CAM/LU, CD239 | Laminin containing the α5 chain, α4β1 integrin |
| LW | CD242, ICAM-4, LW | Leukocyte, endothelial and platelet integrins, including αVβ3, LFA-1 (αLβ2), Mac-1 (αMβ2), αVβ1, αVβ5, αIIbβ3 |
| Nak$^a$ (platelets) | CD36 (reticulocytes only), platelet GPIV, Nak$^a$ (platelets) | Thrombospondin (platelets), LDL |
| Ok$^a$ | CD147, neurothelin | Type IV collagen, fibronectin. Laminin in other tissues |
| None known | VLA-4 (reticulocytes only), α4β1 integrin (CD49d/CD29) | Thrombospondin, VCAM-1, possibly fibronectin |
| None known | CD47, integrin-associated protein (IAP) | Thrombospondin, SIRP-1α |
| None known | CD58, lymphocyte-associated antigen-3 (LFA-3) | CD2 |
| RAPH1 | CD151, *MIC2* gene product | Proposed role in kidney and skin morphogenesis, possibly through adhesion to laminin or collagen |
| Scianna | ERMAP (erythroid membrane-associated protein) | Possible adhesion molecule that localizes to points of cell–cell contact |

stration that CD44 also bound to this component of extra-cellular matrix and basement membranes. On leukocytes, CD44 appears to be involved in the interaction of leukocytes with endothelial cells, including the homing of lymphocytes to peripheral lymphoid organs and sites of inflammation. Ligand binding to CD44 can also induce cytokine release and T-cell activation. However, on erythrocytes the functional significance of CD44 remains unclear, although one report has indicated that CD44 contributes to the ability of early erythroid precursors to bind to bone marrow fibronectin. CD44 also plays an important role in the metastatic behavior of tumor cells.

The molecule that bears Lutheran blood group antigens has been identified as a laminin receptor. Lutheran antigens are expressed by two proteins that arise from alternate splicing of a single gene. These two proteins (sometimes called B-CAM and LU) are identical except for their cytoplasmic domains, and they both appear to function equally well as laminin receptors. Interestingly, B-CAM/LU expression and function are increased on red cells from patients with sickle cell disease, and this function can be activated further by exposure of sickle red cells to epinephrine and other reagents that lead to increased intracellular cyclic AMP. Increase in cyclic AMP leads to activation of protein kinase A, which appears to phosphorylate B-CAM/LU. Genetic studies of red cell adhesion in patients with sickle cell disease have shown that higher adhesion to laminin is associated with specific polymorphisms in the genes encoding the β$_2$-adrenergic receptor and adenylyl cyclase 6, one of the more ubiquitous isoforms of adenylyl cyclase. B-CAM/LU has also been implicated in the abnormal behavior of red cells from patients with polycythemia vera. In this disease, red cells are also abnormally adherent to laminin and bear constitutively phosphorylated B-CAM/LU. Finally, B-CAM/LU has also been shown to mediate adhesion to the α4β1 integrin, also known as VLA-4, which is expressed by reticulocytes and leukocytes, among other cells. However, the contribution of B-CAM/LU-mediated red cell adhesion to the pathophysiology of vaso-occlusion or to the frequent thrombotic complications of polycythemia remains unproven.

The LW protein also appears to be an adhesion receptor, although, unlike CD44 and B-CAM/LU, LW interacts with cell surface proteins rather than extracellular matrix components. LW has also been called intercellular adhesion molecule (ICAM)-4 because it is highly homologous to other members of the ICAM family of adhesion molecules. Like other ICAMs, LW can bind to the leukocyte integrins CD11a/CD18 (LFA-1, αLβ2), CD11b/CD18 (MAC-1, αMβ2) and CD11c/CD18. Recently, it has also been shown that LW can bind to αV integrins, as well as to the αIIbβ3 integrin of platelets. LW contributes to the adhesion of sickle red cells to the endothelium by binding to αVβ3. This interaction appears to be the dominant high-affinity interaction between sickle red cells both *in vitro* and *in vivo*. Interestingly, LW adhesive function is also activated by exposure of red cells to epinephrine, which leads to cyclic AMP- and protein kinase A-dependent LW phosphorylation. In addition, some investigators speculate that LW may be important in facilitating the adhesion of erythroid precursors to bone marrow macrophages in erythroid islands during erythropoiesis.

## Blood group antigen proteins with other functions

Table 22.2 lists blood group antigens associated with functions other than adhesion. As indicated, proteins bearing blood group antigens have a broad diversity of functions. Some, such as the proteins that bear the Kidd and Colton blood group antigens, are transporters. Others, such as those that bear the Cartwright and Kell antigens, are ectoenzymes. In addition, erythrocytes bear receptors for complement components and chemokines. The degree to which polymorphisms and deficiency of these proteins contribute to human disease remains to be further explored.

**Table 22.2** Diverse functions of blood group antigen proteins.

| Blood group | Alternative name(s) | Function |
|---|---|---|
| Cartwright | ACHE | Acetylcholinesterase |
| Colton | Aquaporin-1 (AQP-1) | Water channel |
| Cromer | Decay accelerating factor, CD55 | Promotes the degradation of C3 and C5 convertases |
| Dombrock | DOK | ADP-ribosyltransferase ectoenzyme |
| Duffy | DARC | Chemokine receptor |
| Kell | KEL | Zinc-binding neutral endopeptidase; cleaves big endothelin-3 to endothelin-3 |
| Kidd | UT1 | Urea transporter |
| Knops/McCoy | C3b/C4b receptor (CD35), complement receptor type 1 | Binds C3b and C4b and facilitates immune clearance |
| Kx | | Possibly a neurotransmitter transporter; deficiency causes neuroacanthocytosis or McLeod syndrome |

## Summary

Proteins that bear blood group antigens have diverse functions, and some proteins, such as AE1, encompass several functions within a single protein molecule. Abnormalities of these proteins, in the form of either deficiencies or mutations, can lead to red cell disorders, such as hemolytic anemia, or have more far-reaching effects, as in the association of Kx deficiency with neuroacanthocytosis and mutations of AE1 with renal tubular acidosis. Finally, these proteins undoubtedly contribute both to normal physiology and to the pathophysiology of human diseases, including sickle cell anemia, malaria, and perhaps others.

## Further reading

### AE1

Anderson RA, Marchesi VT. (1985) Regulation of the association of membrane skeletal protein 4.1 with glycophorin by polyphosphoinositide. *Nature*, **318**, 295–298.

Bennett-Guerrero E, Veldman TH, Doctor A *et al.* (2007) Evolution of adverse changes in stored RBCs. *Proceedings of the National Academy of Sciences of the United States of America*, **104**, 17063–17068.

Bruce LJ, Kay MMB, Lawrence C *et al.* (1993) Band 3 HT, a human red-cell variant associated with acanthocytosis and increased anion transport, carries the mutation pro 868 leu in the membrane domain of band 3. *Biochemical Journal*, **293**, 317–320.

Celedon G, Gonzalez G, Pino J, Lissi EA. (2007) Peroxynitrite oxidizes erythrocyte membrane band 3 protein and diminishes its anion transport capacity. *Free Radical Research*, **41**, 316–323.

Chu H, Low PS. (2006) Mapping of glycolytic enzyme-binding sites on human erythrocyte band 3. *Biochemical Journal*, **400**, 143–151.

Chu H, Breite A, Ciraolo P, Franco RS, Low PS. (2008) Characterization of the deoxyhemoglobin binding site on human erythrocyte band 3: implications for $O_2$ regulation of erythrocyte properties. *Blood*, **111**, 932–938.

Cohen CM, Dotimas E, Korsgren C. (1993) Human erythrocyte membrane protein 4.2 (pallidin). *Seminars in Hematology*, **30**, 119–137.

Davis L, Lux SE, Bennett V. (1989) Mapping the ankyrin-binding site of the human erythrocyte anion exchanger. *Journal of Biological Chemistry*, **264**, 9665–9672.

Funder J, Wieth JO. (1966) Chloride and hydrogen ion distribution between human red cells and plasma. *Acta Physiologica Scandinavica*, **68**, 234–245.

Genton B, Al-Yaman F, Mgone CS *et al.* (1995) Ovalocytosis and cerebral malaria. *Nature*, **378**, 564–565.

Guizouarn H, Martial S, Gabillat N, Borgese F. (2007) Point mutations involved in red cell stomatocytosis convert the electroneutral anion exchanger 1 to a nonselective cation conductance. *Blood*, **110**, 2158–2165.

Gutierrez E, Sung LA. (2007) Interactions of recombinant mouse erythrocyte transglutaminase with membrane skeletal proteins. *Journal of Membrane Biology*, **219**, 93–104.

Hassoun H, Wang Y, Vassiliadis J et al. (1998) Targeted inactivation of murine band 3 (AE1) gene produces a hypercoagulable state causing widespread thrombosis *in vivo*. *Blood*, **92**, 1785–1792.

Hess DT, Matsumoto A, Kim S-O, Marshall HE, Stamler JS. (2005) Protein S-nitrosylation: purview and parameters. *Nature Reviews. Molecular Cell Biology*, **6**, 150–166.

Inaba M, Yawata A, Koshino I et al. (1996) Defective anion transport and marked spherocytosis with membrane instability caused by hereditary total deficiency of red cell band 3 in cattle due to a nonsense mutation. *Journal of Clinical Investigation*, **97**, 1804–1817.

Jarolim P, Palek J, Amato D et al. (1991) Deletion in erythrocyte band 3 gene in malaria-resistant Southeast Asian ovalocytosis. *Proceedings of the National Academy of Sciences of the United States of America*, **88**, 11022–11026.

Jarolim P, Rubin HL, Brabec V et al. (1995) Mutations of conserved arginines in the membrane domain of erythroid band 3 protein lead to a decrease in membrane-associated band 3 and to the phenotype of hereditary spherocytosis. *Blood*, **85**, 634–640.

Jia L, Bonaventura C, Bonaventura J et al. (1996) S-nitrosohaemoglobin: a dynamic activity of blood involved in vascular control. *Nature*, **380**, 221–226.

Khositseth S, Sirikanerat A, Wongbenjarat K et al. (2007) Distal renal tubular acidosis associated with anion exchanger 1 mutations in children in Thailand. *American Journal of Kidney Diseases*, **49**, 841–850.

Kindt JT, Woods A, Martin BM et al. (1992) Covalent alteration of the prosthetic heme of human hemoglobin by BrCCl₃ cross-linking of heme to cysteine residue 93. *Journal of Biological Chemistry*, **267**, 8739–8743.

Kittanakom S, Cordat E, Reithmeier RA. (2008) Dominant-negative effect of Southeast Asian ovalocytosis anion exchanger 1 in compound heterozygous distal renal tubular acidosis. *Biochemical Journal*, **410**, 271–81.

Kollert-Jons A, Wagner S, Hubner S et al. (1993) Anion exchanger 1 in human kidney and oncocytoma differs from erythroid AE1 in its NH₂ terminus. *American Journal of Physiology*, **265**, F813–F821.

Ling E, Danilov YN, Cohen CM. (1988) Modulation of red cell band 4.1 function by cAMP-dependent kinase and protein kinase C phosphorylation. *Journal of Biological Chemistry*, **263**, 2209–2216.

Liu SC, Zhai S, Palek J et al. (1990) Molecular defect of the band 3 protein in Southeast Asian ovalocytosis. *New England Journal of Medicine*, **323**, 1558–1560.

Low PS, Allen DP, Zioncheck TF et al. (1987) Tyrosine phosphorylation of band 3 inhibits peripheral protein binding. *Journal of Biological Chemistry*, **262**, 4592–4596.

McMahon TJ, Stone AE, Bonaventura J et al. (2000) Functional coupling of oxygen binding and vasoactivity in S-nitrosohemoglobin. *Journal of Biological Chemistry*, **275**, 16738–16745.

McMahon TJ, Moon RE, Luschinger BP et al. (2002) Nitric oxide in the human respiratory cycle. *Nature Medicine*, **8**, 711–717.

Miki Y, Tazawa T, Hirano K et al. (2007) Clearance of oxidized erythrocytes by macrophages: involvement of caspases in the generation of clearance signal at band 3 glycoprotein. *Biochemical and Biophysical Research Communications*, **363**, 57–62.

Ohanian V, Wolfe LC, John KM et al. (1984) Analysis of the ternary interaction of the red cell membrane skeletal proteins spectrin, actin, and 4.1. *Biochemistry*, **23**, 4416–4420.

Pawloski JR, Stamler JS. (2002) Nitric oxide in RBCs. *Transfusion*, **42**, 1603–1609.

Pawloski JR, Swaminathan RV, Stamler JS. (1998) Cell-free and erythrocyte S-nitrosohemoglobin inhibits human platelet aggregation. *Circulation*, **97**, 263–267.

Pawloski JR, Hess DT, Stamler JS. (2001) Export by red blood cells of nitric oxide bioactivity. *Nature*, **409**, 622–626.

Pawloski JR, Hess DT, Stamler JS. (2005) Impaired vasodilation by red blood cells in sickle cell disease. *Proceedings of the National Academy of Sciences of the United States of America*, **102**, 2531–2536.

Perrotta S, Borriello A, Scaloni A et al. (2005) The N-terminal 11 amino acids of human erythrocyte band 3 are critical for aldolase binding and protein phosphorylation: implications for band 3 function. *Blood*, **106**, 4359–4366.

Rauenbuehler PB, Cordes KA, Salhany JM. (1982) Identification of the hemoglobin binding sites on the inner surface of the erythrocyte membrane. *Biochimica et Biophysica Acta*, **692**, 361–370.

Reynolds JD, Ahearn GS, Angelo M, Zhang J, Cobb F, Stamler JS. (2007) S-nitrosohemoglobin deficiency: a mechanism for loss of physiological activity in banked blood. *Proceedings of the National Academy of Sciences of the United States of America*, **104**, 17058–17062.

Ribeiro ML, Allosio N, Almeida H et al. (2000) Severe hereditary spherocytosis and distal renal tubular acidosis associated with the total absence of band 3. *Blood*, **96**, 1602–1604.

Shingles R, Roh MH, McCarty RE. (1997) Direct measurement of nitrite transport across erythrocyte membrane vesicles using the fluorescent probe, 6-methoxy-n-(3-sulfopropyl) quinolinium. *Journal of Bioenergetics and Biomembranes*, **29**, 611–616.

Singel DJ, Stamler JS. (2005) Chemical physiology of blood flow regulation by red blood cells: the role of nitric oxide and S-nitrosohemoglobin. *Annual Review of Physiology*, **67**, 99–145.

Stamler JS, Jia L, Eu JP et al. (1997) Blood flow regulation by S-nitrosohemoglobin in the physiological oxygen gradient. *Science*, **276**, 2034–2037.

Stamler JS, Toone EJ, Lipton SA et al. (1997) (S)NO signals: translocation, regulation, and a consensus motif. *Neuron*, **18**, 691–696.

Stehberger PA, Shmukler BE, Stuart-Tilley AK, Peters LL, Alper SL, Wagner CA. (2007) Distal renal tubular acidosis in mice lacking the AE1 (band3) Cl⁻/HCO3⁻ exchanger (slc4a1). *Journal of the American Society of Nephrology*, **18**, 1408–1418.

Thevenin BJM, Bicknese SE, Park J et al. (1996) Distance between cys-201 in erythrocyte band 3 and the bilayer measured by single-photon radioluminescence. *Biophysical Journal*, **71**, 2645–2655.

Tsuneshige A, Imai K, Tyuma I. (1987) The binding of hemoglobin to red cell membrane lowers its oxygen affinity. *Journal of Biochemistry*, **101**, 695–704.

Vince JW, Reithmeier RAF. (2000) Identification of the carbonic anhydrase II binding site in the Cl⁻/HCO3⁻ anion exchanger AE1. *Biochemistry*, **39**, 5527–5533.

von Kalckreuth V, Evans JA, Timmann C et al. (2006) Promoter polymorphism of the anion-exchange protein 1 associated with severe malarial anemia and fatality. *Journal of Infectious Diseases*, **194**, 949–957.

Weaver DC, Pasternack GR, Marchesi VT. (1984) The structural basis of ankyrin function. II. Identification of two functional domains. *Journal of Biological Chemistry*, **259**, 6170–6175.

Zhou J, Low PS. (2001) Characterization of the reversible conformational equilibrium in the cytoplasmic domain of human erythrocyte membrane band 3. *Journal of Biological Chemistry*, **276**, 38147–38151.

## Rh

Avent ND, Madgett TE, Lee ZE *et al.* (2006) Molecular biology of Rh proteins and relevance to molecular medicine. *Expert Reviews in Molecular Medicine*, **8**, 1–20.

Callebaut I, Dulin F, Bertrand O *et al.* (2006) Hydrophobic cluster analysis and modeling of the human Rh protein three-dimensional structures. *Transfusion Clinique et Biologique*, **13**, 70–84.

Conroy MJ, Bullough PA, Merrick M, Avent ND. (2005) Modelling the human rhesus proteins: implications for structure and function. *British Journal of Haematology*, **131**, 543–551.

Endeward V, Cartron JP, Ripoche P, Gros G. (2008) RhAG protein of the Rhesus complex is a $CO_2$ channel in the human red cell membrane. *FASEB Journal*, **22**, 64–73.

Khademi S, Stroud RM. (2006) The Amt/MEP/Rh family: structure of AmtB and the mechanism of ammonia gas conduction. *Physiology (Bethesda)*, **21**, 419–429.

Le Van Kim C, Colin Y, Cartron J-P. (2006) Rh proteins: key structural and functional components of the red cell membrane. *Blood Reviews*, **20**, 93–110.

Marini AM, Urrestarazu A, Beauwens R *et al.* (1997) The Rh (rhesus) blood group polypeptides are related to $NH_4^+$ transporters. *Trends in Biochemical Sciences*, **22**, 460–461.

Nicolas V, Mouro-Chanteloup I, Lopez C *et al.* (2006) Functional interaction between Rh proteins and the spectrin-based skeleton in erythroid and epithelial cells. *Transfusion Clinique et Biologique*, **13**, 23–28.

Planelles G. (2007) Ammonium homeostasis and human Rhesus glycoproteins. *Nephron Physiology*, **105**, 11–17.

Polin H, Danzer M, Hofer K, Gassner W, Gabriel C. (2007) Effective molecular RHD typing strategy for blood donations. *Transfusion*, **47**, 1350–1355.

Soupene E, King N, Feild E *et al.* (2002) Rhesus expression in a green alga is regulated by $CO_2$. *Proceedings of the National Academy of Sciences of the United States of America*, **99**, 7769–7773.

Soupene E, Inwood W, Kustu S. (2004) Lack of the Rhesus protein Rh1 impairs growth of the green alga *Chlamydomonas reinhardtii* at high $CO_2$. *Proceedings of the National Academy of Sciences of the United States of America*, **101**, 7787–7792.

Szekely D, Chapman BE, Bubb WA, Kuchel PW. (2006) Rapid exchange of fluoroethylamine via the Rhesus complex in human erythrocytes: $^{19}$F NMR magnetization transfer analysis showing competition by ammonia and ammonia analogues. *Biochemistry*, **45**, 9354–9361.

Wagner FF, Moulds JM, Flegel WA. (2005) Genetic mechanisms of Rhesus box variation. *Transfusion*, **45**, 338–344.

Westhoff CM. (2007) The structure and function of the Rh antigen complex. *Seminars in Hematology*, **44**, 42–50.

Westhoff CM, Ferreri-Jacobia M, Mak DO, Foskett JK. (2002) Identification of the erythrocyte Rh blood group glycoprotein as a mammalian ammonium transporter. *Journal of Biological Chemistry*, **277**, 12499–12502.

## Glycophorins C and D

Chang SH, Low PS. (2001) Regulation of the glycophorin C–protein 4.1 membrane-to-skeleton bridge and evaluation of its contribution to erythrocyte membrane stability. *Journal of Biological Chemistry*, **276**, 22223–22230.

Colin Y, Le Van Kim C, Tsapis A *et al.* (1989) Human erythrocyte glycophorin C. Gene structure and rearrangement in genetic variants. *Journal of Biological Chemistry*, **264**, 3773–3780.

Diakowski W, Grzybek M, Sikorski AF. (2006) Protein 4.1, a component of the erythrocyte membrane skeleton and its related homologue proteins forming the protein 4.1/FERM superfamily. *Folia Histochemica et Cytobiologica*, **44**, 231–248.

Gascard P, Cohen CM. (1994) Absence of high-affinity band 4.1 binding sites from membranes of glycophorin C- and D-deficient (Leach phenotype) erythrocytes. *Blood*, **83**, 1102–1108.

Hemming NJ, Anstee DJ, Mawby WJ *et al.* (1994) Localization of the protein 4.1-binding site on human erythrocyte glycophorins C and D. *Biochemical Journal*, **299**, 191–196.

Kusunoki H, Kohno T. (2007) Structural insight into the interaction between the p55 PDZ domain and glycophorin C. *Biochemical and Biophysical Research Communications*, **359**, 972–978.

Lobo CA, Rodriguez M, Reid M, Lustigman S. (2003) Glycophorin C is the receptor for the *Plasmodium falciparum* erythrocyte binding ligand PfEBP-2 (BAEBL). *Blood*, **101**, 4628–4631.

Maier AG, Duraisingh MT, Reeder JC *et al.* (2003) *Plasmodium falciparum* erythrocyte invasion through glycophorin C and selection for Gerbich negativity in human populations. *Nature Medicine*, **9**, 87–92.

Mayer DC, Jiang L, Achur RN *et al.* (2006) The glycophorin C N-linked glycan is a critical component of the ligand for the *Plasmodium falciparum* erythrocyte receptor BAEBL. *Proceedings of the National Academy of Sciences of the United States of America*, **103**, 2358–2362.

Patel SS, Mehlotra RK, Kastens W *et al.* (2001) The association of the glycophorin C exon 3 deletion with ovalocytosis and malaria susceptibility in the Wosera, Papua New Guinea. *Blood*, **98**, 3489–3491.

Pinder JC, Chung A, Reid ME *et al.* (1993) Membrane attachment sites for the membrane cytoskeletal protein 4.1 of the red blood cell. *Blood*, **82**, 3482–3488.

Takakuwa Y, Tchernia G, Rossi M *et al.* (1986) Restoration of normal membrane stability to unstable protein 4.1-deficient erythrocyte membranes by incorporation of purified protein 4.1. *Journal of Clinical Investigation*, **78**, 80–85.

Telen MJ, Le Van Kim C, Chung A *et al.* (1991) Molecular basis for elliptocytosis associated with glycophorin C and D deficiency in the Leach phenotype. *Blood*, **78**, 1603–1606.

## Adhesion proteins

Bailly P, Tontti E, Hermand P *et al.* (1995) The red cell LW blood group protein is an intercellular adhesion molecule which binds to CD11/

CD18 leukocyte integrins. *European Journal of Immunology*, **25**, 3316–3320.

Brittain JE, Han J, Ataga KI, Orringer EP, Parise LV. (2004) Mechanism of CD47-induced alpha4beta1 integrin activation and adhesion in sickle reticulocytes. *Journal of Biological Chemistry*, **279**, 42393–42402.

El Nemer W, Rahuel C, Colin Y *et al.* (1997) Organization of the human LU gene and molecular basis of the Lu(a)/Lu(b) blood group polymorphism. *Blood*, **89**, 4608–4616.

El Nemer W, Wautier MP, Rahuel C *et al.* (2007) Endothelial Lu/BCAM glycoproteins are novel ligands for red blood cell alpha4beta1 integrin: role in adhesion of sickle red blood cells to endothelial cells. *Blood*, **109**, 3544–3551.

Eyler CE, Jackson T, Elliott LE *et al.* (2008) Beta2-adrenergic receptor and adenylate cyclase gene polymorphisms affect sickle red cell adhesion. *British Journal of Haematology*, **141**, 105–108.

Hermand P, Gane P, Huet M, *et al.* (2003) Red cell ICAM-4 is a novel ligand for platelet-activated alpha IIbbeta 3 integrin. *Journal of Biological Chemistry*, **278**, 4892–4898.

Hines PC, Zen Q, Burney SN *et al.* (2003) Novel epinephrine and cyclic AMP mediated activation of B-CAM/LU-dependent sickle (SS) RBC adhesion. *Blood*, **101**, 3281–3287.

Lee G, Lo A, Short SA *et al.* Targeted gene deletion demonstrates that the cell adhesion molecule ICAM-4 is critical for erythroblastic island formation. *Blood*, **108**, 2064–2071.

Mankelow TJ, Burton N, Stefansdottir FO *et al.* (2007) The Laminin 511/521-binding site on the Lutheran blood group glycoprotein is located at the flexible junction of Ig domains 2 and 3. *Blood*, **110**, 3398–406.

Murphy MM, Evans A, Zayed MA *et al.* (2005) Role of Rap1 in promoting sickle red blood cell adhesion to laminin via BCAM/Lu. *Blood*, **105**, 3322–3329.

Telen MJ, Eisenbarth GS, Haynes BF. (1983) Human erythrocyte antigens. Regulation of expression of a novel erythrocyte surface antigen by the inhibitor Lutheran In(Lu) gene. *Journal of Clinical Investigation*, **71**, 1878–1886.

Telen MJ, Udani M, Washington MK *et al.* (1996) A blood group-related polymorphism of CD44 abolishes a hyaluronan-binding consensus sequence without preventing hyaluronan binding. *Journal of Biological Chemistry*, **271**, 7147–7153.

Udani M, Zen Q, Cottman M *et al.* (1998) Basal cell adhesion molecule/Lutheran protein: the receptor critical for sickle cell adhesion to laminin. *Journal of Clinical Investigation*, **101**, 2550–2558.

Verfaillie CM, Benis A, Iida J *et al.* (1994) Adhesion of committed human hematopoietic progenitors to synthetic peptides from the C-terminal heparin-binding domain of fibronectin: cooperation between the integrin alpha 4 beta 1 and the CD44 adhesion receptor. *Blood*, **84**, 1802–1811.

Wautier MP, El Nemer W, Gane P *et al.* (2007) Increased adhesion to endothelial cells of erythrocytes from patients with polycythemia vera is mediated by laminin alpha5 chain and Lu/BCAM. *Blood*, **110**, 894–901.

Zen Q, Cottman M, Truskey G *et al.* (1999) Critical factors in basal cell adhesion molecule/Lutheran-mediated adhesion to laminin. *Journal of Biological Chemistry*, **274**, 728–734.

Zen Q, Batchvarova M, Twyman CA *et al.* (2004) B-CAM/LU expression and the role of B-CAM/LU activation in binding of low- and high-density red cells to laminin in sickle cell disease. *American Journal of Hematology*, **75**, 63–72.

Zennadi R, Hines PC, De Castro LM, Cartron JP, Parise LV, Telen MJ. (2004) Epinephrine acts via erythroid signaling pathways to activate sickle cell adhesion to endothelium via LW–$\alpha_v\beta_3$ interactions. *Blood*, **104**, 3774–3781.

Zennadi R, Moeller BJ, Whalen EJ *et al.* (2007) Epinephrine-induced activation of LW-mediated sickle cell adhesion and vaso-occlusion in vivo. *Blood*, **110**, 2708–2717.

## Other blood group antigen proteins

Afenyi-Annan A, Kail M, Combs MR, Orringer EP, Ashley-Koch A, Telen MJ. (2008) Lack of Duffy antigen expression is associated with organ damage in patients with sickle cell disease. *Transfusion*, **48**, 917–924.

Karamatic Crew V, Burton N, Kagan A *et al.* (2004) CD151, the first member of the tetraspanin (TM4) superfamily detected on erythrocytes, is essential for the correct assembly of human basement membranes in kidney and skin. *Blood*, **104**, 2217–2223.

Peng J, Redman CM, Wu X *et al.* (2007) Insights into extensive deletions around the XK locus associated with McLeod phenotype and characterization of two novel cases. *Gene*, **392**, 142–150.

Tournamille C, Filipe A, Badaut C *et al.* (2005) Fine mapping of the Duffy antigen binding site for the *Plasmodium vivax* Duffy-binding protein. *Molecular and Biochemical Parasitology*, **144**, 100–103.

# Chapter 23 Autoimmune hematological disorders

## Drew Provan[1] Adrian C Newland[2] & John W Semple[3]

[1] Centre for Haematology, Institute of Cell and Molecular Science, Barts and The London School of Medicine & Dentistry, The Royal London Hospital, London, UK
[2] Department of Haematology, Barts and The London School of Medicine & Dentistry, London, UK
[3] St Michael's Hospital; Department of Laboratory Medicine and Pathobiology, University of Toronto; Canadian Blood Services, Toronto, Ontario, Canada

## Introduction

Autoimmune diseases are disorders where antibodies or cells react against self antigens to cause disease, at which point an adaptive immune response is mounted against the self antigen or antigens. This results in clearance of the antigen from the body. The normal adaptive response results in complete removal of the non-self antigen, whereas in autoimmune disease there is incomplete clearance of the antigen, which leads to perpetuation of the immune response. Autoimmune disorders occur in about 5% of the population, although many individuals have no symptoms. In all, there are more than 70 different disorders, most of which are uncommon, apart from rheumatoid disease and autoimmune thyroiditis. Autoimmune diseases are clinical syndromes mediated by activation of T or B lymphocytes, or both, in the absence of infection or other discernible cause. Until recently, although we could describe the pathological features of autoimmune disease, we had little idea as to their actual cause. Through the development of animal models and the identification of target genes, we have gained considerable insight into the pathogenetic basis of these complex diseases. Autoreactive cells may affect virtually any body tissue, including blood, and blood disorders in which autoantibodies are found include cytopenias such as autoimmune hemolytic anemia, idiopathic thrombocytopenic purpura (ITP) and autoimmune neutropenia, in addition to coagulation disorders such as acquired hemophilia.

Although autoimmune disease is clinically and pathologically diverse, the common end result is damage to antigen, which may result in disease. Factors that play a role in this process include immune dysregulation, genetic factors and triggering events. We discuss all of these after briefly reviewing the structure and function of the immune system.

## The immune system

The immune system comprises cells and molecules whose main role is defense against invading pathogens. The two principal components are the *innate* immune system, comprising skin, mucous membranes, neutrophils, macrophages/dendritic cells that serve as antigen-presenting cells (APCs) and other scavenging cells, in addition to the complement system and natural killer (NK) cells; and the *adaptive* immune system, which involves exclusively B and T lymphocytes (Figure 23.1). The B cells are responsible for secreting antibody, aided by T cells. Key features of the adaptive system include antigen receptor diversity, antigen specificity and immunological memory. This is in sharp contrast to the innate system, which lacks these features.

### The innate immune system

Despite varied challenges by many antigens, because the innate system lacks the ability to develop immunological memory the responses remain the same throughout life. In

*Molecular Hematology*, 3rd edition. Edited by Drew Provan and John Gribben.
© 2010 Blackwell Publishing.

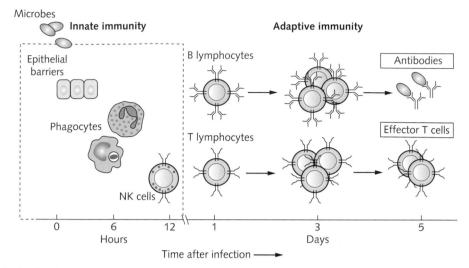

**Fig. 23.1 Innate and adaptive immune systems**
The innate system comprises physical barriers (e.g., skin) along with scavenger cells, while the adaptive system comprises B and T lymphocytes. Temporarily, the innate system is the immediate first line of defense but lacks specificity. The adaptive system comes into play later and possesses immunological specificity and memory. From Abbas AK, Lichtman AH, Pober JS. (2000) *Cellular and Molecular Immunology*, 4th edn. © 2000, with permission from Elsevier.

evolutionary terms, the innate system probably developed before the adaptive system. The innate immune system is composed of physical, chemical and cellular components that act together to mediate the first line of defense against invading microorganisms. These components are intimately linked with inflammatory processes and ultimately lead to the removal of most of the infectious organisms encountered by a host. The innate immune response activates quickly (within seconds) after exposure of foreign infectious agents and is antigen non-specific in that there is no memory associated with the immunity. These characteristics distinguish the innate immune system from the adaptive immune response, which is mediated exclusively by B and T cells, is slower to activate and is exquisitely antigen-specific, generating memory with subsequent exposure to the stimulating antigen.

APCs are key players of innate immunity and physically link innate and adaptive immune responses by presenting antigens to T cells. APCs additionally possess surface receptors for antibody (immunoglobulin) and complement. Microorganisms opsonized by antibody and/or complement are recognized by these receptors, phagocytosed and broken down within the interior of the APCs. Within cells such as neutrophils, killing and digestion of the pathogen involves the generation of superoxide and hydroxyl radicals, nitric oxide and proteolytic enzymes. In addition to the removal of pathogens, the innate system also plays a role in the removal of dead cells and remodeling of tissue during healing. Cells undergoing programmed cell death (apoptosis) express molecules such as phosphatidylserine on their

surface, targeting their removal. Dendritic cells also play a key role in innate immunity, and activation of dendritic cells occurs following exposure to heat-shock proteins, interferon (IFN)-α and other stimuli. Dendritic cells are professional APCs that are able to migrate to lymph nodes, process antigen and present this to T cells in conjunction with major histocompatibility complex (MHC) molecules, of which there are two classes, class I and class II.

## The adaptive immune system

Two requirements of an effective immune system are (i) the ability to recognize millions of potential antigens and (ii) the prevention of self-reacting lymphocytes from causing tissue damage. The former is achieved through irreversible somatic recombination of immunoglobulin and T-cell receptor (TCR) genes, generating many millions of different antibody and TCR molecules.

## B and T cells possess antigen receptors on their surface

The antigen receptor of the B cell is an immunoglobulin and that of the T cell is the TCR. These molecules are expressed on their respective cell surfaces and interact with antigen, either as native (immunoglobulin) or processed (TCR) antigens. The TCR is a transmembrane protein and consists of a heterodimer of either αβ or γδ subunits. TCRs, like immunoglobulins, contain hypervariable regions and in evolutionary terms the two receptors are probably related. Unlike TCRs, antibody molecules are both expressed on the B-cell surface and secreted into body fluids. One feature that both receptors share is the ability to generate enormous diversity through irreversible recombination of germline variable (V), diversity (D) and joining (J) region segments in addition to random mutations within the rearranged genes. Immunoglobulin molecules possess two key regions: the hypervariable region (antigen binding) and the Fc portion at the C-terminal end which, as outlined above, is recognized by the Fc receptor (e.g., FcγR) on macrophages. Antibodies may be of the IgG, IgA, IgM, IgD or IgE class, with subclasses within some of the groups (e.g., there are four IgG subclasses and two IgA subclasses). Having such enormous diversity ensures that there is an antibody for every potential antigen, but the downside of this extreme diversity is that antibodies are generated that recognize self antigens (*autoantibodies*), and it is likely that in normal healthy subjects autoantibodies are generated against a wide variety of antigenic targets. Since autoimmune disease is not common, there must exist a mechanism for removing self-reacting antibodies. In effect, an immunological lack of responsiveness or *tolerance* must exist, whereby self-reactive cells are prevented from causing damage. Recent research has shown this to be the case.

## The major histocompatibility complex

Class I MHC molecules comprise human leukocyte antigen (HLA)-A, -B and -C, and class II molecules consist of HLA-DP, -DQ and -DR. Class II molecules are responsible for presentation of antigen to the TCR on helper T cells.

NK cells have receptors for the immunoglobulin Fc region and are responsible for antibody-dependent cellular cytotoxicity following FcγR linkage of NK cells and antibody-opsonized targets. In addition, NK cells can effect killing using killer-activating receptors, which recognize specific molecules on nucleated cells. An inhibitory molecule (killer inhibitory) recognizes MHC class I on nucleated cells, preventing killing, but if MHC class I is lost (e.g., during infection of the cell by virus or after malignant transformation) the nucleated cell is recognized as being abnormal and is therefore targeted for destruction.

## Soluble molecules: cytokines orchestrate the immune response

The innate system relies on a complex network of soluble molecules, such as cytokines and complement components, that coordinate the entire immune response. We discuss these briefly here since they are implicated in the pathogenesis of autoimmune disease.

Cytokines are mediators secreted by one cell that influence the behavior of other cells. Most cytokines are soluble, apart from interleukin (IL)-1 and tumor necrosis factor

(TNF)-α, which have membrane-bound forms. Cytokines are small molecules of around 15–25 kDa whose actions include promotion of cell growth, inflammation, immunity and repair of tissues. These molecules are responsible for the regulation and orchestration of the entire immune response. Their effects are short-lived and their actions are largely local. In order to exert their effect, cytokines interact with specific receptors and promote signal transduction. Their main routes of action are via the Janus kinase (JAK)/STAT and Ras/MAP pathways. The cytokine profile may be proinflammatory or anti-inflammatory and the cytokine balance will dictate whether a helper T-cell clone engages in a Th1 or Th2 response. In general, Th1 responses are effective against intracellular pathogens and Th2 responses aid B cells.

## Cytokine profiles of Th1 and Th2 responses
(Table 23.1)

Antigen-presenting cells, and in particular dendritic cells, are responsible for T-cell differentiation toward the Th1 or Th2 phenotype; the cytokine IL-12 plays a key role in the Th1 response, IL-4 in the Th2 response. Since cytokines play such a key role in orchestrating an effective immune response, it is likely that dysregulation of cytokine levels may induce an autoimmune response in some disorders. This has been shown to be the case in experimental models and also in human disease. For example, transfection of the gene for IFN-γ on the insulin promoter has been shown to induce inflammation within the pancreas, with aberrant expression of MHC class II and the development of diabetes. In

**Table 23.1** Cytokine profiles of Th1 and Th2 responses.

| Th1 response (activates macrophages) | Th2 response (deactivates macrophages) |
| --- | --- |
| IL-2 | – |
| IL-3 | – |
| – | IL-4 |
| – | IL-5 |
| – | IL-6 |
| – | IL-10 |
| – | IL-13 |
| TNF-α | – |
| TNF-β | TNF-β |
| IFN-γ | – |
| GM-CSF | GM-CSF |

These are the principal cytokines involved in generation of Th1 and Th2 responses. Imbalance in Th1 or Th2 cytokines may play a role in the development of autoimmune disease, allergy and other disorders.

addition, proinflammatory cytokines, such as IL-12, TNF and IFN-γ, can induce organ-specific autoimmunity.

Because of limitations of space, the role of complement is only very briefly discussed here. Following infection, cells of the immune system migrate toward the affected site. Complement component C3b coats the pathogen surface. The molecules C3b, C3a, C4a and C5a, in addition to neutrophil chemoattractant, trigger mast cells to release histamine. This induces smooth muscle contraction and increased blood vessel permeability, allowing neutrophils to pass through the blood vessel walls more easily, an essential requirement for an effective innate response.

## T cells (Figure 23.2)

These develop within the thymus. T cells bearing αβ TCRs recognize processed antigen presented to them by APCs, including dendritic cells. Within the thymus, T cells are selected in order to prevent autoreactivity; that is to say, mechanisms exist whereby T cells are prevented from reacting with self antigens. Positive selection occurs when T cells express TCRs that are able to interact with MHC complexes on thymic cortex epithelial cells. The effect of positive selec-

tion is to prevent apoptosis. T cells expressing TCRs with high or low affinity for self molecules are negatively selected and undergo apoptosis.

## Immunological tolerance prevents damage to self antigens

Tolerance defines the body's ability to recognize, but not react with, self antigens, while retaining the ability to respond to non-self antigens. This process involves the negative selection of T cells, as outlined above. In addition, the process involves the control of autoreactive B cells. The process of selecting T cells and B cells in the thymus and bone marrow respectively is known as *central tolerance*. For autoreactive lymphocytes that escape into the periphery there are additional *peripheral tolerance* mechanisms to provide a safety net for unwanted autoreactivity.

### T-cell tolerance: central mechanisms

Immature T cells from the bone marrow migrate to the thymus, where they complete their development. The T cells within the thymus interact with MHC molecules in low- or

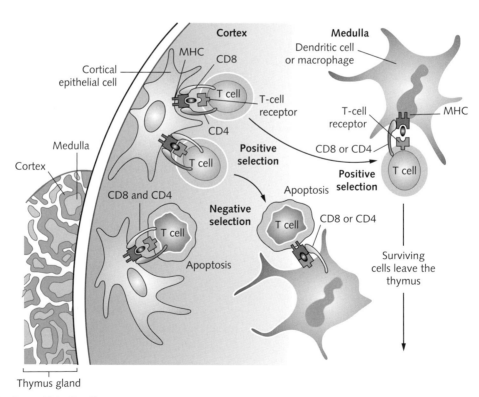

**Fig. 23.2 T-cell selection within the thymus**
T cells undergo positive and negative selection. CD4+CD8+ T cells interact with MHC–peptide complexes. Depending on the strength of the interaction, the T cells either undergo apoptosis (the majority) or survive and leave the thymus (the minority). Reproduced with permission from Delves PJ, Roitt IM. (2000) The immune system. First of two parts. *New England Journal of Medicine*, **343**, 37–49.

high-affinity interactions. If the TCRs have low affinity for the peptide (e.g., self peptide), they receive apoptotic signals and die within the thymus. T cells participating in high-affinity interactions have a similar fate and it is only when the interaction is of intermediate affinity that the T cells survive and migrate to the periphery, a process termed *positive selection*. In general, positive selection occurs when CD4$^+$CD8$^+$ T cells interact with TCR–MHC–peptide complexes. For most T cells the interaction is of low avidity and the T cells die before leaving the thymus. A minority of CD4$^+$CD8$^+$ T cells have intermediate avidity reactions and hence these cells survive, after which they mature into CD4$^+$CD8$^-$ and CD4$^-$CD8$^+$ cells. CD4$^+$ T cells are the main effectors of autoimmune disease.

### T-cell tolerance: peripheral mechanisms

From studies of animal models it is apparent that self-reactive lymphocytes are present peripherally, having escaped central tolerance checkpoints. Furthermore, some form of immunological ignorance is invoked whereby such circulating autoreactive T cells fail to respond to the specific self antigen. The mechanisms for such ignorance are not fully characterized but may involve low levels of circulating antigen (i.e., below a critical threshold), or the antigen may be in a separate compartment from the autoreactive cells (e.g., the blood–brain barrier), or there may be an absence of the costimulatory signals required for T-cell costimulation and activation.

### T-cell activation: role of costimulatory molecules

Antigen reaches lymphoid tissue via the lymphatic system or, in some cases, within dendritic cells that have ingested and processed antigen. In general, antigen in blood is taken to the spleen and tissue antigen is taken to the lymph nodes. Antigen is then processed and presented on MHC molecules by two major routes: (i) the antigen may be produced within the cell itself, for example viral antigens may be expressed within cells and complexed with MHC class I molecules; or (ii) APCs may take up antigen exogenously and then phagocytose, process and express the antigen on MHC class II molecules.

### Recognition of antigen by T cells

Antigen recognition differs between CD4$^+$ and CD8$^+$ T cells. For example, CD4$^+$ cells can only recognize antigen on class II molecules and CD8$^+$ cells recognize antigen in association with MHC class I molecules. In this way the MHC dictates the type of response generated.

### TCR signaling

TCR molecules are found on the T-cell surface complexed with CD3 molecules. CD3 transmits signals intracellularly, with tyrosine phosphorylation of residues in the CD3 cytoplasmic tail. This transmits signals to the nucleus, resulting in T-cell proliferation. Co-receptor molecules on T cells are important since they play a major role in T cell activation following engagement of the TCR. The generation of a specific immune response to a pathogen requires the recognition of the foreign agent by specialized cells in the body, presentation of the foreign antigen to T cells, and the orchestration of the subsequent immune response. T cells must receive two signals from the APCs for a complete immune response to occur. One signal involves the presentation of antigens in context of the MHC on the surface of the APC to the TCR complex on the T cells. This interaction provides the specificity of the immune response. This signal alone is not sufficient to trigger an optimal immune response and a second signal is required. The second, or costimulatory, signal involves the interaction of B7 on the APC with CD28 receptors on the T cells. The interaction of B7 with CD28 is required for the T cells to proliferate, produce lymphokines, and provide help for the induction of antibody- and cell-mediated immune responses directed at the original antigen. The B7-induced CD28 signal is delivered to the T-cell nucleus via several intermediate steps and results in the direct induction of the IL-2 gene and the receptor for this lymphokine. T cells stimulated via their TCR (antigen-specific signal) and the costimulatory signal proliferate, produce many lymphokines and direct the specific immune response against the presented antigen.

The principal co-receptors on APCs are CD80 (B7-1), CD86 (B7-2) and CD40, binding respectively to CD28, cytotoxic T-lymphocyte antigen (CTLA)-4 and CD40 ligand on T cells. Dendritic cells express large quantities of both B7 and CD40, are professional APCs and are the most effective stimulators of naive T cells. Following activation, the T cells undergo clonal expansion, generating effector cells that move toward the site of inflammation after leaving the lymphoid tissue (Figure 23.3).

### Mechanisms for controlling autoreactive T cells

Harmful autoreactive T cells may be eliminated by several mechanisms, including apoptosis, anergy, inhibition, clonal deletion and suppression. Anergy refers to T cells that do not produce IL-2 after their encounter with antigen. Such cells are not activated and may produce IL-10, which further suppresses T-cell activation. Inhibition of T cells is mediated by CTLA-4, also known as CD152. This molecule binds to the B7 family of receptors (B7-1 and B7-2) on APCs, including

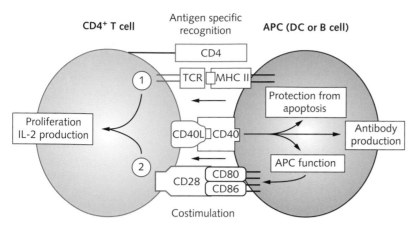

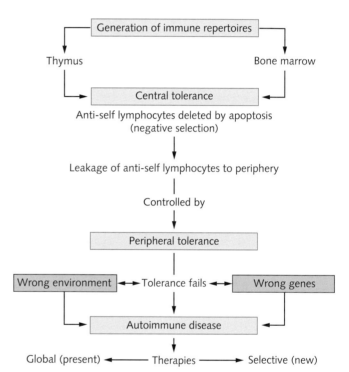

**Fig. 23.3 Interaction between APCs (e.g., dendritic cells or B cells) and CD4⁺ T cells**

The first signal to the T cell is via MHC and T-cell receptor (TCR). This signal is not sufficient for proliferation and IL-2 production and a second signal, such as interaction of B7-1 or B7-2 with CD28, is required. If no second signal is received, the T cells undergo apoptosis. Figure kindly supplied by Dr Masataka Kuwana, Institute for Advanced Medical Research, Keio University School of Medicine, Tokyo.

B cells and dendritic cells, with higher affinity than to CD28, a counter-receptor for B7. CTLA-4 mediates suppression of the T cell.

### Loss of immunological tolerance leads to autoimmunity

In order for autoimmune disease to occur, there must be loss of tolerance to self antigens. This occurs despite central and peripheral T-cell tolerance controls. Possible mechanisms leading to loss of tolerance include variability in intrathymic T-cell deletion and activation of harmful T cells in the periphery, for example by infection. The latter has been postulated to cause type 1 diabetes (insulin-dependent diabetes mellitus) in some individuals (Figure 23.4).

## Beneficial effects of autoimmunity

The concept of clonal deletion has been central to immunology for many years. This process deletes self-reactive lymphocytes in order to prevent the harmful effects that these might otherwise cause. We now know that low-level autoreactivity is found in normal healthy individuals and autoantigens play a role in generating our normal immune repertoire. Self and non-self antigens have few differences and lymphocytes have probably not evolved in order to distinguish between the two; their role is rather to respond to antigen under specific circumstances, for example as directed by the cytokine network. In addition, autoreactive cells are also responsible for the remodeling of tissues, wound healing and other physiological processes. *Autoimmunity* therefore differs from *autoimmune disease*. In fact, transient autoimmune attack of self antigens has been shown to occur when there is tissue damage, but this type of autoimmune response is generally not sustained.

**Fig. 23.4 Autoimmunity is multifactorial**

Central tolerance is achieved within the bone marrow or thymus but some self-reacting cells leak out into the periphery, where peripheral tolerance checkpoints exist. Self-reactive lymphocytes escaping central *and* peripheral tolerance may cause autoimmune disease in predisposed individuals (the "wrong" genes) when they encounter a specific trigger (the "wrong" environment). Reproduced from Mackay IR. (2000) Science, medicine, and the future: tolerance and autoimmunity. *British Medical Journal*, **321**, 93–96.

## The spectrum of autoimmune diseases

For clinical convenience, autoimmune diseases are subdivided arbitrarily into those that are *organ-specific*, such as

Hashimoto thyroiditis, and those that are *non-organ-specific*, such as systemic lupus erythematosus (SLE). Many diseases lie between these two extremes. Conditions in which there are circulating immune complexes tend to be systemic, while conditions associated with autoantibodies or autoreactive T-cell responses are organ-specific. However, in general this classification tells us nothing about the causes of disease and it may be better to classify them into those diseases in which there is disturbed selection, regulation or death of T and B cells (e.g., mediated by Fas or Fas receptor abnormalities), and a second group in which there is abnormal expression of an antigen, for example the demyelination syndrome that follows gut infection with the bacterium *Campylobacter jejuni*. This method of classification may help guide treatment.

The factors that may play a role in the development of autoimmune disease include:
- failure of tolerance to self antigens
- infection
- tissue injury
- abnormalities of APCs
- imbalance between proinflammatory and anti-inflammatory cytokines
- genetic factors
- variable effector mechanisms, for example production of immune complexes, autoantibodies or autoreactive T cells.

## Role of genetic factors

It has long been recognized that genetic factors play a key role in autoimmune disease, the strongest correlation being with MHC genes, especially MHC class II. Support for a genetic basis comes from a variety of observations. For example, autoimmune diseases often cluster within families and twin studies show that there is much higher concordance between monozygotic than dizygotic twins: in monozygotic twins the chance of both twins having autoimmune disease is higher than in dizygotic twins. Examples of diseases with high concordance rates between monozygotic twins include type 1 diabetes, rheumatoid arthritis and SLE; the concordance rate for monozygotic twins is around 20% and for dizygotic twins it is less than 5%. Some disorders are due to mutations in a single gene, for example autoimmune polyglandular endocrinopathy with candidiasis and ectodermal dysplasia (APECED) and the autoimmune lymphoproliferative disorder. In APECED there is a mutation in the gene for an autoimmune regulator protein that is active within the thymus. The mutation leads to autoimmunity and immune deficiency. In the autoimmune lymphoproliferative disorder the autoreactivity is due to an inability to induce apoptosis of activated lymphocytes following encounter with antigen. The disorder is autosomal dominant and involves Fas or its receptor, both of which are involved in the downregulation of activated cells following antigen exposure.

However, most autoimmune diseases are not caused by single gene mutations but rather are multigenic, several genes acting together to cause the disease phenotype. Type 1 diabetes is a prime example of a disease in which multiple genes are implicated. For example, 95% of Caucasians with type 1 diabetes possess HLA-DR3, HLA-DR4 or both (only found in 40% of normal subjects), and 40–50% of patients are heterozygous for HLA-DR3/DR4 (found in 5% of normal subjects). Other non-HLA genes are also implicated in type 1 diabetes, including IL-2 polymorphism and another region that maps close to CTLA-4. Surprisingly, some of these genetic polymorphisms occur in normal individuals who have normal immune function with no evidence of autoimmune disease. So it would appear that there is a need for specific genetic polymorphisms in conjunction with other susceptibility polymorphisms. The MHC is one candidate for this role.

Most autoimmune diseases described to date have linkage with specific MHC class I or II polymorphisms, but again these do not produce the disease phenotype in isolation; rather they require the presence of polymorphisms within other genes, such as those for cytokines (e.g., TNF-α). For diseases such as ankylosing spondylitis, type 1 diabetes and rheumatoid disease, certain HLA subtypes induce disease susceptibility. The link between MHC genotype and disease susceptibility is logical given the fact that autoimmune diseases involve autoreactive T cells. The ability of a T cell to respond to a particular antigen depends largely on the MHC since the MHC determines how the antigen is presented to the autoreactive T cells. In addition, the MHC has a powerful influence on determining the body's T-cell repertoire. Other HLA alleles appear to be able to offer protection from autoimmune disease. For example, when the disease-causing allele HLA-DQB1*0301 or 0302 is present together with HLA-DQB1*0602, the latter appears to offer protection from disease. The mechanism underlying such protection is not known. Some HLA alleles cause disease only within specific populations. For example, HLA-DRB1*0401 and *0402 are associated with rheumatoid disease in Europeans but not in black or Hispanic individuals. Again, the mechanism here is not clearly understood.

## Some autoimmune diseases have strong association with cytokine gene polymorphisms

Since cytokines, through interaction with their ligands, orchestrate the immune response, it is possible that dysregu-

**Table 23.2** Autoimmune diseases in which strong associations with cytokine SNPs have been described.

| Disease | Implicated cytokine polymorphism |
| --- | --- |
| Juvenile chronic arthritis | IL-6 |
| Myasthenia and multiple sclerosis | TGF-β |
| Rheumatoid disease | IL-10 |

Associations have now been reported for many autoimmune disorders and a full database is provided at http://www.bris.ac.uk/pathandmicro/services/GAI/cytokine4.htm

lation of cytokines may play a role in autoimmune disease. Indeed, many single-nucleotide polymorphisms (SNPs) have been described within cytokine or cytokine receptor genes and such SNPs may alter cytokine structure or their expression. This may result in overexpression or underexpression. In the blood disorder ITP and other autoimmune diseases, abnormal cytokine profiles have been described. In chronic ITP, IL-2, IFN-γ and IL-10 levels are increased, suggesting a Th1 activation profile (Table 23.2).

Not only do cytokine gene SNPs predispose to disease, but data from animal models such as the rheumatoid rat indicate that specific polymorphisms may determine disease chronicity and severity. In addition, there are data to suggest that specific genetic polymorphisms may correlate with responses to specific treatments, but it is probably too early to draw firm conclusions from such studies.

## Antibody Fc receptor gene polymorphisms

For autoimmune blood diseases in which autoantibody-opsonized cells are sequestered and destroyed within the reticuloendothelial system, there are data from a number of studies showing that polymorphisms within the Fcγ receptors may influence disease. Antiplatelet antibodies, as with other antibodies, possess two distinct functional components: a Fab end, which binds to the targeted antigen, and an Fc end, which is recognized by scavenger cells (e.g., macrophages) in the spleen, liver and bone marrow. The receptors on the macrophages that sense the presence of antibodies are termed Fc receptors. How well the Fc receptors recognize and bind antibody attached to platelets determines, in part, how aggressively the platelets are destroyed. Polymorphisms of the FcγRIIA (FCGR2A) gene have been implicated in heparin-induced thrombocytopenia, SLE and childhood recurrent bacterial infections.

Intravenous immunoglobulin (IVIg) is effective in ITP, although its mechanisms of action are not fully understood.

However, one of the actions of IVIg is to attach to Fc receptors on the macrophages, thereby blocking the receptor. Once the receptor is blocked it cannot bind antibody bound to platelets and the antibody-coated platelets are spared destruction by the immune system.

Recent reports have highlighted genetic variations in FcγR genes which alter their ability to recognize and bind antibody. The genetics of FcγR genes is complex, but essentially there are three major types: FcγRIA, FcγRIIA and FcγRIIIA. A recent study of FcγRIIA suggests that a polymorphism in the FCGR2A gene may be responsible for causing refractory ITP (ITP that responds poorly to treatment). The polymorphism influences the efficiency of the receptor to bind with antibody molecules. A similar polymorphism in the FCGR2A gene has been shown to alter the function of the receptor and may predispose individuals to autoimmune disease such as ITP, and in those individuals developing ITP the disease is more likely to be chronic. Human FCGR2A-transgenic mice have been shown to have a more severe form of ITP than normal mice, which provides further evidence that FcγRIIA contributes to platelet destruction.

## Mouse models of autoimmune disease

These have provided much insight into autoimmune disease and to date around 25 genes have been shown to play a role in the development of disease, either when the genes are deleted or overexpressed. The genes encode cytokines or their receptors, costimulatory molecules or proteins involved in apoptotic pathways. Whether a mutation within one of these critical genes induces disease depends on the genetic background of the animal, which would tend to imply that other genes can influence the phenotype. One other point worth noting is that mutations within a gene may be involved in more than one clinical disorder.

With respect to hematological autoimmune diseases, there have been several animal models of ITP, including the secondary autoimmune model, where thrombocytopenia is secondary to lupus nephritis; the passive transfer model, where continuous injection of platelet-specific antibodies is required to maintain a steady state of thrombocytopenia; and the viral acute ITP model, where thrombocytopenia develops following a viral infection. Although these models have been important in studying treatments such as IVIg, they are not ideal for pathophysiological studies since the induced thrombocytopenia is either secondary, or there is no endogenous antibody production. Recently, however, a platelet-specific immune model of fetal/neonatal alloimmune thrombocytopenia was developed using CD61

(GPIIIa) knockout mice. In this model, fetal platelet antigen is the cause of the autoimmunity. With the advent of transgenic mice expressing human Duffy and glycophorin antigens, there are now murine models of autoimmune hemolytic anemia.

## Human studies

A number of candidate genes have been studied in human autoimmune disease, including variants of CTLA-4. This molecule is a natural downregulator of activated T cells. One polymorphism within this gene causes a reduction in the inhibitory signal normally induced by the CTLA-4 molecule and this polymorphism has been found to be associated with human type 1 diabetes, thyroid disease and primary biliary cirrhosis.

## Critical events in the generation of autoreactivity

Since autoimmune diseases are multifactorial, there are obviously triggering events within genetically predisposed individuals that lead to the development of autoimmune disease. Animal models show that if animals genetically susceptible to autoimmune disease are injected with self antigens from genetically identical animals with an appropriate adjuvant (e.g., bacterial), the animal will mount an immune response against the self antigen. In humans autoimmune disease usually arises spontaneously, although it is accepted that there must be triggering events giving rise to the disease phenotype. What factors might be responsible for inducing autoimmune disease? Several have been proposed, including infectious and non-infectious triggers.

### Environmental factors in the development of autoimmune disease

If the development of autoimmune disease were entirely genetic, then we would expect complete or near-complete concordance in monozygotic twins. However, the concordance rate for the second twin if the first twin has autoimmune disease is less than 50%, which suggests that additional, possibly external, factors are required for autoimmune disease. Possible external influences might include infection. Evidence for a role of infection in the development of autoimmune disease is provided by disorders such as Lyme disease and its associated arthritis. In this condition there is cross-reactivity between the pathogen and host tissue antigens. The self protein targeted is leukocyte function-associated antigen (LFA)-1, also called CD11a and CD18. LFA-1 shares determinants with protein antigens of *Borrelia*

*burgdorferi*. Another example is Epstein–Barr virus (EBV), which appears to have a role in the development of SLE, from case–control studies using stored serum from patients with SLE. Whether significant or not, there is one antigenic determinant on EBV that is shared with SLE. However, this evidence is fairly circumstantial at present.

### How might infection cause autoimmunity?

Pathogens may be able to induce autoimmunity through a variety of mechanisms:
• production of local inflammation
• change in reticuloendothelial function, e.g., phagocytosis
• production of neoantigens
• molecular mimicry.

Local inflammation can expose costimulatory molecules on APCs and lead to the breakdown of T-cell anergy and the development of autoimmune disease. Tissue injury may result in the production of neoantigens for which an autoantibody may have specificity. Lastly, in molecular mimicry, antigens on microorganisms may resemble those on the host tissues such that antibodies produced against the pathogen will cross-react with the host tissue. Examples may include multiple sclerosis, type 1 diabetes and childhood acute ITP, if the antibody produced in a childhood viral infection by chance cross-reacts with antigen(s) on the platelet surface. Although elegant, there is little apart from circumstantial evidence at present to support the existence of molecular mimicry in humans.

### Non-infectious triggers

Infection may play a role in autoimmune disease, but what non-infectious triggers might there be which could induce autoimmune disease in susceptible individuals? Hormones may play a role since we know that most autoimmune disorders are commoner in women than men, and in mice with SLE the administration of estrogens worsens the disease; this effect is believed to be due to an alteration of the B-cell repertoire. Also in SLE, complement deficiency (e.g., C1 or C4 components) may worsen the disorder. Haptens such as drugs can also induce autoimmune disease. For example, penicillin acts as a hapten when it binds to the red cell membrane, inducing an autoimmune response that leads to autoimmune hemolytic anemia. Complexes formed between two proteins may trigger disease. For example, celiac disease is an autoimmune disorder in which transglutaminase and its substrate gliadin form a complex that induces autoantibody generation against both gliadin and transglutaminase.

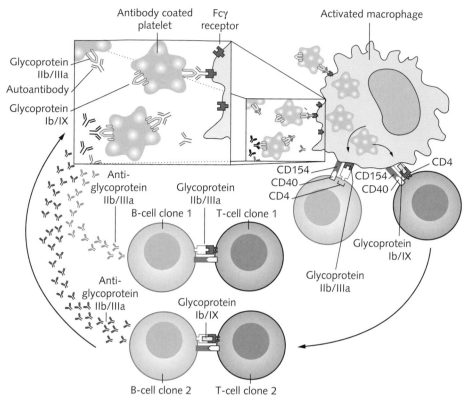

**Fig. 23.5 Epitope spread**

In ITP, for example, platelet glycoproteins are processed and presented to T cells by antigen-presenting cells (APCs). A variety of different peptides may be presented by APCs, resulting in multiple T-cell clones, each targeting distinct epitopes on different glycoprotein molecules. Reproduced from Cines DB, Blanchette VS. (2002) Immune thrombocytopenic purpura. *New England Journal of Medicine,* **346**, 995–1008.

### Epitope spread

This phenomenon may play a role in some autoimmune diseases, and involves the initial generation of autoreactivity with subsequent development of chronic autoimmune disease. During the process there is a gradual increase in the number of autoantigens targeted by T cells; hence there is spread to epitopes beyond the initial triggering epitope (Figure 23.5).

### Hormonal influences

Many autoimmune diseases are more common in females, particularly in the childbearing years, when hormone levels are at their highest. The mechanism whereby the hormonal profile of females influences the development of autoimmune disease is unknown.

## Autoimmune disease is complex and multifactorial

From studies of autoimmune disease, it is clear that ITP and other autoimmune disorders are multifactorial. It is likely that loss of tolerance to a self antigen alone is insufficient to generate the autoimmune disorder. Rather, patients probably require (i) a specific set of genetic determinants (e.g., polymorphisms within MHC, CTLA-4, or other genes); (ii) dysregulation of the immune response (involving dendritic cells, T or B cells, or all three); and (iii) an environmental trigger. Autoimmune disease arises only when all these determinants are present in an individual at one particular time. This is reinforced by the observation that self-reactive lymphocytes are commonly found in normal individuals. For example, siblings of patients who have autoimmune disorders are more likely to have autoantibodies themselves, albeit at lower titers than their affected sibs, but no overt evidence of autoimmune disease *per se*, perhaps because they have not been exposed to the environmental trigger required to tip the balance toward autoimmune disease.

## How do autoreactive cells induce tissue damage in autoimmune disease?

This is a large topic which is discussed only briefly here. In autoimmune disease, since the autoantigen is not cleared completely from the affected individual, the process tends to be prolonged because there is always a supply of autoantigen available to keep the process going. Autoantigens, especially IgG and IgM, may attach to cell membrane antigens on cells and cause local tissue damage. Where the antigens are soluble a more systemic disease profile results. In addition to autoantibody-mediated disease, T cells can themselves directly cause disease. When autoantibodies such as IgG and IgM attach to blood cells, premature destruction of the cells results. Cells involved include red cells, resulting in autoimmune hemolytic anemia, white cells, causing neutropenia (any white cell may be involved but neutropenia is commonest) and platelets, inducing thrombocytopenia. Red cell attack by IgG antibodies results in premature red cell destruction by the macrophages of the reticuloendothelial system, via Fcγ receptors. When the autoantibody is IgM, complement activation occurs and there may be intravascular lysis, although more commonly the complement cascade does not reach the lytic stage but generally stops at the C3d stage because of the presence of complement regulatory proteins. However, even with incomplete complement activation, the presence of molecules such as C5a generates local inflammation and tissue damage through activation of cytokines. Autoimmune blood cell disorders are discussed below.

Rather than cause direct cellular damage, some autoantibodies may activate or block receptors. For example, Graves disease is caused by an autoantibody that stimulates the thyroid-stimulating receptor, leading to elevated levels of thyroid hormones. In myasthenia gravis the autoantibody blocks acetylcholine receptors, preventing neuromuscular transmission. Other mechanisms of autoantibody and T-cell damage also occur, but there is insufficient space to discuss these here.

## Idiopathic thrombocytopenic purpura as a model of autoimmune blood disease

ITP is usually an acquired disorder in which platelets are coated (*opsonized*) with antiplatelet autoantibodies and removed prematurely by the reticuloendothelial system, predominantly the spleen, leading to a reduced peripheral blood platelet count. Of interest, it has been estimated that approximately 40% of patients with chronic ITP have no detectible antibodies yet are thrombocytopenic. CD8+ T cells have been linked to the pathogenesis of many autoimmune diseases such as type 1 diabetes, and recently it was shown that ITP patients have a CD8+ T-cell-mediated cytotoxicity that induces platelet destruction. At present, however, it is unknown whether cell-mediated platelet destruction contributes to the severity of disease or the difficulty of treatment in some patients with ITP.

The etiology of ITP is unknown and the clinical course is variable and unpredictable. ITP has an incidence of around 60 new cases per million population per year in the USA. Childhood ITP is generally termed "acute" since the illness is seasonal, typically follows a trivial viral infection or vaccination, is transient in most cases and requires no treatment, with spontaneous recovery in 80% of cases. One proposed mechanism invoked in childhood ITP is molecular mimicry, in which the antibody directed against an invading pathogen coincidentally cross-reacts with one of the platelet glycoprotein epitopes. As discussed earlier, the normal adaptive immune response ceases once the offending pathogenic antigen is destroyed, and this might account for the acute nature of ITP in childhood. That is to say, once the pathogen is eradicated the source of non-self antigen is removed and cross-reacting antibody levels fall.

In the adult (chronic) form there is usually no obvious antecedent illness and most patients have chronic thrombocytopenia; spontaneous recovery is uncommon. In most cases of adult ITP the platelet glycoprotein (GP) antigen targets are GPIIb/IIIa and GPIb/IX.

## Etiology

It is believed that ITP is most likely due to an inappropriate immune response to an environmental trigger; the nature of this trigger has not yet been identified. The disorder may represent an abnormality of APCs, with an increase in the numbers of CD4+ and CD8+ cells. It has been increasingly recognized that T cells play a significant role in autoantibody production and recent data suggest that, in some instances, T cells may actually mediate platelet destruction in ITP. Furthermore, two new and exciting possibilities have emerged in ITP research related to T-cell abnormalities that may prove be key to unraveling the pathogenesis of the disorder and may also reveal new therapeutic options for ITP. It appears that patients with ITP have functionally reduced numbers of T-regulatory cells that may relieve T-cell tolerance mechanisms and allow platelet autoimmunity to proceed, whereas therapeutic removal of B cells in the disorder by therapies such as rituximab raises platelet counts by actually normalizing these T-cell functional deficiencies. Figure 23.6 highlights the cellular immune abnormalities found in patients with ITP.

As regards causal genetic abnormalities, most attention has focused on the identification of MHC susceptibility genes, given their role in determining the nature and specificity of the adaptive immune response. However, the results of HLA association studies in ITP have not produced clear results. A large analysis focusing on HLA-DR4 gene variations in more than 100 Japanese patients with ITP reported that the DRB1*0410 allele was significantly increased in ITP patients compared with controls. Moreover, this allele was

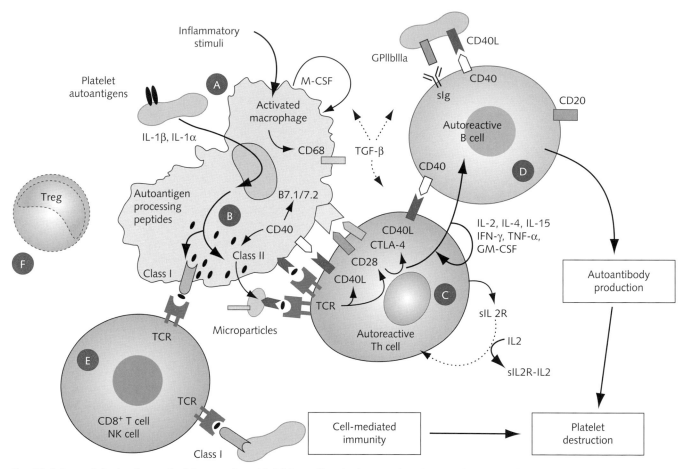

**Fig. 23.6 Potential stimulatory (solid arrows) and inhibitory (hatched arrows) pathways that may affect the pathogenesis of chronic ITP**

This model assumes that a tolerance event has broken down, allowing autoreactive T and B cells to be present. (A) Platelets are normally taken up by macrophages during senescence and are presumably destroyed intracellularly within lysosomes. Inflammatory stimuli can activate macrophages that may alter the way they normally process platelet autoantigens or induce the expression of inflammatory cytokines (e.g., IL-1) that may support autoimmune responses. (B) In the activated APC, platelet autoantigenic peptides can be loaded onto MHC class II molecules for presentation to the T-cell receptor (TCR) of autoreactive Th cells. (C) Once the TCR has been occupied by the MHC class II molecules and platelet autoantigen, it can initiate a series of molecular costimulatory interactions within the T cell. First, CD40L upregulated on the T-cell surface interacts with CD40 on the APC that stimulates B7.1 and B7.2 expression. The TCR–MHC interaction also enhances CD28 expression on the Th cells that then interact with the B7.1, culminating in a strong costimulation response and activation of the Th cell. (D) Th activation leads to the secretion of Th0/Th1 cytokines (e.g., IL-2, IL-10, IFN-γ) that effectively drive autoreactive B cells to divide and differentiate into plasma cells and secrete antiplatelet autoantibodies. Also shown are a number of potential regulatory events that could either enhance or suppress autoimmunity in ITP. For example, macrophage colony-stimulating factor (M-CSF) can activate macrophages within the spleen to enhance their phagocytosis of platelets. Additionally, IFN-γ and TNF-α produced by the autoreactive Th cells can feed back on macrophages, enhancing their expression of MHC class II molecules and potentially aggravate the response. On the other hand, transforming growth factor (TGF)-β (produced by either Th3 cells or platelets) together with the Th cell's soluble IL-2 receptor can control the autoimmune response by inhibiting lymphocyte activation. This may also occur during costimulation via the expression of CTLA-4 on the Th cell. Also shown are the potential interactions of MHC class II- and CD40L-positive platelets with Th and B cells activation respectively. These events may be responsible for initiating and/or aggravating autoimmunity in patients with AITP. (E) Recent evidence suggests that CD8+ T cells are active and present in patients with ITP that do not demonstrate autoantibodies. These cytotoxic cells bind to platelets and mediate cytolysis. (F) It appears that many of the defects shown in the figure may be the result of defective or lack of CD4+CD25+ T regulatory (Treg) cells due to a breakdown in self tolerance. Adapted from Coopamah MD, Garvey MB, Freedman J, Semple JW. (2003) Cellular immune mechanisms in autoimmune thrombocytopenic purpura: an update. *Transfusion Medicine Reviews*, **17**, 69–80, with permission.

significantly decreased in patients who showed a good response to prednisolone. MHC may therefore play a role in some cases of ITP but there are clearly other genes implicated. These include genetic polymorphisms within cytokine and other immune regulatory genes.

## Clinical features

The ITP phenotype is heterogeneous: some patients suffer major bleeding from the outset, while others have few problems apart from an increased tendency to bruise. This may partly be explained by the acquired platelet dysfunction that is seen in some patients with ITP, which in turn may be related to the target antigen involved in the autoimmune process (this is discussed later; *see section Antibodies and their target antigens*). Autoantibodies reacting with GPIIb/IIIa affect platelet aggregation, and anti-GPIb/IX autoantibodies impair platelet adhesion to the subendothelial matrix, causing unexpectedly severe bleeding for the level of platelet count. In general, however, in contrast with thrombocytopenia due to marrow infiltration (e.g., leukemias, lymphomas and other malignancies) or aplasia, patients with ITP are able to tolerate remarkably low platelet counts and to maintain an adequate quality of life. The degree of bleeding is largely dependent on the platelet count, and patients with counts below $10 \times \times 10^9/L$ (and usually below $5 \times 10^9/L$) are at greatest risk of bleeding, including intracranial bleeding.

## Diagnosis

The diagnosis of ITP remains clinical, and one of exclusion. Secondary causes include SLE, lymphoproliferative disease and HIV infection. Standard investigation includes a full blood count (isolated thrombocytopenia), blood film (to ensure no red cell fragments, leukemia, parasitic infections) and autoimmune profile (to exclude secondary cause). A bone marrow examination is often carried out in adults but not usually in children, and will usually show normal or increased megakaryocytes in an otherwise normal marrow. Immunological assays have been devised, including platelet-associated IgG or IgM and monoclonal antibody immobilization of platelet antigens, but these do not alter the management and are of debatable value.

## Antibodies and their target antigens

### Antiplatelet antibodies

Many patients with ITP show elevated levels of platelet-associated IgG, which is believed to be the autoantibody, but

for unknown reasons platelet-associated IgG may be elevated in other non-immunological causes of thrombocytopenia. The autoantibodies involved in ITP are generally IgG, but IgA and IgM autoantibodies have been reported. Opsonized platelets are removed prematurely by the reticuloendothelial system through an Fc-dependent mechanism. However, many patients fail to respond to therapies aimed at inactivation of the reticuloendothelial system, suggesting that other mechanisms of platelet destruction exist.

### Antigenic targets

Using antigen-specific assays, such as the monoclonal antibody-specific immobilization of platelet antigens, platelet-associated IgG and antigen capture assays, several platelet antigens have been characterized. These include GPIIb/IIIa ($\alpha$IIIb$\beta$3, the fibrinogen receptor) and GPIb/IX (the von Willebrand receptor), which appear to be the most frequently involved. Less commonly, GPIa/IIa, GPIV and GPV are involved. Recent reports suggest that possibly 40% of autoantibodies are reactive to both GPIIb/IIIa and GPIb/IX, possibly due to the serum in some patients with ITP containing two different IgG antibodies. In terms of disease chronicity, GP-specific autoantibodies may be important in the pathogenesis of chronic ITP; from available data GPIIb/IIIa appear to play a major role in the development of chronic ITP in 30–40% of cases.

### Which epitopes are involved?

Previous investigators have looked for autoantigenic epitopes on the GPIIb/IIIa molecule using competitive binding between human autoantibodies and mouse monoclonal antibodies. In addition, enzyme-cleaved IIb or IIIa fragments and synthesized peptides corresponding to different sequences of GPIIIa have been used to localize epitopes on the respective glycoprotein.

Kekomaki and colleagues have shown that the 33-kDa chymotryptic core fragment of IIIa is a frequent target. Fujisawa and colleagues, using synthetic peptides corresponding to IIIa sequences, showed that in 5 of 13 sera from patients with chronic ITP binding was to residues 721–744 or 742–762, corresponding to the carboxy terminal of IIIa. Recently, Nieswandt and colleagues have examined the pathogenic effects of IgG monoclonal antibodies of different IgG subclasses against murine GPIIb/IIIa, Ib$\alpha$, Ib/IX, V and CD31. Their data suggest that, at least in mice, the antigenic specificity of the antiplatelet antibodies determines the pathogenic effects rather than the IgG subclass. They also demonstrated that antibodies against GPIb/IX caused thrombocytopenia through an Fc-independent mechanism, while that from autoantibodies against GPIIb/IIIa involved the Fc system. Further work is clearly needed in order to determine the significance of all these findings, which may translate into stratification of patients into those in whom Fc receptor blockade or inactivation is a useful option, and those in whom it is not.

At the T-cell level, it has been demonstrated that T cells from Japanese patients with chronic ITP could proliferate *in vitro* in response to disulfide-reduced GPIIb/IIIa or the molecule's tryptic peptides. This suggested that autoreactive CD4⁺ Th cells in chronic ITP need to recognize a modified GPIIb/IIIa molecule, implying that antigen-processing mechanisms within recipient APCs may be required to present GPIIb/IIIa autoantigens in the context of self HLA-DR molecules. Subsequently, mapping studies using six large (~200 amino acids) recombinant fragments encoding different portions of the GPIIbα and GPIIIa chains showed that the T cells from patients with ITP recognized

primarily the amino-terminal portion of the two chains (GPIIbα 18–259 and GPIIIa 22–262) and that these molecules also stimulated the production of antiplatelet autoantibodies. Ultimately, the GPIIIa molecule has been mapped for CD4⁺ T-cell specificities by using 15-mer peptides of the GPIIIa chain and this has revealed several immunodominant peptides spanning the entire breadth of the molecule. What was particularly intriguing was that despite a lack of HLA association observed in many studies of patients with ITP, some patients apparently recognize common elements on the GPIIIa molecule. This may suggest that either a host (e.g., antigen processing) or environmental (e.g., infection) factor could be responsible for generating a common autoepitope that is presented to T cells across different HLA. If this were true, it would be an efficacious way of developing peptide antigen-specific T-cell therapies for autoantibody production and subsequent platelet destruction in ITP.

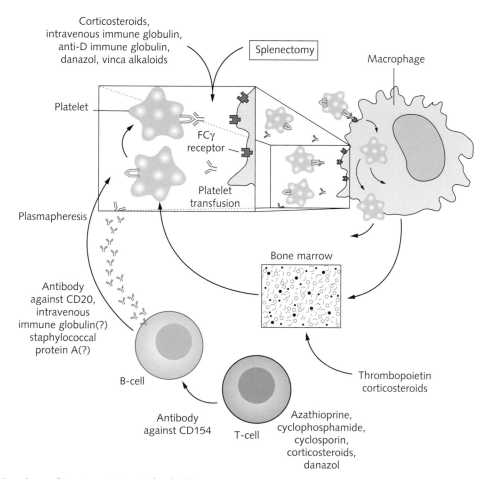

**Fig. 23.7 Standard and novel treatment strategies in ITP**

Standard treatments include corticosteroids, intravenous immunoglobulin, danazol and vinca alkaloids. Their sites and modes of action are illustrated. New therapies include monoclonal antibodies against CD154 (CD40 ligand) and CD20 (on B cells, leading to transient B-cell depletion). Reproduced from Cines DB, Blanchette VS. (2002) Immune thrombocytopenic purpura. *New England Journal of Medicine*, **346**, 995–1008.

## Standard treatment

There is a lack of clinical trial data to help guide treatment and our energies should now be focused on constructing high-quality randomized trials in order to determine the most effective therapy in this disorder. Therapy is seldom necessary for patients whose platelet counts exceed 20–$30 \times 10^9$/L and in whom there are few spontaneous bleeding episodes, unless they are undergoing any procedure likely to induce blood loss. Standard treatments, including oral prednisolone, IVIg and splenectomy, will elevate the platelet count sufficiently in most adults (Figure 23.7). However, some 20–25% of adults with ITP are refractory to first-line therapy.

### Chronic refractory ITP

This defines those patients who fail to respond to first-line treatment or require unacceptably high doses of corticosteroids to maintain a safe platelet count. A number of agents have been used as second-line therapy for ITP, including high-dose steroids, high-dose IVIg, intravenous anti-D, vinca alkaloids, danazol, azathioprine, combination chemotherapy and dapsone.

## Targeted versus untargeted therapies for autoimmune disease

Until now most of our treatments for autoimmune disease have been untargeted and unselective in their modes of action. In disorders such as ITP the therapeutic aim has been to induce global immunosuppression in the hope that, as part of this process, the ITP-related component of the immune system will be suppressed and that this will help reduce the quantity of autoantibody produced. For antibody-mediated autoimmune diseases, what remains unclear is whether the B-cell population that is generating the antiplatelet autoantibody is the primary problem, or whether events downstream, such as those involving antigen presentation or T-cell regulation, are disturbed, and simply driving the passive B cells, resulting in the autoantibody phenotype.

Now that we have a clearer understanding of the immunological mechanisms involved in autoimmune disease, we have started to develop more targeted therapies. We are now developing treatments designed to target T cells, B cells and other effectors within the immune system. For ITP these include Campath-1H and anti-CD20. Although these agents are not entirely specific because they deplete the B-cell compartment, they should reduce the quantity of autoantibody produced. Other therapies which may be of benefit in ITP are mycophenolate mofetil and anti-CD40 ligand.

## Campath-1H

Campath-1H is a humanized IgG monoclonal antibody that targets the CD52 antigen, present on mature human lymphocytes (T and B cells) and monocytes. Campath-1H is effective in the treatment of malignant B-cell disorders, especially B-cell chronic lymphocytic leukemia, in which it has been shown to be effective in clearing lymphocytes from both blood and bone marrow.

Campath-1H has been used in a variety of autoimmune diseases, including rheumatoid arthritis, vasculitis and Wegener granulomatosis. There is ongoing interest in the use of Campath-1H for the treatment of autoimmune hematological disease that is refractory to first- and second-line therapies. One recent study of the use of Campath-1H in autoimmune neutropenia, autoimmune hemolytic anemia, pure red cell aplasia, immune thrombocytopenia and combined hemolytic anemia and ITP (Evans syndrome) has shown responses in 15 of 21 patients treated; in six patients the response was sustained. Campath-1H therefore appears to be an effective agent in severe refractory autoimmune disease. The drug is well tolerated, but because it can precipitate bleeding during administration it should not be given in the presence of active bleeding (or active infection).

## Anti-CD20 monoclonal antibody therapy

Rituximab, a genetically engineered chimeric human/mouse anti-CD20 monoclonal antibody, has been developed as a treatment for B-cell lymphoproliferative disease (non-Hodgkin lymphoma). The antibody is an IgG κ immunoglobulin comprising murine light- and heavy-chain variable-region sequences and human constant-region sequences. The antigen-binding domain binds to the CD20 antigen on B cells while the Fc domain mediates B-cell lysis through recruitment of immune effector cells. Because of its specificity for B cells, rituximab has been viewed as a potential treatment for autoimmune disease, the rationale being the reduction or elimination of autoantibody-producing B cells with concomitant improvement of the autoimmune disease. A recent study by Stasi and colleagues reports on the efficacy of rituximab in the treatment of 25 patients with chronic refractory ITP. Patients were treated if their platelet counts were below $20 \times 10^9$/L irrespective of symptoms, or at higher platelet counts if bleeding or bruising was problematic. All patients had received between two and five previous treatments; eight had failed splenectomy. Rituximab was administered in the same manner and dose as that used in non-Hodgkin lymphoma. After four courses, 40% of patients achieved a platelet count of at least $50 \times 10^9$/L; five achieved complete remission (platelets $>100 \times 10^9$/L) and five partial remission (platelets 50–100 × $10^9$/L). Responses were seen during treatment with rituximab, with a peak response up to 4 weeks after the end of treatment; 28% had responses that lasted for more than 6 months.

The results suggest that the use of rituximab resulted in responses similar to those given by other second-line agents used in ITP (including vinca alkaloids, cyclophosphamide and azathioprine), around 40–50%, but sustained responses to these agents is usually seen in fewer than 20% of patients (i.e., lower than for rituximab). Rituximab would appear to be useful for some patients with chronic symptomatic refractory ITP in whom there is a definite need to elevate the platelet count to a safe level.

The mechanism of action of rituximab in ITP has been assumed to be due to selective depletion of $CD20^+$ B cells that subsequently affects autoantibody development. This concept was recently shattered when it was demonstrated, using a variety of sophisticated techniques to analyze T-cell parameters, that only when the abnormal T-cell subsets were normalized was rituximab therapy effective. The reasons for these results are not clear, but may relate to how B-cell populations may be either important in maintaining autoreactive T-cell activation patterns or, by decreasing the total mass of B cells, may cause a collapse of autoreactive T-cell stimulation and normalization of the T-cell repertoire even as the B cells begin to return months after the therapy. What is perhaps more enlightening is the demonstration that the abnormal Treg populations are indirectly targeted by rituximab therapy; the anti-CD20 treatment reverses the Treg deficiency in patients with ITP and normalizes the autoimmunity. Taken together, these studies truly lend credence to the notion that attacking T cells in ITP, even indirectly by the destruction of B cells, is perhaps the only way to reduce platelet destruction effectively.

## Costimulatory blockade

Therapies such as Campath-1H and anti-CD20 may not produce lasting remission if the autoimmune B cells are driven by dysregulated T cells, and a novel agent, CTLA-4-Ig, has been evaluated in psoriasis in an attempt to block T-cell costimulation, thereby inducing anergy in the T-cell compartment. CTLA-4-Ig, a fusion protein between CTLA-4 and the Fc portion of human immunoglobulin, binds to B7-1 and B7-2, blocking T-cell costimulation (Figure 23.8). This small trial showed that, at least within this group of patients, CTLA-4-Ig was able to improve the disorder and was shown to be safe. CTLA-4-Ig may have applications within other autoimmune disorders, including ITP. If a drug such as CTLA-4-Ig were shown to be effective in ITP, not only would it provide an additional targeted treatment modality, but would also provide useful evidence of T-cell dysfunction in this disease. Interestingly, the CTLA-4 gene has been mapped as a susceptibility gene in autoimmune thyroid disease and type 1 diabetes in humans.

## Other options: *Helicobacter pylori* eradication

This bacterium is the main cause of gastritis and peptic ulcer disease. It has also been implicated in the development of gastric adenocarcinoma and mucosa-associated lymphoid tumors and in some autoimmune disorders. Previous studies of *H. pylori* in ITP showed improvement in platelet counts after eradication of the bacterium in patients shown to be positive for *H. pylori*. More recently, Emilia and colleagues looked for the presence of *H. pylori* in 30 patients with chronic refractory ITP. *Helicobacter pylori* was found in 13 of 30 patients (43.3%). Standard triple therapy for *H. pylori*

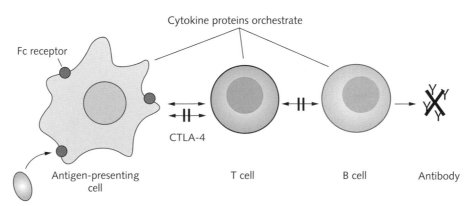

**Fig. 23.8 Costimulatory blockade may be beneficial in some autoimmune diseases**
CTLA-4 linked to human immunoglobulin Fc (CTLA-4-Ig) blocks the critical second signal between antigen-presenting cells and T cells, resulting in T-cell anergy. This should result in a reduction in antibody production and amelioration of disease if the autoimmune disease is antibody-mediated. CTLA-4-Ig treatment has been shown to be of benefit to patients with psoriasis. Similarly, anti-CD40 ligand also blocks the second signal with similar results, and has been shown to be of value in refractory ITP.

eradication resulted in a complete response in 4 of 12 patients in whom the bacterium was eradicated, and partial response in 2 of 12 (16.6%). The responses were maintained for a median of 8.33 months. In addition, there are other anecdotal reports of improvements in platelet counts in adults and children with ITP after eradication of *H. pylori*. Larger studies are required to confirm these earlier findings, but from the available data triple therapy appears to offer a non-immunosuppressive therapy for patients with refractory ITP and possibly other autoimmune diseases.

On the other hand, platelets express Toll-like receptor (TLR)4 and this has been shown to be responsible for the thrombocytopenia induced by lipopolysaccharide administration *in vivo*. It now appears that bacterial products such as lipopolysaccharide together with IgG bound to platelets can significantly enhance Fc-mediated platelet phagocytosis by mononuclear phagocytes. This suggests that infectious agents, in combination with antiplatelet antibodies, could affect platelet destruction *in vivo* and may be at least one explanation of why thrombocytopenia worsens in some patients with ITP during infections and, alternatively, resolves in other patients with ITP who are treated with bacterial eradication therapy.

## Novel therapies for the treatment of other autoimmune diseases

Human and animal studies have been helpful in learning how the immune system works in both health and disease, but can such information be translated into better patient care? Until recently the treatment strategy for autoimmune diseases has been to induce global immunosuppression in the hope that the autoimmune process may be abrogated or stopped. In some cases treatment is effective but it is clear from longitudinal follow-up studies of patients with ITP that there is very significant morbidity and mortality associated with our current treatments. Infection plays a major role in the death of patients with autoimmune disease, and such fatalities are usually induced by immunosuppression. Now that we have a better understanding of the components of the immune system and how these interact in disease, we should be able to develop targeted therapies that aim to modify specific components of the immune system while leaving most of the immune system intact and able to fight infection.

Such therapeutic advances are in fact being made, and many of these have been developed through knowledge concerning specific components of the immune system in disease. We have now been able to develop targeted therapies for rheumatoid disease, multiple sclerosis, psoriasis, diabetes and systemic lupus. We discuss each of these briefly in turn.

## Rheumatoid arthritis and blockade of TNF-alpha

Disease-modifying therapies, designed to reduce deformity in rheumatoid disease, have been around for a number of years. Methotrexate is one of the main agents in this category. Bone destruction in rheumatoid disease is partly mediated by macrophages through an inflammatory process. With our increased understanding of cytokines and their interactions, specific modulators of the immune response have been developed. Because TNF-$\alpha$ plays a key role in the inflammatory response, antibodies against TNF-$\alpha$ have been developed and shown to be of value. To date, two antibodies appear promising: the first is a TNF-$\alpha$ receptor–IgG1 fusion protein, etanercept; the second, infliximab, is a monoclonal antibody directed against TNF-$\alpha$ itself. This form of therapy also appears to have a place in the management of other autoimmune diseases, such as Crohn's disease, psoriatic arthropathy and ankylosing spondylitis.

Another cytokine involved in the pathogenesis of rheumatoid disease is IL-1. Blockade of the IL-1 receptor using a recombinant antagonist may slow down the development of erosive bone disease but from available data this appears to be less effective than TNF-$\alpha$.

## Multiple sclerosis

IFN-$\beta$ has recently been introduced for the treatment of multiple sclerosis and the available study data indicate that it may delay the onset of the disease if started immediately after the patient's first attack of optic neuritis.

## Psoriasis

This autoimmune skin disorder has been treated by TNF-$\alpha$ blockade with and without methotrexate. Other agents used in small clinical trials include IL-10 and CTLA-4-Ig; the latter molecule is a recombinant protein comprising the extracellular domain of CTLA-4 linked to the constant region of IgG1. CTLA-4-Ig downregulates activated T cells and prevents activation of naive T cells. CTLA-4-Ig was well tolerated in a small trial conducted by Bristol-Myers-Squibb and the patients' skin condition improved by more than 50%. Further studies are required to confirm safety and efficacy.

There are studies of other agents used in the treatment of autoimmune disease but there is insufficient space to discuss these here. However, it would appear that our knowledge of immunity and autoimmunity is now being used to design more subtle and specific treatments for patients with autoimmune disease. It is expected that these treatments will reduce immunosuppression, morbidity and mortality and offer modern solutions to these otherwise intractable diseases. No doubt the future will see even more designer drugs being developed for this fascinating group of diseases.

## Conclusions

Autoimmune diseases are complex immunological disorders affecting 5% of the population. Until recently our understanding of the pathogenesis and treatment of these disorders was severely limited. However, with greater understanding of the immune system in health and autoimmune disease we are able to identify underlying abnormalities leading to the develop of autoimmunity. With this new knowledge we have been able to modify our therapies by replacing non-selective immunosuppressive treatment with more subtle targeted therapies.

## Further reading

### General

Janeway CA, Travers P, Walport M, Capra JD. (1999) *Immunobiology: The Immune System in Health and Disease*, 4th edn. New York: Current Biology.

Roitt IM, Delves PJ. (2001) *Roitt's Essential Immunology*, 10th edn. Oxford: Blackwell Science.

### Immune system and HLA

Chien YH, Gascoigne NR, Kavaler J et al. (1984) Somatic recombination in a murine T-cell receptor gene. *Nature*, **309**, 322–326.

Delves PJ, Roitt IM. (2000) The immune system. First of two parts. *New England Journal of Medicine*, **343**, 37–49.

Delves PJ, Roitt IM. (2000) The immune system. Second of two parts. *New England Journal of Medicine*, **343**, 108–117.

Klein J, Sato A. (2000) The HLA system. First of two parts. *New England Journal of Medicine*, **343**, 702–709.

Klein J, Sato A. (2000) The HLA system. Second of two parts. *New England Journal of Medicine*, **343**, 782–786.

Parkin J, Cohen B. (2001) An overview of the immune system. *Lancet*, **357**, 1777–1789.

Tonegawa S. (1983) Somatic generation of antibody diversity. *Nature*, **302**, 575–581.

### Tolerance

Dario A, Vignali A, Collison LW, Workman CJ. (2008) How regulatory T cells work. *Nature Reviews. Immunology*, **8**, 523–532.

Kamradt T, Mitchison NA. (2001) Tolerance and autoimmunity. *New England Journal of Medicine*, **344**, 655–664.

Mackay IR. (2000) Science, medicine, and the future: tolerance and autoimmunity. *British Medical Journal*, **321**, 93–96.

Sarzotti M. (1997) Immunologic tolerance. *Current Opinion in Hematology*, **4**, 48–52.

### Autoimmunity

Davidson A, Diamond B. (2001) Autoimmune diseases. *New England Journal of Medicine*, **345**, 340–350.

Maloy KJ, Powrie F. (2001) Regulatory T cells in the control of immune pathology. *Nature Immunology*, **2**, 816–822.

Sinha AA, Lopez MT, McDevitt HO. (1990) Autoimmune diseases: the failure of self tolerance. *Science*, **248**, 1380–1388.

Taneja V, David CS. (2001) Lessons from animal models for human autoimmune diseases. *Nature Immunology*, **2**, 781–784.

### Role of genetic and other factors in autoimmune disease

Albert LJ, Inman RD. (1999) Molecular mimicry and autoimmunity. *New England Journal of Medicine*, **341**, 2068–2074.

Benoist C, Mathis D. (2001) Autoimmunity provoked by infection: how good is the case for T cell epitope mimicry? *Nature Immunology*, **2**, 797–801.

Choy EH, Panayi GS. (2001) Cytokine pathways and joint inflammation in rheumatoid arthritis. *New England Journal of Medicine*, **344**, 907–916.

Criswell LA, Moser KL, Gaffney PM et al. (2000) PARP alleles and SLE: failure to confirm association with disease susceptibility. *Journal of Clinical Investigation*, **105**, 1501–1502.

Ermann J, Fathman CG. (2001) Autoimmune diseases: genes, bugs and failed regulation. *Nature Immunology*, **2**, 759–761.

Gianani R, Sarvetnick N. (1996) Viruses, cytokines, antigens, and autoimmunity. *Proceedings of the National Academy of Sciences of the United States of America*, **93**, 2257–2259.

Marron MP, Zeidler A, Raffel LJ et al. (2000) Genetic and physical mapping of a type 1 diabetes susceptibility gene (IDDM12) to a 100-kb phagemid artificial chromosome clone containing D2S72-CTLA4-D2S105 on chromosome 2q33. *Diabetes*, **49**, 492–499.

Spielman RS, Ewens WJ. (1996) The TDT and other family-based tests for linkage disequilibrium and association. *American Journal of Human Genetics*, **59**, 983–989.

Wanstrat A, Wakeland E. (2001) The genetics of complex autoimmune diseases: non-MHC susceptibility genes. *Nature Immunology*, **2**, 802–809.

### Idiopathic thrombocytopenic purpura

Aslam R, Speck ER, Kim M et al. (2006) Platelet Toll-like receptor expression modulates lipopolysaccharide-induced thrombocytopenia and tumor necrosis factor-production in vivo. *Blood*, **107**, 637–641.

Bussel JB. (2002) Novel approaches to refractory immune thrombocytopenic purpura. *Blood Reviews*, **16**, 31–36.

Cines DB, Blanchette VS. (2002) Immune thrombocytopenic purpura. *New England Journal of Medicine*, **346**, 995–1008.

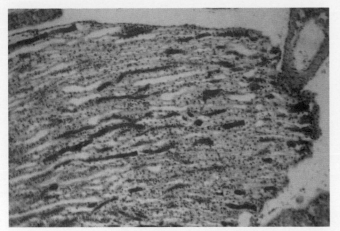

**Plate 15.1 Renal medulla of transgenic mice expressing β$^S$ and β$^{S-Antilles}$**

Note the extensive obstructive aggregation of sickle red cells in the renal medullary vasculature.

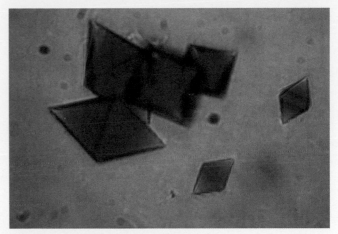

**Plate 15.2 Hb C tetragonal crystals**

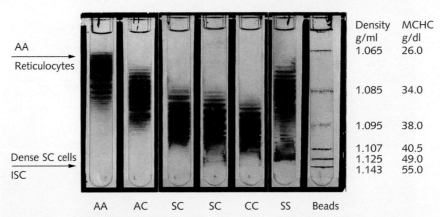

| | Density g/ml | MCHC g/dl |
|---|---|---|
| AA Reticulocytes → | 1.065 | 26.0 |
| | 1.085 | 34.0 |
| | 1.095 | 38.0 |
| Dense SC cells → | 1.107 | 40.5 |
| | 1.125 | 49.0 |
| ISC | 1.143 | 55.0 |

AA   AC   SC   SC   CC   SS   Beads

**Plate 15.3 Percoll density gradients of AA, CC and SC red cells**

This shows the separation of red cells by density. Light-density cells are on top, high-density cells on the bottom. Note that SS blood has normal-density red cells as the largest compartment, then some very dense cells, and some intermediate-density cells between the two. In contrast, all the cells of the CC patients are denser than normal red cells. The SC red cells are intermediate.

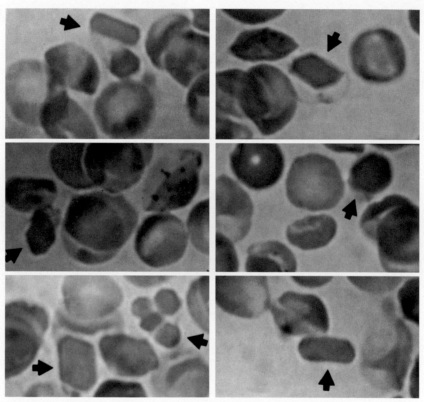

**Plate 15.4 SC red cells from a double-stained smear**
This blood smear is from a patient with Hb SC and is stained with Wright's and reticulocyte stain. Note the flat thin cells (which generate target cells), folded cells and those with intracellular tetragonal crystals (arrows).

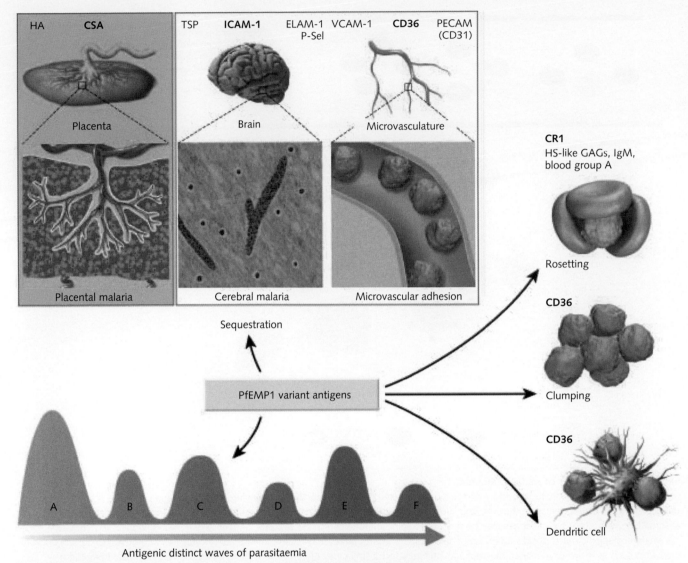

Antigenic distinct waves of parasitaemia

**Plate 16.1** *P. falciparum* **erythrocyte membrane protein (PfEMP)1 and pathology**

PfEMP1 expressed on the surface of mature red blood cells infected with *P. falciparum* undergoes clonal antigenic variation and can bind to many host receptors through its multiple adhesion domains. The different properties of PfEMP1 – sequestration for evading clearance in the spleen and antigenic variation for evading antibody-dependent killing – contribute to the virulence and pathogenesis of *P. falciparum* and are essential for survival of the parasite. Parasite sequestration in the brain and placenta contribute to the complications of cerebral malaria and placental malaria, respectively. Simultaneous binding to several receptors, binding of uninfected erythrocytes (rosetting), and clumping of infected erythrocytes through platelets are associated with the pathogenesis of malaria. Parasite-infected red blood cells binding to dendritic cells downregulates the host immune response. HA, hyaluronic acid; TSP, thrombospondin; ELAM-1, endothelial/leukocyte adhesion molecule 1; P-Sel, P-selectin; VCAM-1, vascular cell adhesion molecule 1; PECAM (CD31), platelet endothelial cell adhesion molecule 1; CR1, complement receptor 1; HS-like GAGs, heparin sulfate-like glycosaminoglycans. From Miller LH, Baruch DI, Marsh K, Doumbo OK. (2002) The pathogenic basis of malaria. *Nature*, **415**, 673–679, with permission.

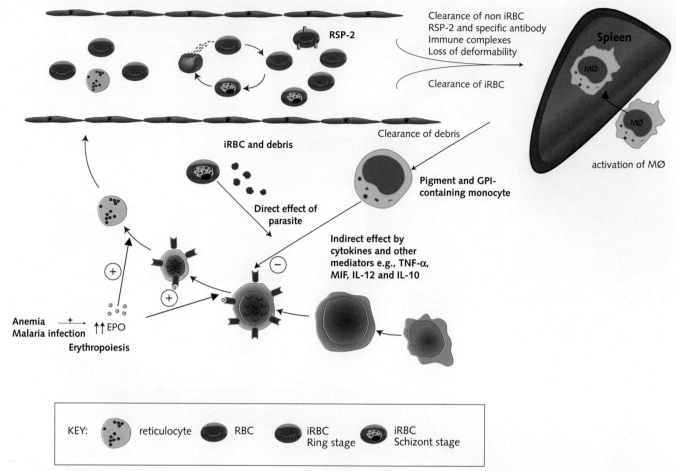

RSP-2

Clearance of non iRBC
RSP-2 and specific antibody
Immune complexes
Loss of deformability

Clearance of iRBC

Spleen

MØ

MØ

activation of MØ

iRBC and debris

Clearance of debris

Pigment and GPI-
containing monocyte

Direct effect of
parasite

Indirect effect by
cytokines and other
mediators e.g., TNF-α,
MIF, IL-12 and IL-10

Anemia
Malaria infection

↑↑EPO

Erythropoiesis

KEY:  ⬤ reticulocyte    ⬭ RBC    ⬬ iRBC
Ring stage    ⬬ iRBC
Schizont stage

**Plate 16.2 Pathogenesis of malarial anemia**
Severe malarial anemia is characterized by destruction of infected red blood cells (iRBC) following schizogony and clearance of both iRBCs and uninfected RBCs. During malarial infection, ring surface protein (RSP)-2 may be deposited on the membrane, immune complexes may be absorbed and senescent-type changes may occur. The resultant immune complexes of RBCs, antigen and immunoglobulin, e.g., RBC:RSP2:Ig, are cleared by splenic macrophages (MØ). Pigment-containing macrophages may release inflammatory cytokines and other biologically active mediators such as 4-hydroxynonenal. Macrophage inhibitory factor (MIF) may be released by macrophages or a plasmodial homolog may suppress erythropoiesis. Malarial pigment or other parasite products may have a direct inhibitory effect on erythropoiesis. Inhibition of erythropoiesis may be at one or more sites in the growth and differentiation of hematopoietic progenitors. Both indirect and direct effects may cause suppression of the bone marrow and spleen, resulting in inadequate reticulocyte counts for the degree of anemia. EPO, erythropoietin; GPI, glycosylphosphatidylinositol anchors of merozoite proteins; Hz, hemozoin.

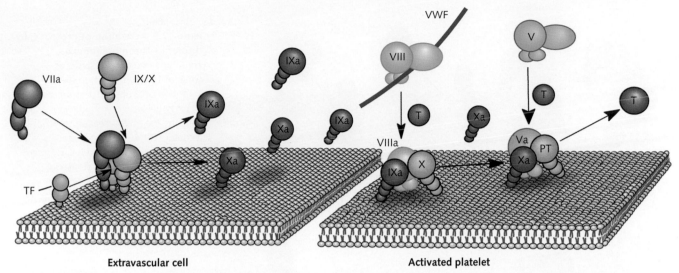

**Extravascular cell**                                         **Activated platelet**

**Plate 17.1 Initiation and propagation of blood coagulation**

Blood coagulation takes place on the surface of cell membranes where enzymes and cofactors form complexes that efficiently convert their respective proenzyme substrates to active enzymes. The exposure of tissue factor (TF) to blood with subsequent binding of FVII/FVIIa and activation of FIX and FX initiates the reaction sequence. The subsequent assembly of tenase (FIXa/FVIIIa) and prothrombinase (FXa/FVa) complexes on the surface of negatively charged phospholipid membranes (mainly provided by platelets) results in amplification, propagation of the process and the generation of high concentrations of thrombin (T). Thrombin feedback activates FVIII (circulates in complex with von Willebrand factor, VWF) and FV.

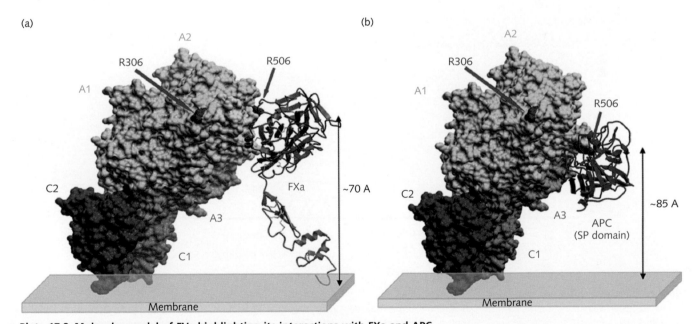

**Plate 17.2 Molecular model of FVa highlighting its interactions with FXa and APC**

FVa is shown as a solid surface (domains A1, green; A2, cyan; A3, brown; C1, pink; C2, purple) and FXa as an orange ribbon. The virtual membrane is represented as a gray box. (a) FVa/FXa complex with FVa residues probed experimentally to be important for FXa binding shown in white. (b) APC approaching the cleavage site at Arg506. The two main cleavage sites of APC (Arg306 and Arg506) are indicated in red. The serine protease domain of APC is shown as a blue ribbon. Segers K, Dahlbäck B, Nicolaes GA. (2007) Coagulation factor V and thrombophilia: background and mechanisms. *Thrombosis and Haemostasis*, **98**, 530–542, with permission.

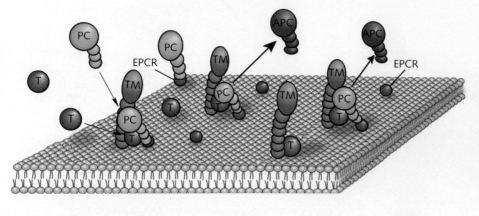

**Plate 17.3 Activation of protein C by thrombin–thrombomodulin**
Thrombomodulin (TM) serves as a cofactor to thrombin (T) in the activation of protein C. It is present on all endothelial cells. Endothelium also contains the endothelial protein C receptor (EPCR) that binds the Gla domain of protein C and helps present protein C to the T/TM complex. Activated protein C (APC) remains in the bloodstream to control coagulation reactions.

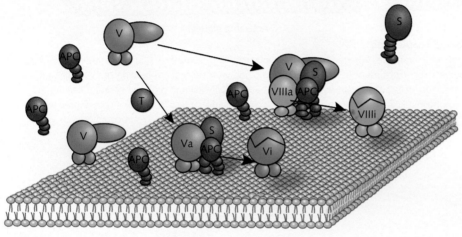

**Plate 17.4 Degradation of FVa and FVIIIa by APC**
Both FVa and FVIIIa are cleaved and inhibited by APC in phospholipid membrane-bound reactions that also involve cofactors to APC. Protein S and APC are sufficient to inhibit FVa, whereas the regulation of FVIIIa additionally includes FV, which in this situation serves as cofactor to APC.

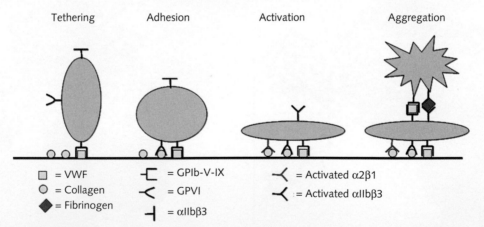

|  | Tethering | Adhesion | Activation | Aggregation |

■ = VWF    ⊏ = GPIb-V-IX    ≺ = Activated α2β1

○ = Collagen    ≺ = GPVI    ≺ = Activated αIIbβ3

◆ = Fibrinogen    ⊤ = αIIbβ3

**Plate 20.1 Platelet thrombus formation**
Following vessel wall injury, the matrix of the subendothelium is exposed. Under high-shear conditions, platelets adhere and become tethered via GPIb–V–IX on platelets binding to von Willebrand factor (VWF) in the matrix. This interaction starts platelet activation but also brings platelets into contact with the subendothelium, allowing other receptors, such as GPVI, to interact with collagen and enhance activation. Under static or low-shear conditions, the GPVI–collagen interaction is mainly responsible for the initial activation. Platelet activation brings additional receptor–ligand interactions into play, such as α2β1–collagen, since this receptor does not bind in the resting state. Platelet activation also leads to shape change, release of granule contents, activation of other receptors, such as αIIbβ3, and exposure of negatively charged phospholipids, critical for procoagulant activity. Binding of VWF and fibrinogen to GPIb–V–IX and αIIbβ3 on adjacent platelets leads to platelet aggregation and the formation of a thrombus.

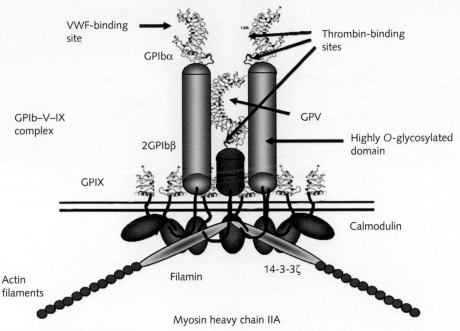

**Plate 20.2 Structure of the GPIb–V–IX complex**
GPIbα is linked via disulfide bridges to two GPIbβ molecules and this complex is non-covalently associated with GPIX and GPV in the ratio of 2:4:2:1. Mutations and deletions leading to Bernard–Soulier syndrome and platelet-type von Willebrand disease are described in the text. Mutations affecting cytoskeletal molecules such as filamin-1 and myosin heavy chain IIA, which interact directly or indirectly with GPIb complex, can also lead to giant platelet syndromes.

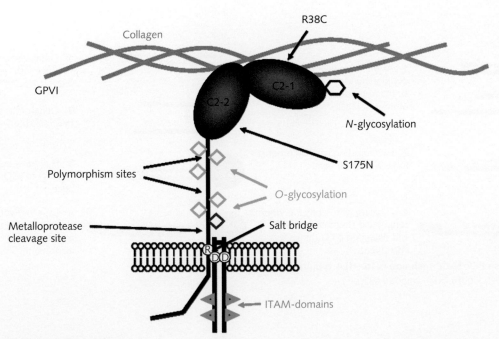

**Plate 20.3 Structure of the GPVI complex**
GPVI is linked via a salt bridge to FcγR, which provides most of the signaling to the platelet cytoplasm. The position of mutations leading to decreased expression and of polymorphisms thought to affect function are indicated. Activation of GPVI by autoantibodies can lead to coactivation of matrix metalloproteases and loss of GPVI by cleavage.

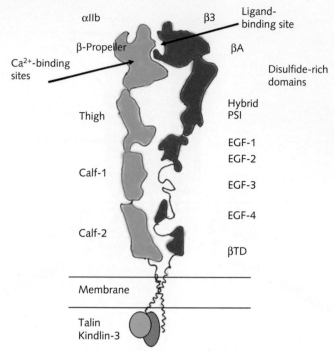

**Plate 20.4 Structure of the αIIbβ3 complex**
This major platelet integrin is shown in the activated state. The various structural domains are labeled. Cytoskeletal proteins associated with the cytoplasmic domain of β3 in the activated state are shown.

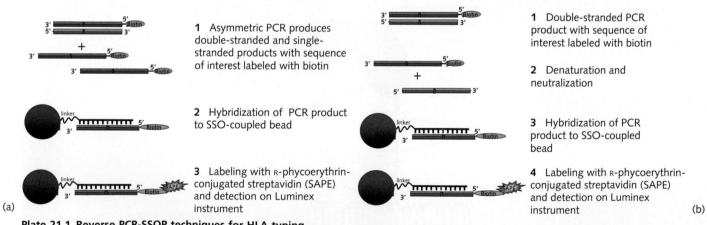

(a)

1  Asymmetric PCR produces double-stranded and single-stranded products with sequence of interest labeled with biotin

2  Hybridization of PCR product to SSO-coupled bead

3  Labeling with R-phycoerythrin-conjugated streptavidin (SAPE) and detection on Luminex instrument

1  Double-stranded PCR product with sequence of interest labeled with biotin

2  Denaturation and neutralization

3  Hybridization of PCR product to SSO-coupled bead

4  Labeling with R-phycoerythrin-conjugated streptavidin (SAPE) and detection on Luminex instrument

(b)

**Plate 21.1 Reverse PCR-SSOP techniques for HLA typing**
(a) Tepnel LIFECODES kit. (b) One Lambda LABType kit.

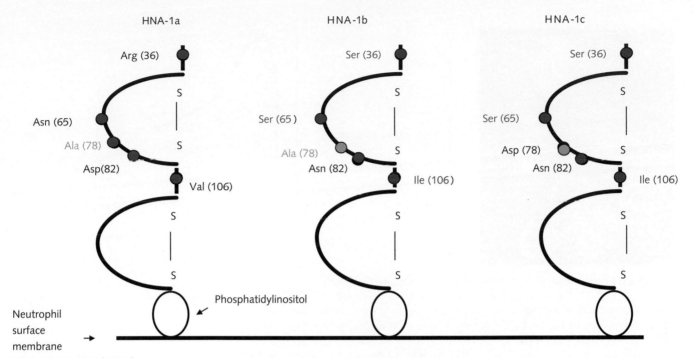

**Plate 21.2 FcγRIII (CD16)**

The low-affinity receptor for aggregated IgG is encoded by the *FCGR3B* gene on chromosome 1.

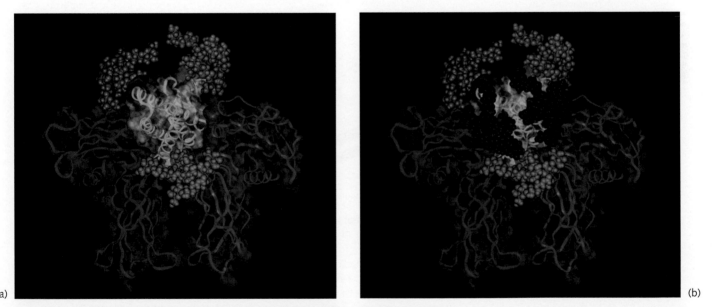

(a)                                                                                                                (b)

**Plate 24.1 Binding of recombinant human EPO and darbepoetin to the EPO receptor**

(a) Epogen (yellow/green helical structure) contains three N-linked carbohydrates (green balls) that are attached to the EPO protein at regions that are not involved in binding to the EPO receptor (blue colored dimer). (b) Aranesp has two additional N-linked glycosylation carbohydrates (red), resulting in an erythropoiesis-stimulating protein with longer half-life and improved *in vivo* efficacy.

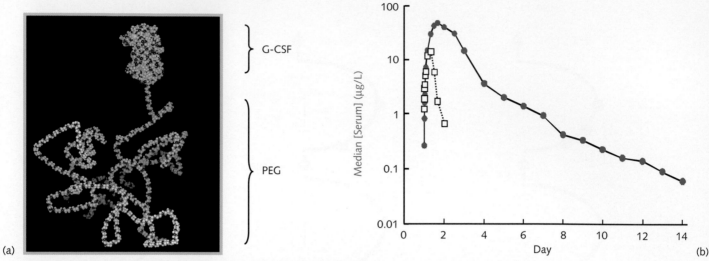

(a)

(b)

**Plate 24.2 Structure and pharmacokinetics of Neulasta (pegfilgrastim)**
(a) Human G-CSF is a 175-amino-acid glycoprotein with a molecular mass of 19 kDa. To extend the half-life of Neupogen in the circulation, a 20-kDa linear polyethylene glycol (PEG) moiety was covalently attached to the N-terminus of the protein. (b) Serum concentrations following a single subcutaneous injection of filgrastim (open squares; 5 μg/kg) or pegfilgrastim (solid circles; 60 μg/kg) in healthy human volunteers (*N* = 8 per group). The longer half-life of pegfilgrastim as a result of increasing its hydrodynamic size to eliminate renal clearance is evident. Adapted from Roskos LK *et al.* (1999) A cytokinetic model describes the granulopoietic effects of r-metHuG-CSF-SD/01 and the homeostatic regulation of SD/01 clearance in normal volunteers. *Clinical Pharmacology and Therapeutics*, **65**, 196, with permission.

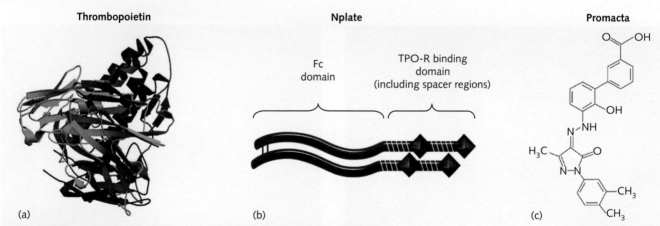

**Thrombopoietin**

**Nplate**

**Promacta**

(a)

(b)

(c)

**Plate 24.3 Structures of thrombopoietin (TPO) and synthetic c-mpl ligands**
(a) Native TPO is a 332-amino-acid glycoprotein with a molecular mass of 60–70 kDa. It is the major humoral regulator of platelet production. (b) Nplate (romiplostim) is a 60-kDa synthetic "peptibody" that does not share any amino acid homology to native TPO. It comprises a human immunoglobin Fc domain linked via polyglycine to two divalent mpl-binding peptide regions. The Fc component extends the half-life of the drug in the circulation, while the peptide "warhead" binds to the TPO receptor, c-mpl, and activates signaling. (c) Promacta (eltrombopag) is an orally bioavailable hydrazone small molecule with a molecular mass of 546 Da. Unlike TPO and Nplate, which bind the extracellular domain of c-mpl, Promacta is reported to bind to the transmembrane region of c-mpl. From Kuter DJ. (2007) New thrombopoietic growth factors. *Blood*, **109**, 4607–4616. © American Society of Hematology.

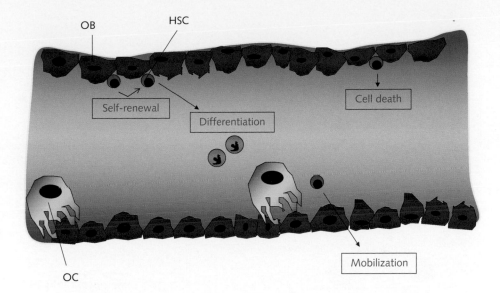

**Plate 30.1 Hematopoiesis: niche and mobilization**
HSC, hematopoietic stem cells; OB, osteoblast; OC, osteoclast.

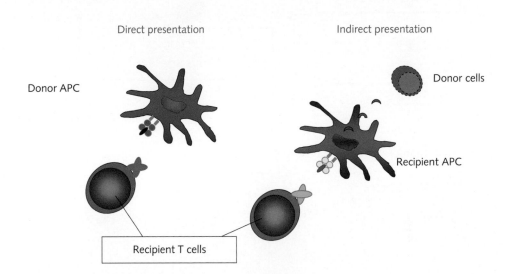

**Plate 30.2 Mechanisms of allorecognition**

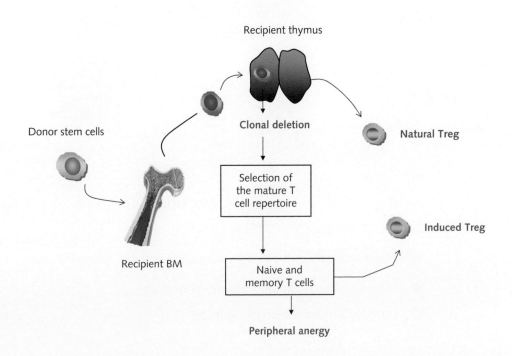

**Plate 30.3 Mechanisms of transplantation tolerance**

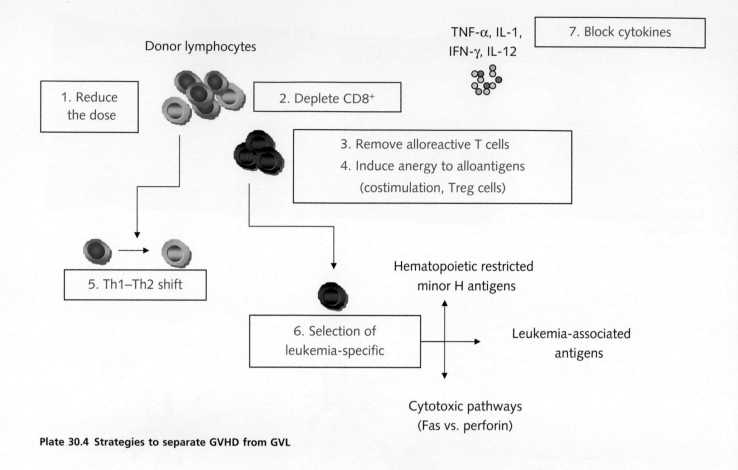

**Plate 30.4 Strategies to separate GVHD from GVL**

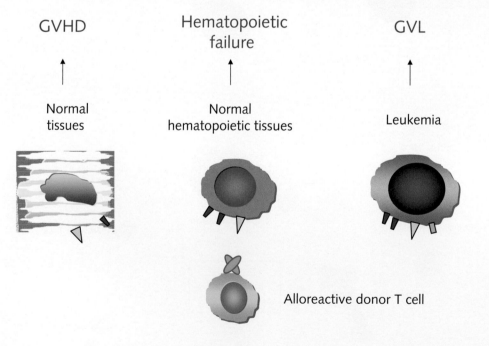

Polymorphisms expressed on all normal and malignant tissues

Hematopoietic-restricted polymorphisms

Leukemia-restricted polymorphisms

**Plate 30.5 Minor histocompatibility antigens in GVHD and GVL**

Coopamah MD, Garvey MB, Freedman J, Semple JW. (2003) Cellular immune mechanisms in autoimmune thrombocytopenic purpura: an update. *Transfusion Medicine Reviews*, **17**, 69–80.

de Luis DA, Varela C, de La Calle H *et al.* (1998) *Helicobacter pylori* infection is markedly increased in patients with autoimmune atrophic thyroiditis. *Journal of Clinical Gastroenterology*, **26**, 259–263.

Emilia G, Longo G, Luppi M *et al.* (2001) *Helicobacter pylori* eradication can induce platelet recovery in idiopathic thrombocytopenic purpura. *Blood*, **97**, 812–814.

Fujisawa K, Tani P, O'Toole TE *et al.* (1992) Different specificities of platelet-associated and plasma autoantibodies to platelet GPIIb-IIIa in patients with chronic immune thrombocytopenic purpura. *Blood*, **79**, 1441–1446.

Gasbarrini A, Franceschi F, Tartaglione R *et al.* (1998) Regression of autoimmune thrombocytopenia after eradication of *Helicobacter pylori*. *Lancet*, **352**, 878.

Kekomaki R, Dawson B, McFarland J *et al.* (1991) Localization of human platelet autoantigens to the cysteine-rich region of glycoprotein IIIa. *Journal of Clinical Investigation*, **88**, 847–854.

Kuwana M, Kaburaki J, Ikeda Y. (1998). Autoreactive T cells to platelet GPIIb-IIIa in immune thrombocytopenic purpura. Role in production of anti-platelet autoantibody. *Journal of Clinical Investigation*, **102**, 1393–1402.

Nieswandt B, Bergmeier W, Rackebrandt K *et al.* (2000) Identification of critical antigen-specific mechanisms in the development of immune thrombocytopenic purpura in mice. *Blood*, **96**, 2520–2527.

Portielje JE, Westendorp RG, Kluin-Nelemans HC *et al.* (2001) Morbidity and mortality in adults with idiopathic thrombocytopenic purpura. *Blood*, **97**, 2549–2554.

Provan D, Newland A. (2002) Fifty years of idiopathic thrombocytopenic purpura (ITP): management of refractory ITP in adults. *British Journal of Haematology*, **118**, 933–944.

Semple JW, Freedman J. (2006) Mechanisms underlying autoimmunity in hematology. *Drug Discovery Today: Disease Mechanisms*, **3**, 231–235.

Stasi R, Pagano A, Stipa E *et al.* (2001) Rituximab chimeric anti-CD20 monoclonal antibody treatment for adults with chronic idiopathic thrombocytopenic purpura. *Blood*, **98**, 952–957.

Sukati H, Watson HG, Urbaniak SJ *et al.* (2007) Mapping helper T-cell epitopes on platelet membrane glycoprotein IIIa in chronic autoimmune thrombocytopenic purpura. *Blood*, **109**, 4528–4538.

Zentilin P, Savarino V, Garnero A *et al.* (1999) Is *Helicobacter pylori* infection a risk factor for disease severity in rheumatoid arthritis? *Gastroenterology*, **116**, 503–504.

## Therapeutic advances

Abrams JR, Lebwohl MG, Guzzo CA *et al.* (1999) CTLA4Ig-mediated blockade of T-cell costimulation in patients with psoriasis vulgaris. *Journal of Clinical Investigation*, **103**, 1243–1252.

Bell S, Kamm MA. (2000) Antibodies to tumour necrosis factor alpha as treatment for Crohn's disease. *Lancet*, **355**, 858–860.

Brandt J, Haibel H, Cornely D *et al.* (2000) Successful treatment of active ankylosing spondylitis with the anti-tumor necrosis factor alpha monoclonal antibody infliximab. *Arthritis and Rheumatism*, **43**, 1346–1352.

Kremer JM. (2001) Rational use of new and existing disease-modifying agents in rheumatoid arthritis. *Annals of Internal Medicine*, **134**, 695–706.

Kuwana M, Kawakami Y, Ikeda Y. (2003) Suppression of autoreactive T-cell response to glycoprotein IIb/IIIa by blockade of CD40/CD154 interaction: implications for treatment of immune thrombocytopenic purpura. *Blood*, **101**, 621–623.

Maini RN, Taylor PC. (2000) Anti-cytokine therapy for rheumatoid arthritis. *Annual Review of Medicine*, **51**, 207–229.

Mease PJ, Goffe BS, Metz J *et al.* (2000) Etanercept in the treatment of psoriatic arthritis and psoriasis: a randomised trial. *Lancet*, **356**, 385–390.

Semple JW, Aslam R, Kim M, Speck ER, Freedman J. (2007) Platelet-bound lipopolysaccharide enhances Fc receptor-mediated phagocytosis of IgG opsonized platelets. *Blood*, **109**, 4803–4805.

Stasi R, Cooper N, Del Poeta G *et al.* (2008) Analysis of regulatory T cell changes in patients with idiopathic thrombocytopenic purpura receiving B-cell depleting therapy with rituximab. *Blood*, **112**, 1147–1150.

# Chapter 24 Hematopoietic growth factors: a 40-year journey from crude "activities" to therapeutic proteins

## Graham Molineux & Stephen J Szilvassy

*Hematology-Oncology Research, Amgen Inc., Thousand Oaks, CA, USA*

## Introduction

Blood cell generation, or hematopoiesis, is one of the most well-studied physiological processes and serves as a paradigm for stem cell biology and the regulation of self-renewing tissues. The primary function of blood cells is oxygenation of tissues but an important secondary function is combating infection via both cell-based and humoral mechanisms. During normal hematopoiesis in humans, approximately 250 billion new blood cells are produced each day to replace those lost through natural aging processes. During "stress hematopoiesis," which can be stimulated for example by hypoxia, traumatic blood loss or disease, the number of cells required to meet physiological demands can expand rapidly by more than 10-fold. The capacity for this remarkable expansion while maintaining the appropriate balance between the various types of specialized blood cells resides in a complex hierarchy of cellular elements found mainly in the bone marrow. At the apex of this hierarchy lies a relatively small population of around 50 million pluripotent hematopoietic stem cells (HSCs). Upon execution of a series of asymmetric cell divisions and fate decisions, HSCs give rise to a heterogeneous pool of differentially committed progenitor cells. At one extreme, these progenitor cells may retain the potential to develop into any of the eight major blood cell lineages (Figure 24.1). At the other extreme, they may be capable of responding in one of only two ways, either by dying (a process referred to as apoptosis) or by differentiating into a single type of mature blood cell. The key difference between hematopoietic stem and progenitor cells is the ability of stem cells to maintain an adequate supply of mature blood cells throughout adult life by balancing their production with the process of self-renewal, thus preventing exhaustion of the stem cell pool. At the level of an individual stem cell, other than the decision to undergo self-renewal (which is regulated predominantly by intracellular transcription factors that control the expression of an array of "stemness" genes), the probability of executing any one of these developmental options is tightly regulated by a complex network of humoral regulators, variously called hematopoietic growth factors (HGFs), interleukins or cytokines.

## Isolation and characterization of hematopoietic growth factors

In the current era of recombinant proteins and regenerative medicine it is worth recalling that the concepts that (i) blood is composed of many different cell types, (ii) its cellular composition may be subject to change in response to environmental variation, and (iii) humoral factors may be the mediators of such changes originated from the work of scientists such as Carnot and Viault early in the last century. However, it was another 60–70 years before experimental systems were developed to facilitate the quantitation and detailed functional characterization of hematopoietic stem and progenitor cells. These novel methods underpinned the development of a deeper understanding of the cellular diversity of blood and represented the first steps toward unraveling the complexity of the regulation of blood cell production. Although the spleen colony-forming units (CFU-S) first described by Till and McCulloch were ultimately demonstrated to exhibit only some of the hallmark properties that characterize the most primitive HSCs (i.e., most CFU-S lacked lymphoid differentiation potential and had only a

*Molecular Hematology*, 3rd edition. Edited by Drew Provan and John Gribben.
© 2010 Blackwell Publishing.

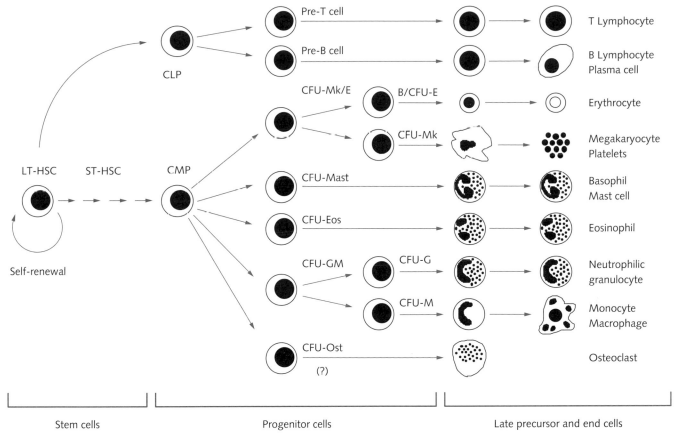

**Fig. 24.1 General model of the hematopoietic cell hierarchy**
The most primitive HSCs (LT-HSC) with self-renewal potential can maintain hematopoiesis long term (>6 months). These give rise to short-term stem cells (ST-HSC) that, while multipotent, have lost the ability to self-renew and produce clones with shorter lifespan. Common lymphoid progenitor (CLP) and common myeloid progenitor (CMP) cells are oligopotent precursors of the lymphoid and myeloid compartments. These mature into cohorts of committed progenitor cells with progressively restricted differentiation potential, culminating in the non-replicating late-stage precursors and end cells of the major hematopoietic lineages. Note that this model is continually evolving and readers should consult the latest papers describing precursor/progeny and lineage relationships.

limited capacity for self-renewal), this assay and the cell it detected is viewed by many to have ushered in the modern era of stem cell biology. The first *in vitro* colony-forming unit (CFU) assays (later known as colony-forming cell or CFC assays when it was demonstrated that individual colonies were derived from single cells) for hematopoietic progenitor cells were described in the mid-1960s and offered a practical end point for identifying factors that stimulate myelopoiesis. The extent to which development of these clonal hematopoietic cell assays represented a critical prerequisite to the identification of HGFs is underscored by the fact that the first such regulators were named colony-stimulating factors (CSFs).

CFU assays were used initially to identify and guide purification of the active components from crude preparations of body fluids, tissue extracts, or medium "conditioned" by various cell types that stimulated the proliferation of other-

wise unrecognizable precursor cells. Throughout the 1970s and 1980s, the "activities" in these complex biological fluids were resolved into pure proteins. In 1977, macrophage (M)-CSF (also known as colony-stimulating factor-1, CSF-1) was the first HGF to be purified, initially from human urine and later from medium conditioned by a murine fibroblast cell line. This was followed in the same year by the isolation of granulocyte/macrophage (GM)-CSF from medium conditioned by tissues from the lungs of mice previously treated with bacterial lipopolysaccharide, and a few years later by the identification of a third myeloid growth factor, granulocyte (G)-CSF. Cloning was a relatively new technology at that time and it was some years before the genes that encoded these proteins were cloned. However, following the cloning of the first hematopoietic cytokine, murine interleukin (IL)-3, in 1984, progress was rapid and soon thereafter a flurry of papers reported the cloning of human M-CSF, erythropoietin (EPO), GM-CSF, G-CSF, IL-3 and IL-5. Over the following two decades as many cytokines became available in very large quantities in recombinant form, they were characterized biochemically and studies of their effects on highly enriched subpopulations of hematopoietic stem and progenitor cells contributed to the evolution of an increasingly refined understanding of the humoral control of hematopoiesis.

HGFs were found to comprise either single subunit proteins or two identical subunits in which the tertiary structure that facilitates their association with specific cell surface receptors is maintained by essential disulfide bonds. The natural versions of most hematopoietic cytokines were found to be glycosylated, for example IL-3, IL-5, IL-6 , IL-7, GM-CSF, G-CSF, M-CSF, stem cell factor (SCF), and EPO. In several cases the carbohydrate was shown to be unnecessary for the maintenance of biological activity (e.g., the O-linked carbohydrate at threonine 133 on natural G-CSF). In the case of EPO, however, the carbohydrate component enhances the stability and serum half-life of the molecule and, while dispensable for activity *in vitro*, is obligatory for *in vivo* action. Carbohydrate content is increased in several novel erythropoiesis-stimulating agents (ESAs) with improved pharmacokinetic properties, such as darbepoetin alfa and AMG 114. Of these agents, only darbepoetin alfa, which contains two additional sialic acid-containing N-linked carbohydrate chains, has been commercialized (Plate 24.1). Many cytokines undergo additional post-translational modifications such as sulfation and proteolytic cleavage, and are thus frequently both structurally and functionally heterogeneous to some degree. From a drug development perspective, this has presented both complex regulatory challenges and opportunities to develop new molecular entities with improved drug properties, as discussed below.

## Production and biological functions of hematopoietic growth factors

Because of the high level of blood flow through the kidney, it represents an ideal organ to both sense and respond to the level of blood oxygenation. The kidney is the main source of EPO which is released into the bloodstream where it can then manifest its action on erythroid progenitor cells that reside mainly in the bone marrow. This remote control of blood cell production also holds true for platelet production, which is stimulated by thrombopoietin (TPO) that is produced constitutively mainly in the liver. However, with these exceptions, hematopoiesis is subject largely to local control within the bone marrow. Most HGFs are produced by marrow "stromal" cells such as macrophages, fibroblasts,

osteoblasts and endothelial cells. Stromal cells also express adhesion molecules that facilitate the retention of hematopoietic cells within the bone marrow, thus colocalizing them with factors that regulate the earliest events in stem cell development (i.e., cell cycle initiation, lineage commitment and differentiation). Within so-called "niches," the action of the HGFs to promote proliferation and differentiation is balanced by that of various inhibitory factors, which are not discussed here. The opposing activities of these positive and negative regulators on various cell types can be further modulated in a concentration-dependent manner and depending on the context in which they are presented to the target cell (i.e., either alone or in combination with other cytokines) and whether the growth factor is soluble or bound to the cell membrane or extracellular matrix of stromal cells.

Some HGFs act on relatively primitive cells with multilineage differentiation potential (e.g., IL-3 and SCF), while others act only on more committed cells in the later stages of blood cell production (e.g., EPO). In this regard, HGFs exhibit a general hierarchical organization in their actions that mirrors the organization of the hematopoietic stem and progenitor cell hierarchy (Figure 24.2). There is a surprising degree of overlap in target cell populations and some of those cytokines that were originally thought to act only on lineage-committed progenitor cells or their differentiated progeny have now been shown to have multiple levels of biological activity including on the most primitive HSCs (e.g., TPO). Thus pleiotropy and redundancy have emerged as dominant themes. This has presented significant challenges for drug development and more lineage-restricted cytokines have, in general, proven the more useful, as exemplified by the clinical utility of EPO, G-CSF and GM-CSF and the promise of TPO-mimetics.

HGFs transmit signals to their target cells by binding to cognate receptors that share a number of structural features. The type I cytokine receptors are composed of either dimers of a single protein subunit (e.g., receptors for EPO, TPO and G-CSF) or are heterodimers of a unique ligand-binding (or α) chain and one of three possible signaling subunits: the common β chain, used by receptors for GM-CSF, IL-3 and IL-5; the gp130 receptor, used by receptors for IL-6, IL-11 and leukemia inhibitory factor (LIF) among others; or the common γ chain, used by receptors for IL-2, IL-4, IL-7, IL-9, IL-13, IL-15 and IL-21 (as reviewed by Robb). HGFs bind to their receptors with extremely high affinity, as exemplified by dissociation constants ($K_d$) in the picomolar range. Ligand binding initiates receptor homodimerization (e.g., G-CSFR), heterodimerization (e.g., GM-CSFR), or induces changes in the conformation of preformed homodimers (e.g., EPOR) resulting in the activation of various signal transduction pathways. Most cytokine receptors transmit their signals via the Janus (JAK) family of tyrosine kinases. JAK proteins are

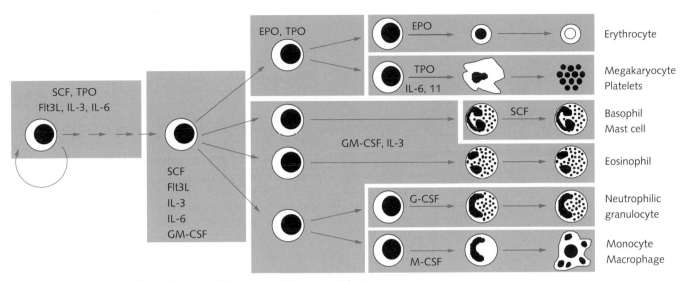

**Fig. 24.2 Major target cells of the myeloid hematopoietic growth factors**
Stem and progenitor cell types and late-stage cells of each lineage are reproduced from Fig. 24.1. The gray boxes depict the earliest target cell type and its progeny upon which the indicated HGF has been shown to act by stimulating proliferation and/or differentiation. SCF and Flt3L promote the survival of the most primitive HSCs but also synergize with most later-acting factors to increase their potency. Not shown are reported activities of some HGFs on other cell types when used at very high concentrations under experimental conditions.

constitutively associated with the membrane proximal intracellular portion of cytokine receptors and, upon ligand binding, phosphorylate themselves and the associated receptor. Experiments in which defined regions of the intracellular domain of some HGF receptors have been mutated demonstrate that phosphorylation of distinct tyrosine residues results in transmission of different signals for cell survival, proliferation and/or differentiation. In some cases, (e.g., the receptors for G-CSF and Flt3 ligand) acquired mutations in these regions that result in constitutive receptor activation have been shown to be the underlying genetic lesion that induces dysregulated growth and the development of malignant hematological diseases such as leukemia. Similarly, the V617F mutation in Jak2 that results in its constitutive activation was recently shown to be important for 99% of myeloproliferative disorders. Phosphorylation of the JAK/receptor complex triggers the binding, phosphorylation and dimerization of additional downstream signaling proteins, such as the signal transducer and activator of transcription (STAT) proteins. STAT dimers then translocate to the nucleus where they bind to the promoter regions and activate transcription of a number of genes that play a role in cell survival and proliferation. As noted above, hematopoiesis is subject to exquisite regulation and these stimulatory signals rapidly induce various mechanisms for their attenuation, such as JAK inhibition and signaling component degradation. These are mediated by phosphotyrosine phosphatases (e.g., SHP) and suppressors of cytokine signaling (SOCS) proteins, among others. HGF receptors also serve as a sink for circulating growth factors and, as discussed in detail below, facilitate downmodulation of the proliferation response as mature cells accumulate in sufficient numbers to consume the ligand that initiated their production.

## Clinical exploitation of hematopoietic growth factors

The first phase of the development and clinical application of recombinant human cytokines that stimulate hematopoiesis is now complete. Since their regulatory approval and commercial launch in the early 1990s, the first-generation recombinant HGFs have been administered to millions of patients; recombinant EPO has revolutionized the treatment of anemia associated with chronic kidney disease, and G-CSF and GM-CSF have proven to have immense practical value in promoting the recovery of neutrophils in patients receiving cancer chemotherapy either alone or in conjunction with HSC transplantation. However, not all the attempts to translate a detailed understanding of the preclinical biology of HGFs into therapeutic applications have been successful. The clinical development of TPO was a notable failure in this regard and the unenthusiastic uptake of IL-11 (oprelvekin, Neumega) in thrombocytopenia suggests its limited usefulness. However, even these less satisfactory experiences have proven valuable in igniting the current era of hematopoietin therapies in which molecularly engineered versions of native factors that offer improved pharmacodynamic properties, or molecular entities with no sequence homology to natural cytokines, are finding clinical application. In the following sections, we highlight key aspects of the biology of the major HGFs, with particular emphasis on those with proven clinical utility, and review some interesting new developments that offer a glimpse into how these drugs may be used in the future.

## Recombinant human EPO for the treatment of anemia

EPO, a 35-kDa glycoprotein, is the primary humoral regulator of erythropoiesis and acts by stimulating the differentiation and maturation of erythroid progenitor cells. When EPO concentrations decrease, erythroid colony-forming units (CFU-E) undergo apoptosis. A normal 70-kg human produces on the order of $2.5 \times 10^{11}$ erythrocytes daily and this rate of production is maintained by a basal EPO level of around 10–20 mU/mL. In patients with chronic kidney disease, a decrease in the number of renal peritubular interstitial cells, which produce about 90% of circulating EPO, frequently leads to anemia and fatigue, dramatically impairing the capacity to conduct daily life activities. The cloning of the EPO gene in 1985 facilitated the expression of recombinant human (rHu)EPO (epoetin alfa, Epogen) in Chinese hamster ovary cells. Clinical studies were conducted to evaluate its efficacy as a hormone-replacement therapy for the treatment of anemia in chronic kidney disease. Pharmacological administration of rHuEPO at a dose intended to sustain a three times per week dosing cycle (150 U/kg) or a weekly treatment cycle (40 000 U/kg) yielded a maximum plasma concentration of 150 or 850 mU/mL respectively, emphasizing that erythropoiesis driven by administered rHuEPO is analogous to "stress erythropoiesis" more typically associated with serious blood loss. Circulating reticulocyte counts increase within about 5 days after starting rHuEPO therapy, followed by a change in hemoglobin concentration that is normally discernible by day 8. Detailed studies of the pharmacokinetics and pharmacodynamic response to EPO have shown that the erythropoietic response is driven by drug exposure: the accumulated time during which EPO serum concentration exceeds the threshold level required to stimulate erythropoiesis is the sole driver of efficacy. Longer-acting analogs of EPO with improved serum half-life, such as Aranesp (darbepoetin alfa) and Mircera (methoxy polyethylene glycolepoetin beta), have been developed that are able to sustain up to 3 or 4 weeks between injections. Certain of these molecules have been deployed in millions of patients with chronic kidney disease and in recent years the utility of some has been extended to use as a supportive care agent to promote the regeneration of red blood cells depleted in cancer patients undergoing chemotherapy. It is curious, however, that despite around two decades of clinical use and the development of at least three longer-acting ESAs (the third being Hematide, a synthetic peptide-based ESA), the dominant route of drug clearance is still not well defined. However, small amounts of native and recombinant EPO are excreted intact in the urine and this has been exploited in the development of biochemical tests that betray the unapproved use of ESAs for the purpose of performance enhancement by athletes (*see below*).

## Recombinant human G-CSF for the treatment of neutropenia

G-CSF is an "emergency" cytokine. Although mice in which G-CSF has been genetically ablated or neutralized with a specific antibody survive with normal lifespan, they have about 20–30% of normal neutrophil numbers and are impaired in their ability to respond to infection. This activity and the impressive lineage fidelity of G-CSF spurred its development as a supportive care agent in cancer patients who have been rendered neutropenic due to the relatively non-specific cytotoxic effects of many conventional chemotherapeutic agents. In response to such myelosuppressive regimens, patients overproduce G-CSF to stimulate neutrophil regeneration. However, the endogenous G-CSF response is rather modest and rather late, from a baseline of less than 30 pg/mL to 100 pg/mL around 16 days after chemotherapy. In contrast, Takatani *et al.* showed that patients administered daily therapeutic G-CSF (filgrastim, Neupogen) starting 1 day after chemotherapy attain levels exceeding 100 pg/mL from day 3 (the first day measured) onwards, and peak G-CSF levels approach 10 000 pg/mL at around days 11–12. The effect of this potent stimulatory signal is a return of neutrophil counts to above $5 \times 10^9$/L by day 17. In comparison, only one in three untreated patients (i.e., relying on endogenous G-CSF) saw this neutrophil count by day 23 and one never recovered to this level during the observation period. The timing of administration of recombinant cytokine therapies is an interesting and important component of such clinical studies and is particularly notable in the early studies of G-CSF. In comparing two additional dosing regimens in the previous study – one that relied on monitoring neutrophil counts daily and beginning G-CSF treatment on the first day that neutropenia was documented, and the other in which G-CSF treatment was initiated on a standard day 8, about a week before the nadir might be expected – it was found that all regimens were more effective than relying on endogenous G-CSF. Prophylactic therapy, starting 1 day after chemotherapy, produced the shortest duration of severe neutropenia when patients would be expected to be at risk of infection. However, this regimen also showed the lowest absolute neutrophil count at nadir. The other therapeutic regimens also improved counts at nadir and shortened the period of danger associated with serious neutropenia, but not as effectively as early prophylaxis. In every tested regimen, the common factor in effective treatment of neutropenia appeared to be early (in this sense meaning before the endogenous response could be mounted by the body) and high exposure to exogenous G-CSF. How precisely to dose G-CSF to provide the maximum benefit while guarding against futile dosing and unnecessary exposure is something of a conundrum, and G-CSF is not unique in this regard. At the root of the problem is the rapid clearance of G-CSF, which drives the need for repeated daily injections. To address this issue, pegfilgrastim (Neulasta), a second-generation G-CSF therapeutic, was engineered to offer improved utility in chemotherapy-induced neutropenia. It is a long-acting form that evades renal clearance due to its increased hydrodynamic size resulting from the covalent attachment of a polyethylene glycol (PEG) molecule to the N-terminus of the protein (Plate 24.2a). This form stimulates neutrophil production (Plate 24.2b) and is still sensitive to neutrophil-mediated clearance. In normal use pegfilgrastim is administered as a 6-mg dose, irrespective of patient body weight, 1 day after chemotherapy. Pegfilgrastim serum levels quickly rise to a level far in excess of those attainable with the recommended dose of Neupogen (5–10 μg/kg daily, depending on indication) and provide a strong stimulus for neutrophil production. Prior to neutrophil recovery, the blockade of renal clearance prevents serum pegfilgrastim levels from falling and the maximum stimulus for neutrophil production is maintained. As neutrophil recovery begins, the newly generated G-CSFR-expressing cells begin to consume the available drug, ultimately eliminating the stimulator as their numbers approach normal. These pharmacokinetics and pharmacodynamics are schematically illustrated in Figure 24.3. This pegylated form of G-CSF thus removes the need for weight-based dosing, repeated injections, determining the starting day for treatment and monitoring neutrophil counts. It also accounts for idiosyncratic responses as it adapts itself to the individual patient's response to chemotherapy and ability to recover.

## C-mpl agonists for the treatment of thrombocytopenia

Despite being named in 1958, TPO was not isolated until 1994 when five groups simultaneously reported cloning the gene and expression of the protein. TPO is the seminal stimulator of platelet production and is consumed by megakaryocytes and platelets expressing the c-mpl receptor. Deficiency in the level of circulating TPO has not been documented

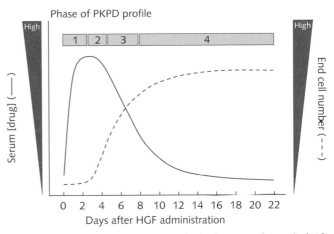

**Fig. 24.3 General pharmacokinetic (PK)/pharmacodynamic (PD) profile for a therapeutic hematopoietic growth factor with end cell-mediated clearance**
Four phases are depicted by the gray bars. In phase 1, low numbers of target cells define the cytopenia being treated. Intravenously administered drug disseminates rapidly in the blood and reaches $C_{max}$ within hours. In phase 2, receptor-positive target cells bind the stimulator and begin to proliferate. In phase 3, drug is consumed as the target cell compartment is repopulated. In phase 4, all drug has been consumed and end-cell numbers have been restored. The schedule of subsequent dosing is determined in part by the lifespan of the cell type in question.

frequently. Nevertheless, numerous clinical conditions characterized by thrombocytopenia represent potential indications for the use of thrombopoietic factors. Two forms of recombinant human TPO were initially evaluated for their therapeutic potential in treatment of chemotherapy-induced thrombocytopenia in cancer patients: a full-length glycosylated molecule (rHuTPO) that is equivalent to the native growth factor, and a truncated and pegylated version known as megakaryocyte growth and development factor (PEG-rHuMGDF). Between 3 and 4 days after administration of MGDF, reticulated platelets (a measure of early platelet increases) could be detected in the circulation and platelet counts peaked after 13–15 days. This delayed response probably reflects the indirect nature of c-mpl agonism on thrombocytopoiesis, the main action being confined to an increase in megakaryocyte ploidy and maturation rather than platelet formation itself. Despite their efficacy, neither of these first-generation agents attained regulatory approval due mainly to the production of antibodies by the human immune system that were directed against the administered therapeutic. These antibodies were also capable of neutralizing endogenous TPO, resulting in an extended-term thrombopoietin-refractory thrombocytopenia.

This failure spurred the creation of several novel next-generation c-mpl ligands, all of which have the feature of no

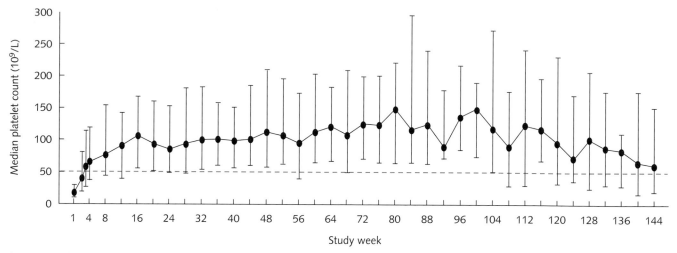

**Fig. 24.4 Nplate corrects thrombocytopenia in patients with immune thrombocytopenic purpura (ITP)**
Shown are the median peripheral blood platelet counts over 144 weeks in ITP patients administered Nplate subcutaneously at an initial dose of 1 μg/kg, adjusted individually to a maximum of 10 μg/kg (N = 142 at week 1, N = 11 on week 144, excluding those who received rescue therapies such as platelet transfusions). The horizontal dashed line indicates a clinically relevant threshold of 50 × 10⁹/L circulating platelets. From Bussel JB et al. (2007) Long-term dosing of AMG 531 in thrombocytopenic patients with immune thrombocytopenic purpura: 2-year update. Blood, 113, 2161–2171. © American Society of Hematology.

overlap in amino acid sequence with endogenous TPO. One such molecule is Nplate (romiplostim), a completely synthetic "peptibody" protein that contains four agonistic c-mpl-specific peptide regions covalently attached to the Fc region of human immunoglobulin (Plate 24.3). The c-mpl-specific "warhead" stimulates proliferation of receptor-positive target cells and the immunoglobulin scaffold enhances the pharmacokinetic properties of the molecule. Nplate was recently approved for the treatment of idiopathic thrombocytopenic purpura (ITP), an autoimmune disease associated with antiplatelet antibodies that mediate platelet destruction (ITP patients exhibit a mean platelet count of 41 ± 7 × 10⁹/L compared with normal counts of 150–450 × 10⁹/L) and thus an increased risk of bleeding events. The constitutive production of TPO by the liver is unaffected by this process, but as platelets are produced and destroyed in excess, TPO is also consumed. So although TPO deficiency is not part of the development of the disease, functional TPO deficiency is an indirect consequence and a rational point of therapeutic intervention with a replacement stimulator (Figure 24.4). The clinical development of c-mpl agonists is not yet complete and it remains to be seen for what uses they may ultimately gain regulatory approval. Other potential indications include the thrombocytopenia associated with myelodysplastic syndromes (MDS), aplastic anemia, cancer chemotherapy treatment, thrombotic thrombocytopenic purpura, and chronic or viral liver disease.

## Unforeseen applications

### Hematopoietic stem and progenitor cell mobilization by G-CSF

As described above, the dominant clinical effect of G-CSF action is neutrophilia, though minor or sporadic effects on other blood cells have been reported. Most notably, G-CSF is well documented as increasing monocyte proliferation, which may also be linked to reports of increased osteoclast-mediated bone turnover. However, from the early preclinical studies of G-CSF in mice it was noted that part of the pharmacodynamic response to this cytokine is an increase in the number of hematopoietic stem and progenitor cells present in the peripheral blood, a phenomenon known a little imprecisely as stem-cell mobilization. These primitive cells normally circulate only transiently and in very low numbers. However, following G-CSF administration, their numbers can increase by several hundred-fold, the magnitude of the effect being dependent on the genetic background in inbred strains of laboratory mice. Similar interindividual differences in mobilization efficiency are well documented in humans and about 10% of individuals fail to mobilize at all. Quantitative trait locus analysis of recombinant inbred mouse strains generated by interbreeding parental strains that are phenotypically "good" (e.g., DBA) or "poor" (e.g., C57BL/6) mobilizers has enabled the identification of specific loci that confer the capacity for efficient

G-CSF-mediated mobilization. Mobilization has revolutionized the field of HSC transplantation as it enables large numbers of primitive cells (typically defined in humans by their expression of the CD34 cell surface antigen) to be harvested from the blood by apheresis, a process that is less invasive and bears a lower risk to the donor than conventional bone marrow aspiration. The rate of hematological reconstitution following mobilized peripheral blood (MPB) cell transplantation is also significantly faster than with bone marrow-derived cells (9–10 vs. ~20 days to reach a neutrophil count of $500 \times 10^6/L$ in the autologous transplant setting) and MPB has become the gold standard for this therapy. Interestingly, mobilization is not a direct effect of G-CSF, but occurs as a consequence of neutrophil proliferation in the marrow. Neutrophil-derived proteases such as elastase and cathepsin G cleave many of the adhesion molecules that tether stem and progenitor cells within the bone marrow stroma, facilitating their release into the circulation. Several days of rHuG-CSF treatment is required for efficient mobilization by G-CSF alone, though a potential "fix" for this delay has recently been exploited in the development of plerixafor (Mozobil), a small-molecule inhibitor of the chemokine receptor CXCR4, which in combination with G-CSF can induce more rapid emigration of CD34$^+$ cells from the marrow to the blood.

## GM-CSF in immunotherapy

The two dominant myeloid growth factors are G-CSF and GM-CSF. Their names would suggest that they are closely related to one another and some would even use the agents interchangeably. However, the scale and manner of their use in clinical practice betrays profound differences between the two cytokines beyond the first stimulating neutropoiesis and the second neutropoiesis plus monocytopoiesis, activities ascribed to each factor through their effects on isolated progenitor cells, but only peripherally related to the full spectrum of their effects *in vivo*.

Shortly after it was cloned, normal blood-derived monocytes were cultured with GM-CSF and found to develop into tumoricidal effector cells capable of killing a malignant melanoma cell line. In an attempt to exploit this effect observed *in vitro* for potential clinical benefit, GM-CSF was later administered to cancer patients whose harvested monocytes were then found to mount an enhanced antibody-dependent cellular cytotoxic response against antibody-coated chicken erythrocytes and to overproduce tumor necrosis factor (TNF)-α. Interestingly, a somewhat different slant is more commonly exploited today whereby GM-CSF is used to provoke an immune response by stimulating the development of dendritic cells that ingest, process and present antigens to the immune system. Though quite different from modulating effector function of the type discussed above, this is a very important observation and underpins numerous modern applications of GM-CSF in immunotherapy, even while an imperfect understanding of its biology means that its optimal deployment for this purpose remains under investigation. Nevertheless, these effects of GM-CSF could hardly have been imagined by the investigators who were cloning the gene for human GM-CSF in the mid-1980s.

## Non-hematopoietic effects of EPO

Since its approval for the treatment of anemia in 1989, a number of pleiotropic actions for EPO and next-generation ESAs have been reported, including beneficial effects in stroke, nerve crush injury, heart failure, myocardial infarction, immunomodulation and cognitive function. However, this area is highly controversial for a number of reasons. First, despite some enticing reports, numerous studies have failed to demonstrate a beneficial effect of ESAs in animal models of renal ischemia, immunomodulation, lipopolysaccharide-induced myocardial depression, neuroprotection and endotoxemia-induced organ damage. This suggests that the putative cytoprotective effects of ESAs may be restricted to certain animal models or clinical conditions. Second, the simple and attractive hypothesis that cytoprotective mechanisms may be mediated through the expression of a "non-hematopoietic" EPOR is not well supported. For example, EPOR mRNA is expressed at very low levels in non-hematopoietic tissues and the antibodies frequently used to detect EPOR protein have been shown to yield false-positive results. Therefore the presence of functional EPOR in non-hematopoietic tissues remains unclear. Finally, it is possible that some of the beneficial effects reported may be due to on-target effects of ESAs through modulation of erythropoiesis, elevation of hemoglobin or changes in iron metabolism, which have not been well investigated. Nevertheless, functional effects of EPO and ESAs have been noted in some preclinical models and in some early clinical studies, though the mechanisms and general applicability of ESAs to cytoprotection remain unclear.

## Blood doping

Athletes have sought ways to enhance their performance since ancient times. Expansion of erythrocyte mass by transfusion of whole blood or packed red cells to increase muscle tissue oxygenation has been one approach used by participants of endurance events in particular. With the dawn of the era of recombinant DNA technology came new opportunities for blood "doping," including the use of erythropoietic proteins. As athletes adopted rHuEPO as a more convenient means of inducing erythrocytosis than cell

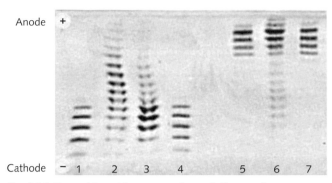

Anode +

Cathode −  1      2      3      4        5      6      7

**Fig. 24.5 Recombinant human erythropoietins can be distinguished from endogenous EPO by differences in their isoform content**

Shown is an electropherogram of recombinant human EPO standards (Epogen, epoetin alfa; lanes 1 and 4 and Aranesp, darbepoetin alfa; lanes 5 and 7), and extracts of human urine obtained from a healthy control (lane 2) and individuals treated with Epogen (lane 3) or Aranesp (lane 6). Evident are the unique isoform signatures of the drugs compared with native EPO, and the higher content of negatively charged isoforms in Aranesp resulting from the addition of two extra N-linked glycosylation sites in the coding sequence of the protein. Adapted from Catlin DH, Breidbach A, Elliott S *et al.* (2002) Comparison of the isoelectric focusing patterns of darbepoetin alfa, recombinant human erythropoietin, and endogenous erythropoietin from human urine. *Clinical Chemistry*, **48**, 2057–2059.

transfusions, sporting regulatory organizations responded by developing tests to identify its presence in the urine and to distinguish it from native EPO. The first direct test for EPO abuse was developed in 1995 and deployed in a practical form in 2000, 13 years after epoetin alfa was approved by the US Food and Drug Administration. It is based on the fact that endogenous EPO is biochemically heterogeneous and comprises a number of differentially charged isoforms that can be resolved by isoelectric focusing and immunoblotting using an EPO-specific antibody. The spectrum of these isoforms differs from that of the injected forms (epoetin alfa or darbepoetin alfa), which are more acidic. By analyzing these isoelectric patterns it is possible to determine if the excreted EPO is of natural or recombinant origin (Figure 24.5). This test enables detection of epoetin alfa in the urine of all samples for 2 days, and about 50% remain positive 4 days after a 3-week course of drug administered at 150 U/kg per week. Consistent with its longer serum half-life, darbepoetin alfa can be detected in the urine for up to 12 days after a modest single dose of 0.4 μg/kg. Though useful, the ultimate utility of this and other tests for controlling abuse of recombinant proteins depends on the relationship between the drug's pharmacokinetic profile and clearance, which is defined by such tests, and its pharmacodynamics, in this case increased hematocrit and $Vo_{2max}$ (the maximal oxygen-carrying capacity of the blood). Several studies have shown that the enhancing effects of rHuEPO persist for 3–4 weeks after the last dose. This highlights the advantage of random testing and the need to further refine these assays to enable detection of illicit EPO use for longer periods after cessation of dosing.

## Disposition of therapeutic hematopoietic growth factors in the body

In common with many protein therapeutics, HGFs must be administered via intravenous or subcutaneous injection since orally administered proteins tend to be destroyed in the gut and the skin is relatively impermeable to topical application. Alternative means of delivery such as pulmonary (inhaled), buccal and intradermal routes have been tested but have yet to realize significant potential, presently yielding low relative bioavailability and high variability in delivered dose. Predictably, intravenous injection results in high maximum plasma concentrations measured shortly after administration. Initial dissemination of the injected material rarely exceeds blood volume but subsequently injected material can concentrate in tissues with large numbers of target cells. Subcutaneous injection can slow absorption to the plasma and prolong resultant exposure. This has been exploited in clinical practice, whereby subcutaneous administration increases the apparent "efficiency" of EPO compared with intravenous administration, resulting in a reduction in the dose required for efficacy. However, subcutaneous administration can also result in deposition of the drug or its degradants in immunologically sensitive areas. Exposure levels to exogenously administered cytokines are generally much higher than would be encountered during normal hematopoiesis. As described above, the peak level of endogenous G-CSF is about 100 pg/mL, whereas the level attained therapeutically can be up to 200 times higher. However, this peak therapeutic level of rHuG-CSF is only approximately threefold higher than has been recorded in bacterial infection. Thus short-term pharmacological dosing of rHuG-CSF is in fact only marginally supraphysiological at peak concentrations. This lends some comfort over concerns that pharmacological amounts of G-CSF may pose additional risks through, for example, changes in chromosome replication or gene expression in normal MPB donors, as has been suggested.

The effect of administered HGFs on target cell kinetics has been studied in detail. G-CSF has been shown to insert a relatively modest number of extra amplification divisions into the granulocyte progenitor compartment and to accelerate neutrophil release from the marrow. The cells produced appear to have normal function and lifespan. These effects combine to produce the marked pharmacodynamic effect of the drug. The other myeloid growth factors, GM-CSF and IL-3, have rather more modest effects on cell production kinetics. Administration of rHuEPO produces a similar imbalance in normal red cell production which is often described as "stress erythropoiesis." In this situation reticulated erythrocytes are released prematurely from the bone marrow and spend a longer proportion of their otherwise unchanged lifespan in the blood rather than the marrow.

An interesting phenomenon exemplified by EPO is the mismatch between persistence of the drug (i.e., its pharmacokinetics) and persistence of its biological (or pharmacodynamic) effect, in this case an increase in hemoglobin concentration. Recombinant EPO is cleared from the body with a half-life of approximately 8 hours, so within 2 days drug would be expected to be undetectable. However, erythrocytes produced in response to EPO survive for approximately 3 months. Thus a brief exposure to EPO can have a very long-lasting effect, in marked contrast to the majority of drugs (e.g., antibiotics or statins) which must actually be present to have an effect. This has at least one beneficial effect: it is relatively simple to understand the pharmacokinetic/pharmacodynamic relationship of all ESAs. As defined several years ago, the presence of the drug in the body determines the increment in hemoglobin elevation, which in turn determines the interval between EPO doses. This model has proven remarkably applicable to all the current ESAs and suggests that the same constraints are likely to be placed on any ESA dosed in humans. In a less exaggerated manifestation of the same phenomenon, the production kinetics of platelets suggest that all c-mpl agonists, excepting any conflicting factors like indirect mechanism of action or dose constraints placed by off-target activities, will ultimately produce a similar pharmacodynamic response. That pharmacodynamic response is in turn constrained by the underlying biology. Although TPO, like EPO, is the major regulator of its cell lineage, neither hormone controls the latter stages of end-cell production. Proplatelet formation is independent of c-mpl and the final stages of erythrocyte production are independent of EPO, so a lag between the action of these drugs and their desirable clinical effects is inevitable and constant. There is no treatment regimen that uses TPO, its mimics, or EPO that will produce a pharmacodynamic response in less than 4 or 5 days.

Clearance of HGFs is often associated with end-cell response. M-CSF was the first HGF for which this mechanism was elucidated in detail. Mice normally have detectable M-CSF in the serum and studies performed using radiolabeled M-CSF demonstrated that the serum half-life was about 10 min. Approximately 96% of the cleared M-CSF could be accounted for by splenic or hepatic macrophages,

the remainder being eliminated in the urine. On analysis of a number of parameters, including the effect of lysosomal protease inhibitors, it was apparent that internalization and degradation in macrophages via the cell surface M-CSF receptor, c-fms, was the predominant mechanism of M-CSF clearance. The implications of this mechanism are clear. Firstly, the clearance of physiological amounts of cytokines can be quite rapid, mediated by the normal population of receptor-positive cells. Second, pharmacological levels of exogenous cytokine can quickly saturate this clearance mechanism, leading to prolonged exposure and increasing the relative contribution of non-specific clearance mechanisms, if applicable (e.g., renal filtration). Third, as the pharmacodynamic response to the cytokine accumulates over time, the capacity of the selective clearance mechanism will increase, reducing the relative role of the non-specific pathways. Fourth, in the absence of a target cell response, the clearance of cytokine might be rather slow, increasing as the response mounts. This model is very attractive for explaining homeostatic regulation of cytokine and target cell populations, and has ramifications for therapeutic administration of recombinant cytokines that share much of their biology with their endogenous prototypes. Indeed this exact mechanism was used to develop therapeutically enhanced versions of G-CSF (i.e. Neulasta) as outlined above.

## Emerging issues

Although the era of novel discoveries in the field of hematopoietic cytokines would appear to have peaked in the 1980s and 1990s, their clinical use and refinement through molecular engineering continues to evolve. The large and increasing number of patients who have received recombinant cytokines has meant that, almost inevitably, unforeseen events have occurred. First, thrombocytopenia in some recipients of PEG-rHuMGDF (*see above*), then pure red cell aplasia that occurred as a rare event associated with a manufacturing change in Europe for epoetin alfa (Eprex) alerted the world to the potential evolution of anti-cytokine antibodies that could cross-neutralize the endogenous protein leading to drug-refractory cytopenias. However, although these represented major setbacks at the time, such failures were followed by the inception of new cytokine mimics such as Nplate and Hematide with different immunogenic profiles.

Safety events such as thromboembolic risks have been emphasized recently in association with the use of high doses of ESAs (epoetin alfa, epoetin beta and darbepoetin alfa), and in certain subsets of cancer patients (receiving radiotherapy alone and with relatively high hemoglobin levels) the risk of adverse events is now thought to outweigh the potential benefits. The effect sizes are admittedly small and sometimes not statistically significant, and a valid question may be whether such safety signals would even have been identifiable without access to high-quality meta-analysis of clinical trial data arising from the widespread use of HGFs. An illustrative example here is the use of rHuG-CSF for the treatment of severe congenital neutropenia (Kostmann disease). Originally described in 1956 in a Swedish family, this autosomal recessive disorder is typified by low neutrophil counts, persistent infections and, if left untreated, 70% mortality in the first year of life. Recombinant G-CSF has revolutionized the treatment of this disease and patients can expect to be spared from life-threatening infections (<1% mortality per year due to sepsis) for many years. However, after 6 years of G-CSF therapy there was a 2.9% incidence of acute myeloid leukemia or myelodysplasia (AML/MDS) per year, a risk that increased to 8% per year after 12 years on G-CSF. In addition, in a subgroup of patients who received higher doses of G-CSF because they had poorer neutrophil responses, as many as 40% developed AML/MDS after 10 years and 14% died of sepsis. One could argue that it would not have been possible to reveal the perhaps inevitable progression of severe congenital neutropenia to AML/MDS had patients not been protected from lethal infections earlier in life. So did G-CSF *cause* the leukemias? It is true that the leukemia would not have developed without G-CSF but this perhaps misrepresents the underlying mechanism.

While safety issues have emerged with HGF use in patients, so also has the breadth of diseases treated with these agents grown and continues to grow. GM-CSF in immunotherapy is a new and exciting therapeutic possibility, as is its possible use in Crohn's disease. Some early studies that as yet lack any definitive understanding of the mechanisms involved have suggested the use of ESAs in schizophrenia and stroke, as well as the use of G-CSF to mobilize stem cells that mediate tissue repair for heart attacks or ischemic limb disease.

Many of the earliest commercialized HGFs have emerged, or will soon do so, from patent protection, presenting the potential for diverse sourcing and cost savings, but perhaps offset to a degree by concerns over manufacturing processes, comparability assessment and regulatory approval processes. With respect to the clinical development and subsequent consideration of therapeutic proteins by regulatory agencies, it has been suggested that the protein product represents in essence the process used to manufacture it, with efficacy and safety intimately tied to the proprietary host cell systems used to express the protein, the culture media components, purification processes and final formulations for each drug. This perspective presents a considerable hurdle in comparing related products like follow-on biologicals (also referred to as "subsequent entry biologicals" or "biosimilars") intended to offer alternative products after innovator patent expiry. Thus, the term "generic" is difficult to apply given the non-identity of proteins produced by different entities (see Figure 24.6 for example with epoetin alfa). This presents an interesting challenge for regulatory authorities for which differing solutions are being developed in different countries.

| Sample ID | Concentration (IU/mL) | Origin |
|---|---|---|
| IA | 2000 | Korea |
| IB | 4000 | Korea |
| IIA | 2000 | Korea |
| IIB | 10000 | Korea |
| IIIA | 2000 | Korea |
| IIIB | 10000 | Korea |
| IV | 2000 | Argentina |
| V | 10000 | Argentina |
| VI | 4000 | India |
| VII | 10000 | China |
| VIII | | China |

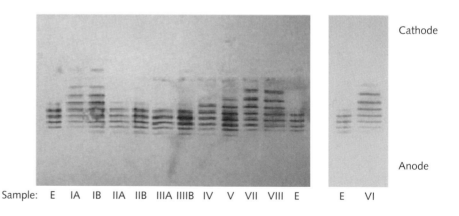

**Fig. 24.6 Different epoetin alfa products can vary widely**

Shown is a comparison of the isoform content of recombinant human EPO (Eprex, epoetin alfa; designated E in the right panel) and biosimilars obtained from various sources as identified in the table. The differences in the electrophoretic patterns underscore the point that due to the complexity of these molecules and the processes used to manufacture them, biosimilar drugs are never identical to originator products. Adapted from Schellekens H. (2004) Biosimilar epoetins: how similar are they? *EJHP*, vol. 3, pp. 43–47.

Novel points of intervention have also been discovered that may lead us away from protein-based cytokines. The inhibition of hypoxia-inducible factor prolyl hydroxylase (HIF-PH) by small molecules (the conventional drug modality of the pharmaceutical industry) has been shown to increase the physiological production of EPO, perhaps obviating the need for an injectable agent to treat EPO deficiency. In addition, several non-peptidyl small-molecule mimics of TPO have been recently developed that offer the advantage of oral dosing and one of them (eltrombopag, Promacta; see Plate 24.3) was recently approved for human use. In this case the mechanism would appear to be more direct than HIF-PH inhibition in anemia by binding directly to the cell surface receptor c-mpl. The ingenuity shown in devising these agents attests not only to the creativity of medicinal chemists, but also illustrates the continued excitement over making drugs that act like cytokines. However, the target remains mimicry of hematopoietic cytokine biology so the use of these agents is thus largely limited to correcting blood cell deficiencies and the associated biology, an application often disparaged as supportive care rather than curative therapy. Though this dismissal may not comport with patients' perception of value in a medicine, it is often used in the context of discussions about the cost of biological therapies to argue against their use, the contention being that these are complex drugs that are expensive to make and develop, but do not actually "cure" disease.

Protein-based cytokine mimics have also emerged of late. Agonistic antibodies, non-natural antibody-like constructs and peptide-based semisynthetic constructs that exhibit a progressively lower likelihood of off-target interactions have all been recently divulged. As described above, the c-mpl agonist Nplate is the first such molecule to be commercialized and exemplifies an approach used to eliminate the possibility of neutralizing the natural cytokine in the event that antibodies are produced against the drug. Many of these present interesting new aspects to cytokine biology such as partial agonism, bell-shaped dose–response curves, evasion of known clearance mechanisms and altered targeted tissue disposition. Thus the future holds many exciting possibilities for utilizing molecularly modified factors or even completely synthetic mimics of native HGFs that should lead to improvements in the therapeutic application of this fascinating family of cell growth stimulators.

## Further reading

Bartley TD, Bogenberger J, Hunt P *et al.* (1994) Identification and cloning of a megakaryocyte growth and development factor that is a ligand for the cytokine receptor Mpl. *Cell*, **77**, 1117–1124.

Bradley TR, Metcalf D. (1966) The growth of mouse bone marrow cells in vitro. *Australian Journal of Experimental Biology and Medical Science*, **44**, 287–299.

Burgess AW, Camakaris J, Metcalf D. (1977) Purification and properties of colony stimulating factor from mouse lung conditioned medium. *Journal of Biological Chemistry*, **252**, 1998–2003.

De Sauvage FJ, Hass PE, Spencer SD *et al.* (1994) Stimulation of megakaryocytopoiesis and thrombopoiesis by the c-mpl ligand. *Nature*, **369**, 533–538.

Fung MC, Hapel AJ, Ymer S *et al.* (1984) Molecular cloning of cDNA for murine interleukin-3. *Nature*, **307**, 233–237.

Grigg AP, Roberts AW, Raunow H *et al.* (1995) Optimizing dose and scheduling of filgrastim (granulocyte colony-stimulating factor) for mobilization and collection of peripheral blood progenitor cells in normal volunteers. *Blood*, **86**, 4437–4445.

Jacobs K, Shoemaker C, Rudersdorf R *et al.* (1985) Isolation and characterization of genomic and complementary DNA clones of human erythropoietin. *Nature*, **313**, 806–810.

James C, Ugo V, Le Couedic JP *et al.* (2005) A unique clonal JAK2 mutation leading to constitutive signalling causes polycythaemia vera. *Nature*, **434**, 1144–1148.

Jelkmann W. (2007) Erythropoietin after a century of research: younger than ever. *European Journal of Haematology*, **78**, 183–205.

Kawasaki ES, Ladner MB, Wang AM *et al.* (1985) Molecular cloning of a complementary DNA encoding human macrophage-specific colony-stimulating factor Csf-1. *Science*, **230**, 291–296.

Metcalf D. (2008) Hematopoietic cytokines. *Blood*, **111**, 485–491.

Molineux G, Pojda Z, Hampson IN *et al.* (1990) Transplantation potential of peripheral blood stem cells induced by granulocyte colony-stimulating factor. *Blood*, **76**, 2153–2158.

Nagata S, Tsuchiya M, Asano S *et al.* (1986) Molecular cloning and expression of cDNA for human granulocyte colony-stimulating factor. *Nature*, **319**, 415–418.

Orlic D, Kajstura J, Chimenti S *et al.* (2001) Mobilized bone marrow cells repair the infarcted heart, improving function and survival. *Proceedings of the National Academy of Sciences of the United States of America*, **98**, 10344–10349.

Robb L. (2007) Cytokine receptors and hematopoietic differentiation. *Oncogene*, **26**, 6715–6723.

Rosenberg PS, Alter BP, Bolyard AA *et al.* (2006) The incidence of leukemia and mortality from sepsis in patients with severe congenital neutropenia receiving long-term G-CSF therapy. *Blood*, **107**, 4628–4635.

Souza LM, Boone TC, Gabrilove J *et al.* (1986) Recombinant human granulocyte colony-stimulating factor: effects on normal and leukemic myeloid cells. *Science*, **232**, 61–65.

Sun CH, Ward HJ, Paul WL *et al.* (1989) Serum erythropoietin levels after renal transplantation. *New England Journal of Medicine*, **321**, 151–157.

Takatani H, Soda H, Fukuda M *et al.* (1996) Levels of recombinant human granulocyte colony-stimulating factor in serum are inversely correlated with circulating neutrophil counts. *Antimicrobial Agents and Chemotherapy*, **40**, 988–991.

Wong GG, Witek JS, Temple PA *et al.* (1985) Human granulocyte–macrophage colony-stimulating factor molecular cloning of the complementary DNA and purification of the natural and recombinant proteins. *Science*, **228**, 810–815.

# Chapter 25 Molecular therapeutics in hematology: gene therapy

## Jeffrey A Medin

*Department of Medical Biophysics and the Institute of Medical Science, University of Toronto, Ontario, Canada*

## Introduction

Approved clinical investigation of gene transfer into humans began with the seminal trial of Rosenberg and colleagues, which involved transplantation of genetically altered lymphocytes into patients. This landmark trial was closely followed by studies of therapeutic gene transfer using other hematopoietic cells. Studies involving the blood system have therefore been central to the development of human gene therapy. Gene marking or gene therapy protocols are under increasingly intensive investigation worldwide, with 300 approved clinical trials by the end of 1997 and more than 1300 approved clinical trials by the end of 2008. Importantly, some of the first successes in the entire field of gene therapy have recently been realized. Since hematology has contributed so much to the genesis and progression of human gene therapy, it is the purpose of this chapter to reiterate both the inherent promise and revisit some of the remaining obstacles posed by the application of gene transfer into humans employing hematopoietic cells.

Pluripotent hematopoietic stem cells (HSCs) are attractive targets for gene therapy in humans because of their capacity for self-renewal and the systemic multilineage distribution of their progeny (Figure 25.1). Sustained expression of transgenes at clinically relevant levels in the progeny of HSCs would result in novel and potentially curative treatments for a wide range of blood diseases, including, for example, hemophilia A and B, hemoglobinopathies, hereditary immune deficiencies, and some lysosomal storage disorders. Even the partial correction of such blood disorders would have substantial impact on the transfusion needs of the affected populations. Nevertheless, despite the inherent promise of HSC gene transfer, successful long-term engraftment of genetically modified HSCs in humans has proven to be a difficult and often elusive goal. Other hematopoietic cell subpopulations are also important targets for gene therapy. This discussion examines some of the targets of gene therapy involving the hematopoietic system and outcomes mediated by a variety of gene transfer mechanisms.

## General comments on gene transfer/therapy

An array of techniques has been described to facilitate gene transfer into blood cells. These techniques can be broadly grouped as *physical methods* or *viral vectors*. An important point to note here is that most gene therapy as practiced is actually gene augmentation, involving co-expression or even amplified overexpression of wild-type cDNA sequences. Indeed, selective repair of the genetic defects themselves within the host genome has proven to be a very difficult end point. Some studies are underway to develop reproducible systems with appreciable efficiencies that lead to actual gene repair but clinical protocols to date are not of this nature.

Physical methods of gene transfer are generally of low efficiency and provide only transient gene expression in the absence of selection. The advantages of these systems are that genes are transferred without viral sequences, which may affect the biology of the target cell or the host. In addition, large or multiple genes can be transferred and gene transfer is independent of the proliferative status and cell-surface receptor profile of the target cell. Those methods of physical gene transfer that have been used in the clinical setting include *electroporation* (electric fields that create channels in cell

*Molecular Hematology*, 3rd edition. Edited by Drew Provan and John Gribben.
© 2010 Blackwell Publishing.

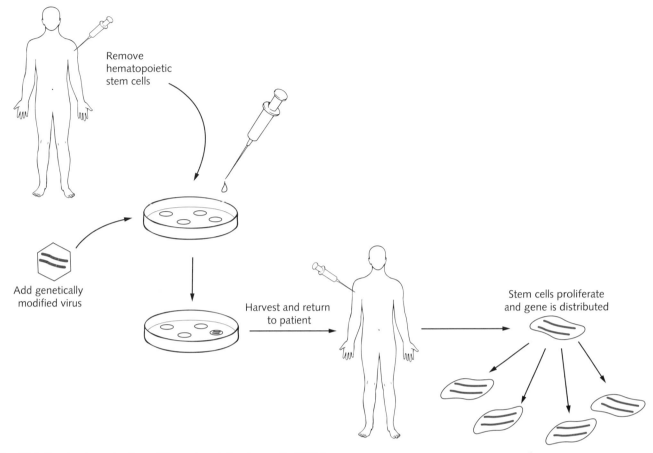

**Fig. 25.1** *Ex vivo* **transduction of hematopoietic stem cells (HSCs)**
HSCs can be harvested from patients and retrovirally transduced. The transduced cells are returned to the patient, where all blood cells maturing from the gene-modified stem cells retain a copy of the transgene. In theory, this gene transfer method could help distribute the gene product throughout the body at clinically relevant levels.

membranes allowing passage of DNA into the cell), *particle bombardment* (microscopic gold beads labeled with DNA, which are forced through the cell membrane by $CO_2$-driven pressure) and *liposomal encapsulation* of DNA. Liposomal-mediated gene delivery has gained most acceptance in the clinical arena, driven by the higher gene transfer efficiencies obtained with newer liposomal formulations and by safety considerations as an alternative to viral vector-mediated gene delivery. Other non-viral gene delivery systems include the use of plasmid DNA alone (so-called "naked" DNA), the use of synthetic polymers, transposons, and the adaptation of bacterial gene delivery systems. The use of plasmid DNA alone is particularly efficacious in specific tissues such as muscle. Thus DNA-based gene delivery is gaining in popularity for use in malignancy and infectious disease, and in applications directed toward the vascular bed. In cancer, DNA-based vaccines have been used in clinical trials where the immunogenic antigen is encoded by the plasmid itself with or without an added immunostimulatory gene. Yet,

while this approach is promising, clearly more work on modulating the biology of the immune response is needed.

Physical methods such as electroporation, direct DNA transfer, and liposome-mediated DNA transfer have been used with varying levels of success for transferring genes into hematopoietic cells. However, transgenes rarely integrate with physical methods of transfer, except transposons, and the vectors are diluted in dividing daughter cells, and thus are generally of little value to long-term stable gene transfer applications. Nevertheless, when transient gene expression is sufficient, such as in cancer immunotherapy applications, physical methods of gene transfer may find a niche.

## Viral vectors for gene transfer

The most commonly used viral backbones in clinical gene therapy trials to date are based on murine oncoretroviruses and human adenoviruses; however, herpes simplex virus, poxvirus, vaccinia virus, adeno-associated virus (AAV), and lentiviruses (among others) are also being developed and evaluated. The relative merits and disadvantages of some of these vector systems are outlined in Table 25.1. The particular nuances of the acquired or inherited disorder to be corrected determines which delivery system is more appropriate.

Viral gene transfer methods take advantage of facets of the normal virus life cycle to facilitate transfer of genetic material into target cells. For synthesis of recombinant retrovirus-based gene transfer systems for example, the wild-type viral genome is modified by deletions of most viral genes and insertion of therapeutic or marker sequences in their place. The viral gene products necessary for the production of recombinant virions are then provided in *trans* by transfections or by established packaging cell lines, which have been transfected with plasmids that engineer expression of the missing viral factors. Recombinant viral vector plasmids containing appropriate packaging signals are then transfected into the packaging cells, and replication-incompetent virions are produced. In this aspect, replication-incompetent virions are deemed safe for clinical applications because they transduce target cells only once; they are unable to cause a subsequent infection because of the absence of secondary expression of viral genes required for replication and virion packaging (Figure 25.2).

## Oncoretroviral gene transfer systems

Oncoretroviruses are double-stranded RNA viruses belonging to the gammaretrovirus genera of the family *Retroviridae*. The viral RNA genome is reverse-transcribed into double-stranded DNA, which integrates into the genome of target cells in a fairly random manner, although regions of active gene transcription are seemingly preferred. Currently, oncoretroviral vectors derived from the Moloney murine leukemia virus (MMLV) and other murine oncoretroviruses are used for clinical gene transfer protocols targeting hematopoietic cells.

For gene transfer vectors, the wild-type oncoretroviral genome is modified by deleting most of the *gag*, and all *pol* and *env* sequences. Viral sequences that are retained in the oncoretroviral vector include the packaging signal and the long terminal repeats (LTRs), which are necessary for viral integration and often drive transcription of the marking or therapeutic transgene in the absence of an added heterologous promoter. These deletions render the vectors replication-incompetent while making approximately 6–8 kb of space available for the insertion of desired transgene sequences. Stable oncoretroviral packaging cell lines have been engineered to minimize the chance of accidental replication-competent retrovirus (RCR) production. Plasmids

used to create these stable packaging cell lines engineer expression of key components of the parental virus but have extensive deletions along with split genes and promoters. These modifications have minimized recombination-prone homologous sequences between the added gene transfer vector encoding the transgene of interest and the stable packaging cells, thereby significantly reducing the chance of RCR being generated. Another measure of safety is naturally present in oncoretroviral gene transfer systems as these vectors, when packaged in murine-based packaging cell lines at least, are rapidly inactivated by human serum. Recently, taking a lesson from commonly used lentiviral gene transfer systems (*see below*), investigators have generated recombinant oncoretroviruses with self-inactivating 3′ LTRs. Thus upon reverse transcription, this promoter unit is modified, making it unable to drive transcription itself if productive recombination should occur and also making it unable to drive transcription in the presence of viruses that may encode cross-promoting functions. Lastly, along with the inherent safety features described above, all viral supernatants and patient cell samples that have been exposed to clinical-grade oncoretroviral supernatants are extensively tested for the presence of RCR and other possible contaminants prior to infusion into patients.

In addition to the relative safety of oncoretroviral vectors for gene therapy, another advantage of this delivery system over some others includes the stable integration of the vector into the host cell genome, allowing long-term transgene expression in the target cell and its progeny. These vectors also generate minimal immune responses in themselves due to the extensive deletions of wild-type coding subunits that they have undergone. Disadvantages of oncoretroviral vectors include the requirement of target cells to be in cycle for genomic integration, the randomness of the integration event itself, and the specificity of virion/receptor binding, which can reduce infection rates into some target cells depending on the *env* pseudo-typing employed. Another issue is that oftentimes extensive periods of *ex vivo* culturing is required to obtain efficient gene transfer into key target cells such as human HSCs.

Since long-term expression of transgenes is a requirement for most HSC-based gene therapies, oncoretroviral vectors use viral promoters, such as the endogenous MMLV/LTR, which can direct high levels of expression. Nevertheless, a few studies, mainly using embryonic stem cells for analyses, have shown that such promoters can be shut down or silenced *in vivo*. There are several potential mechanisms of such downregulation. These include cytokine-mediated promoter suppression, DNA methylation, an unstable integration environment, or an adverse contextual position of the cistronic unit within the oncoretroviral vector (internal promoter competition). Another potentially overriding possibility is that perhaps culture conditions for *ex vivo* cell

**Table 25.1** Some viral vectors used in the application of gene therapy.

| | Oncoretrovirus | Adenovirus | Helper-dependent adenovirus | Adeno-associated virus | Herpes virus | Lenti-retrovirus | Pox viruses |
|---|---|---|---|---|---|---|---|
| Advantages | Well-studied Integrates | Very efficient gene transfer High transgene expression | Large cloning capacity Not immunogenic | Cell-cycle independent Safe | Very efficient gene transfer Cell-cycle independent | Integrates Efficient gene transfer Large capacity | Efficient gene transfer |
| Disadvantages | Cell-cycle dependent Promoter silencing Safety issues | Immunogenic Transient expression Pre-existing immunity | Technically cumbersome Helper-virus contamination Transient expression | Limited cloning capacity Helper-virus contamination Production | Transient Cytotoxic | Production Public perception | Transient expression Immunogenic |
| Potential applications | Many involving hematopoietic cells | Cancer immunotherapy | Gene augmentation therapy | Cancer immunotherapy Gene augmentation therapy via muscle | Cancer immunotherapy Pain management | Many involving hematopoietic cells Non-dividing targets | Cancer immunotherapy |

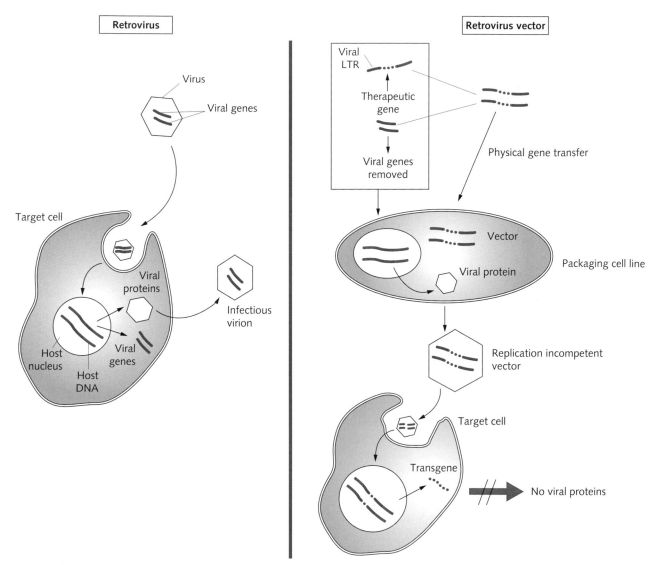

**Fig. 25.2 Biology of retroviruses and the development of packaging cell lines**
For wild-type retroviruses, after binding and entry the provirus integrates into the genome of infected cells. Viral proteins and new mRNA molecules are produced. Virions are then assembled for the next round of infection. For recombinant retroviral vectors the *gag*, *pol* and *env* genes have been removed to allow space for cloning of the gene of interest. To make an infectious virus, the vector is introduced into a packaging cell line engineered to express these *gag*, *pol* and *env* genes as separate cistronic units. The resulting virions can then bind to, and be internalized by, a target cell where integration into the host genome occurs and the vector transgene product is synthesized. Since the infected target cell lacks the genes necessary to form a new virion, the vector is not secondarily infectious.

transductions have caused primate HSCs to fully differentiate, and therefore transgene expression is really lost by maturation and death of provirus-positive cells over time. Thus, even if efficient gene transfer is achieved, transgene expression, and thus therapeutic impact, may be low. However, newer-generation oncoretroviral vectors and improved *ex vivo* transduction methods have led to significantly higher and longer transgene expression than was observed previously. For example, MSCV, MND, and MFG vectors have been designed with multiple modifications to the MMLV

backbone that enable genes to be expressed more efficiently in murine, non-human primate, and human hematopoietic cells.

Oncoretrovirally encoded marking and therapeutic transgenes can also be expressed in a cell-specific manner using specific virion pseudotyping and/or internal cellular promoters, which allow for regulated expression. For example, expression in leukocytes can be directed by CD11b, CD18, or major histocompatibility complex (MHC) class I promoters, while expression in erythroid cells can be greatly enhanced by the β-globin promoter and locus control region. Furthermore, viral transgene expression may be regulated by inducible promoter systems such as the *tet* operon system, which uses exogenous tetracycline to specifically transactivate a promoter leading to ordered expression of the gene of interest. Such regulated and cell-specific systems may have utility in therapeutic applications by providing an additional control mechanism for the expression of potentially toxic gene products for example.

## Lentiviral gene transfer systems

As discussed above, oncoretroviral vectors only integrate into cells actively undergoing mitosis, which precludes their use for delivery to target cells that are non-dividing or slowly dividing, such as the majority of HSCs. Among other considerations, this has led to the development of replication-incompetent viral vector systems based on lenti-retroviruses (lentiviruses, LVs) and human foamy virus, for example, which can integrate into these and other key non-dividing target cells. LVs and human foamy virus are also members of the family *Retroviridae*. They are sometimes termed "complex" retroviruses, in contrast to oncoretroviruses which are termed "simple" retroviruses. Foamy viruses have a large genome (and hence a large transgene carrying capacity), do not cause any known disease, and can be used for *in vivo* gene transfer because they are not effectively inactivated by human serum. LVs also show significant promise as gene transfer vehicles and many laboratories around the world are adopting this alternative delivery system. Current LVs contain less than 25% of the HIV-1 genome and seem to be much less susceptible to "shutdown" effects compared with recombinant oncoretroviruses. To further increase safety, many laboratories now use third-generation recombinant LVs that have a self-inactivating 3′ LTR. To further minimize the chance of recombination leading to the production of replication-competent lentivirus, some laboratories even use up to seven separate plasmids in transient transfections of packaging cell lines to generate recombinant virions (although three separate plasmids is more the norm). LVs can be readily pseudotyped with alternative envelope proteins, such as VSV-g, which expands the tropism of the virions and also allows stable concentration of effective viral titer by ultracentrifugation. There is thus considerable optimism that recombinant LVs will overcome some of the shortcomings of MMLV-based oncoretroviruses by facilitating delivery of transgenes of interest to a wide spectrum of cell types, including HSCs. Preliminary studies show that this may indeed be the case, although this needs to be further substantiated by a number of independent laboratories in long-term, large animal, and clinical studies. Furthermore, due to a marked increase in LV-mediated transduction effi-

ciencies over previous methods, it may be possible to now better manage other secondary components of the *ex vivo* gene therapy procedure, such as enhancing engraftment of transduced cells in recipients by minimizing culture periods and exposure to differentiation-inducing cytokines for example. Alterations have also been made to LV backbones such as the addition of a central polypurine tract and a WPRE element to possibly enhance nuclear import or enhance transgene expression levels, respectively.

Important results have been presented lately that LV genomic integration patterns differ from oncoretroviral integration patterns. It has been found that LVs tend to distribute throughout open chromatin, whereas oncoretroviral vectors show a propensity to integrate into promoter-proximal regions. That said, due to their increased efficiency, LVs tend to integrate into permissive cells in higher copy numbers than oncoretrovirus-based vectors. This increase can be good in order to generate higher levels of transgene products for correction but it also necessitates careful planning concerning effective multiplicity of infections (MOIs) and the tolerance of the infected cell population to multiple proviral copies. Indeed, it may turn out that MOIs with LVs actually need to be reduced to minimize this multiplicity effect in some protocols. One clinical protocol using LVs has been completed to date (*see below*) and others are under way. In that landmark first study in HIV-AIDS patients, no detectable recombination occurred between the gene transfer vector and wild-type HIV-1 even when the latter was present in very high copy numbers in patient blood.

## Other viral gene transfer systems

Recombinant adenoviral gene transfer systems are commonly used for some gene therapy applications, especially in immunotherapy protocols. Adenoviruses infect cells efficiently *in vitro* and *in vivo*, express high levels of transgene products, can infect both cycling and stationary cells, and exhibit wide tissue tropisms. They can also be produced at very high titers and have a large carrying capacity for foreign cDNAs. Adenoviral vectors have been used to efficiently transfer genes into a variety of human tumors by direct injection and into circulating hematopoietic progenitor and malignant cells in *ex vivo* transduction procedures. Nevertheless, circulating B and T lymphocytes have generally proven relatively resistant to adenoviral-mediated gene transfer. So have CD34$^+$ hematopoietic cells until it was found that serotype 35 fiber knob domains can help overcome this blockade. Furthermore, many patients have pre-existing immunity to common adenoviral serotypes used in clinical protocols. This can lead to a strong immune response to the vector and also severely restricts readministration efficacy.

The receptor for most adenoviruses used in gene transfer applications has been identified as the coxsackie-and-adenovirus receptor protein and has been useful in determining the mechanism of adenovirus binding and cell entry. Adenoviral vectors do not integrate into the genome at an appreciable frequency and are lost from most cycling target cells within weeks of transduction. First-generation adenoviral vectors may also incite potent immune responses due to viral genes encoded by the vectors, resulting in the elimination of transduced cells and further minimizing the chances of successful vector readministration. Adenoviruses are therefore ideal vectors if an immune response and/or short-term high levels of transgene expression are desired; however, they are not suitable for therapies that require long-term expression or integration of the transgene. In an attempt to overcome some of these limitations, newer generations of adenoviral vectors have retained immunosuppressive sequences in the E3 region, eliminated all viral sequences except the necessary inverted terminal repeats, or are based on a helper-dependent systems with low levels of contaminating helper virus. Oncolytic adenovirus vectors, which replicate only in permissive cancer cells, have been developed and hold promise for the treatment of solid tumors and leukemic cells. For example, one such vector system only replicates in cells harboring defective p53 tumor-suppressor gene function.

Versions of the human parvovirus, AAV, are also being used more frequently as a vehicle for therapeutic gene transfer. AAVs are non-pathogenic in humans and establish a latent infection in the absence of adenovirus itself or helper functions provided by other viruses. Wild-type AAV integrates at some frequency into a specific site on human chromosome 19q13.3–qter, which appears to be a relatively benign location. Only the AAV inverted terminal repeats are required as transcriptional units for recombinant AAV vectors, which allows about 4 kb for foreign inserts given the size of the parental viral genome. However, both the efficiency and specificity of integration are lost without the wild-type genes; recombinant AAV integrates at a very low frequency. As usually produced, AAVs have titers of approximately $10^6$ particles/mL and can be concentrated to greater than $10^9$ particles/mL, although in each preparation a number of non-infectious particles are generated. Human CD34$^+$ hematopoietic stem/progenitor cells have been transduced with recombinant AAV vectors, with up to 80% of colony-forming units (CFU) carrying the transgene. Interestingly, the optimal use of recombinant AAV-based gene transfer vectors to impact the hematopoietic system may actually be in secondary manifestations. In a landmark study, Kay and colleagues injected recombinant AAV vectors that engineered expression of factor IX into skeletal muscles of severely afflicted hemophilia B patients. Long-term vector persistence was observed in that study as were slight increases in the circulating levels of the corrective proenzyme.

## Gene-marking studies involving hematopoietic cells

Genetic marking of hematopoietic cells facilitates study of the long-term distribution and survival of transplanted cells *in vivo*. In many applications, the cells to be tagged are incubated *ex vivo* with a replication-defective retrovirus bearing a reporter gene. The reporter gene that has been used most often in clinical studies is the bacterial *neomycin phosphotransferase* (*neo$^R$*) gene which, when expressed, confers resistance to the neomycin analog G418. Other marker genes are now available and include those encoding for the murine heat stable antigen, the human CD24 and CD25 antigens, the truncated nerve growth factor receptor, modified CD4 or CD19 or CD34 antigens, and an array of fluorescent proteins. The stable and unique integration pattern of proviral DNA in the genome of marked cells can provide a permanent marker for individual hematopoietic or malignant cells and their clonal descendants. This marking pattern can be established using a polymerase chain reaction (PCR)-based analysis that has been developed called ligation-mediated PCR, which provides information on the actual site of integration of the provirus. Clinical applications in which gene marking has provided new and important information include the infusion of oncoretrovirally marked, autologous, tumor-infiltrating lymphocytes into patients with advanced melanoma and the infusion of oncoretrovirally marked bone marrow or peripheral blood into patients with myeloid leukemia, myeloma, and neuroblastoma. The study of such patients offers three important lines of investigation.

1 Is retroviral-mediated gene transfer relatively safe?
2 Do genetically altered bone marrow or blood stem cells contribute to long-term hematopoiesis?
3 Do malignant cells or their precursors contribute to the high relapse rates observed after myeloablative therapy and autologous HSC transplantation?

A number of groups have reported the consequences of infusing gene-marked bone marrow cells into humans and the contribution of contaminating tumor cells in the graft to disease recurrence. The first important observation from these studies is that oncoretrovirus-mediated gene transfer as currently practiced appears relatively safe. No detrimental effects, either on the autograft or in patients, have been reported in these studies. Replication-competent oncoretrovirus has also not been detected at appreciable levels in patients participating in clinical trials. That said, in two recent clinical gene therapy protocols for an inherited disorder, the possibility exists that T-cell leukemias that developed in five patients resulted from the integration of a therapeutic provirus into the regulatory region of a certain oncogene (*see below*). The second important observation from earlier gene-marking studies is that multiple HSCs contribute to long-term hematopoiesis, albeit at relatively low levels. Interestingly, rather than all daughter hematopoietic cells being derived from a single HSC, it thus appears that in actuality multiple stem cells contribute to formation of the renewing blood system.

In the first gene-marking studies in children reported by Brenner and colleagues, 2–15% of clonogenic hematopoietic progenitor cells were marked after autologous bone marrow transplantation. The marker gene was detectable for up to 4 years after transplant and was found in granulocytes, B cells and T cells, at least by PCR. In the earlier adult gene-marking studies, however, oncoretroviral transduction of marrow or peripheral blood HSCs has resulted in detection of integrated vector in only a very low percentage of peripheral blood cells. For example, in one study, although the marker gene persisted for up to 2 years, *neoR*-positive cells could only be detected intermittently with analyses employing PCR. Work by a number of groups suggested that modification of the transduction protocols would result in a significant improvement in the engraftment of genetically modified HSCs. Along these lines, since preclinical experience indicated that the use of bone marrow stroma enhances gene transfer into HSCs, this approach was evaluated in clinical trials. However, the results of this adaptation proved to be no better than those discussed above and, in general, are very similar to those observed in the pediatric gene transfer studies. In another generation of primate gene-marking studies, novel cytokine combinations have been employed to induce HSC cycling and yet maintain some level of the "primitiveness" and "engraftability" of the transduced cell population. In addition, a fragment of the fibronectin protein has been utilized in the past few years to colocalize lower titer virus with target cells and alternatively pseudo-typed oncoretroviruses have shown promise in infecting more primitive hematopoietic cells. Indeed, levels of marking are now more encouraging and are reaching a point where some hematological disorders may actually be ameliorated. For example, one study in baboons by Horn and colleagues, using vectors that engineer expression of fluorescence proteins, demonstrated stable, multilineage, functional marking of up to 25% of peripheral blood cells derived from transduced and transplanted CD34+ hematopoietic cells. This, along with improved vectors and recent clinical results mentioned below, has led to a renewed sense of optimism in the field using stable integrating viruses and suggests that the successful application of human therapeutic gene transfer will eventually be achieved for a variety of disorders that interface with the hematopoietic system.

In total, data on more than 40 patients enrolled in gene-marking studies during bone marow transplantation for acute myeloid leukemia, neuroblastoma, chronic myeloid leukemia, breast cancer, myeloma, acute leukemia, or non-Hodgkin lymphoma have been presented. Of the relapsed patients, gene-marked tumor cells have been detected in a high percentage in many studies. In one patient with acute myeloid leukemia, the simultaneous detection of a cytogenetic marker along with the *neoR* gene confirmed that gene-marked cells contributed to relapse. A second critical observation was made a number of years ago when Rill and colleagues reported that a multiplicity of neuroblastoma cells in the graft contributed to relapse. The high frequency of gene-marked relapse, despite the very low frequency of transfused malignant cells, strongly suggests that a large percentage of tumor cells in the graft contribute to relapse or, alternatively, that tumor cells susceptible to retroviral gene marking are uniquely capable of engraftment and clonal expansion.

The gene-marking studies mentioned above set the stage for the investigation of multiple maneuvers designed to increase long-term gene transfer efficiency into HSCs. Some of the strategies being pursued are described in Table 25.2. These include increasing the true direct target cell-to-virus contact ratio by incorporating prior HSC enrichment, altering retroviral envelope utilization, or increasing colocalization of vector and cell in gene transfer protocols. Newer vector systems improving on both oncoretroviral and lentiviral backbones and incorporating alternative envelope pseudotyping may also increase gene transfer efficiency, while refinement of growth factor combinations may more efficiently induce HSC cycling in shorter time periods, thus improving retroviral integration without compromising engraftment. Many of these approaches have now been incorporated into clinical protocols and have likely contributed to some of the recent successes in this field as described below.

## Therapeutic trials for inherited disorders

The first human clinical gene transfer trials for inherited single-gene disorders focused on adenosine deaminase (ADA) deficiency and are summarized in Table 25.3. Recombinant oncoretroviruses containing the normal human *ADA* cDNA were transferred into either peripheral blood T lymphocytes, bone marrow cells, or cord blood cells from ADA-deficient patients. T-lymphoid cells expressing the normal *ADA* gene have a selective growth and survival advantage over ADA-deficient cells, even though patients are maintained on pegylated-ADA enzyme replacement therapy

**Table 25.2** Strategies for optimization of stable gene transfer into HSCs.

| Strategy | Method |
| --- | --- |
| Inducing recipient cells to cycle | Optimization of *ex vivo* cytokine stimulation<br>Collection of cells during recovery phase after myeloablation or mobilization<br>Culture on stromal layers |
| Increased cell–virus contact | Centrifugation of cells and virus during transduction (spinoculation)<br>Viral supernatant flow-through systems<br>Coat dishes with fibronectin fragment<br>Higher viral titers and multiple exposures |
| Increase viral receptor levels on target cells | Increase levels of amphotropic receptor by phosphate depletion<br>Transfer viral receptor into cell by adenovirus or adeno-associated virus<br>Target subpopulations of cells that have high levels of receptors |
| Alternatively pseudotyped recombinant retroviruses | Exploiting GALV, RD114, 10A1 receptors for entry<br>VSV-G envelope to expand tropism and allow virion concentration |
| Modified retroviral vectors to increase efficiency and infect non-cycling cells | Lentivirus- and foamy virus-based vectors |
| Positive selection of transduced cells | Add positive selectable marker to vector: metabolic, fluorescent, cell-surface |

**Table 25.3** Early gene therapy trials for ADA deficiency.

| Center | Cells | Protocol | *In vitro* gene transfer | *In vivo* results |
| --- | --- | --- | --- | --- |
| NIH | PB supernatant | 9–12 hours | | Increased immune repertoire<br>Number of T cells normalized after 2 years |
| Italy | PB, BM | Coculture 72 hours or supernatant | 2.5–50% cells<br>30–40% CFU | Multilineage repopulation with marked cells<br>Increased immune repertoire for 2 years |
| The Netherlands | CD34⁺ BM | Coculture + IL-3 | 5–12% CFU | Transduced cells detected 3–6 months after transplant |
| St Jude Children's Hospital | CB CD34⁺ | Supernatant + IL-3 + IL-6 + SCF | 12.5–21.5% CFU | Multilineage repopulation with transduced cells |
| Japan | PB | Supernatant + IL-2 | 3–7% cells | Improvement in immune function; 10–20% of blood cells carrying provirus > 1 year |

BM, bone marrow; CB, cord blood; NIH, National Institutes of Health; PB, peripheral blood.

(ERT) for ethical reasons. In these early studies, patients who had received multiple infusions of autologous *ADA*-transduced blood cells had increased levels of enzyme in their serum, and up to 20% of their peripheral blood T cells were found to carry provirus for some period. Indeed, long-term follow-up has revealed that one patient has maintained this level of marking for over 10 years. In two of the three initial trials in which patients received autologous marrow or cord blood cells transduced with *ADA* cDNA-containing oncoretroviruses, between 12 and 40% of CFUs were transduced, and genetically marked cells were found for greater than 1 year after infusion. In the one study, by Hoogerbrugge and colleagues, in which provirally marked cells were not maintained for greater than 6 months, there was lower *in vitro* gene transfer efficiency of 5–12% CFU prior to transplant. In the cord blood study there was evidence for a selective growth advantage of T cells as there were higher levels of marked T cells than myeloid cells even while the patients were maintained on progressively lower doses of PEG-ADA therapy. ERT was withdrawn from one patient and the number of T cells carrying the provirus increased to 30%; however, the total number of B lymphocytes and natural killer cells dropped and the patient had reduced immune function. That patient subsequently resumed PEG-ADA treatment.

Inherited immunodeficiencies, such as severe combined immunodeficiency (SCID) of ADA (*see above*) and X-linked SCID (*see below*), have become focal points for the potential benefits and some of the potential hazards of gene therapy. The above studies in ADA-SCID likely represent the first tangible correction of an inherited disorder by stable transfer of a therapeutic gene into primitive hematopoietic cells and their progeny, although it is difficult to state this unequivocally due to the simultaneous administration of ERT. However, these initial results have been surpassed recently for ADA-SCID in a study published by Aiuti and colleagues, where productive transfer of the *ADA* gene was effected into CD34⁺ cells of non-myeloablated recipients for whom ERT was not available. Many of the incremental improvements in the gene transfer protocols mentioned above were adapted in this protocol and high levels of gene marking (up to 25% of CFU-C initially) and functional correction were demonstrated. Long-term multilineage hematopoietic cell marking was also found in both patients. This study demonstrated, without the confounding implications of ERT, that stable long-term correction of this immune deficiency could be accomplished using this therapeutic approach. Indeed, these patients are presently at home, have normal growth and development parameters, and respond effectively to immune challenge from a variety of agents.

Impressive results have also been demonstrated in efforts to correct another inherited immunodeficiency, X-linked SCID. X-linked SCID (SCID-X1) is caused by a deficiency of the common γ-chain subunit of the receptors for the cytokines interleukin (IL)-2, IL-4, IL-7, IL-9, and IL-15 and is thereby not a candidate for soluble factor augmentation therapy. Expression of γ-chain was also expected to offer a growth advantage to productively transduced cells. This was indeed the case and in this first report in 2000, two patients were shown to have fully corrected immune function as a result of the gene therapy. Since this landmark first description of this beneficial outcome, other X-linked SCID patients have also been treated by this method. In fact, to date approximately 20 patients have received this gene therapy and the majority of these individuals retain improved and stable immune function. Yet even with these impressive results, this study highlights areas where the field of gene therapy must still progress in its understanding. This is because of reports that five of the patients receiving the corrective γ-chain gene in two separate clinical gene therapy protocols for SCID-X1 employing similar vectors and transduction protocols have gone on to develop acute T-cell lymphoblastic leukemia-like disease approximately 3 years after the transplantation of oncoretrovirally transduced cells. In at least two of these patients the development of this proliferative disorder has debatably been ascribed to a deleterious integration event that may have caused dysregulated expression of a proto-oncogene called *LMO2*. Yet while these findings are worrisome, and are causing regulatory agencies to re-examine protocols, the position of most seems to be that this outcome may be specific for this disorder given the dramatic proliferative advantage that is conferred on the productively transduced cells in this case. More study on this topic is definitely required and risks versus benefits for each clinical gene therapy protocol are being evaluated in greater detail given these findings. To reiterate, however, it should be emphasized that since analogous vector backbones and transduction conditions have been used for other studies, such as the ADA-SCID trials mentioned above without the emergence of adverse events, the possibility exists that these leukemia-like diseases are a specific consequence of overexpression of the γ-chain gene itself, since it impacts many diverse signaling pathways that affect a number of cellular functions *in vivo*.

Results from another study involving the hematopoietic system have also generated some close scrutiny recently. Clonal dominance of cells with specific integration events has been observed in a recombinant oncoretrovirus-based clinical gene therapy trial for the X-linked form of chronic granulomatous disease. Here patients have impaired immune function and cannot sufficiently resist bacterial and fungal infections due to an inability of neutrophils to generate superoxide ions; expression of the *CYBB* gene can abrogate this. Interestingly, the amplified integration locus involved the *MDS1* and *EVI1* genes in this case, which differs from that mentioned in the SCID-X1 trials above and may reflect alterations in the activity of myeloid cells post-transduction with this cDNA rather than a specific sequence preference for vector integration.

With regard to Gaucher disease, a lysosomal storage disorder resulting from a deficiency in the enzyme glucocerebrosidase that is manifested mainly in macrophages, it has also been proposed that this defect may be especially amenable to treatment by therapeutic gene transfer into HSCs. Results from two earlier clinical gene transfer studies targeting this disorder have been reported. Mobilized peripheral blood or marrow CD34⁺ cells from Gaucher patients were transduced with an oncoretroviral vector that engineered expression of glucocerebrosidase and then infused into non-myeloablated autologous recipients. In both studies, transduced cells were detected at low levels in blood and/or marrow leukocytes. One patient who received cells transduced with an MFG-based oncoretroviral vector manifested increased levels of enzyme activity corresponding to 50% of normal, which was maintained for 12 months after infusion. No therapeutic benefit or increased enzyme activity was detected in other patients or in the other study. The recent development of a viable murine model for this lysosomal storage disorder will be very beneficial for the testing and implementation of novel gene therapy strategies involving some of the conditional manipulations mentioned above or employing newer vectors.

Collectively, the results from the gene transfer studies for genetic disease described above (and others not directly mentioned) illustrate several points that will likely impact on the clinical success of gene transfer protocols for other single gene inherited disorders.

**1** The presence in patients of cells carrying the provirus for greater than 1 year has demonstrated the feasibility of gene therapy and newer vector systems may further enhance this.

**2** The transfer of genes that provide a growth or survival advantage can provide long-term expression and maintenance of transduced cells.

**3** A selective advantage of transduced cells can compensate for a modest gene transfer efficiency and yet, if too strong, may lead to amplification of deleterious transformation events.

**4** Using the incrementally optimized protocols, gene delivery using oncoretroviruses and subsequent transgene expression levels may presently be sufficient to correct a number of disorders that are directly or indirectly manifested in the hematopoietic system.

Clinical gene therapy trials for other inherited single-gene disorders such as Wiskott–Aldrich syndrome, leukocyte adhesion deficiency, sickle cell disease, Fanconi anemia, mucopolysaccharidosis type I, and Fabry disease among others are completed, ongoing, or proposed.

## Therapeutic trials for acquired disorders

### Chemoprotection

The above results suggest that normal bone marrow cells could be removed, transduced with a recombinant retroviral vector engineering expression of a drug resistance gene, and returned to patients with no toxicity. Theoretically, such protected cells would then expand clonally after chemotherapy treatment and confer relative resistance to a cytotoxic or cytostatic agent, allowing further dose escalation and a potential cure of some patients. Furthermore, such drug resistance genes, if expressed in a multi-cistronic format with a second therapeutic gene product, may even serve as selectable markers allowing *ex vivo* or *in vivo* enrichment or "preselection" of functionally gene-marked cells, which may further enhance observed clinical outcomes.

Numerous potential mechanisms of induction of cellular resistance to chemotherapy agents have been described. Some candidate gene products for chemoprotection schemas include P-glycoprotein, MRP, cytidine deaminase, ribonu-

cleotide reductase, topoisomerase II, aldehyde dehydrogenase, $O^6$-methylguanine-DNA-methyltransferase (MGMT), glutathione S-transferase, dihydrofolate reductase, thymidylate synthase, and tubulin. The cDNA for the human *MDR-1* gene (P-glycoprotein) has been subcloned and expressed in both mouse and human cells in culture. Transfer of the *MDR-1* gene into mouse and human bone marrow cells using oncoretroviral constructs leads to drug resistance *in vitro*. Transduced and transplanted cells engraft and confer drug resistance to bone marrow cells *in vivo* and also allow for positive selection of *MDR-1* transduced cells, for example by chemotherapy (Figure 25.3). Mutant forms of MGMT are also currently drawing substantial interest in the field as chemotherapeutic agents, and pharmacological inhibitors can be combined to allow selection of primitive hematopoietic cells transduced with these cDNAs *in vitro* and *in vivo*. While this is promising, more work needs to be performed to ensure that the resulting enriched hematopoietic cell population maintains appropriate lineage variability in correct ratios upon differentiation and that clonal dominance of selected cells does not lead to leukemia-like disease.

Clinical trials of *MDR-1* gene transfer into hematopoietic cells for chemoprotection in cancer therapy have been performed. The approach used for gene transfer is generally similar to that used for human gene-marking trials. Preliminary results indicated that infusion of *MDR-1*-modified cells is safe and no deleterious effects of infusing such gene-modified cells have been observed. In a landmark study by Abonour and colleagues concerning this approach, a combination of some of the incremental improvements in gene transfer protocols (*see above*) yielded fairly efficient transfer of the human *MDR-1* gene into long-term repopulating hematopoietic cells. Indeed, of the 12 subjects enrolled and transplanted in that protocol, appreciable levels of gene marking (up to 15% positive) were observed at 1 year after transplantation by PCR analyses on soft-agar colonies of cells from six recipients. Furthermore, in three of these patients, functional expression of the *MDR-1* gene was ultimately demonstrated by productive growth of colonies in the presence of paclitaxel.

### Genetic immunotherapy

A number of potential approaches using gene therapy for hematological malignancies can be considered (Table 25.4). Proof of concept for immunotherapy as a valid approach to the treatment of hematological malignancy has been provided by clinical studies that demonstrated that infusion of allogeneic T cells can eradicate minimal disease in patients relapsing after allogeneic transplant. Unfortunately, these encouraging allogeneic responses require a haploidentical T-cell donor, which is not available to the vast majority

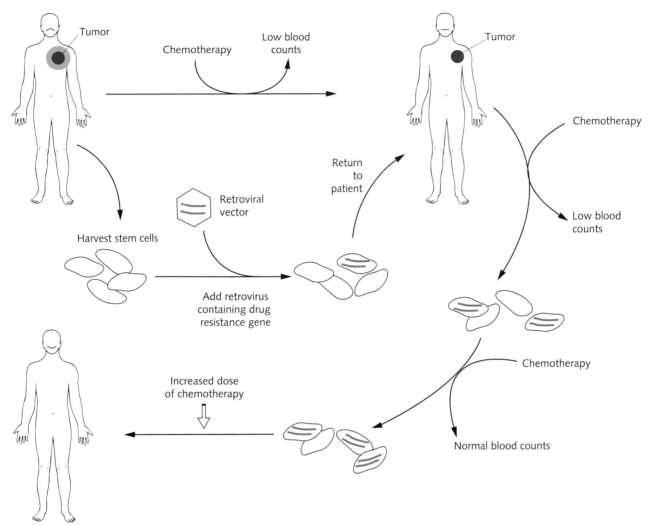

**Fig. 25.3 Hematopoietic stem cells removed from the patient can be genetically engineered to express a drug resistance gene**
Theoretically, after return to the patient, the cells are selected by chemotherapy (normal stem cells survive chemotherapy less well than cells expressing the drug resistance gene). At a certain point the number of drug-resistant bone marrow cells rises to a degree that protects bone marrow from the effects of chemotherapy and thus higher doses of chemotherapy can be given without all the usual side effects. Note, however, that systemic side effects not related to bone marrow will persist. This method could also be used to select for a second gene product expressed in concert with the drug resistance gene.

**Table 25.4** Approaches to gene therapy targeting hematological malignancies.

| Strategy | Genes employed | Problems and merits |
| --- | --- | --- |
| Gene replacement | p53, p16, Rb | Gene delivery to every cell required<br>Specific to defective cancer cell |
| Gene inhibition | BCR-ABL, MYC, CCND1 (cyclin D1), BCL-2 | Gene delivery to every cell required |
| Suicide genes | Thymidine kinase, cytosine deaminase | Immunogenicity and bystander effect contribute |
| Drug resistance genes | MDR-1, DHFR, MGMT | Stem cell gene delivery required |
| Immunotherapy | IL-2, IL-12, B7-1, CD40L, GM-CSF, tumor-associated antigens (TAAs) | Systemic response, autoimmunity a theoretical problem<br>For TAAs, requires that tumors express foreign antigen |

of patients. Another more widely applicable approach is the use of autologous tumor cells that have been genetically engineered to express immunostimulatory cytokines. Trials using this strategy in myeloma, low-grade lymphoma, leukemia, and chronic lymphocytic leukemia are being pursued.

Many tumor cells express unique antigens on their cell surface, either alone or as proteolytically cleaved peptides in association with MHC class I molecules. The specificity and sheer quantity of these tumor-associated antigens (TAAs) may allow immune effector cells to distinguish tumor from normal tissue (Figure 25.4). Some of these TAAs have been isolated and shown to be recognized by T-cell receptor (TCR) complexes on human cytotoxic T lymphocytes. This has engendered gene therapy strategies to augment T-cell-mediated eradication of tumors. Indeed, while to date cancer has been the primary target of the bulk of clinical gene therapy protocols, this area has seen limited success. That is until the results of a landmark study were published in 2006 by Morgan and colleagues demonstrating definitive success in this area. The cDNAs for the α and β chains of a TCR against a melanoma antigen were subcloned into an

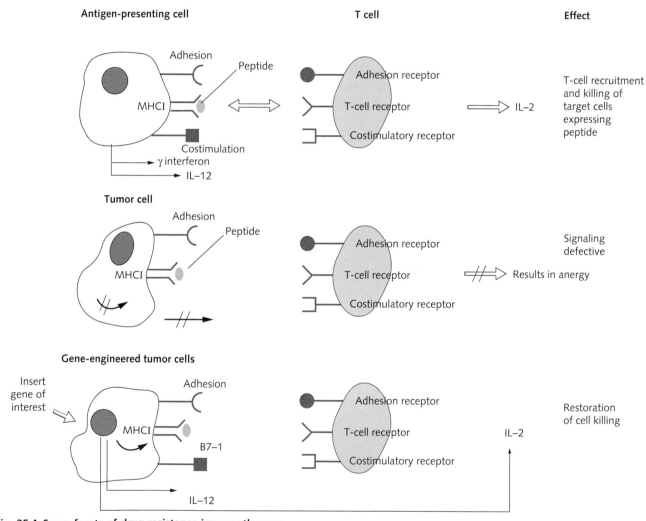

**Fig. 25.4 Some facets of drug resistance immunotherapy**
Efficient signaling of T cells occurs following adhesion, engagement of the major histocompatibility complex (MHC) class I/T-cell receptor signal, and after a costimulatory signal is received. Under normal circumstances, professional antigen-presenting cells (APCs) present processed peptides in the groove of the MHC class I complex to T cells. Tumor cells are often deficient in one or all of the components required to function as APCs because they lack an appropriate tumor antigen, cannot process the antigen, or are deficient in adhesion molecules, MHC class I or costimulatory molecules required to generate a T-cell response. These missing components can be provided or expression enhanced using gene transfer techniques. By overcoming the deficiencies of the tumor cell, the gene-engineered cells can serve as autologous cancer vaccines presenting foreign antigen to the host T cells.

oncoretroviral vector and used to transduce peripheral blood lymphocytes of melanoma patients. Following infusions of the transduced cells into 17 patients, two patients demonstrated actual sustained tumor regressions as determined by standard criteria. Furthermore, 1 year after infusions both of the responding patients had high levels of gene-transduced cells in their circulation (20–70% of peripheral blood mononuclear cells). Multiplexing TCR complexes to broaden the immune response and overcoming antigen drift and subsequent tumor evasion, adaptation of recombinant LVs to increase gene transfer frequencies, along with incorporation of methods to overcome immune dampening mechanisms driven by the tumors themselves may increase the potency of this strategy in future protocols.

Another facet of immunotherapy for cancer that has received substantial interest is the application of gene delivery techniques to induce specific immune responses in patients by directing efficient antigen presenting cells (APCs) to present peptides from such TAAs to T cells. Where patients have sufficient immune capacity for this kind of manipulation, this can cause upregulation of the immune response against that specific TAA. The most immunologically powerful (so-called *professional*) APCs are bone marrow-derived dendritic cells. Dendritic cells express MHC class I and II, B7-1, B7-2, CD40, ICAM-1, and LFA-3. They are capable of presenting processed antigen for days, and are potent stimulators of immunity when administered as vaccines to animals. Dendritic cells modulate immune responses in part by secretion of IL-12 (hence the notion of converting tumor cells into APCs by introduction of IL-12 and B7-1 sequences). Dendritic cells can be readily expanded from bone marrow progenitors *in vitro* using cytokine-supplemented medium (useful cytokines include Flt3L, TNF-α, GM-CSF, IL-4). Such cells may also be genetically engineered by a variety of methods to express TAAs, thereby presenting peptides in a proper context; this holds promise for the immunotherapy of hematological malignancies and for some solid tumors. Clinical trials have been performed in this area targeting a number of TAAs. Results have indicated that immune responses can be generated in patients. Current work is focused on enhancing that immune outcome and capitalizing on that facet to decrease tumor burdens.

As alluded to above, tumor cells known to express potentially antigenic peptides manage to evade host immunosurveillance and proliferate *in vivo*. Thus, tumor cells may lack or downmodulate expression of the necessary accessory signals required to induce expression by immune effector cells of cytokines that are necessary for activation and directed *in vivo* expansion of cytotoxic T lymphocytes. The end result is anergy, a failure of T cells to respond to the tumor antigen. In addition to optimal presentation of antigen to the TCR, efficient activation of naive T cells requires a second costimulatory signal. It is now appreciated that molecules of the B7 family (B7-1/CD80, B7-2/CD86) on APCs engaging CD28/CTLA-4 receptors on T cells play a key role in this process, inducing autocrine IL-2 production and T-cell proliferation. Murine models have demonstrated that T-cell-mediated rejection of tumors can be induced by transduction of tumor cells with such costimulatory molecules. In the absence of costimulatory signals, it is possible to bypass this requirement by ectopic expression of cytokines and thus overcome or prevent anergy of the immune effector cells. Proof-of-principle that cytokine gene-transduced tumor cells can prevent tumor engraftment has been obtained. Such models have also shown that transduction of the genes for various cytokines, such as IL-2, IL-4, IL-6, IL-7, IL-12, IFN-γ, GM-CSF and TNF-α, into murine tumors not only led to primary rejection of the modified cells but often elicited protective immunity against subsequent tumor challenge with unmodified tumor cells. Furthermore, in such models, synergy has been demonstrated between molecules with varying mechanisms of action, for example IL-2, IL-12 and B7-1.

## Genetic inhibition: antisense RNA, ribozymes, and siRNA

A number of oncogenes, for example *RAS*, *MYC*, *CCND1* (cyclin D1) and *BCR-ABL*, are overexpressed in hematological malignancies and in many cases are pivotal to the progression of disease. RNAs with enzymatic activity (*ribozymes*) that possess highly sequence-specific RNA-cleaving potential have been used to decrease expression of such oncogenes. Another gene therapy approach directed against such malignancies is the use of antisense mRNAs to bind to, and prevent translation of, the sense target sequence. An analogous study using antisense RNA has been performed in the clinic for treatment of HIV-AIDS by Levine and colleagues. This was the first protocol in humans to employ recombinant LVs. Here T cells were transduced with a conditionally replicating LV that engineered expression of an antisense sequence to the HIV envelope. Cells were infused a single time into five subjects. One recipient demonstrated a sustained decrease in HIV load and immune function improved in four patients. No insertional mutagenesis was observed, nor was recombination between the gene transfer vector and wild-type HIV. Lastly, RNA interference (RNAi), which entails the use of small double-stranded RNAs to elicit downmodulation of target gene expression, is also being developed by a number of groups to be used in this context. Indeed, many investigators have demonstrated that this technique can modulate expression of a variety of important factors in hematopoietic cells, and such procedures are now being pursued in the clinical context.

## Safety

### Suicide gene therapy

With the obvious importance of stably integrating vectors in gene therapy protocols involving the hematopoietic system, and given the deleterious outcomes in clinical trials for one inherited disorder (*see above*), it is appropriate that the field is now directing much more attention to studying the safety of such gene delivery agents. Extensive sequencing analyses have revealed that LVs and oncoretroviral vectors have different integration patterns. Yet, in both cases, such integrations are still fairly random. Efforts are underway to tether the viral integrases to specific sequences in the genome, thereby directing proviral integration into specific areas of chromatin; however, such studies are still in their infancy. Another method under scrutiny is to use gene transfer to endow target cells of interest with factors that may allow their selective eradication should deleterious outcomes arise. This approach certainly has applications in hematological transplantation, and also in numerous other developing research fields employing different candidate populations such as embryonic stem cells and induced pluripotent stem cells.

The so-called "suicide genes" encode enzymes which, when expressed by transduced target cells, confer susceptibility to drug-induced cell death by specifically converting normally non-toxic prodrugs into potent cytolytic or cytostatic molecules. At least three general applications of suicide gene therapy can be envisioned. One is direct tumor therapy, where the vector is injected into the tumor mass and patients are given the prodrug, which is activated only in the tumor. The second application is in reduction of graft-versus-host disease (GVHD) after donor lymphocyte infusion. Here, if symptoms of GVHD appear, productively transduced and transplanted cells can be selectively removed by addition of prodrug. Lastly, if a truly portable system exists, such safety elements could conceivably be incorporated into any cell transplanted out of its normal context or into any gene therapy vector in order to protect transduced cells from genotoxicity and the development of leukemias should such outcomes occur.

The gene most commonly employed in clinical trials in this context is the *human herpes simplex virus (HSV) type 1 thymidine kinase* gene, which confers sensitivity to the drugs ganciclovir and aciclovir, among others. Use of thymidine kinase is further enhanced for some direct tumor applications by diffusion of the converted prodrug into neighboring cells and thus a *bystander effect* occurs that is mediated largely via gap junctions between connecting cells (Figure 25.5). The obvious limitations of this treatment approach are that not all cells targeted will be successfully gene modified and thus, even with the bystander effect, only a fraction of malignant cells will be destroyed. Nevertheless, applications of this type are in clinical trials for treatment of solid tumors. Another proven clinical application of this suicide approach, which may actually have a higher probability of success, is in the prevention of GVHD following transplantation. These trials were first performed by Bonini and colleagues in patients who first received T-cell-depleted allogeneic bone marrow transplantation followed by infusions of oncoretrovirally transduced lymphocytes. The transduced cells demonstrated antitumor activity in five patients. Three patients developed GVHD, which was controlled by addition of ganciclovir.

Further refinements of the suicide approach have also been described recently. These were necessary due to inherent issues with the HSV thymidine kinase system. In this context, HSV thymidine kinase converts ganciclovir to ganciclovir monophosphate. This molecule is eventually converted into ganciclovir triphosphate by other cellular kinases and incorporated into DNA, causing chain termination in dividing cells. Yet HSV thymidine kinase is not all that efficient at converting ganciclovir to ganciclovir monophosphate. In addition, this reaction is only one of the rate-limiting reactions in this cascade, such substrate conversion merely transferring the rate-limiting step on to the next enzyme in the pathway, guanylate kinase. HSV thymidine kinase is also a foreign protein and anti-thymidine kinase immune responses have been reported in patients receiving such transduced cells. This can lead to premature clearing of the transplanted cell population. Lastly, it should be noted that many transplant patients are already on prophylactic ganciclovir to reduce the possibility of cytomegalovirus infection.

The system developed by Sato and colleagues abrogates many of the above issues. Here, a human enzyme (thymidylate kinase) has been minimally modified to direct it to efficiently convert azidothymidine monophosphate to azidothymidine diphosphate. Toxicity profiles for azidothymidine are well known. This system also allows for killing of non-cycling cells through mitochondrial membrane disruption. *In vitro* and *in vivo* testing of such a suicide safety system has been completed and recombinant LV that engineers expression of this variant enzyme is being produced for eventual clinical trials.

## Conclusions

While still a relatively young field, some successes have been observed in clinical gene therapy trials. Some concerns have also been raised. Development and implementation of gene

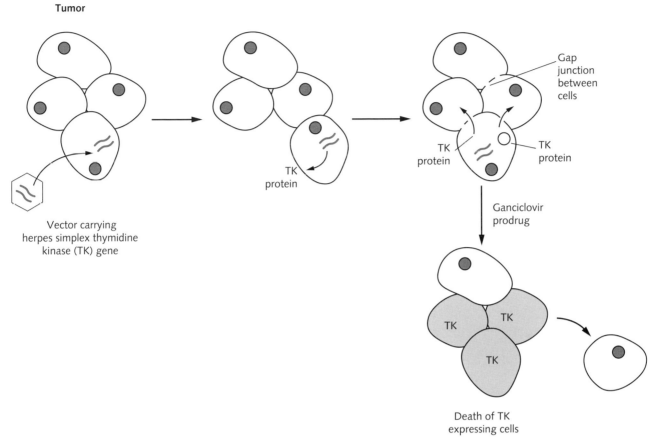

**Fig. 25.5 Basis of suicide gene therapy**
The metabolic product of the activity of the thymidine kinase suicide gene appears capable of diffusing into neighboring cells via gap junctions, which join the cells together. This non-specific diffusion allows a greater effective cell killing percentage than might be predicted using direct gene transfer efficiency alone. Because cells are dying and releasing tumor antigen into the local milieu of the tumor, it is possible that such suicide gene therapies will synergize with immune-based treatment strategies.

delivery systems has also led to accumulation of important secondary knowledge. For example, gene delivery methods are now routinely used in most basic biology laboratories to study many different processes. Viral entry mechanisms are now much better understood and immune responses initiated following viral infections are better characterized. As a result of the use of integrating vectors it has also now been demonstrated that some T cells in humans are actually very long-lived and that multiple HSCs contribute to hematopoiesis. Much more has also been learned concerning mechanisms that contribute to the development of leukemias. Some concepts and approaches to molecular therapy of diseases that interface with the blood system have been described in this chapter; many other therapeutic strategies are also being developed. Indeed, the advent and success of human gene therapy trials combined with rapid advances in gene transfer technology and implementation of differential delivery systems, along with the full sequencing of the human

genome, are setting the stage for a new era in human medicine. The field of human molecular medicine will surely continue to expand and make inroads in a therapeutically relevant way. It seems likely that study of the blood system, both in the laboratory and in patients, will continue to play a pivotal role in the further development of this field.

## Further reading

### Introduction

Brenner MK. (2001) Gene transfer and the treatment of hematological malignancy. *Journal of Internal Medicine*, **249**, 345–358.

Brenner MK, Rill DR, Holladay MS *et al.* (1993) Gene marking to determine whether autologous marrow infusion restores long term haemopoiesis in cancer patients. *Lancet*, **342**, 1134–1137.

Brenner MK, Rill DR, Moen RC *et al.* (1993) Gene-marking to trace origin of relapse after autologous bone-marrow transplantation. *Lancet*, **341**, 85–86.

Miller AD. (1992) Human gene therapy comes of age. *Nature*, **357**, 455–460.

Rosenberg SA, Aebersold P, Cornetta K *et al.* (1990) Gene transfer into humans: immunotherapy of patients with advanced melanoma, using tumor-infiltrating lymphocytes modified by retroviral gene transduction. *New England Journal of Medicine*, **323**, 570–578.

Williams DA, Smith FO. (2000) Progress in the use of gene transfer methods to treat genetic blood diseases. *Human Gene Therapy*, **11**, 2059–2066.

## Gene transfer systems

Bergelson JM, Cunningham JA, Droguett G *et al.* (1997) Isolation of a common receptor for Coxsackie B viruses and adenoviruses 2 and 5. *Science*, **275**, 1320–1323.

Crystal RG. (1995) Transfer of genes to humans: early lessons and obstacles to success. *Science*, **270**, 404–410.

Dilloo D, Rill D, Entwistle C *et al.* (1997) A novel herpes vector for the high-efficiency transduction of normal and malignant human hematopoietic cells. *Blood*, **89**, 119–127.

Horn PA, Topp MS, Morris JC *et al.* (2002) Highly efficient gene transfer into baboon marrow repopulating cells using GALV-pseudotype oncoretroviral vectors produced by human packaging cells. *Blood*, **100**, 3960–3967.

Miller AD, Buttimore C. (1986) Redesign of retrovirus packaging cell lines to avoid recombination leading to helper virus production. *Molecular and Cellular Biology*, **6**, 2895–2902.

Miller DG, Adam MA, Miller AD. (1990) Gene transfer by retrovirus vectors occurs only in cells that are actively replicating at the time of infection. *Molecular and Cellular Biology*, **10**, 4239–4242.

Mitchell RS, Beitzel BF, Schroder AR *et al.* (2004) Retroviral DNA integration: ASLV, HIV, and MLV show distinct target site preferences. *PLoS Biology*, **2**, E234.

Mulligan RC. (1993) The basic science of gene therapy. *Science*, **260**, 926–932.

Naldini L, Blomer U, Gallay P *et al.* (1996) *In vivo* gene delivery and stable transduction of nondividing cells by a lentiviral vector. *Science*, **272**, 263–267.

Pawliuk R, Bachelot T, Wise RJ *et al.* (1999) Long-term cure of the photosensitivity of murine erythropoietic protoporphyria by preselective gene therapy. *Nature Medicine*, **5**, 768–773.

Qin G, Takenaka T, Telsch K *et al.* (2001) Preselective gene therapy for Fabry disease. *Proceedings of the National Academy of Sciences of the United States of America*, **98**, 3428–3433.

Thornhill SI, Schambach A, Howe SJ *et al.* (2008) Self-inactivating gammaretroviral vectors for gene therapy of X-linked severe combined immunodeficiency. *Molecular Therapy*, **16**, 590–598.

## Gene-marking studies involving hematopoietic cells

Deisseroth AB, Zu Z, Claxton D *et al.* (1994) Genetic marking shows that Ph⁺ cells present in autologous transplants of chronic myelog-

enous leukemia (CML) contribute to relapse after autologous bone marrow transplant in CML. *Blood*, **83**, 3068–3076.

Dunbar CE, Cotter-Fox M, O'Shaughnessy JA *et al.* (1995) Retrovirally marked CD34-enriched peripheral blood and bone marrow cells contribute to long term engraftment after autologous transplantation. *Blood*, **85**, 3048–3057.

Rill DR, Santana VM, Roberts WM *et al.* (1994) Direct demonstration that autologous bone marrow transplantation for solid tumors can return a multiplicity of tumorigenic cells. *Blood*, **84**, 380–383.

## Therapeutic trials for inherited disorders

Aiuti A, Slavin S, Aker M *et al.* (2002) Correction of ADA-SCID by stem cell gene therapy combined with nonmyeloablative conditioning. *Science*, **296**, 2410–2413.

Blaese RM, Culver KW, Miller AD *et al.* (1995) T lymphocyte-directed gene therapy for ADA-SCID: initial trial results after 4 years. *Science*, **270**, 475–480.

Cavazzana-Calvo M, Hacein-Bey S, de Saint Basile G *et al.* (2000) Gene therapy of human severe combined immunodeficiency (SCID)-X1 disease. *Science*, **288**, 669–672.

Hoogerbrugge PM, van Beusechem VW, Fischer A *et al.* (1996) Bone marrow gene transfer in three patients with adenosine deaminase deficiency. *Gene Therapy*, **3**, 179–183.

Kay MA, Manno CS, Ragni MV *et al.* (2000) Evidence for gene transfer and expression of factor IX in haemophilia B patients treated with an AAV vector. *Nature Genetics*, **24**, 257–261.

Kohn DB, Weinberg KI, Nolta JA *et al.* (1995) Engraftment of gene-modified umbilical cord blood cells in neonates with adenosine deaminase deficiency. *Nature Medicine*, **1**, 1017–1023.

Onodera M, Ariga T, Kawamura N *et al.* (1998) Successful peripheral T-lymphocyte-directed gene transfer for a patient with severe combined immune deficiency caused by adenosine deaminase deficiency. *Blood*, **91**, 30–36.

Ott MG, Schmidt M, Schwarzwaelder K *et al.* (2006) Correction of X-linked chronic granulomatous disease by gene therapy, augmented by insertional activation of MDS1-EVI1, PRDM16 or SETBP1. *Nature Medicine*, **12**, 401–409.

## Therapeutic trials for acquired disorders

Abonour R, Williams DA, Einhorn L *et al.* (2000) Efficient retrovirus-mediated transfer of the multidrug resistance 1 gene into autologous human long-term repopulating hematopoietic stem cells. *Nature Medicine*, **6**, 652–658.

Hesdorffer C, Ayello J, Ward M *et al.* (1998) Phase I trial of retroviral-mediated transfer of the human MDR1 gene as marrow chemoprotection in patients undergoing high-dose chemotherapy and autologous stem-cell transplantation. *Journal of Clinical Oncology*, **16**, 165–172.

June CH. (2007) Adoptive T cell therapy for cancer in the clinic. *Journal of Clinical Investigation*, **117**, 1466–1476.

Levine BL, Humeau LM, Boyer J *et al.* (2006) Gene transfer in humans using a conditionally replicating lentiviral vector. *Proceedings of the National Academy of Sciences of the United States of America*, **103**, 17372–17377.

Morgan RA, Dudley ME, Wunderlich JR *et al.* (2006) Cancer regression in patients after transfer of genetically engineered lymphocytes. *Science*, **314**, 126–129.

Mossoba ME, Medin JA. (2006) Cancer immunotherapy using virally transduced dendritic cells: animal studies and human clinical trials. *Expert Review of Vaccines*, **5**, 717–732.

Sorrentino BP, Brandt SJ, Bodine D *et al.* (1992) Selection of drug-resistant bone marrow cells *in vivo* after retroviral transfer of human MDR1. *Science*, **257**, 99–103.

Zielske SP, Reese JS, Lingas KT *et al.* (2003) In vivo selection of MGMT (P140K) lentivirus-transduced human NOD/SCID repopulating cells without pretransplant irradiation conditioning. *Journal of Clinical Investigation*, **112**, 1561–1570.

## Safety

Bonini C, Ferrari G, Verzeletti S *et al.* (1997) HSV-TK gene transfer into donor lymphocytes for control of allogeneic graft-versus-leukemia. *Science*, **276**, 1719–1724.

Montini E, Cesana D, Schmidt M *et al.* (2006) Hematopoietic stem cell gene transfer in a tumor-prone mouse model uncovers low genotoxicity of lentiviral integration. *Nature Biotechnology*, **24**, 687–696.

Sato T, Neschadim A, Konrad M *et al.* (2007) Engineered human tmpk/AZT as a novel enzyme/prodrug axis for suicide gene therapy. *Molecular Therapy*, **15**, 962–970.

# Chapter 26 Pharmacogenomics

## Leo Kager[1] & William E Evans[2]

[1] St Anna Children's Hospital, Vienna, Austria
[2] St Jude Children's Research Hospital, Memphis, TN, USA

## Introduction

It has long been recognized that there is great heterogeneity in the way people respond to medications. For example, when a standard dose of a certain drug is given to a cohort of patients, some will respond and some will not respond, some will respond only partially, and some will experience adverse drug reactions (ADRs) that can be life-threatening. This variation in both host toxicity and treatment efficacy can have many different causes, including environmental (e.g., nutrition, cigarette smoking, other medications), physiological (e.g., age, gender, nutritional status, renal and liver function), pathophysiological (e.g., pathogenesis and severity of the disease being treated), and genetic factors. Overall, genetic factors are estimated to account for 15–30% of interindividual differences in drug metabolism and response. For certain drugs, however, genetic factors are of the utmost importance and can account for up to 95% of interindividual variability in drug disposition and effects.

The science of pharmacogenomics, which aims to define the genomic determinants for drug disposition and effects, has a long tradition in the field of hematology. In the 1950s, the relationship between hemolysis after antimalarial therapy and the inherited glucose 6-phosphate dehydrogenase (G6PD) activity in erythrocytes was identified. This discovery explained why the ADR of hemolysis is observed mainly in Africans, where up to 10% of individuals are deficient in G6PD, but is rarely seen in other ethnic groups like Caucasians, in whom G6PD deficiency is uncommon. In 1959, Friedrich Vogel defined pharmacogenetics as "the study of the role of genetics in drug response." Until 2000,

efforts were mainly concentrated on mapping highly penetrant monogenic loci for drug-metabolizing enzymes that strongly influence the effects of medications. Interestingly, two of the most important clinical examples of Mendelian pharmacogenetics – polymorphisms in the thiopurine S-methyltransferase (*TPMT*) gene that affect the efficacy and toxicity of thiopurines, and polymorphisms in the cytochrome P4502C9 (*CYP2C9*) and vitamin K epoxide reductase complex 1 (*VKORC1*) that affect efficacy and toxicity of warfarin – were again discovered in the field of hematology, namely in the treatment of acute lymphoblastic leukemia (ALL) and oral anticoagulant therapy, respectively. However, it is well recognized that most pharmacological effects result from the interplay of numerous gene products, and now that the human genome has been sequenced and the human haplotypes of the most common form of genetic variation, namely single-nucleotide polymorphisms (SNPs), have been mapped, genome-wide approaches (i.e., pharmacogenomics) are increasingly used to elucidate the genomic contributors of variability in drug effects. The terms "pharmacogenetics" and "pharmacogenomics" are synonymous for all practical purposes, and we herein use the term pharmacogenomics.

In this short chapter, validated clinically relevant examples are presented to illustrate how pharmacogenomics can be used to improve current drug therapy in hematological diseases and to identify novel targets for developing new therapeutic approaches in hematological diseases.

## Principles of pharmacogenomics

The effects of drugs are determined by the interplay of many gene products that influence the pharmacokinetics and pharmacodynamics of medications. Whereas pharmacokinetics describes the absorption, distribution, metabolism, and excretion of drugs (so-called "ADME"), pharmacody-

*Molecular Hematology*, 3rd edition. Edited by Drew Provan and John Gribben.
© 2010 Blackwell Publishing.

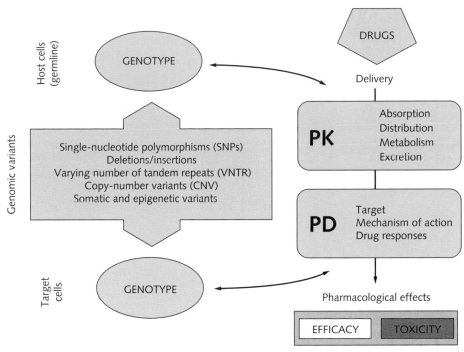

**Fig. 26.1 General principles of pharmacogenomics**
The goal of pharmacogenomics is to elucidate genomic determinants that influence pharmacokinetics (PK) and pharmacodynamics (PD) of delivered drugs, thereby influencing both efficacious and toxic effects. Investigating these functionally important variants in the human population can help to explain some differences in drug effects.

namics studies the relationship between the pharmacokinetic properties of drugs and their pharmacological effects, which can be desired or adverse. The ultimate goal of pharmacogenomics is to elucidate functionally relevant genomic determinants for drug disposition (germline variants) and response (variants in target cells) to select medications and dosage of medications on the basis of each patient's inherited ability to metabolize, eliminate, and respond to specific drugs (Figure 26.1). Many variants in the human genome have been identified that influence the expression and activity of pharmacologically relevant proteins.

## Variation in the human genome

The human genome consists of about $3 \times 10^9$ bp (3 Gb). Although any two humans are thought to be up to 99.9% identical in their DNA sequence, the remaining small fraction of the genome, which constitutes the genetic diversity among individuals, contains many forms of variation, ranging from large microscopically visible chromosome anomalies to single nucleotide changes. Variants that are about 3 Mb or more in size are referred to as microscopic variants. The smaller, and much more abundant, variants

include SNPs, small (<1 kb) insertions and deletions (*indels*) of nucleotides, variation in the number of repeats of a specific motif (i.e., variable number tandem repeats, minisatellites and microsatellites), duplications, and variants of DNA segments 1 kb or larger that are collectively defined as copy number variations (CNVs). Common DNA variants, often defined as greater than 1% in a given population, are named polymorphisms, whereas rare DNA variants are named mutations.

### Single-nucleotide polymorphisms

The most common and most extensively studied inherited genomic variations are SNPs, positions in the genome where individuals have inherited a different nucleotide. SNPs are found approximately every 300 bp in both the coding and non-coding regions of the human genome. About 18 million SNPs have been identified (of which about 40% are currently validated) and are in the public domain at http://www.ncbi.nlm.nih.gov/SNP/snp_summary.cgi. SNPs that cause amino acid changes in the encoded protein are named non-synonymous coding SNPs, whereas SNPs that do not change the amino acid composition are named synonymous (or silent) SNPs. Amino acid substitutions have the potential to change the function of a protein, and have more relevance in functionally important domains of the protein (e.g., the catalytic cleft of an enzyme). However, it has recently been demonstrated for the ATP-binding cassette transporter ABCB1 (or P-glycoprotein) that a silent or synonymous SNP can also affect *in vivo* protein folding and function. Moreover, SNPs in genomic regions that influence the expression of functionally relevant genes like transcription factors or microRNA binding sites can also have pharmacological consequences. For example, a so-called microRSNP (defined as a functional SNP that can interfere with microRNA function and which results in loss of the microRNA-mediated regulation of a drug target gene) was recently found to be associated with antifolate resistance by influencing the expression of the antifolate target dihydrofolate reductase (*DHFR*) gene.

### Haplotypes, linkage disequilibrium, and haplotype map

SNPs and other genomic variants are not inherited independently, but rather belong to segments of DNA that are inherited as units, with each unit referred to as a haplotype. Genome-wide haplotypes can be constructed by linkage disequilibrium (LD) analysis, a statistical measure of the extent to which particular alleles or SNPs at two loci are associated with each other in the population. LD occurs when haplotype combinations of alleles or SNPs at different loci occur more frequently than would be expected from random association. SNPs and alleles of interest are presumably inherited together if they are physically close to each other (typically 50 kb apart or closer), producing strong LD.

By studying 3.1 million SNPs in 270 individuals from four geographically diverse populations, the international HapMap consortium recently created a genome-wide map of haplotypes, the phase II HapMap (http://www.hapmap.org). The HapMap project has revealed a block-like structure of LD, as well as the existence of areas of low or high recombination rate, leading to the identification of so-called tagging (tag) SNPs. Tag SNPs can be used to predict with high probability the alleles at other cosegregating "tagged" SNPs. Phase II HapMap results show that the vast majority of common SNPs in the 3-Gb human genome can be reduced to about 500 000 tag SNPs for individuals of European and Asian ancestry and to about 1 million tag SNPs for individuals of African ancestry, with a prediction accuracy of $r^2 \geq 0.8$. Recently, ultra-high-throughput genotyping has become possible, with the ability to analyze more than 1 million SNPs using oligonucleotide SNP arrays. This high-throughput genotyping method and the relatively manageable number of tag SNPs will help to establish genome-wide pharmacogenomic models.

### Copy number variants

DNA segments 1 kb or larger and which are present at variable copy number in comparison with a reference genome are defined as CNVs. Recently, a first-generation CNV map of the human genome revealed a total of about 1500 CNV regions covering 360 Mb (12%) of the genome. Because common CNVs affect approximately 12% of the human genome, any variation in copy number will affect a wide spectrum of genomic sequences (from the kilobase up to the megabase range), and possibly many pharmacologically relevant genes. Although CNVs have been reported to influence the activity of certain drug-metabolizing enzymes like CYP isoenzymes and glutathione *S*-transferases, CNVs have not been widely investigated in pharmacogenomics yet, but may be of upmost importance for genome-wide investigations in the near future.

### Somatic and epigenetic variations

Non-random genetic abnormalities, including gains and losses of chromosomes, can be found in the majority of hematological malignancies. This can create allele-specific copy number differences between normal host cells (i.e., germline genotype) and cancer cells, and such differences can have pharmacologically relevant consequences. For example, it has been demonstrated that the cellular acquisition of an additional chromosome can cause discordance between germline and leukemia cell genotypes and phenotypes that can influence antimetabolite therapy.

Epigenetic modifications, mainly DNA methylations at CpG dinucleotides, can affect the expression of genes. Aberrant methylation of CpG islands is a common feature of cancer cells and, as demonstrated in childhood ALL, such aberrant methylation can also have pharmacologically relevant consequences.

Collectively, insights from recent investigations point to the potential necessity of qualitative and quantitative genomic analyses, as well as the integration of genomic and epigenomic data to establish accurate pharmacogenomic models in hematological malignancies.

### Genetic variation among ethnic groups

It is well known that differences in the frequency and nature of genetic variants among ethnic groups must also be recognized when attempting to extrapolate research from one population to another. For example, allele frequencies and types of polymorphisms in the *TPMT* gene, which influence efficacy and toxicity of thiopurine therapy, vary greatly among different ethnic groups. Therefore, pharmacogenomic relations must be validated for each therapeutic indication within different ethnic groups.

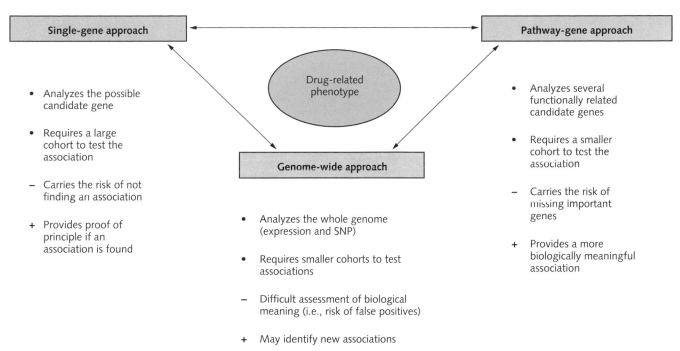

**Fig. 26.2 Comparison of single-gene, candidate pathway-gene and genome-wide pharmacogenomic approaches to the analysis of drug-related phenotypes**
The main characteristics (•), disadvantage (–) and advantage (+) of each approach is indicated. The arrows between the three approaches indicate that any approach can lead to another and that a combination of approaches might be considered. SNP, single-nucleotide polymorphism. From Cheok MH, Evans WE. (2006) Acute lymphoblastic leukaemia: a model for the pharmacogenomics of cancer therapy. *Nature Reviews. Cancer*, **6**, 117–129, with permission.

## Approaches for establishing pharmacogenomic models

Pharmacogenomics is a broad strategy for establishing models by integrating information from functional genomics, high-throughput molecular analyses, pharmacokinetics, and pharmacodynamics. These models can be used to further optimize existing drug therapy or identify novel therapeutic targets. As described above, there is a bewildering array of human genomic variation, and a central issue in pharmacogenomics is to elucidate those genomic determinants that are pharmacologically relevant, namely which genomic variants are associated with certain drug-related phenotypes. Pharmacogenomic models can be established using two strategies: candidate gene strategies, which focus on either the analysis of single genes or sets of related genes in functional metabolic or biochemical pathways, and genome-wide strategies (Figure 26.2). A few clinically relevant examples of candidate gene and genome-wide approaches are presented to illustrate how these strategies can be used to improve drug therapy in hematology.

## Candidate gene approaches

Candidate gene approaches can either study the correlation between single genes and drug-related phenotypes or investigate the correlation between a set of functionally related genes and drug-related phenotypes (i.e., candidate pathway gene approach) (Figure 26.2). The main advantage of the single-gene strategy is that it focuses on genes with known biological function, and provides proof of principle if an association with a certain pharmacological phenotype is found. However, this strategy requires a large cohort to test the association and carries the risk of not finding an association. The candidate pathway gene strategy offers the advantage of combining information on several genes that are common to a pathway, thereby requiring smaller cohorts to test the association. Moreover, it minimizes the *noise* of a non-targeted genome-wide approach, although it potentially excludes genes of importance. Many candidate gene investigations have focused on functionally relevant SNPs in genes encoding proteins that play an important role in the generation of a clinical drug reaction in the treatment of

hematological malignancies, in the prevention of thrombosis, and in the prevention of ADRs manifesting as hematological disorders (e.g., hemolysis, myelosuppression). Examples of these genes and their products are listed below.
• Drug-metabolizing enzymes that modify the functional part of drugs, such as cytochrome P450 enzymes (e.g., *CYP2C9*) and dihydropyrimidine dehydrogenase (*DPD*).
• Conjugate drugs with endogenous substituents, such as *TPMT*, glutathione *S*-transferases (*GSTM1*) and UDP-glucuronosyltransferases (*UGT1A1*).
• Proteins that protect cells against free radicals and toxic oxygen metabolites produced by drugs, such as *G6PD* and NADPH quinone oxidoreductase (*NQO1*).
• Proteins that have important functions in pathways targeted by drugs, like *VKORC1*, prothrombin (*FII*) and factor V (*FV*), or the folate metabolism pathway that includes dihydrofolate reductase (*DHFR*), methylenetetrahydrofolate reductase (*MTHFR*) and thymidylate synthetase (*TYMS*).
• Variants in genes that encode important drug transporters, such as the major methotrexate transporter reduced folate carrier (*RFC* or *SLC19A1*) and the ATP-binding cassette transporters that include *ABCB1* (or P-glycoprotein), *ABCC2* (or MRP2), and *ABCG2* (or breast cancer resistant protein).

A few selected examples are given below which illustrate how results from the candidate gene approach can be used to improve drug therapy in hematology.

## Antimetabolite therapy in childhood ALL

The cure rate in children with ALL, now exceeding almost 80% in most treatment protocols in industrialized countries, has mainly been achieved empirically. To further boost event-free survival rates in this disease and to reduce the risk of short- and long-term side effects of antileukemic medications, a better understanding of ALL pathogenesis and the underlying mechanisms of drug resistance in leukemia blast cells and drug-induced toxicity in normal host cells is necessary. Antimetabolites are key elements in the treatment of many hematological malignancies including ALL, and many candidate gene approaches have focused on the improvement of antimetabolite therapy in childhood ALL.

### Thiopurines

The thiopurine antimetabolites mercaptopurine and thioguanine are essential components in childhood ALL treatment protocols. To exert cytotoxicity, the prodrugs have to undergo anabolism to form active cytotoxic thioguanine nucleotides (TGNs). These anabolic reactions are in competition with direct drug inactivation (*S*-methylation) via TPMT. TPMT activity determines how much thiopurine is inactivated and how much remains for conversion to cyto-

toxic TGNs. Variations in TPMT activity are regulated primarily by variants in the *TPMT* gene. Three non-synonymous SNPs account for more than 95% of the relevant *TPMT* variants, namely *TPMT*2* (238G→C), *TPMT*3C* (719A→G), and *TPMT*3A* (460G→A + 719A→G). One in 300 persons carries two variant *TPMT* alleles and does not express functional TPMT activity (due to lesser stability of the variant protein); about 5–10% are heterozygous and have intermediate levels of enzyme activity, whereas 95% of individuals are homozygous for the wild-type allele (*TPMT*1/TPMT*1*) and have normal TPMT activity (Figure 26.3). Population studies have shown significant differences in TPMT pharmacogenetics among ethnic groups. For example, *TPMT*3A* is the most common variant allele in Caucasians, whereas *TMPT*3C* accounts for more than 50% of variants in Africans. *TMPT*3C* is also the major variant allele in East Asian populations, populations that generally lack the *TPMT*3A* allele.

Patients who carry two non-functional *TPMT* alleles experience severe hematotoxicity if treated with conventional doses of thiopurines. Depending on the dose (e.g., $60\,mg/m^2$ daily) and the comedications, many patients with one non-functional TPMT allele can tolerate mercaptopurine therapy at full doses. However, these patients might be at higher risk of dose-limiting hematotoxicity with slightly higher mercaptopurine doses (e.g., $75\,mg/m^2$ daily), but may experience better leukemia control than do those who have two wild-type *TPMT* alleles. Moreover, patients with one non-functional *TPMT* allele may be at increased risk of epipodophyllotoxin-related acute myeloid leukemia and irradiation-induced brain tumors as a result of thiopurine therapy, and of veno-occlusive disease of the liver following thioguanine therapy. Most importantly, results from the St Jude Children's Research Hospital Total XIIIB childhood ALL treatment trial provide proof of principle that prospective mercaptopurine dose adjustment based on *TPMT* genotypes can decrease toxicity without a compromise in treatment efficacy. Based on a US Food and Drug Administration (FDA) advisory committee recommendation, a change in labeling for mercaptopurine, with *TPMT* testing and dosage recommendations provided for TPMT-deficient patients, was implemented in 2004. Of note, there is evidence that *TPMT* genotyping before initiation of mercaptopurine treatment can be cost-effective in children with ALL.

Because patients who share the same *TPMT* genotypes still exhibit considerable variations in their response to mercaptopurine, other unidentified genetic variations may contribute to the toxicity and response to mercaptopurine. Indeed, a genetic polymorphism of inosine triphosphate pyrophosphatase was recently identified to be a significant determinant of mercaptopurine metabolism and of severe

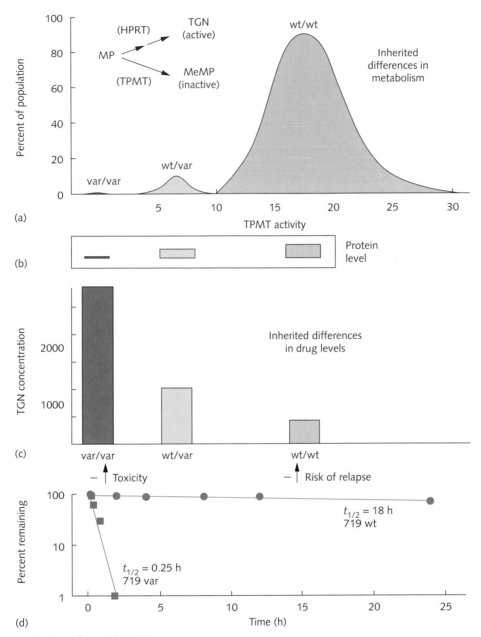

**Fig. 26.3 Thiopurine methyltransferase (TPMT)**

(a) Mercaptopurine (MP) can be activated to thioguanine nucleotides (TGN) by hypoxanthine phosphoribosyltransferase (HPRT) or inactivated to methylmercaptopurine (MeMP) via TPMT. The genetic polymorphism in *TPMT* results in a trimodal population frequency distribution in TPMT activity, with deficient activity caused by inheritance of two variant (var) alleles, intermediate activity caused by heterozygosity, and high activity associated with homozygote wild-type (wt) genotypes. (b) TPMT activity is directly proportional to the amount of TPMT protein and (c) is inversely related to intracellular concentrations of active TGN metabolites in hematopoietic cells following MP therapy. (d) The biochemical basis for low protein conferred by the most common var polymorphism (719A→G) is illustrated by the longer half-life for *in vitro* expressed wt TPMT when compared with the rapidly degraded var protein. From Jones TS, Yang W, Evans WE, Relling MV. (2007) Using HapMap tools in pharmacogenomic discovery: the thiopurine methyltransferase polymorphism. *Clinical Pharmacology and Therapeutics*, **81**, 729–734, with permission.

febrile neutropenia after combination chemotherapy for ALL in which mercaptopurine doses were individualized on the basis of *TPMT* genotypes.

Besides single-gene approaches, candidate pathway gene approaches and genome-wide approaches including HapMap analyses have provided important additional novel insights into the cellular pharmacology of thiopurines. For example, it has been shown that ALL blast cells containing the *TEL–AML1* fusion gene have lower expression of genes involved in purine metabolism and lower *de novo* purine synthesis compared with other ALL subtypes, and that the expression of genes encoding mercaptopurine metabolic enzymes and transporters (e.g., *SLC29A1*) was significantly associated with the *in vivo* accumulation of TGNs. Clearly, further studies are necessary to translate these interesting results from bench to bedside.

### Methotrexate

The antifolate drug methotrexate (MTX) is widely used in hematology to treat patients with ALL and lymphomas. Folates are essential cofactors in cellular one-carbon metabolism, pyrimidine and *de novo* purine synthesis, and the structural analog MTX inhibits steps in these pathways (Figure 26.4).

MTX pharmacokinetics exhibit large interindividual and intraindividual variability that is often unexplained in patients with normal renal function and sufficient hydration, and functional polymorphisms in MTX transporters may help to explain some of the observed differences. Indeed, a severe impairment in MTX excretion in an adult lymphoma patient was recently reported to be associated with a heterozygous 1271A→G (Arg412Gly) mutation in the *ABCC2* gene that results in non-functionality of the encoded ATP-binding cassette class transporter 2 or MRP2. If confirmed, these results may help to identify patients at very high risk for impaired MTX excretion.

Cellular uptake of MTX is mainly mediated by the reduced folate carrier (*RFC* or *SLC19A1*), whereas its efflux is mediated by ATP-binding cassette transporters. Putative relevant polymorphisms in these genes have been identified (e.g., 80G→A non-synonymous SNP in *SLC19A1*) but their clinical relevance remains to be validated. Intracellulary, the prodrug MTX is converted into poly(γ-glutamate) forms (MTXPGs) via folylpolyglutamate synthetase (*FPGS*). Interestingly, *FPGS* polymorphisms have not been definitely linked to MTX metabolism yet. Compared with MTX, MTXPGs are retained longer in cells because they are not readily effluxed by ATP-binding cassette transporters. MTX exerts its cytotoxic effects through inhibition of its primary target enzyme dihydrofolate reductase (*DHFR*), whereas MTXPGs also target other folate-dependent enzymes such

as thymidylate synthetase (*TYMS*) or glycinamide ribonucleotide transformylase. The interaction with key enzymes of *de novo* purine synthesis and pyrimidine synthesis leads to the inhibition of DNA synthesis and causes cell death.

MTXPGs can be converted back into the parental drug in lysosomes via γ-glutamylhydrolase (*GGH*). A so-called "substrate-specific" polymorphism was identified in the *GGH* gene (452C→T), with 67% lower catalytic activity in the degradation of long-chain MTXPGs but normal activity in the degradation of short-chain MTXPGs.

Genetic variants in key enzymes of the folate metabolism pathway, such as 5,10-methylene-tetrahydrofolate reductase (*MTHFR*) and thymidylate synthetase (*TYMS*), have been identified, and these variants may influence MTX therapy. An analysis of 520 children with ALL who were treated on Children's Cancer Group 1891 protocol showed that patients who carried the *MTHFR* 677C→T variant allele, which decreases enzymatic activity, had significantly higher risk of relapse. As this variant was not reported to be associated with a higher risk of toxicity and infection, if confirmed in other trials the *MTHFR* 677C→T variant may be a potential candidate for optimizing MTX therapy.

Associations between variants of the *TYMS* promoter and outcome were investigated in children with ALL treated on Dana-Farber Cancer Institute (DFCI) protocols. These studies showed that patients who were homozygous for a triple (3R) 28-bp repeat element (associated with higher *TYMS* expression) had a significantly higher risk of relapse or risk of an event. Moreover, in two investigations that examined the combined effects of different polymorphisms in different genes in children who were treated on DFCI or St Jude Total XIIIB protocols, patients (high-risk patients in Total XIIIB) who carried the *TYMS* 3R/3R genotype were found to have poorer outcomes. Because in neither the St Jude Total XIIIB nor DFCI protocols were *TYMS* polymorphisms associated with higher risk of toxicity, increased MTX dosage may be a strategy to improve outcome in patients who carry the *TYMS* 3R/3R genotype and are treated on similar protocols.

A pathway-directed candidate gene approach was used to elucidate genomic determinants of MTXPG accumulation in ALL blast cells. *In vivo* MTXPG accumulation was found to differ significantly among ALL subtypes, and expression data showed a significant pattern of folate-related genes significantly associated with ALL subtypes and cellular MTXPG accumulation. This study allowed researchers to identify mechanisms explaining subtype-specific differences in MTXPG accumulation and such insights may help to individualize MTX therapy in ALL.

More recently, genome-wide association studies have identified genomic determinants for MTXPG accumulation and *in vivo* response to MTX in childhood ALL. In an

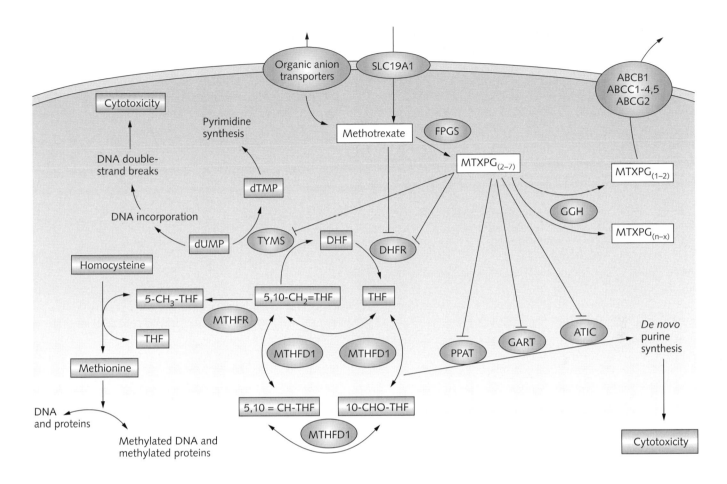

**Fig. 26.4 The folate pathway**

Methotrexate enters cells through the reduced folate carrier (SLC19A1) or other transport systems. Its main intracellular target is dihydrofolate reductase (DHFR), inhibition of which results in accumulation of dihydrofolate (DHF) and depletion of cellular folates. Cytosolic folylpolyglutamyl synthase (FPGS) adds glutamate residues to methotrexate to produce methotrexate polyglutamates (MTXPGs). Because these larger and more hydrophilic metabolites are not substrates of folate-transport systems, they are retained by the cell, and the resulting increase in the intracellular MTXPG concentration increases the efficacy of methotrexate. The addition of glutamate residues to methotrexate also increases its affinity for other target enzymes, i.e., thymidylate synthetase (TYMS) and enzymes of the *de novo* purine synthesis pathway: phosphoribosylpyrophosphate amidotransferase (PPAT), phosphoribosylglycinamide formyltransferase (GART), and IMP cyclohydrolase (ATIC). Other enzymes that are indirectly affected by methotrexate include 5,10-methylenetetrahydrofolate reductase (MTHFR) and methylenetetrahydrofolate dehydrogenase (MTHFD1). dTMP, deoxythymidine monophospate; dUMP, deoxyuridine monophospate; THF, tetrahydrofolate. From Cheok MH, Evans WE. (2006) Acute lymphoblastic leukaemia: a model for the pharmacogenomics of cancer therapy. *Nature Reviews. Cancer*, **6**, 117–129, with permission.

investigation at the St Jude Children's Research Hospital, gene expression, CNV, and SNP profiles were analyzed and seven genes were identified that were significantly associated with MTXPG accumulation in leukemia cells. In another investigation, gene expression in ALL blast cells was correlated with the *in vivo* response to MTX therapy in children with ALL; 48 genes (including *TYMS* and *DHFR*) were identified whose expression was significantly related to the reduction of circulating leukemia cells and cell proliferation. This measure of initial MTX *in vivo* response and the associ-

ated gene expression pattern were predictive of long-term disease-free survival, thereby providing new insights into the genomic basis of MTX resistance and interpatient differences in MTX response, pointing to new strategies to overcome MTX resistance in childhood ALL.

## Oral anticoagulant therapy

The oral anticoagulants of the coumarin type, warfarin (used in the UK and the USA), acenocoumarol and phenprocoumon (preferentially used in continental Europe), have similar pharmacodynamic properties but differences in half-life (phenprocoumon, 156–172 hours; warfarin, 32–43 hours; acenocoumarol, 2–8 hours), and act by inhibiting the activation of vitamin K-associated clotting factors. Each year, millions of patients take coumarins to prevent thromboembolic events in chronic conditions such as atrial fibrillation, deep venous thrombosis, pulmonary emboli, acute myocardial infarction, stroke, and disease and/or replacement of heart valves. A very narrow therapeutic index, with risk of serious hemorrhage if over-coagulated and thrombosis if under-coagulated, and inter-individual variability in response to coumarins necessitates individualization of treatment, which is based primarily on monitoring prothrombin time and calculation of the International Normalized Ratio (INR). Whereas INR is helpful in tailoring coumarin maintenance therapy, prospective studies have identified coumarin induction therapy as the period when the INR is most likely to be out of range and when the rate of iatrogenic ADRs is greatest. For example, because warfarin is the leading cause of hospital admissions for ADRs in the UK and the USA, there is an urgent need for establishing algorithms to estimate the coumarin dose a priori.

Many factors have been identified as affecting the degree of anticoagulation achieved by coumarins, including patient age (less dose requirement in elderly), gender, body size, ethnicity, diet (particularly vitamin K intake), cigarette smoking, disease (e.g., liver diseases, blood loss during surgery), and coadministration of other drugs (particularly those which inhibit the activity of CYP2C9). More recently, however, polymorphisms in genes that affect pharmacokinetics and pharmacodynamics of coumarins have been shown to act as major determinants of coumarin dosage requirements.

Coumarins are a racemic mixture of R and S enantiomers that differ in their patterns of metabolism and in their potency of pharmacodynamic effect. For example, it has been suggested that s-warfarin accounts for up to 70% of the overall anticoagulation response of warfarin. After oral administration, warfarin is completely absorbed and bound to albumin (99%) in plasma. Free warfarin is taken up into liver cells where it is biologically active and either inhibits VKORC1 or is catabolized by cytochrome P450 isoenzymes (Figure 26.5).

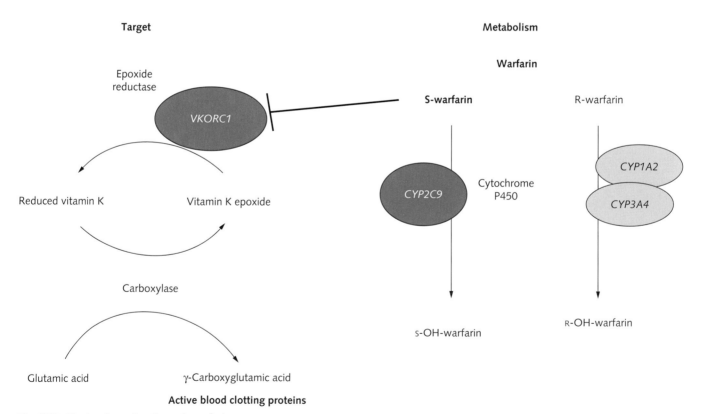

**Fig. 26.5 Mechanism of action of warfarin**

The racemic mixture of r- and the more potent s-warfarin inhibits the reductase in the vitamin K cycle, impairing the synthesis of active vitamin K-dependent clotting factors in liver cells and causing bleeding. The cytochrome P450 isoenzyme *CYP2C9* (and to a lesser extent *CYP3A4* and *CYP1A2*) and vitamin K epoxide reductase complex 1 (*VKORC1*) genotypes influence warfarin dose requirement.

**Cytochrome P450 2C9**

A number of CYP isoforms contribute to warfarin metabolism; however, hydroxylation by CYP2C9 is the most important inactivation pathway of the pharmacologically more relevant s-warfarin. CYP2C9 is the principal CYP2C isoenzyme in the human liver, and it is involved in the oxidative metabolism of several clinically important drugs, including oral anticoagulants, phenytoin, and various non-steroidal anti-inflammatory drugs. To date, numerous polymorphic alleles (*CYP2C9*1* to *CYP2C9*30*) have been identified for the known *CYP2C9* gene, at least half of which are associated with diminished enzyme activity. The two most common *CYP2C9* variants are *CYP2C9*2* and *CYP2C9*3*. *CYP2C9*2* has a cytosine to thymine transversion at nucleotide 430 (430C→T) that leads to the substitution of cysteine by arginine at amino acid residue 144 (Arg144Cys); *CYP2C9*3* has an adenine to cytosine transversion at nucleotide 1075 (1075A→C) that encodes isoleucine instead of leucine at amino acid residue 359 (Ile359Leu). As with most polymorphisms, there are differences in the frequency of polymorphic *CYP2C9* alleles among different ethnic groups. In Caucasians, the overall allelic frequency of *CYP2C9*2* is about 10–20%, and that of *CYP2C9*3* is about 5–10%. The *2 and *3 variants are very rare in African-Americans and Asians; 95% of these persons express the wild-type genotype *1/*1 (i.e., extensive metabolizers). Compared with wild-type enzyme activity of *CYP2C9*1*, the enzyme activity of the *CYP2C9*2* variant is reduced about 30–50%, and the *CYP2C9*3* variant activity is reduced by 90% *in vitro*.

Both *CYP2C9*2* and *CYP2C9*3* are important in the metabolism of warfarin, as well as of other coumarin anticoagulants, and it is well established that the *CYP2C9* genotype is correlated with coumarin metabolism and dose requirement. However, because interindividual variability in the dose requirement occurs within the various *CYP2C9* groups, genotyping for additional polymorphic genes that encode clotting factors, transporters and warfarin target could possibly further improve anticoagulation therapy. Indeed, a pharmacodynamic mechanism underlying warfarin resistance has been elucidated with the discovery of sequence variants in the warfarin target gene *VKORC1*, which encodes the vitamin K epoxide reductase complex 1.

**Vitamin K epoxide reductase complex 1**

This complex regenerates reduced vitamin K for another cycle of catalysis, essential for the γ-carboxylation of the vitamin K-dependent clotting factors II, VII, IX, and X (Figure 26.5). The identification of common variants in *VKORC1* has emerged as one of the most important genetic factors determining coumarin dose requirements. Main

*VKORC1* haplotypes include the reference haplotype (wild-type) *VKORC1*1*, the low-dose coumarin haplotype *VKORC1*2* (which includes an SNP in the promoter region −1639/3673G→A), and the high-dose coumarin haplotypes *VKORC1*3* and *VKORC1*4*. There are major differences in the distribution of *VKORC1* haplotypes among ethnic groups, and this may explain inter-ethnic differences in coumarin requirement. For example, the significantly higher average warfarin requirement in Africans is in line with the significantly lower occurrence of the low-dose coumarin *VKORC1*2* haplotype in Africans. Overall, the hereditary pharmacodynamic factor *VKORC1* may explain about 25% of the variance in coumarin dose requirement, compared with 5–10% for the hereditary pharmacokinetic factor *CYP2C9* alone.

Pharmacogenomic dosing algorithms for coumarins have been developed, and have for example identified the *VKORC1* promoter SNP −1639/3673G→A as the most important factor in predicting warfarin dose requirement. In a recent investigation, the pharmacogenomic equation explained 54% of the variability in the warfarin dose; this dosing algorithm is available at a non-profit website (http://www.WarfarinDosing.org). Several companies have developed genotyping platforms to facilitate pharmacogenomic dosing of coumarins, and the US FDA has also changed warfarin labeling to encourage lower initial doses in patients who have the *VKORC1* −1639/3673G→A (or *VKORC1*2*), *CYP2C9*2*, or *CYP2C9*3* alleles. The International Warfarin Pharmacogenetics Consortium recently provided a pharmacogenetic algorithm (including clinical factors) that can be used as a robust basis for a prospective clinical trial of the efficacy of genetically informed dose estimation for patients who require warfarin.

## Genome-wide approaches

Robust high-throughput whole-genome technologies like global gene expression profiling using DNA microarrays or global SNP analyses using oligonucleotide SNP arrays are increasingly used to establish pharmacogenomic models. An advantage of the unbiased genome-wide strategy is that it includes most genes or SNPs of potential importance and therefore may help to identify new therapeutic and diagnostic targets. A disadvantage of this non-targeted genome-wide approach is that it will inevitably be influenced by noise (i.e., expression signals of irrelevant genes or SNPs) and that functionally unimportant genes or SNPs will be identified by chance alone (i.e., false-positive results). The successful implementation of this genome-wide strategy has been achieved rather easily in hematological diseases like leukemias, because these malignancies are rather homogeneous liquid tumors and because leukemia blast cells can be easily isolated and characterized.

Here we give some selected examples on how genome-wide approaches have been used to elucidate genomic determinants for drug resistance mechanisms in childhood ALL, and how the insights obtained from these investigations can be used to develop strategies to circumvent drug resistance mechanisms and to identify novel therapeutic targets in ALL cells that are resistant to conventional antileukemic drugs.

## Overcoming drug resistance and identification of novel therapeutic targets

Genome-wide assessment of gene expression has been used to identify gene expression profiles that are significantly associated with sensitivity or resistance to individual antileukemic agents and/or treatment outcome (Fig. 26.6). This work began in human tumor cell lines, but has moved rapidly to the assessment of primary ALL cells. For example, in order to elucidate resistance mechanisms for antileukemic agents in primary ALL cells, *in vitro* sensitivity was used to identify gene expression patterns that differed significantly between sensitive and resistant ALL cells. This investigation

revealed distinctive sets of genes associated with drug resistance for each of four structurally different and widely used antileukemic agents (prednisolone, vincristine, L-asparaginase and daunorubicin). Of note, there was very little overlap among resistance genes for the four agents, supporting the concept of multiagent combination chemotherapy for ALL. Importantly, the identified gene expression patterns were significantly related to treatment response in a multivariate analysis, and this four-drug gene profile was subsequently validated in an independent cohort of children with ALL treated with the same agents but on a different protocol at a separate institution.

In further investigations, a unique set of 49 genes was found to be associated with multidrug cross-resistance to these four antileukemic agents, and the cross-resistance gene expression profile was able to identify a subgroup of ALL patients with a markedly inferior treatment outcome (38% event-free survival). Recently, genome-wide gene expression in ALL blast cells was correlated with the *in vivo* response to MTX therapy in children with ALL, and 48 genes (including *TYMS* and *DHFR*) were identified whose expression was significantly related to the reduction of circulating leukemia cells and treatment outcome. Collectively, this series of

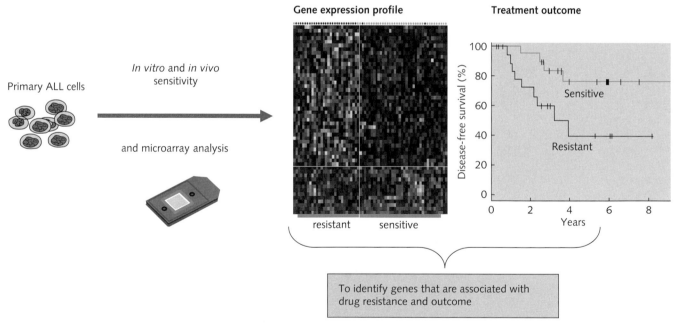

### Fig. 26.6 A gene expression signature associated with drug resistance

A large set of primary acute lymphoblastic leukemia (ALL) cells are subjected to gene expression analysis and sensitivity to individual medications to identify gene expression patterns that are related to *in vitro* drug sensitivity and potentially to treatment outcome. After prospective validation, these gene expression patterns might identify patients at high risk of treatment failure and treatment can subsequently be adjusted. In addition, by linking genes to resistance to individual anticancer agents, this might provide insights into the mechanisms of resistance and point to strategies for overcoming drug resistance. From Cheok MH, Evans WE. (2006) Acute lymphoblastic leukaemia: a model for the pharmacogenomics of cancer therapy. *Nature Reviews. Cancer*, **6**, 117–129, with permission.

experiments have thus shown that the expression of a relatively small set of less than 50 genes can identify ALL cells resistant to widely used antileukemic agents and that this is related not only to *in vivo* and *in vitro* drug resistance but importantly to the outcome of patients treated with these medications.

These findings also point to potential new targets for the development of new medications to modulate resistance to current chemotherapy. For example, a novel approach was used to computationally connect disease-associated gene expression signatures (e.g., ALL blast cells intrinsically sensitive or resistant to glucocorticoid-induced apoptosis *in vitro*) to drug-associated gene expression profiles, the so-called Connectivity Map, in order to identify molecules that reverse a drug resistance signature. This strategy builds on prior findings that antileukemic drugs can induce treatment-specific changes in gene expression in leukemia cells *in vivo*. Indeed, the profile induced by the mTOR inhibitor rapamycin was found to match the signature of glucocorticoid sensitivity in ALL cells, and it was shown that rapamycin sensitized a resistant leukemia cell line to glucocorticoid-induced apoptosis via modulation of the anti-apoptotic protein MCL-1. These findings are consistent with earlier work revealing MCL-1 overexpression in steroid-resistant ALL. Collectively, this series of experiments suggests that glucocorticoid in combination with rapamycin could be an effective approach for overcoming intrinsic glucocorticoid resistance in ALL, thereby providing evidence that such a gene expression-based chemical genomic approach might be useful for identifying molecules with the potential to overcome intrinsic drug resistance in leukemia.

Using genome-wide gene expression analyses, the FMS-like tyrosine kinase 3 (*FLT3*) gene was recently identified as being overexpressed in certain ALL subtypes (i.e., MLL-rearranged and hyperdiploid ALL). Small-molecule inhibitors of FLT3 (e.g., CEP-701 and PKC412) have been shown to inhibit growth in cells that overexpress *FLT3*. Thus, the inclusion of FLT3 inhibitors seems worthy of being investigated in the therapy of the poor-prognostic ALL subtype with MLL rearrangements, especially infant ALL, and perhaps of hyperdiploid ALL that also overexpress *FLT3*. The Interfant Study Group is already planning to include FLT3 inhibitors in future clinical trials for infants with MLL-rearranged ALL.

## Summary and challenges for the future

As there are numerous non-genetic factors that influence drug effects (e.g., compliance, nutritional factors, concur-

rent medications), it is clear that pharmacogenomics will never explain all interindividual variability in drug effects. However, there is evidence that pharmacogenomic models can help to improve drug treatment in hematology by facilitating appropriate dose individualization, optimal treatment selection, and drug discovery. For example, candidate gene approaches have identified functionally important variants in the *TPMT*, *CYP2C9*, and *VCORC1* genes, and the *TPMT* and *CYP2C9/VCORC1* models can now be used to individualize thiopurine and coumarin therapy a priori, thereby reducing the risk of severe ADRs.

However, in general many of the published candidate gene studies have non-negligible limitations, such as the retrospective nature of some studies and the relatively low number of patients included. An example on how to assess the relationship between candidate polymorphisms and clinical phenotypes in a prospective clinical trial was recently provided by the Scottish Randomized Trial in Ovarian Cancer. Using different statistical approaches (false-discovery rate, univariate and multivariate models), their study served as a filter for determining which SNPs had sufficiently robust associations with relevant phenotypes.

It is clearly recognized that most drug responses are influenced by many genes, so polygenic models will be required to fully elucidate the genomic determinants of drug responses. Besides candidate pathway gene approaches, genome-wide approaches are of increasing importance. Future investigations will therefore focus on the use of large-scale public genetic databases, such as the HapMap project, to elucidate linkage of genetic markers and drug effects in different populations, leading to the identification of new genes and the elucidation of polygenic determinants of drug responses. Recently, ultra-high-throughput genotyping became possible, with the ability to analyze more than 1 million SNPs using oligonucleotide SNP arrays. This high-throughput genotyping method, and the relatively manageable number of tag SNPs, will help to establish genome-wide pharmacogenomic models.

The final important challenge will be to integrate information obtained from ultra-high-throughput genomics (e.g., genome-wide human SNP arrays), proteomics (the large-scale study of proteins), and pharmaco-metabonomics (the prediction of efficacy or toxicity of a drug or xenobiotic intervention in an individual based on a mathematical model of pre-intervention metabolite signatures) to elucidate causes of interpatient variability in drug response. Collectively, the remaining challenges in pharmacogenomics, though partly daunting, are better than continuing to stumble in the dark by using medications on the principle of trial and error.

# Further reading

## Principles of pharmacogenomics

Cheng Q, Yang W, Raimondi SC, Pui CH, Relling MV, Evans WE. (2005) Karyotypic abnormalities create discordance of germline genotype and cancer cell phenotypes. *Nature Genetics*, **37**, 878–882.

Cheng Q, Cheng C, Crews KR *et al.* (2006) Epigenetic regulation of human gamma-glutamyl hydrolase activity in acute lymphoblastic leukemia cells. *American Journal of Human Genetics*, **79**, 264–274.

Cheok MH, Evans WE. (2006) Acute lymphoblastic leukaemia: a model for the pharmacogenomics of cancer therapy. *Nature Reviews. Cancer*, **6**, 117–129.

Cheok MH, Pottier N, Kager L, Evans WE. (2009) Pharmacogenetics in acute lymphoblastic leukemia. *Seminars in Hematology*, **46**, 39–51.

Evans WE, McLeod HL. (2003) Pharmacogenomics: drug disposition, drug targets, and side effects. *New England Journal of Medicine*, **348**, 538–549.

Evans WE, Relling MV. (1999) Pharmacogenomics: translating functional genomics into rational therapeutics. *Science*, **286**, 487–491.

Evans WE, Relling MV. (2004) Moving towards individualized medicine with pharmacogenomics. *Nature*, **429**, 464–468.

Huang RS, Ratain MJ. (2009) Pharmacogenetics and pharmacogenomics of anticancer agents. *CA. A Cancer Journal for Clinicians*, **59**, 42–55.

Ingelman-Sundberg M, Sim SC, Gomez A, Rodriguez-Antona C. (2007) Influence of cytochrome P450 polymorphisms on drug therapies: pharmacogenetic, pharmacoepigenetic and clinical aspects. *Pharmacology and Therapeutics*, **116**, 496–526.

Kimchi-Sarfaty C, Oh JM, Kim IW *et al.* (2007) A "silent" polymorphism in the MDR1 gene changes substrate specificity. *Science*, **315**, 525–528.

Marsh S, Paul J, King CR, Gifford G, McLeod HL, Brown R. (2007) Pharmacogenetic assessment of toxicity and outcome after platinum plus taxane chemotherapy in ovarian cancer: the Scottish Randomised Trial in Ovarian Cancer. *Journal of Clinical Oncology*, **25**, 4528–4535.

Mishra PJ, Humeniuk R, Longo-Sorbello GS, Banerjee D, Bertino JR. (2007) A miR-24 microRNA binding-site polymorphism in dihydrofolate reductase gene leads to methotrexate resistance. *Proceedings of the National Academy of Sciences of the United States of America*, **104**, 13513–13518.

Roden DM, Altman RB, Benowitz NL *et al.* (2006) Pharmacogenomics: challenges and opportunities. *Annals of Internal Medicine*, **145**, 749–757.

Weinshilboum R. (2003) Inheritance and drug response. *New England Journal of Medicine*, **348**, 529–537.

## Variation in the human genome

Beckmann JS, Estivill X, Antonarakis SE. (2007) Copy number variants and genetic traits: closer to the resolution of phenotypic to genotypic variability. *Nature Reviews. Genetics*, **8**, 639–646.

Feuk L, Carson AR, Scherer SW. (2006) Structural variation in the human genome. *Nature Reviews. Genetics*, **7**, 85–97.

Frazer KA, Ballinger DG, Cox DR *et al.* (2007) A second generation human haplotype map of over 3.1 million SNPs. *Nature*, **449**, 851–861.

Hinds DA, Kloek AP, Jen M, Chen X, Frazer KA. (2006) Common deletions and SNPs are in linkage disequilibrium in the human genome. *Nature Genetics*, **38**, 82–85.

Redon R, Ishikawa S, Fitch KR *et al.* (2006) Global variation in copy number in the human genome. *Nature*, **444**, 444–454.

## Candidate gene approaches

Aplenc R, Thompson J, Han P *et al.* (2005) Methylenetetrahydrofolate reductase polymorphisms and therapy response in pediatric acute lymphoblastic leukemia. *Cancer Research*, **65**, 2482–2487.

Gage BF, Eby C, Johnson J *et al.* (2008) Use of pharmacogenetic and clinical factors to predict the therapeutic dose of warfarin. *Clinical Pharmacology and Therapeutics*, **84**, 326–331.

Hulot JS, Villard E, Maguy A *et al.* (2005) A mutation in the drug transporter gene ABCC2 associated with impaired methotrexate elimination. *Pharmacogenetics and Genomics*, **15**, 277–285.

International Warfarin Pharmacogenetics Consortium. (2009) Estimation of the warfarin dose with clinical and pharmacogenetic data. *New England Journal of Medicine*, **360**, 753–764.

Kager L, Cheok M, Yang W *et al.* (2005) Folate pathway gene expression differs in subtypes of acute lymphoblastic leukemia and influences methotrexate pharmacodynamics. *Journal of Clinical Investigation*, **115**, 110–117.

Kishi S, Cheng C, French D *et al.* (2007) Ancestry and pharmacogenetics of antileukemic drug toxicity. *Blood*, **109**, 4151–4157.

Krajinovic M, Costea I, Primeau M, Dulucq S, Moghrabi A. (2005) Combining several polymorphisms of thymidylate synthase gene for pharmacogenetic analysis. *Pharmacogenomics Journal*, **5**, 374–380.

Lennard L, Richards S, Cartwright CS, Mitchell C, Lilleyman JS, Vora A. (2006) The thiopurine methyltransferase genetic polymorphism is associated with thioguanine-related veno-occlusive disease of the liver in children with acute lymphoblastic leukemia. *Clinical Pharmacology and Therapeutics*, **80**, 375–383.

Oldenburg J, Bevans CG, Fregin A, Geisen C, Muller-Reible C, Watzka M. (2007) Current pharmacogenetic developments in oral anticoagulation therapy: the influence of variant VKORC1 and CYP2C9 alleles. *Thrombosis and Haemostasis*, **98**, 570–578.

Relling MV, Hancock ML, Rivera GK *et al.* (1999) Mercaptopurine therapy intolerance and heterozygosity at the thiopurine S-methyltransferase gene locus. *Journal of the National Cancer Institute*, **91**, 2001–2008.

Relling MV, Pui CH, Cheng C, Evans WE. (2006) Thiopurine methyltransferase in acute lymphoblastic leukemia. *Blood*, **107**, 843–844.

Rocha JC, Cheng C, Liu W *et al.* (2005) Pharmacogenetics of outcome in children with acute lymphoblastic leukemia. *Blood*, **105**, 4752–4758.

Rodriguez-Antona C, Ingelman-Sundberg M. (2006) Cytochrome P450 pharmacogenetics and cancer. *Oncogene*, **25**, 1679–1691.

Stanulla M, Schaeffeler E, Flohr T *et al.* (2005) Thiopurine methyltransferase (TPMT) genotype and early treatment response to mercaptopurine in childhood acute lymphoblastic leukemia. *Journal of the American Medical Association*, **293**, 1485–1489.

Stocco G, Cheok MH, Crews KR *et al.* (2009) Genetic polymorphism of inosine triphosphate pyrophosphatase is a determinant of mercaptopurine metabolism and toxicity during treatment for acute lymphoblastic leukemia. *Clinical Pharmacology and Therapeutics*, **85**, 164–172.

Wang L, Weinshilboum R. (2006) Thiopurine S-methyltransferase pharmacogenetics: insights, challenges and future directions. *Oncogene*, **25**, 1629–1638.

## Genome-wide approaches

Brown P, Levis M, Shurtleff S, Campana D, Downing J, Small D. (2005) FLT3 inhibition selectively kills childhood acute lymphoblastic leukemia cells with high levels of FLT3 expression. *Blood*, **105**, 812–820.

Cheok MH, Yang W, Pui CH *et al.* (2003) Treatment-specific changes in gene expression discriminate in vivo drug response in human leukemia cells. *Nature Genetics*, **34**, 85–90.

French D, Yang W, Cheng C *et al.* (2009) Acquired variation outweighs inherited variation in whole genome analysis of methotrexate polyglutamate accumulation in leukemia. *Blood*, **113**, 4512–4520.

Holleman A, Cheok MH, den Boer ML *et al.* (2004) Gene-expression patterns in drug-resistant acute lymphoblastic leukemia cells and response to treatment. *New England Journal of Medicine*, **351**, 533–542.

Lamb J, Crawford ED, Peck D *et al.* (2006) The Connectivity Map: using gene-expression signatures to connect small molecules, genes, and disease. *Science*, **313**, 1929–1935.

Lugthart S, Cheok MH, den Boer ML *et al.* (2005) Identification of genes associated with chemotherapy crossresistance and treatment response in childhood acute lymphoblastic leukemia. *Cancer Cell*, **7**, 375–386.

Sorich M, Pottier N, Pei D *et al.* (2008) In vivo response to methotrexate forecasts outcome of acute lymphoblastic leukemia and has a distinct gene expression profile. *PLoS Medicine*, **5**, e83.

Stam RW, den Boer ML, Schneider P *et al.* (2005) Targeting FLT3 in primary MLL-gene-rearranged infant acute lymphoblastic leukemia. *Blood*, **106**, 2484–2490.

Wei G, Twomey D, Lamb J *et al.* (2006) Gene expression-based chemical genomics identifies rapamycin as a modulator of MCL1 and glucocorticoid resistance. *Cancer Cell*, **10**, 331–342.

Yang JJ, Cheng C, Yang W *et al.* (2009) Genome-wide interrogation of germline genetic variation associated with treatment response in childhood acute lymphoblastic leukemia. *Journal of the American Medical Association*, **301**, 393–403.

Yeoh EJ, Ross ME, Shurtleff SA *et al.* (2002) Classification, subtype discovery, and prediction of outcome in pediatric acute lymphoblastic leukemia by gene expression profiling. *Cancer Cell*, **1**, 133–143.

# Chapter 27 Gene expression profiling in the study of lymphoid malignancies

## Ulf Klein & Riccardo Dalla-Favera

*Herbert Irving Comprehensive Cancer Center, Columbia University, New York, NY, USA*

## Introduction

Lymphoid malignancies have long been studied using immunohistochemical, biochemical and genetic approaches to dissect their phenotype and genotype and identify their cellular derivation. Gene expression profiling (GEP) analysis provides another potent tool for analyzing the pathogenesis of these tumors. By allowing simultaneous screening of thousands of parameters in the form of expressed genes, GEP analysis has had a major impact on our understanding of lymphoid neoplasia.

The platforms of GEP analysis, DNA microarrays, contain a large number (tens of thousands) of either polymerase chain reaction (PCR) products or shorter oligonucleotides representing distinct mRNA sequences that are spotted on glass slides. RNA transcripts from the cells under study are labeled with fluorescent tags, hybridized to the microarrays, and the respective fluorescent signals are acquired by scanning the gene chip. The normalized data generated from the hybridizations of various samples are then comparatively analyzed by applying biostatistical methods to determine gene expression differences.

The enormous number of data points resulting from GEP experiments, especially in a large study, called for the development of hierarchical clustering algorithms that can identify patterns of gene expression among the cell types under study (Figure 27.1). With these algorithms, unsupervised clustering can be used to identify cell types which have not been classified a priori, whereas supervised analysis allows the identification of differentially expressed genes between

samples defined a priori according to a given criterion, for example cell type or genotype.

The pattern of expressed genes identified by supervised or unsupervised clustering that specifies a cell type is conventionally called a "signature." These signatures are then used for a number of goals in the study of disease pathogenesis, and eventually for the development of novel clinical approaches for these diseases. Thus, gene expression signatures may help to distinguish novel tumor subtypes that are not currently identifiable by other diagnostic means based on single marker analysis. It would be especially desirable to identify subtypes of tumors that cannot be distinguished by current methods but which differ in their clinical outcome. Second, the comparative analysis of gene expression profiles derived from lymphoid malignancies versus those from healthy lymphocytes may help to identify the normal cellular counterparts of the tumors, and provide insight into the molecular mechanisms responsible for malignant development. Third, the comparative analysis of a large number of samples, especially when using supervised analysis tools, allows the identification of genes that are specifically upregulated or downregulated in B-cell malignancies. Following validation of the corresponding gene products in tumor biopsies, such molecules may represent potential diagnostic or therapeutic targets. Finally, GEP may allow the activity of certain signaling pathways to be monitored in the cell type under study. To this end, the respective profiles are either scanned for concerted changes in the expression of genes known to be associated with a particular signaling pathway or transcriptional response, or the gene expression signatures specific for a certain signaling or transcriptional activation are generated *in vitro* and then tracked for their occurrence in the respective *in vivo* signatures. These results may provide insights into the specific stimuli to which a cell is subjected.

*Molecular Hematology*, 3rd edition. Edited by Drew Provan and John Gribben.
© 2010 Blackwell Publishing.

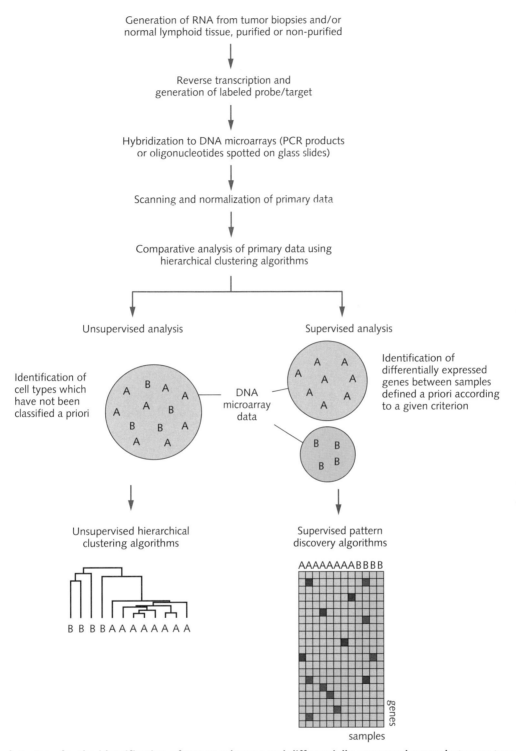

**Fig. 27.1 General strategy for the identification of tumor subtypes and differentially expressed genes between tumor subtypes by GEP analysis**

In the matrix (lower right), the dark and light tints identify upregulated and downregulated genes, respectively. Columns represent individual samples and rows correspond to genes.

Microarray platforms and other detection mechanisms have already been developed to assay for microRNAs and could identify cell type-specific microRNA signatures. In the future, GEP experiments will undoubtedly complement the analysis of a cell type-specific transcriptome with that of the corresponding miRnome.

## Identification of tumor subtypes

Certain categories of lymphoid malignancies, such as diffuse large B-cell lymphoma (DLBL), exhibit marked clinical heterogeneity, suggesting that what is presently recognized as single disease entity may in fact include distinct pathological conditions. By enabling the simultaneous screening of thousands of parameters, GEP analysis substantially enhances the sensitivity of analyses that are aimed at identifying tumor subtypes, which may eventually lead to improved diagnostic approaches that can predict clinical outcome with higher confidence.

The feasibility of the molecular classification of cancer by GEP was first demonstrated by its ability to distinguish acute myeloid leukemia (AML) and acute lymphoblastic leukemia (ALL). Without previous knowledge about the origin of tumor specimens, GEP could determine whether new leukemia cases were derived from ALL or AML. The principal steps of this approach are summarized in Figure 27.2a.

As mentioned above, DLBLs represent a category of lymphoid malignancies that appears very heterogeneous. Using a gene chip enriched for genes and expressed sequence tag (ESTs) expressed in B-lymphocytes ("lymphochip"), a panel of DLBL cases could be separated into two subgroups, one that has characteristics of germinal center B cells (GC-type DLBL) and another that resembles *in vitro*-activated B cells (ABC-type DLBL). Significantly, the clinical data from these two subgroups suggested that the GC-type DLBL has a more benign clinical course. Subsequent studies, using either the same or a different type of DNA microarray, found that DLBLs can be subdivided into three major groups by GEP. The observation from GEP analysis that DLBL cases can be classified into biologically distinct subgroups has fueled new hypotheses about the pathogenic mechanisms of this disease that are currently being investigated.

Compared with other B-cell malignancies, B-cell chronic lymphocytic leukemia (B-CLL) was long considered to be a relatively homogeneous disease, primarily because of the uniform morphology of the tumor cells. Genetic analyses could identify subgroups of B-CLLs that show particular genomic lesions, which most frequently represent deletions. Furthermore, unlike other tumor types, B-CLL cases can be subdivided into those that harbor somatic hypermutations in their rearranged immunoglobulin variable (IgV) genes, and those with germline IgV sequences. Notably, the two subgroups also differ in their clinical prognosis, IgV-mutated B-CLLs showing a more benign disease course. On this background, it was surprising to find that global gene expression analyses performed independently by two laboratories revealed few gene expression differences among the two B-CLL subgroups (approximately 100 among more than 10 000 genes). Nonetheless, the small set of genes distinguishing IgV-mutated and -unmutated B-CLL cases could assign unclassified panels of B-CLL cases into either of the two subgroups with high confidence. Based on the example of B-CLL, Figure 27.2b summarizes the use of a set of genes identified by pattern discovery analysis in the class prediction of unrelated cases. At present, the relatively laborious and costly GEP analysis is not widely used in clinical practice to distinguish B-CLL subtypes. However, gene products that have been identified in GEP-based analyses to correlate with subtypes of B-CLL are either being tested for their potential value in, or have already found their way into, clinical diagnosis of B-CLL. For example, a flow-cytometric assay has been developed to measure the tyrosine kinase ZAP-70, which is predominantly expressed in B-CLL with an IgV-unmutated genotype and which correlates with poor prognosis. Today, ZAP-70 expression in a newly diagnosed B-CLL case is often determined together with the IgV gene hypermutational status and the cytogenetic profile. In the future, the set of genes separating IgV-mutated and -unmutated cases may be helpful in clarifying the diagnosis of ambiguous cases (e.g., those showing a low level of IgV somatic hypermutation), either by performing gene chip hybridization or by establishing biochemical or immunohistochemical assays to detect the most informative B-CLL subtype-specific molecules.

## Normal cellular counterparts and mechanism of transformation

Ever since it became possible to classify lymphoid tumors as B-cell- or T-cell-derived malignancies, the focus has shifted to further elucidate the stage of differentiation from which each tumor type derives within each lymphoid lineage. To understand the precise developmental stage of a B-cell malignancy has obvious implications for understanding its pathogenesis: it may become possible to dissociate the components of the malignancy that represent the normal cellular stage of development from which the tumor arose from truly disease-associated genes, providing potential insights into the mechanism of transformation. Also, tumor-specific gene products thus identified can further be studied for their involvement in the pathogenesis of the malignancy.

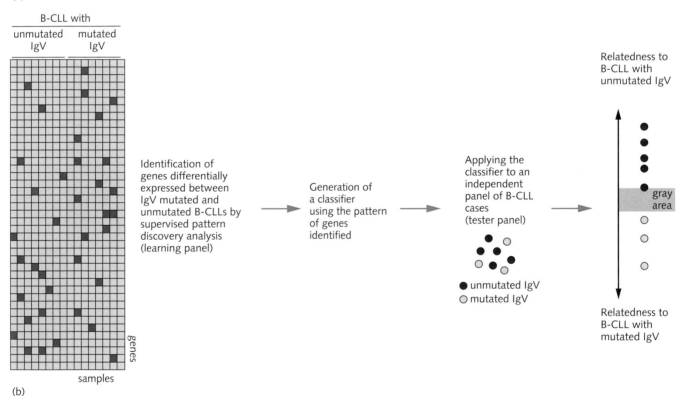

Generation of gene expression profiles
from a number of samples from two (or
serveral) distinct lymphoid malignancies

Generation of a class predictor based on
the DNA microarray data

Testing the suitability of the class predictor
by cross validation using the original tumor
panel

Applying the class predictor to an independent
panel of cases, verifying its suitability
by independent methods

(a)

B-CLL with

unmutated    mutated
IgV          IgV

genes

samples

(b)

Identification of
genes differentially
expressed between
IgV mutated and
unmutated B-CLLs by
supervised pattern
discovery analysis
(learning panel)

Generation of
a classifier
using the pattern
of genes
identified

Applying the
classifier to an
independent
panel of B-CLL
cases
(tester panel)

● unmutated IgV
○ mutated IgV

Relatedness to
B-CLL with
unmutated IgV

gray
area

Relatedness to
B-CLL with
mutated IgV

**Fig. 27.2 Class predictors (classifiers)**
(a) Generation and testing of a class predictor by GEP to identify tumor subtypes. (b) Generation of a class predictor by supervised pattern
discovery. Genes differentially expressed between two tumor subtypes that differ in the level of IgV gene somatic hypermutation are identified
by supervised analysis. A classifier is generated using these genes and applied to an unclassified panel. The relatedness of the respective cases
to either subtype is scored and quantified. Upregulated genes are identified by the dark tint, downregulated genes by the light tint. Columns
represent samples and rows correspond to genes. The arrows in the diagram to the right denote increasing relatedness to either B-CLL
subtype; the relatedness of cases outside the gray area to either of the CLL subtypes is statistically significant. B-CLL, B-cell chronic lymphocytic
leukemia.

Early studies relied on morphological and histological comparison with normal lymphoid tissue to determine the derivation of lymphoid tumors. Subsequently, these analyses were refined by the use of monoclonal antibodies against lymphoid-derived cell surface antigens. This phase was followed by the effort to determine the presence of somatic hypermutation in the rearranged IgV genes of B-cell malignancies as well as B-cell subpopulations isolated from healthy individuals as a marker of mature antigen-experienced B cells. The combination of cell surface markers used to isolate the phenotypically diverse normal B-cell subsets and the concomitant analysis of the IgV genes led to the establishment of a B-cell developmental scheme that was used to assign various B-cell tumor subtypes to defined differentiation stages.

These undertakings clarified the derivation of several tumor entities, as exemplified by the case of Burkitt lymphoma which, based on the expression of markers associated with bone marrow development, was long thought to be derived from an early B cell with actively rearranging antigen receptor genes, but was eventually classified as a germinal center-derived B-cell tumor based on the presence of hypermutated IgV genes. Still, these methods could not conclusively determine the derivation of various tumor entities, most notably DLBL and B-CLL. However, since GEP substantially increases the parameters available for comparing tumor and normal B cells, it should permit a decidedly more conclusive assignment of a tumor to a normal B-cell subpopulation, also by way of outnumbering ectopically expressed genes whose expression could mar such comparisons. A notable advantage of GEP conducted with a common DNA microarray is that comparisons are relative in nature, such that the actual identities of the gene products are irrelevant; genes are simply scored as upregulated or downregulated. Instead, it is the quantity of the gene expression changes between cell subsets that is measured and used to determine developmental relatedness (Figure 27.3).

Based on IgV gene mutation studies, DLBL was early on shown to be derived from B cells residing in the germinal center of the peripheral lymphoid organs. However, as detailed in the previous section, this tumor group is extremely heterogeneous, both in morphological/histological presentation and clinical prognosis. Using genome-wide GEP, DLBL cases could be classified into three main subtypes, including one related to germinal center B cells (GC-type DLBL) and one related to *in vitro*-activated B cells (ABC-type DLBL). While the relationship between the GC-type DLBL subtype and germinal center B cells is strongly suggested by the comparison to *ex vivo* cells, the precise normal cellular counterpart is not so evident for ABC-type DLBL. This is because the existence and localization of such cells in the lymphoid tissues is unclear as no B cell with such a phe-

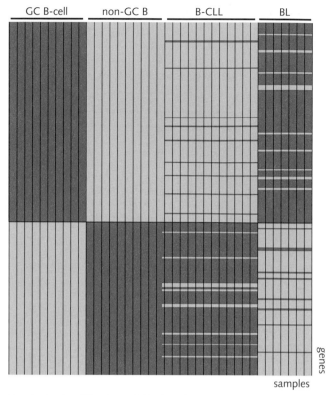

**Fig. 27.3 Identification of the histological derivation of B-cell malignancies**

Genes differentially expressed between normal B-cell subpopulations are identified by supervised pattern discovery analysis. The expression level of the respective genes in different subtypes of B-cell malignancy [B-cell chronic lymphocytic leukemia (B-CLL) and Burkitt lymphoma (BL)] is shown along with the differentially expressed genes. The relatedness of the B-CLL cases to the non-germinal center (GC) B cells and that of the BL cases to the GC B cells is visible from the color-coded expression values and can be quantitatively expressed by statistical analysis. Upregulated genes are identified by the dark tint and downregulated genes by the light tint.

notype has yet been described. However, when discussing the cellular derivation of lymphoid malignancies, one has to consider that the phenotype of a particular B-cell tumor is the product of both the gene expression of the normal cellular counterpart and the changes in gene expression induced by the specific transforming event. Nevertheless, although questions remain regarding the cellular origin of the individual DLBL subtypes, this example represents a first demonstration for the successful use of GEP in assigning lymphoid malignancies to normal B-cell developmental stages.

A methodologically different approach was employed in an attempt to identify the normal cellular counterpart of B-CLL. This malignancy is unique among B-cell-derived tumors in that B-CLL cases carry either somatically mutated or unmutated IgV genes in almost equal fractions, suggesting that only a subset of cases is derived from cells that have passed the germinal center (*see previous section*). Also, the surface marker expression (CD5$^+$CD23$^+$CD27$^+$) of B-CLL tumors is inconsistent with that of any known normal B-cell subpopulation. To define the normal counterpart of B-CLL, specific expression profiles were first established by supervised pattern discovery analysis for each of the developmentally distinct B-cell subpopulations, followed by the tracking of the respective profiles in the B-CLL gene expression data. The relatedness of a given B-CLL biopsy to the subset-specific profile can be quantitatively expressed by a measure of the statistical significance (*P*-value). Using this approach, a relationship of B-CLL to a particular post-germinal center developmental stage, the antigen-experienced (memory or marginal zone) B cell, was uncovered, a result that is consistent with other phenotypic and genotypic properties, suggesting that B-CLL is derived from the malignant transformation of an antigen-experienced B cell. Similarly, a comparative GEP analysis between hairy cell leukemia (HCL) cases and normal B-cell subsets suggested that the tumor cell precursor of HCL is also related to an antigen-experienced B cell, possibly of marginal zone derivation. The examples of B-CLL and HCL demonstrates that GEP has contributed substantially to the emerging concept that certain B-cell malignancies originate from the oncogenic transformation of post-germinal center memory/marginal zone B cells.

A subtype of ALL that carries a translocation involving the mixed-lineage leukemia gene (*MLL*) has a particularly poor prognosis. GEP of this subgroup versus ALLs without the respective translocation and AML showed that the ALL subgroup with *MLL* translocation displays a unique gene expression profile with characteristic features of a distinct early hematopoietic progenitor. The latter cell type is clearly distinct in its phenotype from both the presumed normal cellular counterparts of ALL without translocations and the one giving rise to AML. Therefore, ALL with *MLL* translocation has been proposed to represent a distinct disease.

Another finding of the *MLL* analysis has possible implications for the mechanism of transformation of this tumor entity. Among the genes appearing in the *MLL*-specific signature, a subset, namely the *HOX* genes, represent known target genes of the *MLL* fusion gene product that has been generated by the chromosome translocation. Since one of the *HOX* genes, *HOXA9*, is known to induce leukemia in mice on overexpression, its gene product (or other family members) might represent an important component of *MLL* tumorigenesis. The example of *MLL* demonstrates that a chromosomal translocation can determine a unique gene expression program. A comparative GEP analysis of different subtypes of T-cell-derived leukemias and normal T-cell subsets could identify gene products that are critically involved in the transformation of the respective subgroups, such as the transcription factor HOX11L2. From this analysis, the concept emerged that the overexpression of transcription factors characterizing the leukemia subtypes was not associated with chromosomal translocations, as previously assumed, suggesting the involvement of other genetic mechanisms in deregulating their expression. Taken together, the case of the pediatric leukemias demonstrates that GEP analysis has been very successful in identifying key oncogenic pathways that may be exploited in new therapeutic approaches.

## Identification of tumor-specific genes

GEP-based approaches are especially valuable in the identification of novel diagnostic markers or potential therapeutic targets of a tumor. Comparative GEP analysis between a particular lymphoid malignancy and various normal and malignant cell populations (Figure 27.4) truly represents an unbiased way to identify tumor-specific genes, provided that all samples are processed in the same way. The obvious advantage of this approach over large-scale sequencing strategies, such as EST sequencing or serial analysis of gene expression (SAGE), lies in the circumstance that tumor-specific genes are directly identified by the comparative nature of the GEP approach, namely the simultaneous analysis of a large number of gene chips representing the various subsets. The other approaches require laborious and costly generation of EST or SAGE profiles from the respective cell populations, or specific screening for potential tumor-specific genes by traditional analysis methods in a large panel of normal and malignant cell populations. Clearly, the parallel use of multiple samples of each cell population in a comparative GEP analysis, as opposed to pooling of RNA derived from several samples, allows the identification of differences that would otherwise be lost in procedures involving the pooling. Although gene chips already cover the vast majority of the transcribed genome of several organisms, an advantage of EST sequencing and SAGE over GEP is that these approaches allow the identification of previously unidentified mRNAs.

The expression of potential tumor-specific genes identified through comparative GEP analyses should be verified by PCR or, preferably, Northern blot analysis. This is absolutely required, as the regions representing a specific gene on the DNA microarray generally cover only part of that gene, and because these sequences have not always been tested for the detection of their corresponding RNA transcript. The existence of cell type-specific splice variants of many genes adds another level of complexity to this issue. Ideally, an attempt should also be made to detect the presumed gene

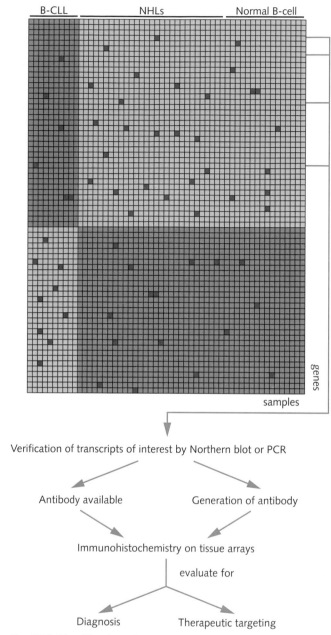

**Fig. 27.4 Identification of tumor-specific genes by supervised analysis**

Genes specifically upregulated or downregulated in a B-cell malignancy [B-cell chronic lymphocytic leukemia (B-CLL)] relative to the various subtypes of non-Hodgkin lymphoma (NHL) and normal B cells are identified by supervised pattern discovery analysis. The expression of genes of potential interest for diagnosis or therapy, such as cell surface receptors or molecules involved in signaling, is verified by Northern or PCR analysis, and eventually by immunohistochemistry. Upregulated genes are identified by the dark tint and downregulated genes by the light tint. Columns represent individual samples and rows correspond to genes.

product in tissue sections by immunohistological analysis or flow-cytometric analysis of cell suspensions.

## Tracking cellular pathways

Because of the large number of genes whose expression in a particular cell type can be monitored simultaneously, GEP experiments are bound to have a profound impact on the analysis of cellular signaling pathways and the cellular response to the activation of transcriptional activators or repressors. The most straightforward way to assess the activity of certain signaling pathways in a cell population is to examine GEP data for changes in the expression of known downstream targets of the respective pathway (Figure 27.5). While this approach relies on previous knowledge about the genes activated in the pathway under study, experimental *in vitro* or *in vivo* systems that recapitulate the activation of a particular signaling pathway can also be used to identify new target genes. For example, cells can be activated through a surface receptor *in vitro*, or cells differing genetically at defined loci (e.g., corresponding wild-type and gene knock-out cells) can be studied for differences in their response following activation (Figure 27.5). Likewise, pharmacologically active compounds can be tested in a cell type or in an *in vitro* system in which the relevant signaling pathway has been activated. Transcription factors can be ectopically expressed in a cell, either in a constitutive or inducible fashion. Regardless of the approach taken, the effects of the stimuli (i.e., the gene expression changes) are determined by comparison with a negative or uninduced control. The identified gene expression profiles can then be tracked within the gene expression data derived from normal or malignant cell populations, potentially providing information about the activity of a particular signaling pathway or transcriptional response in a given cell population. Of note, the interpretation might be obscured by the connectivity of cell signaling pathways *in vivo*, and tackling this problem clearly represents a new task for the field of computational biology, which allows study of the complex network interactions of specific cell types.

Various types of *in vitro* approaches have already been employed in identifying the functional consequences of the activity of transcription factors or cell surface receptors with suggested roles in the development of lymphomas, including the transcription factors c-Myc and BCL6, as well as stimulation through the CD40 cell surface receptor. The exogenous expression of the proto-oncogene c-Myc in an *in vitro* system led to the identification of previously unknown c-Myc target genes involved in cellular proliferation and growth. Expression of the BCL6 transcriptional repressor and proto-oncogene, which is a key player in germinal center B-cell

**Approach 1**

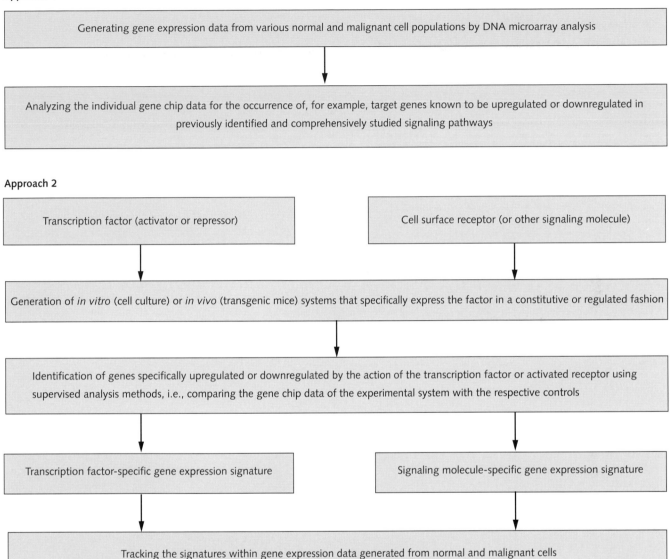

**Approach 2**

**Fig. 27.5 Tracking cellular pathways in normal and malignant cells using GEP approaches**
Approach 1: GEP data of normal and malignant cells are screened for characteristic gene expression changes of a known transcriptional response or signaling pathway. Approach 2: a factor-specific gene expression signature is generated *in vitro* or *in vivo*, followed by tracking of the respective profile in normal or malignant cells. Approach 2, in contrast to approach 1, also results in the identification of previously unidentified genes associated with the activation of the particular response or pathway.

development, is frequently deregulated in lymphomas. A GEP-based approach could identify the transcriptional response of BCL6 in an *in vitro* system, which included the repression of genes involved in differentiation and cell cycle control. The findings provided novel insights into the cellular differentiation and physiology of normal and malignant germinal center B cells. Stimulation through CD40, which results in the translocation of NF-κB, was long known to be essential for B-cell activation and differentiation proc-

esses. In a study aimed at identifying the B-cell subsets that show evidence of CD40 activation, the CD40 signature was first generated in an *in vitro* system. The resulting signature was then tracked in GEP data derived from normal B-cell subsets. Contrary to the previously held view, the results demonstrated that the highly proliferating germinal center B cells are not subjected to CD40 stimulation and activation of the NF-κB pathway, and that CD40 activation instead occurs specifically in the developmental windows prior to and immediately after the proliferative phase of germinal center B cells.

In the future, GEP data will be funneled into algorithms that go far beyond the scope of merely extracting the upregulation and downregulation of specific genes to a certain activation stimulus. Thus, reverse engineering of gene regulatory networks can reconstruct cellular networks solely based on GEP data of cell populations that differ in the activity of a signaling pathway or transcription factor.

## Acknowledgments

We thank Andrea Califano, Gustavo Stolovitzky, Yuhai Tu, Katia Basso and Vladan Miljkovic for their constant input in some of the gene expression profiling experiments described here, and Richard Baer for comments on the manuscript. Work in the authors' laboratory was supported by the National Cancer Institute, the Leukemia Research Fund, and the Human Frontiers Science Program.

## Further reading

### Introduction

Brown PO, Botstein D. (1999) Exploring the new world of the genome with DNA microarrays. *Nature Genetics*, **21**, 33–37.

Califano A, Stolovitzky G, Tu Y. (2000) Analysis of gene expression microarrays for phenotype classification. *Proceedings of the International Conference on Intelligent Systems in Molecular Biology*, **8**, 75–85.

Calin GA, Ferracin M, Cimmino A *et al.* (2005) MicroRNA signature associated with prognosis and progression in chronic lymphocytic leukemia. *New England Journal of Medicine*, **353**, 1793–1801.

Eisen MB, Spellman PT, Brown PO, Botstein D. (1998) Cluster analysis and display of genome-wide expression patterns. *Proceedings of the National Academy of Sciences of the United States of America*, **95**, 14863–14868.

Lockhart DJ, Dong H, Byrne MC *et al.* (1996) Expression monitoring by hybridization to high-density oligonucleotide arrays. *Nature Biotechnology*, **14**, 1675–1680.

Lu J, Getz G, Miska EA *et al.* (2005) MicroRNA expression profiles classify human cancers. *Nature*, **435**, 834–838.

Tamayo P, Slonim D, Mesirov J *et al.* (1999) Interpreting patterns of gene expression with self-organizing maps: methods and application to hematopoietic differentiation. *Proceedings of the National Academy of Sciences of the United States of America*, **96**, 2907–2912.

### Identification of tumor subtypes

Alizadeh AA, Eisen MB, Davis RE *et al.* (2000) Distinct types of diffuse large B-cell lymphoma identified by gene expression profiling. *Nature*, **403**, 503–511.

Crespo M, Bosch F, Villamor N *et al.* (2003) ZAP-70 expression as a surrogate for immunoglobulin-variable-region mutations in chronic lymphocytic leukemia. *New England Journal of Medicine*, **348**, 1764–1775.

Golub TR, Slonim DK, Tamayo P *et al.* (1999) Molecular classification of cancer: class discovery and class prediction by gene expression monitoring. *Science*, **286**, 531–537.

Klein U, Tu Y, Stolovitzky GA *et al.* (2001) Gene expression profiling of B cell chronic lymphocytic leukemia reveals a homogeneous phenotype related to memory B cells. *Journal of Experimental Medicine*, **194**, 1625–1638.

Rassenti LZ, Huynh L, Toy TL *et al.* (2004) ZAP-70 compared with immunoglobulin heavy-chain gene mutation status as a predictor of disease progression in chronic lymphocytic leukemia. *New England Journal of Medicine*, **351**, 893–901.

Rosenwald A, Alizadeh AA, Widhopf G *et al.* (2001) Relation of gene expression phenotype to immunoglobulin mutation genotype in B cell chronic lymphocytic leukemia. *Journal of Experimental Medicine*, **194**, 1639–1647.

Rosenwald A, Wright G, Chan WC *et al.* (2002) The use of molecular profiling to predict survival after chemotherapy for diffuse large-B-cell lymphoma. *New England Journal of Medicine*, **346**, 1937–1947.

Rosenwald A, Wright G, Leroy K *et al.* (2003) Molecular diagnosis of primary mediastinal B-cell lymphoma identifies a clinically favorable subgroup of diffuse large B-cell lymphoma related to Hodgkin lymphoma. *Journal of Experimental Medicine*, **198**, 851–862.

Savage KJ, Monti S, Kutok JL *et al.* (2003) The molecular signature of mediastinal large B-cell lymphoma differs from that of other diffuse large B-cell lymphomas and shares features with classical Hodgkin lymphoma. *Blood*, **102**, 3871–3879.

Shipp MA, Ross KN, Tamayo P *et al.* (2002) Diffuse large B-cell lymphoma outcome prediction by gene-expression profiling and supervised machine learning. *Nature Medicine*, **8**, 68–74.

## Normal cellular counterparts and mechanism of transformation

Alizadeh AA, Eisen MB, Davis RE *et al.* (2000) Distinct types of diffuse large B-cell lymphoma identified by gene expression profiling. *Nature*, **403**, 503–511.

Armstrong SA, Staunton JE, Silverman LB *et al.* (2002) MLL translocations specify a distinct gene expression profile that distinguishes a unique leukemia. *Nature Genetics*, **30**, 41–47.

Basso K, Liso A, Tiacci E *et al.* (2004) Gene expression profiling of hairy cell leukemia reveals a phenotype related to memory B-cells with altered expression of chemokine and adhesion receptors. *Journal of Experimental Medicine*, **199**, 59–68.

Ferrando AA, Armstrong SA, Neuberg DS *et al.* (2003) Gene expression signatures in MLL-rearranged T-lineage and B-precursor acute leukemias: dominance of HOX dysregulation. *Blood*, **102**, 262–268.

Klein U, Tu Y, Stolovitzky GA *et al.* (2001) Gene expression profiling of B cell chronic lymphocytic leukemia reveals a homogeneous phenotype related to memory B cells. *Journal of Experimental Medicine*, **194**, 1625–1638.

Küppers R, Klein U, Hansmann ML, Rajewsky K. (1999) Cellular origin of human B-cell lymphomas. *New England Journal of Medicine*, **341**, 1520–1529.

Stevenson F, Sahota S, Zhu D *et al.* (1998) Insight into the origin and clonal history of B-cell tumors as revealed by analysis of immunoglobulin variable region genes. *Immunological Reviews*, **162**, 247–259.

## Tracking cellular pathways

Basso K, Klein U, Niu H *et al.* (2004) Tracking CD40 signaling during germinal center development. *Blood*, **104**, 4088–4096.

Basso K, Margolin AA, Stolovitzky G *et al.* (2005) Reverse engineering of regulatory networks in human B-cells. *Nature Genetics*, **37**, 382–390.

Coller, HA, Grandori C, Tamayo P *et al.* (2000) Expression analysis with oligonucleotide microarrays reveals that MYC regulates genes involved in growth, cell cycle, signaling, and adhesion. *Proceedings of the National Academy of Sciences of the United States of America*, **97**, 3260–3265.

Feske S, Giltnane J, Dolmetsch R *et al.* (2001) Gene regulation mediated by calcium signals in T lymphocytes. *Nature Immunology*, **2**, 316–324.

Glynne R, Akkaraju S, Healy JI *et al.* (2000) How self-tolerance and the immunosuppressive drug FK506 prevent B-cell mitogenesis. *Nature*, **403**, 672–676.

Jeong H, Tombor B, Albert R *et al.* (2000) The large-scale organization of metabolic networks. *Nature*, **407**, 651–654.

Shaffer AL, Yu X, He Y *et al.* (2000) BCL-6 represses genes that function in lymphocyte differentiation, inflammation, and cell cycle control. *Immunity*, **13**, 199–212.

# Chapter 28 History and development of molecular biology

## Paul Moss

*School of Cancer Sciences, University of Birmingham, Birmingham, UK*

## Evolution is the central tenet of biology

It is entirely fitting that a new edition of *Molecular Hematology* is being developed in 2009, the bicentenary of the birth of Charles Darwin and 150 years since the publication of *On the Origin of Species by Means of Natural Selection* (Figure 28.1a). Darwin's far-reaching insights placed natural variation and adaptation as the prime determinants of population change. Evolution is now recognized as the unifying theme of all biology, including hematology and medicine, and these landmark observations can perhaps be recognized as the initiation of the modern discipline of molecular genetics.

However, despite his unique vision and imagination, Darwin was never able to understand the nature of genetic inheritance. It was clear that phenotypic characteristics were passed from one generation to the next but usually these characteristics were "blended," so that a combination of tall and short parents would produce a child of medium height. Darwin proposed his own model for heredity which he termed *pangenesis* in which cells of the body shed gemmules that collect in the reproductive organs. The concept was that all the tissues in the body thus had some impact on inheritance but this concept has clearly been superseded. At this time there was no concept of the distinction between the germline and somatic tissue, and it is therefore not surprising that even brilliant scientists such as Jean-Baptiste de Lamarck believed that acquired phenotypic features could be passed, through reproduction, into the subsequent generation. However, despite his somewhat imperfect conclusions, Lamarck was actually an extremely important figure

in evolutionary theory as he developed the concept that a species can change *between* different generations, a view entirely in contrast to the prevailing view that all species had been placed on the earth by a divine Creator.

Even in Darwin's time there were fierce arguments about the nature of biological inheritance. Samuel Butler, later to become a celebrated novelist, emigrated to New Zealand to make his fortune in sheep breeding. Whilst there, he read Darwin's work and, through his own highly successful breeding experiments, came to understand the concept that "information" was flowing from one generation to the next. His ideas were taken further by William Bateson, a Cambridge geneticist who introduced the term *genetics* in 1906 to describe the science of inheritance and variation. The units of this information were subsequently termed *genes* by Wilhelm Johannsen.

## The understanding of monogenic and polygenic inheritence

The modern concept of genetic inheritance began with the work of Gregor Mendel, an Austrian priest who had undergone training as a science teacher and is famous for his pea breeding experiments published in 1866 (Figure 28.1b). Mendel used true-breeding varieties of pea to show that the crossing of two dissimilar strains led to a uniform first generation ($F_1$). However, the crossing of the $F_1$ generation with an $F_2$ generation produced a population where three-quarters of the peas had the same (dominant) parental characteristic and one-quarter had the other (recessive) parental form. In the course of over 30 000 observations, Mendel went on to breed subtypes of $F_2$ and laid the rules for dominant and recessive inheritance. He postulated that each characteristic was determined by two elements from the parents and that these were both retained and appeared in the germ-

*Molecular Hematology*, 3rd edition. Edited by Drew Provan and John Gribben.
© 2010 Blackwell Publishing.

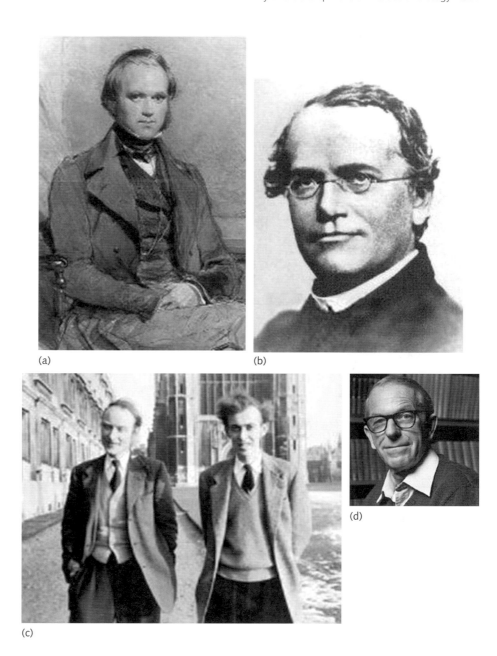

**Fig. 28.1 (a) Charles Darwin. (b) Gregor Mendel. (c) Francis Crick and James Watson. (d) Fred Sanger**

line as single forms in equal proportions. The final expression in each plant was dependent on the combination of dominant or recessive elements. These experiments were hugely influential to the development of molecular biology as they showed that heritable characteristics are *particulate* and not "blended." His work was largely ignored for the next 35 years until it was rediscovered in the early 20th century and widely supported by Bateson and colleagues. The particulate element became known as the gene and the modern basis of genetics was established.

A huge problem in these early days was how to link the clear biological results of Mendelian experiments with the discontinuous phenotypes seen in everyday life. For instance, how can single pieces of information determine such variables such as height or intelligence? It was left to the work of R.A. Fisher in 1918 to show that the inheritance of multiple different single genes could produce a phenotype that displayed discontinuous properties and the concept of *polygenic* inheritance of characteristics was thus borne.

## DNA as the conduit of genetic information

From this time, the science of genetics became firmly established and rooted in all aspects of biological investigation. However, the nature of the genetic material was completely unknown until the pioneering work of Oswald Avery in 1944. Avery trained as a medical doctor and was 67 at the time of his most famous scientific contribution. He had been working on the inheritance of S and R strains of *Streptococcus pneumoniae* and was able to show that, contrary to the current view, the use of proteases could not prevent transmission of genetic information between strains. In contrast, deoxyribonuclease was highly effective in preventing transmission and this work therefore established DNA as the medium for genetic inheritance. Avery died in 1955 and is often regarded as one of the most deserving scientists never to have been awarded the Nobel Prize in Medicine or Physiology. Having established DNA as the physical basis of heritability, genetic research then proceeded to dominate biological investigation for the next 50 years.

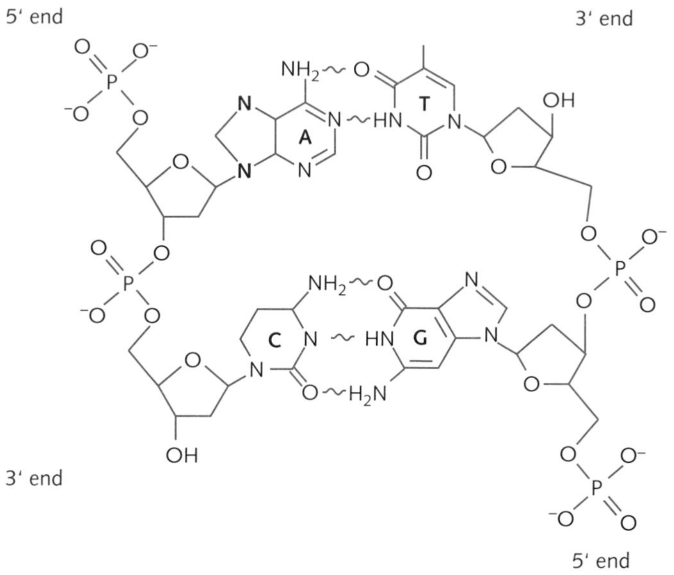

### Elucidation of the structure of DNA

The elucidation of the structure of DNA has become perhaps the most memorable biological achievement of the last century. The story is well known, and involves the outstanding X-ray crystallography of Maurice Wilkins and Rosalind Franklyn combined with the imagination and intelligence of James Watson and Francis Crick (Figure 28.1c). Their paper, published in 1953, took advantage of a wealth of previous information from other investigators, and this was instrumental in allowing a final elucidation.

In 1919 Levene had demonstrated that DNA consisted of three components: the bases (of which there were four types), a sugar (which was either ribose or deoxyribose) and a phosphate group. He showed that these were linked together in a unit that he called a *nucleotide*. The work of Irwin Chargaff defined the so-called *Chargaff ratio*, which relates to the base composition of DNA. This showed that the amount of guanine equals that of cytosine, and the amount of adenine equals that of thymine. Structural analysis revealed that the hydrogen bonds between guanine and cytosine and between adenine and thymine were of similar structure and led to a model in which the hydrophobic bases were on the inside of the double helix, leaving the hydrophilic components on the outside (Figure 28.2).

The structure of DNA has now been well characterized and comprises three different subunits, a sugar, a base and a phosphate group; together these form a nucleotide. DNA is a polymer of nucleotides and it is the sequence of bases

**Fig. 28.2 The structure of DNA**
The deoxyribose pentose sugars are joined by phosphodiester bonds at C-3 or C-5 to phosphate groups. The four bases, adenine (A), thymine (T) , cytosine (C) and guanine (G), are attached to this backbone and the double helix is stabilized by hydrogen bonds (represented by zig-zag lines).

that determines the genetic information. Certain aspects of the nucleotide component are worth looking at in more detail. The backbone of the strand is made from phosphate and sugar residues, the latter being a 2-deoxyribose five-carbon (pentose) sugar. Importantly, these sugars are joined either at their third or fifth carbon atom and this asymmetry gives a *polarity* to the DNA strand, with the 5′ end having a terminal phosphate group and the 3′ end a terminal hydroxyl residue. The phosphate groups form phosphodiester bonds, which contain a phosphorus atom that allows strong covalent linkage through an ester bond. These groups are negatively charged and this plays a role in forcing phosphates away from the center of the DNA helix, as well as combining with positively charged proteins termed *histones* that package the DNA. The core genetic complexity of the DNA molecule comes from the composition of bases at the center of the helix. These bases are of two types, *purines* and *pyrimidines*, the former comprising adenine and guanine, fused heterocyclic compounds of five- and six-membered rings, the latter cytosine and thymidine, which are more simple six-membered rings. The pairing of guanine with cytosine provides greater strength of interaction due to optimal hydrogen bonding.

The mechanism by which DNA replicates was a further question that needed to be resolved. Watson and Crick had ended their paper with the famous words " it has not escaped our notice that the specific pairing we have postulated immediately suggests a possible copying mechanism for the genetic material." This implied that the two helices could separate and allow copying of each strand. In 1958 Matthew Meselson and Franklin Stahl showed that the replication of DNA was *semi-conservative*. That is, when a copy is made of a double-stranded DNA template, a complementary sequence is made against each of the two original strands rather than production of a completely new double strand with retention of the original duplex.

## Decoding the sequence of DNA

Later work by Francis Crick predicted that "adapter" intermediates would be found which decoded the DNA sequence into the synthesis of proteins. *Transfer RNA* was subsequently isolated and found to comprise a triplet anticodon attached to a specific amino acid. In this way the DNA code can be translated into a protein sequence. There are 20 different subtypes of amino acid and these are encoded by a range of different triplet sequences on transfer RNA. This is the *genetic code* that was elucidated in the early 1960s and was set out by Crick in the form in which it is now used. Translation usually commences with an AUG triplet, which codes for methionine. Protein synthesis occurs within the cellular cytoplasm on *ribosomes*, which are complex mixtures of RNA and protein components.

This flow of genetic information from DNA to RNA to protein became known as the *central dogma* of molecular biology. Although never meant to be as truly closed to critical evaluation as the term implies, this observation was highly influential in understanding the centrality of germline DNA in evolutionary processes and essentially contradicted the concept that somatic information could flow back into the germline, as envisaged in the original Lamarckian theory of evolution.

RNA is a major component of the cellular nucleus and three main forms were distinguished in the early days of molecular biology. *Messenger RNA* (mRNA) copies the DNA genetic code into transcripts that travel to the cytoplasm for protein translation. This process of *transcription* allows different cells, all of which carry the same gene content, to utilize their genome in differential ways and transcriptional regulation lies at the heart of cell differentiation programs. The initial concept that one gene gives rise to a single mRNA species, and subsequently a single protein molecule, has been challenged in several ways over the last few decades. The first observation was that genes are split into discrete units of expressed code, termed *exons*, and these DNA segments are

separated by intervening sequences of intronic DNA. Most of the genes within the human genome have this intron–exon structure and although the selective advantage of this development is unknown, it does allow increased flexibility for decoding genetic information into a range of protein transcripts. In order for an initial mRNA species to encode an accurate representation of the exon structures, the transcript must be *spliced* by splicing enzymes within the nucleus by a process that removes intervening intronic RNA segments. Many genetic diseases have now been revealed as due to aberrations in splicing mechanisms and the thalassemia syndromes, which arguably have told us more about the principles of molecular regulation than any other genetic disease, are commonly inactivated by mutations in this mechanism.

*Ribosomal RNA* (rRNA) is complexed with ribosomal proteins to produce the large number of ribosomes that are scattered around the cytoplasm and which act as the principal sites for *protein translation*. There are four different rRNA molecules within the ribosome, 18S, 5.8S, 28S and 5S, and together they constitute over 80% of RNA within the cell. The combination of transcription and translation can be surprisingly slow. It has been estimated that it can take 21 hours to produce a molecule of dystrophin, the largest gene in the genome and the one responsible for Duchenne muscular dystrophy.

Recently, several new classes of RNA species have been discovered and are likely to play very important roles in the genetic regulation of eukaryotic cells. A particularly important discovery has been the finding that RNA can have catalytic activity, demonstrating that it is more than simply a passive scaffold. *MicroRNA* species are approximately 21 nucleotides in length and do not code for proteins but, on the contrary, carry complementary sequences that are able to bind to mRNA species and regulate the rate of protein production. This is done by either binding to mRNA species and preventing translation on ribosomes or via recruitment of ribonucleases that degrade double-stranded RNA species and thus reduce the half-life of the targeted RNA species. Current estimates suggest that there are over 1000 microRNA transcripts within the human genome and it is currently believed that mutations or deregulation of microRNA expression can be implicated in a range of malignant diseases; involvement of deletions of microRNAs in the etiology of chronic lymphocytic leukemia secondary to chromosome 13q deletions is one such example. The net overall effect of these systems is that the cell thus produces not only mRNA for protein translation, but also species of RNA with complementary sequence to mRNA transcripts that serve to limit information derived from each mRNA transcript. This feedback control is, of course, a commonly identified mechanism in many biological systems.

A range of other RNA species are now being identified. These include *small nuclear RNAs* (snRNA), which are involved in processes such as mRNA splicing, and *small nucleolar RNAs*. Many *long non-coding RNA* species of over 200 nucleotides in length are also produced and their functions are largely unknown. They are often very highly conserved in evolution and found in gene-poor regions of the genome. It is likely that they play important and indispensible roles in embryonic development.

## Regulation of transcriptional activity

The DNA genome encodes the information from which our complex multicellular structure can be assembled. However the code is deciphered in a highly complex process involving the interaction of many different proteins and nucleic acids.

DNA is copied into RNA by the *RNA polymerase II* enzyme, which recognizes a *promoter* sequence at the 5′ end of the gene. The organization of promoter sequences is highly disparate, although many contain the TATAAA sequence known as the TATA box. Promoter sequences attract a large number of proteins called *transcription factors*, which serve to activate or repress transcription at that gene. These proteins all contain a DNA-binding domain and attract an additional set of proteins involved in chromatin remodeling that also regulate transcriptional activity (*see section on epigenetics below*).

A further set of DNA regulatory elements are *enhancer* sequences that regulate the transcriptional activity of genes which are often many kilobases away. Their precise mechanism of action is uncertain but is likely to involve processes such as "looping out" of DNA and colocalization of transcription factors.

## The rough guide to the human genome

The human genome contains a sequence of 3000 million bases of DNA from each parent, equating to some 6 billion bases in a diploid cell. The Human Genome Project started in 1990 and 99.3% of the sequence was completed by 2003. Indeed the genome has now been fully sequenced for several individuals, and this is likely to rise substantially by the time this book is published. Large-scale sequencing has revealed a number of surprises about the human genome. The first of these is that the gene content is much lower than was initially estimated. Current estimates suggest a gene content of around 25000, whereas early proposals placed this nearer 100000. In addition, only 2% of the

genome actually codes for protein. The additional 98% has a complex regulatory function and its importance is still largely unknown. During the early days of molecular biology, these regions were rather arrogantly termed "junk DNA" but they have since turned out to be extremely important in factors such as determining speciation and regulation of gene expression.

Different individuals show considerable variation within the genome. This natural polymorphism is typically seen as a base change of around 1 in every 1300 bases, equating to over 4 million differences between individuals. These variants are known as *single-nucleotide polymorphisms* (SNPs) and as well as their intrinsic value in understanding issues such as natural selection and evolutionary change, they are also very valuable in determining genetic linkage of genes in a variety of human diseases. Indeed, SNP-based disease association studies are currently the most popular approach for determining the polygenic basis of disease and around 50% of these variants are in non-coding regions of the genome. Interestingly, most of these variants are quite common in the human population and there is less variation between humans than there is between other great apes. This is believed to reflect the fact that the current human population of some 6 billion people has grown rapidly over 3000 generations from a founder size "bottleneck" of only 10000 individuals.

Sequencing has also revealed that *copy number variation* is a common finding in the human genome. We seem to have a dynamic genome in which relatively large areas of deletion and insertion are seen and this may underlie a range of disorders that may involve cryptic gene inactivation and translocations. It may be that this high level of genomic instability has contributed to our rapid evolution but clearly there also appears to be a price to pay.

## The packaging of genetic material

One fact that we almost all remember is that each cell in the human body contains approximately 1m of double-stranded DNA, if it were stretched out from end to end. Given that we have some $10^{14}$ cells within our body, the whole content of our somatic DNA would stretch for some $10^{14}$ m. It is no surprise therefore that this length of DNA must be packed very accurately and densely into a typical cell of around 8μm. The first order of packaging is the *nucleosome*, in which two loops of DNA are wrapped round a histone protein. As we shall see later, this structure is critical not only for efficient mechanical packaging but also for controlling gene regulation. The second-order structure is coiling of nucleosomes into a rope-like structure, but further order packaging beyond this is currently unknown.

## Epigenetic regulation adds a new dimension of complexity

Additional complexities to understanding the transcriptional regulation of the DNA code are being identified on a regular basis. It is now clear that protein-induced modifications of histone structure play an important role in determining the transcriptional regulation of individual genes. The two major processes involved are *methylation of cytosine bases* at CpG dinucleotides and *acetylation of histone tails*. A wide range of methylases, demethylases, acetylases and deacetylases are involved in dynamic modification of histone structures and this process is now being targeted in clinical practice. Around 75% of all CpG dinucleotides are methylated and unmethylated forms are often grouped at the 5′ end of genes in areas known as *CpG islands*. In general, methylation serves to downregulate transcription from a gene and demethylating agents are used in the management of diseases such as myelodysplasia or acute myeloid leukemia. In contrast, acetylation encourages transcriptional activity and deacetylation inhibitors are therefore also used in a range of hematopoietic disorders. Given the widespread modifications of methylation and acetylation in the human genome, it is perhaps surprising that the non-specific activity of these pharmacological agents can prove of value without engendering significant side effects. However, current practice suggests that they may be relatively well tolerated. Epigenetic regulation also represents one example in which somatic tissues may influence transcription of the germline. Gender, in particular, can have an important impact on transcriptional activity of individual genes. This process of imprinting can be broadly summarized as revealing that males tend to encourage fetal growth whereas the maternal influence is to restrict fetal developmental. Aberrations of epigenetic imprinting results in disorders such as Prader–Willi or Angelman syndrome.

## Experimental techniques and molecular biology

Here I review some of the milestones that have led to the development of the experimental discipline known as molecular biology. This is a field which is moving perhaps more rapidly than any other within biology and while it offers unparalleled opportunities for clinical practice, it is challenging for clinicians to maintain their knowledge base within this area.

## The extraction of nucleic acids

A good place to begin is the extraction of nucleic acids from cells. Nucleic acids are soluble in water but can be precipitated by the addition of ethanol. In one method the cell or tissue of interest is lysed to destroy cell membranes and the protein component degraded by proteinase K or extraction with phenol and chloroform. The latter approach generates an aqueous phase containing RNA and an organic phase that retains protein and lipid, with DNA being trapped at the interface.

The next step is to purify and concentrate the nucleic acid and this can be done by *ethanol precipitation*. Because DNA is charged, it is highly soluble in water but the addition of non-polar ethanol to at least 66% of the final volume draws it out of solution. The precipitate of nucleic acids can then be centrifuged, the ethanol drawn off and the nucleic acid resuspended in water. Genomic DNA is quite stable in this form, perhaps not surprising given its natural physiological role. However, RNA is highly unstable and susceptible to RNases, which are ubiquitous enzymes within the environment. Inhibitors of RNases and rapid cooling of RNA solutions are needed for downstream analysis of ribonucleic acids. Although these chemical steps are effective, and have been in use for many decades, many laboratories now use disposable cartridge methodology for extraction of nucleic acids. These are rapid, often cost-effective, and generally much easier to use.

## Restriction enzymes and expression cloning

Having isolated DNA in an aqueous solution, there is not a great deal that you can usefully do with it in its native state. If it is run on an electrophoresis gel, it will be of such high molecular weight that it will not migrate into the gel to any extent and is therefore not suitable for downstream analysis. A major advance in molecular biology was the development and utilization of bacterial *restriction endonucleases*. These are a large family of enzymes that are present in bacteria and which have evolved to digest double-stranded DNA. They are important in protecting bacteria from invading bacteriophages and thus they "restrict" the vulnerability of the cell to infection. The critical finding about restriction endonucleases was that they cut DNA at specific DNA sequence motifs. For instance, the enzyme *Eco*RI will only cut DNA at positions that have the sequence 5′-GAATTC. Note that this sequence is a palindrome when double stranded and it is in this form that the DNA is cleaved, after the G on both strands. If sufficient enzyme is used in a digestion reaction, every individual site within the target DNA will be cut. These enzymes opened up the field of modern molecular biology because they led to the development of *DNA cloning*. In this procedure, the DNA of interest is digested with a particular endonuclease and then a *vector* DNA sequence, usually in the form of a bacterial plasmid or a virus, is also digested with the same enzyme. Providing that the vector has only two of these restriction sites, a portion of the vector will be excised and then, by combining the digests of the target DNA and vector, the two populations can be ligated such that single copies of DNA are cloned into the vector. Typically these vectors have strong promoters that drive expression of the cloned gene, as well as genes coding for antibiotics, which allow selection for vectors containing an insert. In this way a *library* of the original DNA is made.

This library can then be introduced into cells for propagation and functional analysis. Vectors can be transformed into a bacterial host that can be multiplied using culture medium to a potentially unlimited population size. Lysis of the bacterial colony, followed by recovery of the plasmid or phage, can lead to isolation and analysis of large amounts of individual target DNA sequences. This is a core technique in molecular biology and has led to most of the subsequent development within the field. Libraries can also be introduced into eukaryotic cells through the process of *transfection*, which typically involves incubation with cold cations such as calcium or the use of liposomes.

## Electrophoresis and blotting of nucleic acids

Once DNA has been digested with endonucleases it is broken up into smaller pieces, the exact size and pattern of which will depend on the endonuclease that has been used. Edwin Southern published a technique whereby this DNA was initially subjected to electrophoresis on an agarose gel, thus separating individual pieces on the basis of their size and charge. If a nitrocellulose filter is then applied on top of the agarose gel and moderate pressure applied, the DNA will migrate into the nitrocellulose where it can be fixed using heat or a cross-linking agent. If the DNA filter is then hybridized to a labeled nucleic acid probe, the probe will bind only to that section of the DNA containing a complementary sequence. When genomic DNA from different individuals is

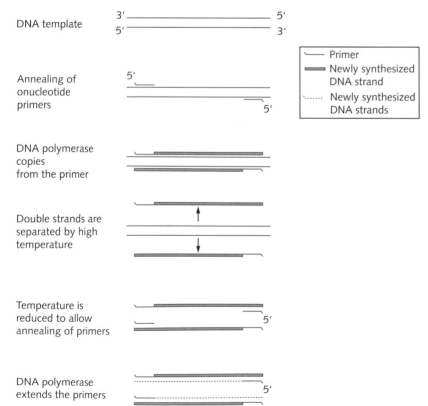

**Fig. 28.3 The polymerase chain reaction**
Typical temperatures for annealing, extension and denaturation are 50–60°C, 72°C and 96°C, respectively.

digested with the same nuclease, all the resulting DNA fragments will be of comparable size, notwithstanding the natural variation found within the human genome. Thus the hybridization band should be similar in different individuals. This technique became known as the *Southern blot* and was widely applied to the detection of chromosomal abnormalities such as deletions, linkage studies, and gene rearrangement identification. It is somewhat less widely used today due to the advent of more modern technologies such as SNP mapping and DNA sequencing.

Southern blot technology has been adopted for use in other ways and a memorable nomenclature has been built up, albeit based on a mischievous interpretation of the derivation of "Southern." The *Northern blot* refers to a technique in which RNA is run on an agarose gel and blotted in the same way as the DNA in a Southern blot. This approach was widely used to examine differential expression of DNA between tissues but has largely been replaced by microarray analysis. *Western blotting* refers to the technique of separating protein molecules by electrophoresis prior to blotting onto a membrane. This membrane is then probed with an antibody for detection of the presence, size and amount of individual protein species.

## The polymerase chain reaction

The development of the polymerase chain reaction (PCR) in the 1980s led to the award of a Nobel Prize to Kary Mullis in 1993 and its value in medical practice is perhaps reflected by the relative swiftness of the Nobel Committee in rewarding the inventor. The idea is, like most powerful innovations, relatively straightforward and involves repetitive cycles of DNA synthesis and dissociation (Figure 28.3). DNA polymerases are used to copy a specific DNA segment and this step is followed by an increase in reaction temperature to dissociate DNA double strands and provide further templates for the amplification process. Mullis performed his initial work using a hot water bath and had to combine DNA polymerase with free nucleotides for the initial synthesis, heat the reaction to "melt" the double strands, and allow the mixture to cool for reannealing of the original primer mix, before then adding further polymerase enzyme as the original aliquot had been killed by the high temperatures used in the melting process. Since then, the technique has been dramatically simplified through the use of thermostable DNA polymerases isolated from bacteria that live at high temperatures. Solid-phase technology, which allows very rapid shifts in temperature, have led to a dramatic reduction in incubation and extension times. The technique utilizes short oligonucleotide primers that anneal to the target gene of interest. The DNA polymerase extends the DNA sequence beyond the primary sequence and, as the primers are directed toward

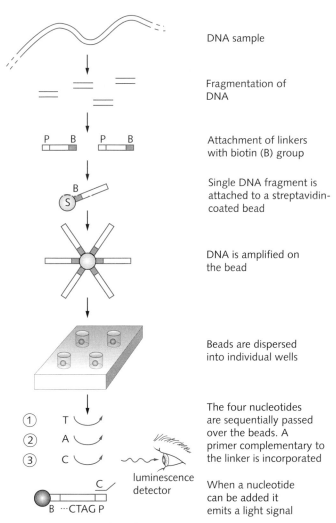

**Fig. 28.4 The principles of 454 next-generation sequencing**

one another on complementary strands of DNA, the result is a complete double-stranded copy of the target gene. Typical PCR reactions might allow amplification of between 500 and 2000 bp of DNA, but innovations do exist that can extend these values. Once a gene has been amplified in this way it can be sequenced, subjected to enzymatic digestion or used in a range of downstream applications.

## DNA sequencing

Although the physical structure of DNA was defined in the 1960s, it would be many years before it became possible to sequence the bases in order to reveal the genetic code. Interestingly, protein sequencing had been reported many years earlier but the technology of DNA sequencing has now advanced so much that its capability far exceeds current abilities to sequence amino acids.

The two original methodologies were developed by Fred Sanger and Walter Gilbert, who shared the Nobel Prize for Chemistry in 1980 (Figure 28.1d). The techniques involved the use of DNA polymerases to sequence DNA from an oligonucleotide primer. However, within the mix of nucleotides needed for the building blocks of the new chains, Sanger's approach incorporated a small quantity of nucleotides that have dideoxy modifications of their sequence such that they cannot be extended. Four separate reactions were used for each DNA sequence, incorporating dideoxy reagents for the A, T, C or G bases respectively. If radioactivity or fluorescence is used to label the newly extended chains, these can then be run on a high-resolution acrylamide gel and from this a ladder of chains is derived which shows the stop positions that occur when each base terminator is used. These bands can then be read off and a DNA sequence can be deduced. This technology was of tremendous value in initial efforts to understand molecular biology and has played a large role in driving the discipline forward over the last 20 years.

## Microarray analysis

Although sequence information of germline DNA provides highly valuable information, in many situations it is more valuable to know how this information is utilized within individual cells or tissues. One approach to this is to use systems which determine the *quantitative profile of mRNA expression* within tissues. Microarrays achieve this by a technique which relies on the synthesis of a huge number of oligonucleotides that are complementary to each of the approximately 25 000 human genes. These oligonucleotides are placed individually on microarray slides and are then hybridized to sample tissue. mRNA from the sample is reversed transcribed to cDNA with the use of fluorescent primers and then this material is hybridized to the oligonucleotides; after washing, the amount of hybridized material is assayed using laser detection. This approach is a highly accurate and reproducible means of measuring the distribution of mRNA species within cells or tissues. Of course, there is no simple correlation between mRNA levels and protein expression and proteomic analysis allows additional understanding of cellular differentiation control. Microarray systems are used widely in diagnostic and investigational approaches to hematopoietic malignancy.

## Next-generation sequencing

Over the last couple of years new technologies have been developed that have dramatically altered the capability of DNA sequencing. Two broad platforms are currently available and are known as 454 pyrosequencing and the Illumina/

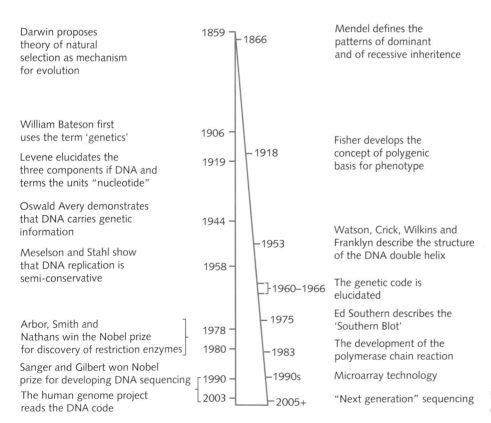

Darwin proposes theory of natural selection as mechanism for evolution — 1859

1866 — Mendel defines the patterns of dominant and of recessive inheritance

William Bateson first uses the term 'genetics' — 1906

1918 — Fisher develops the concept of polygenic basis for phenotype

Levene elucidates the three components if DNA and terms the units "nucleotide" — 1919

Oswald Avery demonstrates that DNA carries genetic information — 1944

1953 — Watson, Crick, Wilkins and Franklyn describe the structure of the DNA double helix

Meselson and Stahl show that DNA replication is semi-conservative — 1958

1960–1966 — The genetic code is elucidated

1975 — Ed Southern describes the 'Southern Blot'

Arbor, Smith and Nathans win the Nobel prize for discovery of restriction enzymes — 1978

1980

1983 — The development of the polymerase chain reaction

Sanger and Gilbert won Nobel prize for developing DNA sequencing — 1990

1990s — Microarray technology

The human genome project reads the DNA code — 2003

2005+ — "Next generation" sequencing

**Fig. 28.5 Some of the key developments in molecular biology**

Solexa systems. Both technologies commence with fragmentation of DNA and then small DNA fragments are captured individually onto beads prior to an amplification step. In the 454 system, these beads are then centrifuged into small wells such that each well contains only one bead and these are sequenced individually. The 454 system is based on luminescence, each base generating a different color; the cameras used for color detection are based on those developed for the Hubble telescope and have very high sensitivity (Figure 28.4).

These technologies have led to a step change in the ability to rapidly sequence DNA and they produce almost frightening levels of information. A single machine run can generate 500 million base pairs of sequence and most of the challenges relate to the bioinformatic analysis of the information or simple storage of data. The 454 system sequenced the entire genome of James Watson in 2 months and in time it is likely that many of our patients, and indeed perhaps ourselves, will undergo full genome sequencing. Our current capabilities are probably only limited by our imagination and they allow experiments such as comparative analysis of the complete sequence of germline DNA in comparison with tumor cells or study of the evolution of infectious organisms in a human host almost in real time.

*Ultra-deep sequencing* refers to the ability to sequence many different copies of an individual sequence in one run, also known as in parallel. As such it can be very powerful for detecting rare mutations in tissue samples or for following genetic variation within populations of viruses.

*Transcriptome sequencing* is the sequence analysis of the mRNA population in a cell or tissue. There is the possibility that this approach could replace some of the uses of microarray analysis as it simultaneously provides information on the number of mRNA species in the sample as well as determining their complete nucleotide sequence.

## Conclusion

The dramatic developments in molecular biology over the last 50 years represent one of the most exciting stories of scientific development (Figure 28.5). Refreshingly, they have also been applied quickly and effectively to human health and are now integral to the clinical practice of hematology. A more detailed analysis of the molecular basis of a wide range of conditions is discussed more fully in subsequent chapters.

## Further reading

Ansorge WJ. (2009) Next-generation DNA sequencing techniques. *Nature Biotechnology*, **25**, 195–203.

Crick F, Watson J. (1962) On the genetic code. http://nobelprize.org/nobel_prizes/medicine/laureates/1962/crick-lecture.html

Reichard P. (2002) Osvald T. Avery and the Nobel Prize in Medicine. *Journal of Biological Chemistry*, **19**, 277, 13355–13362.

Sanger F. (1980) Determination of the nucleotide sequences in DNA. http://nobelprize.org/nobel_prizes/chemistry/laureates/1980/sanger-lecture.html

Siomi H, Siomi MC. (2009) On the road to reading the RNA-interference code. *Nature*, **457**, 396–404.

# Chapter 29 Cancer stem cells

## David C Taussig[1] & Dominique Bonnet[2]

[1] Department of Medical Oncology, Barts and The London School of Medicine & Dentistry, London, UK
[2] Haematopoietic Stem Cell Laboratory, Cancer Research UK London Research Institute, London, UK

## Introduction

Gross anatomy and histology reveal the basic architecture of a tissue. However, there is a functional structure to cells that is not always apparent from the morphology. Within many (if not all) organs, cells are structured functionally as a hierarchy. At the top of the hierarchy are adult stem cells. Adult stem cells give rise to all the cells of the tissue and also make copies of themselves (a process termed *self-renewal*). At the bottom of the hierarchy are differentiated cells. Within the middle ranks of the hierarchy are progenitor cells that give rise to the differentiated cells but which lack the ability to self-renew. The tissues in which this functional structure has been described include the bone marrow, skin, bowel, breast and brain. These studies involve functional studies of subpopulations of cells within a tissue. As little as one adult stem cell from a tissue can be shown to result in the formation of the tissue in functional assays in the laboratory.

The cancer stem cell hypothesis proposes that malignant tissues are organized in a similar manner to normal tissues in terms of having a functional hierarchy. At the top of the hierarchy are cancer stem cells (CSCs), with the ability to produce all the clonal cells that comprise the tumor as well as the ability to self-renew. The bottom of the hierarchy comprises tumor cells with a variable degree of differentiation, but without the ability to self-renew. The cancer stem cell hypothesis does *not* propose the idea that all CSCs are derived from adult stem cells of the relevant tissue (the cell of origin of CSCs will be dealt with later in this chapter).

The CSC hypothesis has important implications for the way researchers approach malignant disease. Elimination or effective suppression of CSCs is thought to be crucial to eradicate or control malignant disease. Therefore, we need to understand how CSCs proliferate and survive, rather than the cells that comprise the bulk of the tumor. The pathways utilized by CSCs will in many cases be different to those utilized by the rest of the tumor cells. Data derived from studies on bulk tumor may not be reflective of events within CSCs. Efforts need to be directed toward understanding CSCs specifically, so that therapies may be developed to target them.

## Evidence for the existence of CSCs

In the 1960s Chester Southam performed studies on humans with advanced cancer in which autologous tumor cells were implanted subcutaneously in varying doses. He noted that no tumors grew where less than 1 million tumor cells were implanted. One interpretation of this observation is that there are rare CSCs whose frequency is in the order of 1 in 1 million tumor cells or less. The group led by John Dick has generated similar data using xenograft studies. Human malignancies are transplantable into immunodeficient animals, such as the non-obese diabetic/severe combined immunodeficiency (NOD/SCID) mouse. For acute myeloid leukemia (AML), more than 1000 cells need to be transplanted to generate a detectable leukemic graft in NOD/SCID mice, although there is large intersample variation in terms of cell numbers required to generate a graft. Similar numbers of unsorted solid tumor cells are required to induce tumor in NOD/SCID mice (e.g., 57 000 colon cancer cells).

The figures for CSC frequency determined using xenografts are likely to be underestimates. The mice tested probably do

*Molecular Hematology*, 3rd edition. Edited by Drew Provan and John Gribben.
© 2010 Blackwell Publishing.

not provide all the necessary supportive signals and there is evidence of residual immunity in NOD/SCID mice. For example, we have observed that some AML samples cannot engraft in NOD/SCID mice but do engraft in the more immunodeficient NOD/SCID/$\beta_2$- microglobulin null strain (which lack natural killer cell activity).

Further evidence for the existence of CSCs comes from the heterogeneity of cells within a given tumor. There are morphological and phenotypic differences between tumor cells, for example AML M5b comprises two populations with different morphological features: immature blast cells and partially differentiated monocytic cells. Another example is chronic myeloid leukemia (CML), where differentiation of malignant cells approaches that of normal hematopoiesis. Leukemic neutrophils or their immediate precursors predominate while immature blast cells make up a minority of cells. The immunophenotype correlates with the morphology; CD34, a marker of normal human hematopoietic stem and progenitor cells, is expressed on a minority of chronic phase CML cells and the proportion increases with increasing blast percentage.

These differences are not simply cosmetic but translate into functional differences *in vitro* and *in vivo*. CD133 is expressed by normal human hematopoietic stem and progenitor cells. It is also expressed on subpopulations of tumor cells. Peter Dirk's group have tested the function of brain tumor cells expressing this marker *in vitro* and *in vivo*. The CD133$^+$ cells from brain tumors form tumor spheres *in vitro*, while CD133$^-$ cells do not. Similar results were generated using NOD/SCID mice as a host for sorted primary brain tumor cells; only the CD133$^+$ fraction initiates tumor when injected into mice brains. The same marker has been used to identify colon cancer cells that can initiate tumor growth *in vivo*. Again, CD133$^-$ cells do not induce tumor growth. The CD133-expressing cells produce not only more CD133$^+$ cells but also CD133$^-$ cells. The tumors that grow in the mice from the CD133$^+$ fractions resemble the primary colon tumors. CD133$^+$ cells could also be taken from mice with tumor and transplanted successfully into other mice, indicating the ability to self-renew. The earliest such experiments were performed with AML. CD34 is a marker of normal human hematopoietic stem and progenitor cells, and for most samples the CD34$^+$ fraction alone contains the cells capable of inducing leukemia when transplanted into mice. Thus not all tumor cells are equal.

Recent work has challenged the CSC hypothesis, at least in terms of the frequency of CSCs. Using mice with a genetic propensity to develop lymphomas or leukemias, one group showed that 10 unselected tumor cells could reliably initiate tumor in congenic recipients. In this model the CSCs were thus a significant proportion of the tumor cells (at least 10% and possibly the majority of cells in some tumors). The

authors question whether it is meaningful to talk about CSCs if they are such a large percentage of the tumor. A CSC frequency of 25% of all cells was reported in which normal cells were transformed by the *MLL* gene and passaged though methylcellulose. These studies relied on synthetic tumors in mice that may not fully resemble spontaneous human tumors. Alternatively, there may be greater heterogeneity with regard to CSC frequency in primary human tumors than previously realized; some human tumors may consist of a significant proportion of CSCs. A recent study on human melanoma utilized an improved xenograft model and showed that the CSC frequency was 27% of all cells.

## The origin of hematological CSCs

The remainder of this chapter focuses on CSCs in hematological malignancies, with an emphasis on leukemia.

### The cell of origin

CSCs arise by the transformation of normal cells. One common misconception is that all hematological CSCs derive from hematopoietic stem cells (HSCs). There is good evidence that this is not the case. Some CSCs derive from HSCs while others derive from progenitors and other more differentiated cells (Figure 29.1). The phenotype of CSCs can indicate the identity of the normal hematopoietic cell from which they originated. Acute lymphoblastic leukemia (ALL) CSCs with *TEL-AML1* or *BCR-ABL* (p190) have a pro-B-cell phenotype (CD34$^+$CD19$^+$), suggesting an origin from B-cell progenitors, whereas ALL CSCs with *BCR-ABL* (p210) have an HSC phenotype consistent with an origin from HSCs (CD34$^+$CD38$^-$CD19$^-$).

HSCs and AML CSCs both have a primitive phenotype with expression of CD34 and absence of CD38, CD71 and HLA-DR, are quiescent most of the time, and show heterogeneity within engrafting populations. These similarities have led some authors to conclude that AML derives from an HSC that is locked into the myeloid lineage by the transforming events. However, the phenotypes of AML CSCs and HSCs are not identical, with discordant expression of c-kit and the interleukin (IL)-3 receptor α chain (IL-3R; CD123).

Recent data from our laboratory suggest that some AML CSCs, including those with a translocation involving the *MLL* oncogene, have a progenitor phenotype (CD34$^+$CD38$^+$) (Figure 29.1). This work is consistent with data showing that mouse myeloid progenitors can be transformed into AML by transduction with the oncogene *MLL-ENL* or *MOZ-TIF2*. These oncogenes confer self-renewal ability on the myeloid

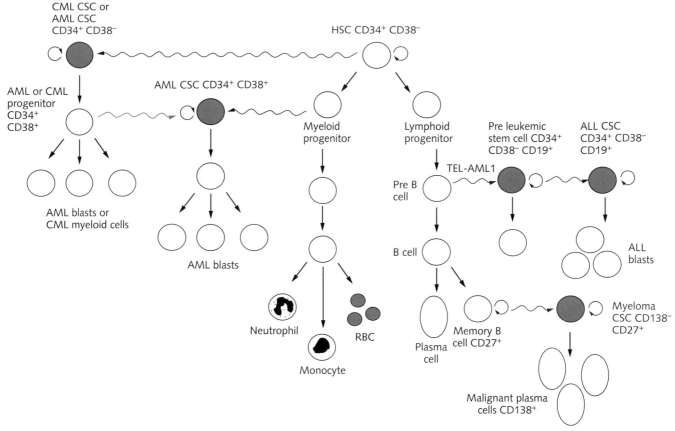

**Fig. 29.1 Origin of cancer stem cells (CSCs)**
The normal hematopoietic hierarchy is shown in the center with the hematopoietic stem cell (HSC) at the apex. The normal hematopoietic cells from which various hematological CSCs are derived are indicated. CSCs are shown as filled circles. Cells capable of self-renewal are shown with an arrow circling back on itself. Transforming events are shown by the wavy arrows. The colored wavy arrow signifies transformation of malignant progenitors to give rise to a second generation of CSCs. See text for definition of other abbreviations.

progenitors. This variability in phenotype of CSCs is unsurprising given the heterogeneity of AML in terms of karyotype, immunophenotype and outcome.

Myeloma CSCs have restricted light chain expression and share surface markers with normal memory B cells (e.g., CD27). Additionally, myeloma cells have clonal somatic hypermutation of the immunoglobulin gene. These data suggest that myeloma CSCs arise from a normal memory B cell. Normal memory T and B cells, in contrast to myeloid progenitors and mature myeloid cells, can self-renew to allow very long-lived immunity. This feature may make these cells more vulnerable to transformation and may explain the relatively high incidence of lymphoid tumors with a mature cell phenotype.

## The evolution of hematological malignancy

However, the origin of CSCs may be more complicated than the above scheme indicates. In a recent study human cord blood cells were transformed to acute leukemia when transduced with the *MLL* oncogene. The original CSCs that were formed were derived from primitive cells with germline immunoglobulin genes. There was evidence that a second generation of CSCs evolved with the passage of time. The second generation of CSCs was derived from malignant progenitor cells (the immunoglobulin genes were rearranged in these cells) that had acquired self-renewal ability. With time these second-generation CSCs came to dominate. This model suggests that for acute leukemia two or more types of CSC may be present (Figure 29.1). We have observed two types of cell that could initiate leukemia in immunodeficient mice, one with a progenitor phenotype (CD34⁺CD38⁺) and one with a more primitive phenotype (CD34⁺CD38⁻) from one AML sample.

The evolution of a second generation of CSCs is thought to underlie some cases of transformation of follicular lymphoma (see below) as well as progression of CML to blast crisis.

## Preleukemic stem cells

The existence of leukemia-associated fusion oncogene sequences in neonatal blood spots has been identified in samples taken years before the onset of leukemia in children. These sequences were also found in children who did not develop leukemia. Indeed, only a minority of children with leukemia-associated sequences developed leukemia. Recent work suggests that the source of this DNA may be preleukemic stem cells, cells that contain the leukemia-associated sequences and which have self-renewal potential but without the ability to induce leukemia. Twins were identified, one who had ALL with the *TEL-AML1* fusion oncogene and one who was healthy but had a long-lived population of progenitor B cells with the same *TEL-AML1* oncogene and an abnormal phenotype ($CD34^+CD38^-CD19^+$). This is the same phenotype as the CSCs from ALL with t(12;21). Transduction of normal human cord blood cells with *TEL-AML1* conferred the ability to self-renew on progenitor B cells (as well as altering the phenotype to $CD34^+CD38^-CD19^+$). Presumably, preleukemic stem cells lack the additional DNA hits to allow full leukemic transformation.

Although *TEL-AML1* confers phenotypic and functional changes, there is no reason to think that all preleukemic stem cells would be phenotypically and functionally different to the normal HSCs. A number of oncogenes, such as *BCR-ABL*, have been introduced into hematopoietic cells without apparent functional effects. Thus many preleukemic stem cells may not be readily detectable, as occurred in the twin study.

Clonal tracking studies in follicular lymphoma indicate that some cases of transformation to diffuse large B-cell lymphoma occur by mutation of clones causing the indolent phase of the disease (analogous to the second generation of CSCs in acute leukemias). However, other cases of transformed disease arise independently of the indolent clone. These studies are consistent with the existence of a common pre-lymphoma stem cell that gives rise to independent clones that cause the indolent and transformed phases. The existence of a common (*JAK2* wild type) preleukemic stem cell would explain the *JAK2* wild-type secondary AMLs that arise in patients with *JAK2* mutated myeloproliferative disorders (the *JAK2* mutation being a later event). A common (Philadelphia chromosome negative) preleukemic stem cell may also be the cause of the Philadelphia-negative chromosomal abnormalities seen in patients with CML treated successfully with imatinib.

Malignant disease may recur many years after remission has been attained. This is difficult to explain with conventional models of tumor growth. In some cases of ALL with *TEL-AML1*, the clones responsible for recurrence are detectable as minority populations at the time of diagnosis of leukemia. Although the clones responsible for recurrence respond poorly to chemotherapy at diagnosis, the main clone responds well. One explanation is that the minor population detectable at diagnosis comprises preleukemic stem cells and their progeny and is resistant to therapy. Between diagnosis and recurrence further mutations occur in the preleukemic stem cells that transform them into fully malignant cells. Rather than terming the process "recurrence," it might be more accurate to describe it as "re-evolution from a surviving preleukemic stem cell." Re-evolution from precancerous stem cells may explain the very late recurrences seen in other types of leukemia and solid tumors such as breast cancer. Eliminating these precancerous stem cells may be important for true cure.

## Translocations and transcription factors in CSC generation

A number of genes have been implicated in the generation and maintenance of HSCs, for example *AML-1*, *SCL*, *TEL*, *MLL*. Disruption of these genes results in a failure of definitive hematopoiesis. These genes are frequently involved in translocations in hematological malignancy. The translocation products have been introduced into normal hematopoietic cells to assess the effects. *AML1-ETO* does not induce leukemia by itself, but only in combination with other mutations (e.g., *FLT3*). However, cells expressing *AML1-ETO* alone do have enhanced replating capacity in methylcellulose and enhanced survival in long-term culture assays. In the study by Higuchi and colleagues, the cells could be passaged at least 10 times, whereas wild-type cells could only be passaged twice. This suggests that progenitor cells had gained self-renewal ability through *AML1-ETO*. Other translocation products (e.g., *MLL-ENL*, *TEL-AML1*) that involve genes critical in generation and maintenance of HSCs can confer the ability to self-renew on progenitors (*see above*). Thus, one of the fundamental features of a CSC, the ability to self-renew, is endowed or enhanced by some leukemogenic translocation products. Another gene crucial for HSC development is *Bmi-1*. Although not a classic target of leukemic translocations, it is expressed at enhanced levels in some AML cases, and is necessary for the self-renewal of HSCs and AML CSCs.

Hematopoietic differentiation is regulated by a number of transcription factors. These transcription factors guide differentiation down specific lineages by upregulating the expression of genes associated with that lineage and by repressing the expression of genes from rival lineages, for example *Pax5* upregulates CD19 and CD79a (genes associated with B lymphocytes) and represses macrophage colony-stimulating factor (associated with myeloid cells) and *NOTCH 1* (associated with T cells) and induces B-cell development from progenitors. Genes for these transcription factors are frequently mutated in hematological malignancy. *Pax5* is mutated or deleted in some cases of pre-B-cell ALL and is thought to result in loss of function. From studies of *Pax5*$^{-/-}$ mice it is known that loss of *Pax5* results in a blockage of B-cell differentiation at the pre-B-cell stage. *Pax5*$^{-/-}$ pre-B cells have self-renewal capacity and can repopulate the bone marrow of recipients in the long term, unlike wild-type pre-B cells. *Pax5* mutation may have a similar effect on pre-B cells, blocking differentiation and conferring self-renewal. Another example of a lineage-specific differentiation factor that is mutated in leukemia is *NOTCH 1* (mutated in more than 50% of T-cell ALL). Mutations in *NOTCH 1* allow proliferation and survival of cell lines derived from T-cell ALL and γ-secretase inhibitors (which block NOTCH signaling) block the cycling of these cells.

JunB forms part of the activator protein-1 transcription factor complex. JunB represses genes like cyclin D1 that are involved in cell cycling and upregulates genes such as p16/INK4α that inhibit progression through the cell cycle. The expression of JunB is downregulated in CML, with the lowest levels found in blast crisis. Deletion of *JunB* in a mouse model induced a CML-like disease. The effect was only seen where *JunB* was deleted in HSCs; no CML-like disease was seen where *JunB* was deleted from myeloid progenitors.

These genetic lesions are almost certainly working in conjunction with other mutations and thus the above models of action are probably too simplistic. Even so they give clues as to the types of genetic events that underlie the transformation of normal hematopoietic cells into CSCs.

## The CSC niche

Normal HSCs require support from non-hematopoietic cells for their survival and function. The supportive microenvironment of the stem cell is termed the stem cell niche. The HSC niche is thought to reside within the endosteal region of the bone marrow (the region lining the inner surface of the bone). Bone marrow stromal cells (non-hematopoietic cells derived from mesenchymal stem cells) such as osteoblasts form part of the niche. Stromal derived factor (SDF)-1 is secreted by bone marrow stromal cells and is involved in the homing and retention of HSCs within the bone marrow (via its interaction with CXCR4 on the HSCs). SDF-1 antagonists mobilize HSCs. The physical tethering of HSCs to a locus within the bone marrow is one key function of the niche (Figure 29.2).

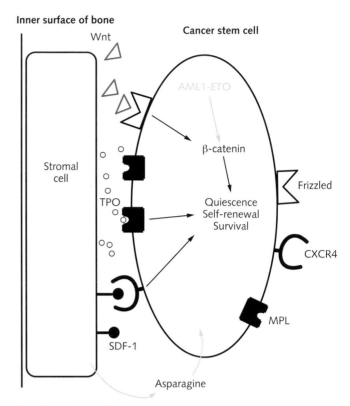

**Fig. 29.2 Stem cell niche**
The niche is composed of stromal cells lining the bone (endosteal region). Stem cells are anchored to the niche via the interaction of CXCR4 and stromal derived factor (SDF)-1. Niche cells signal to adjacent stem cells via thrombopoietin (TPO), Wnt and SDF-1 and their respective receptors on stem cells (MPL, Frizzled and CXCR4). These mediators induce quiescence, survival and self-renewal of stem cells. Some AML translocation products activate the Wnt/β-catenin pathway directly. Stromal cells support ALL CSCs by providing asparagine. See text for definition of other abbreviations.

In addition, the niche regulates proliferation and differentiation of HSCs. The SDF-1/CXCR4 interaction not only anchors HSCs but also induces quiescence. Other stromal cell products have similar roles. Thrombopoietin is produced by osteoblasts and its receptor, MPL, is expressed on HSCs. Ligation of MPL by agonist results in increased quiescence and maintenance of HSCs. In contrast, antagonizing the thrombopoietin–MPL interaction results in cycling of HSCs and depletion of HSCs. The niche supplies HSCs with key signals in the form of Wnt; antagonism of Wnt signaling by expression of Dickkopf-1 (an antagonist of the Wnt receptor) in osteoblasts results in HSC cycling and a decline in transplantability. Wnt agonists activate the β-catenin pathway and β-catenin is required for HSC self-renewal (Figure 29.2). The amount of Wnt signaling from the microenvironment appears to be crucial, as constitutional activation of this pathway results in loss of HSCs (i.e., too much or too little Wnt signaling results in loss of HSCs).

Oncogenic events can replicate some of the signals HSCs get from the niche. *AML1-ETO* and other AML translocation products induce the Wnt/β-catenin pathway and downstream transcription factors. This independence from niche signals is likely to be only partial because a number of signals and molecular pathways are necessary for self-renewal. In addition, leukemia cells appear to depend on the bone marrow microenvironment for survival. Leukemia cells from the peripheral blood of patients with AML are transplantable into immunodeficient mice, indicating that CSCs circulate. Yet many of these patients have no extra-hematopoietic organ involvement. This suggests that the circulating CSCs cannot seed all organs. One explanation is that CSCs are dependent on survival signals from the bone marrow. Blast clearance occurs after chemotherapy first from the peripheral blood and then from the bone marrow and recurrence is usually within bone marrow, again confirming the idea of a supportive CSC niche in the bone marrow. Direct evidence for the protective effect of stromal cells comes from *in vitro* studies. AML blasts undergo less apoptosis in response to chemotherapy if in contact with stromal cells. Stromal cells protect ALL cells (which have low levels of the enzyme asparagine synthetase) from asparaginase by secreting asparagine.

Xenograft experiments provide additional evidence for a supportive CSC niche; few primary leukemias seed organs other than the bone marrow and related hematopoietic organs (e.g., spleen). In immunodeficient mice, leukemia CSCs home to the endosteal region of bone marrow, and leukemia cells spread from here to the rest of the marrow. SDF-1 may be important for CSC homing because antagonists of the SDF-1/CXCR4 interaction reduce homing of leukemia cells. The CSCs within the endosteal region survive treatment by cytarabine chemotherapy, while cells within the central cavity undergo apoptosis.

Quiescence is one property shared by HSCs and CSCs (from both AML and CML). The niche induces quiescence in HSCs (via SDF-1/CXCR4 interaction and other signals) and this is one mechanism that protects stem cells from chemotherapy (which acts on dividing cells). Similar events are likely to induce quiescence in CSCs; the prognosis is worse in AML patients where the CD34$^+$ cells express high levels of CXCR4. Leukemia CSCs may well depend on the same niche as HSCs given the similarities, though this has not been proven and remains an area of active investigation.

## Implications of the CSC hypothesis for cancer drug testing

Laboratory tests for preclinical assessment of potential cancer treatments have generally relied on short-term culture systems that assess the effect of drugs on the proliferation or survival of malignant cells. Many drugs that have activity in preclinical assessments proceed to clinical trials. There is, however, a low success rate of anticancer drugs in clinical trials, suggesting that current preclinical models are inadequate. This may be explained by the hierarchical ordering of cancers. The conventional short-term assays will assess malignant progenitor or other cells in the middle and bottom ranks of the hierarchy, but not CSCs. Only long-term assays will be able to assess the effects of drugs on CSCs. NOD/SCID mice have increasingly been used to assess oncology drugs. These have the advantage that they can test the effect of a drug on long-term growth of malignant cells to see whether drug is truly eliminating CSCs in a microenvironment that approaches that of the patient bone marrow (i.e., with stromal cells that provide proper support for CSCs). Investigators must test the effects of drugs on leukemia that is already engrafted rather than treating the tumor cells *in vitro* and then injecting them into mice because this latter approach inappropriately circumvents the protective effects of bone marrow stroma. Although these new models appeal on rational grounds, no one has yet shown that efficacy of anticancer drugs in xenotransplant models correlates with efficacy in patients.

## Targeting CSCs

CSCs need to be eliminated to allow control of malignant disease. CSCs from hematological malignancies must be targeted selectively to avoid hematopoietic toxicity, but this is not the only type of "friendly fire" that is possible. CSCs also share features in common with non-hematopoietic adult stem cells and care must be taken to spare these vital cells.

Surface antigens that are not present on HSCs or other adult stem cells are an attractive target to deliver a selective hit to CSCs. Monoclonal antibodies against B-lineage antigens such as CD20 have been used successfully to improve the outcome of lymphoma, with relatively little toxicity (presumably the lymphoma CSCs express CD20, although this has not been formally demonstrated). The advent of engineered bispecific antibodies may allow improved selectivity, particularly where CSCs express an aberrant combination of antigens not found in normal tissues.

Cell signaling pathways are frequently activated in cancer cells and components of these pathways are often subject to mutation in cancer. The mutant proteins themselves are an apparent Achilles' heel for cancer and can be effectively inhibited by small molecules in patients where there is a consistent genetic lesion. Even where there are no mutations within the signaling pathway components, overactive pathways may be selectively inhibited for therapeutic benefit where tumor growth is dependent on the pathways (so long as key normal cells do not depend on these same pathways for survival).

Other approaches for targeting CSCs are under investigation but the rest of this section focuses on therapies aimed at surface antigens and signaling pathways as these have yielded effective treatments in the clinic.

## Targeting cell surface antigens

Cell surface antigens have been used to isolate CSCs in a range of conditions. These surface antigens are a potential target for therapy. CD123 and CD33 are both expressed on AML CSCs and therapies that target these antigens are undergoing clinical trials. One therapy comprises diphtheria toxin fused to IL-3. IL-3 binds to its receptor (CD123), which is expressed on AML CSCs but not on most normal bone marrow HSCs. This compound inhibits growth of AML *in vivo* while having a limited effect on normal hematopoietic cells.

Monoclonal antibody against CD33 has been conjugated to a cytotoxic agent to form gemtuzumab ozagamicin (GO). Antibody to CD33 is internalized on binding to the cell surface and so brings the cytotoxic agent into the cell. GO can induce remission in AML when given as a sole agent. However, recurrence is inevitable unless further therapies are given, suggesting that GO fails to kill AML CSCs. The problem appears to be due to resistance of AML CSCs to the cytotoxic agent (i.e., the antibody is delivering toxin to the right cells but the toxin is not killing them); those AML cases that are clinically resistant to GO express multidrug resistance pumps and these are thought to eliminate the cytotoxic agent.

The problem of CSC resistance is critical. Resistance may partly depend on the cell of origin of a CSC. Many CSCs are thought to derive from transformed HSCs (see above). HSCs themselves are very durable cells; they need to provide life-long hematopoiesis through a range of insults. They express many membrane pumps that allow them to expel toxins and possess detoxifying enzymes such as aldehyde dehydrogenase. These features make HSCs highly resistant to toxic insult, including chemotherapy; patients undergoing intensive chemotherapy survive because the HSCs endure the insult and regenerate the bone marrow. Diseases thought to be derived from HSCs such as CML, Philadelphia chromosome-positive ALL (p210) and many cases of AML are all notoriously difficult to eradicate with chemotherapy. The same pumps and enzymes that confer resistance on HSCs have been detected in CSCs.

Overcoming these defensive mechanisms is likely to be key to our ability to kill CSCs. Unless targeting is truly selective, this may lead to catastrophic damage to HSCs. Care must be taken to assess antigen expression on normal HSCs (and other key organs such as vasculature that may be exposed to drugs) when designing targeted therapies to ensure they are selective for CSCs. Many ALL CSCs express CD19 while normal HSCs do not and therefore this makes a potentially attractive surface antigen to target. Another surface marker that may allow selective targeting of leukemia is CD44. Antibody against CD44 was effective at reducing the amount of leukemia in the bone marrow of NOD/SCID mice but spared normal hematopoietic cells. For some diseases the CSCs share a number of features in common with HSCs and the task of identifying antigens specific for the CSC is difficult. Myeloid markers were thought not to be expressed on HSCs and therefore thought to be a good target for therapies against AML CSCs, but recent data from our laboratory and others challenge this notion.

## Targeting CSC signaling pathways

Fusion oncoproteins are an attractive target for therapy. The tyrosine kinase produced by the *BCR-ABL* oncogene is inhibited by a number of relatively selective tyrosine kinase inhibitors (TKIs). These induce complete cytogenetic responses in the majority of patients with CML and result in long-term disease control. However, the disease recurs if the drug is withdrawn. This suggests that TKIs do not eliminate CML CSCs. The CML CSC appears to be resistant to killing by TKIs even where there is no mutation in *BCR-ABL* leading to TKI resistance. A number of mechanisms may be involved in resistance, including membrane pumps that remove TKIs from CSCs, expression of high levels of *BCR-ABL* in CSCs (relative to other CML cells) and quiescence of CSCs.

Another approach is to target signal transduction pathways that are active in CSCs. Phosphatidylinositol 3-kinase (PI3K) belongs to a family of enzymes involved in signal transduction. PI3K generates lipid second messengers and these activate downstream effectors such as AKT, which is important in regulation of cell survival. Components of the PI3K/AKT pathway are a frequent target for mutation in malignant disease. Moreover, the pathway is activated in some malignancies where there are no mutations within the components. In 50% of AML cases there is constitutive activation of the PI3K/AKT pathway. Activation of this pathway is seen not just in blast cells but also in the CD34$^+$CD123$^+$CD38$^-$ fraction that is enriched in CSCs. Inhibiting PI3K pathways *in vitro* enhances chemotherapy-induced cytotoxicity. There are a number of isoforms of PI3K and it is the p110 δ isoform that is expressed in AML. Mice with disrupted p110 δ have only mild hematopoietic defects, suggesting a relatively limited role in HSC function. Targeting p110 δ with specific inhibitors would be predicted to be selective for AML and target the CSCs.

Other pathways are activated in CSCs but not within normal HSCs and these may present themselves as appropriate targets for selective inhibition. The nuclear factor (NF)-κB is constitutively expressed in the CD34$^+$CD38$^-$ fraction of AML (where most AML CSCs reside). It is not expressed in normal HSCs. An inhibitor of NF-κB, parthenolide, has been developed by Craig Jordan's group. Parthenolide reduces engraftment of AML in NOD/SCID mice while having no significant effect on normal hematopoietic cells. Parthenolide derivatives are undergoing clinical trial.

## Conclusions

Our understanding of CSCs is in its infancy. Their existence provides a challenge to researchers in the field of oncology. CSCs form only a minority of cells within a tumor and their interactions with their microenvironment are complicated. This necessitates the use of new methods to assay these cells, including the use of xenograft models. These techniques are expensive and technically demanding. With improved understanding of microenvironmental signals it may be possible to construct the necessary supporting elements to allow the growth of human primary CSCs for prolonged periods *in vitro*.

The durability of CSCs is daunting: many survive harsh myeloablative chemoradiotherapy regimens, graft-versus-leukemia effect and specific targeting by TKIs. Finding vulnerabilities in the armor of CSCs is a difficult task but one that is likely to be rewarding in the clinic. Potential targets of therapy include the supportive interaction of the niche and the CSC, the molecular pathways specific to the CSCs, and the surface molecules that are aberrantly expressed on CSCs. Ultimately, we will need to deal with the driver of malignant disease if we are to control it.

## Acknowledgments

Dr Taussig is supported by an MRC Clinician Scientist Fellowship and Dr Bonnet is supported by Cancer Research UK.

## Further reading

### Evidence for the existence of CSCs

Bonnet D, Dick JE. (1997) Human acute myeloid leukemia is organized as a hierarchy that originates from a primitive hematopoietic cell. *Nature Medicine*, **3**, 730–737.

Brunschwig A, Southam CM, Levin AG. (1965) Host resistance to cancer. Clinical experiments by homotransplants, autotransplants and admixture of autologous leucocytes. *Annals of Surgery*, **162**, 416–425.

Kelly PN, Dakic A, Adams JM, Nutt SL, Strasser A. (2007) Tumor growth need not be driven by rare cancer stem cells. *Science*, **317**, 337.

O'Brien CA, Pollett A, Gallinger S, Dick JE. (2007) A human colon cancer cell capable of initiating tumor growth in immunodeficient mice. *Nature*, **445**, 106–110.

Pearce DJ, Taussig D, Zibara K *et al.* (2006) AML engraftment in the NOD/SCID assay reflects the outcome of AML: implications for our understanding of the heterogeneity of AML. *Blood*, **107**, 1166–1173.

Quintana E, Shackleton M, Sabel MS, Fullen DR, Johnson TM, Morrison SJ. (2008) Efficient tumour formation by single human melanoma cells. *Nature*, **456**, 593–598.

Singh SK, Hawkins C, Clarke ID *et al.* (2004) Identification of human brain tumor initiating cells. *Nature*, **432**, 396–401.

Somervaille TC, Cleary ML. (2006) Identification and characterization of leukemia stem cells in murine MLL-AF9 acute myeloid leukemia. *Cancer Cell*, **10**, 257–268.

### Origin of hematological CSCs

Barabe F, Kennedy JA, Hope KJ, Dick JE. (2007) Modeling the initiation and progression of human acute leukemia in mice. *Science*, **316**, 600–604.

Blair A, Hogge DE, Sutherland HJ. (1998) Most acute myeloid leukemia progenitor cells with long-term proliferative ability in vitro and in vivo have the phenotype CD34(+)/CD71(−)/HLA-DR. *Blood*, **92**, 4325–4335.

Castor A, Nilsson L, Astrand-Grundstrom I *et al.* (2005) Distinct patterns of hematopoietic stem cell involvement in acute lymphoblastic leukemia. *Nature Medicine*, **11**, 630–637.

Cozier A, Passegue E, Ayton PM *et al.* (2003) Similar MLL-associated leukemias arising from self-renewing stem cells and short-lived myeloid progenitors. *Genes and Development*, **17**, 3029–3035.

Guan Y, Gerhard B, Hogge DE. (2003) Detection, isolation, and stimulation of quiescent primitive leukemic progenitor cells from patients with acute myeloid leukemia (AML). *Blood*, **101**, 3142–3149.

Hope KJ, Jin L, Dick JE. (2004) Acute myeloid leukemia originates from a hierarchy of leukemic stem cell classes that differ in self-renewal capacity. *Nature Immunology*, **5**, 738–743.

Huntley BJ, Shigematsu H, Deguchi K *et al.* (2004) MOZ-TIF2, but not BCR-ABL, confers properties of leukemic stem cells to committed murine hematopoietic progenitors. *Cancer Cell*, **6**, 587–596.

Jordan CT, Upchurch D, Szilvassy SJ *et al.* (2000) The interleukin-3 receptor alpha chain is a unique marker for human acute myelogenous leukemia stem cells. *Leukemia*, **14**, 1777–1784.

Matsui W, Wang Q, Barber JP *et al.* (2008) Clonogenic multiple myeloma progenitors, stem cell properties, and drug resistance. *Cancer Research*, **68**, 190–197.

## Preleukemic stem cells

Bumm T, Muller C, Al-Ali HK *et al.* (2003) Emergence of clonal cytogenetic abnormalities in Ph– cells in some CML patients in cytogenetic remission to imatinib but restoration of polyclonal hematopoiesis in the majority. *Blood*, **101**, 1941–1949.

Carlotti E, Wrench D, Matthews J *et al.* (2009) Transformation of follicular lymphoma to diffuse large B-cell lymphoma may occur by divergent evolution from a common progenitor cell or by direct evolution from the follicular lymphoma clone. *Blood*, **113**(15), 3553–3557.

Gale KB, Ford AM, Repp R *et al.* (1997) Backtracking leukemia to birth: identification of clonotypic gene fusion sequences in neonatal blood spots. *Proceedings of the National Academy of Sciences of the United States of America*, **94**, 13950–13954.

Hong D, Gupta R, Ancliff P *et al.* (2008) Initiating and cancer-propagating cells in TEL-AML1-associated childhood leukemia. *Science*, **319**, 336–339.

Jelinek J, Oki Y, Gharibyan V *et al.* (2005) JAK2 mutation 1849G→T is rare in acute leukemias but can be found in CMML, Philadelphia chromosome-negative CML, and megakaryocytic leukemia. *Blood*, **106**, 3370–3373.

Konrad M, Metzler M, Panzer S *et al.* (2003) Late relapses evolve from slow-responding subclones in t(12;21)-positive acute lymphoblastic leukemia: evidence for the persistence of a preleukemic clone. *Blood*, **101**, 3635–3640.

Schessl C, Rawat VP, Cusan M *et al.* (2005) The AML1–ETO fusion gene and the FLT3 length mutation collaborate in inducing acute leukemia in mice. *Journal of Clinical Investigation*, **115**, 2159–2168.

## Translocations and transcription factors in CSC generation

Higuchi M, O'Brien D, Kumaravelu P *et al.* (2002) Expression of a conditional AML1–ETO oncogene bypasses embryonic lethality and establishes a murine model of human t(8;21) acute myeloid leukemia. *Cancer Cell*, **1**, 63–74.

Lessard J, Sauvageau G. (2003) Bmi-1 determines the proliferative capacity of normal and leukaemic stem cells. *Nature*, **423**, 255–260.

Mullighan CG, Goorha S, Radtke I *et al.* (2007) Genome-wide analysis of genetic alterations in acute lymphoblastic leukemia. *Nature*, **446**, 758–764.

Mulloy JC, Cammenga J, Berguido FJ *et al.* (2003) Maintaining the self-renewal and differentiation potential of human CD34⁺ hematopoietic cells using a single genetic element. *Blood*, **102**, 4369–4376.

Nutt SL, Heavey B, Rolink AG, Busslinger M. (1999) Commitment to the B-lymphoid lineage depends on the transcription factor Pax5. *Nature*, **401**, 556–562.

Passegue E, Wagner EF, Weissman IL. (2004) JunB deficiency leads to a myeloproliferative disorder arising from hematopoietic stem cells. *Cell*, **119**, 431–443.

Schaniel C, Gottar M, Roosnek E, Melchers F, Rolink AG. (2002) Extensive in vivo self-renewal, long-term reconstitution capacity, and hematopoietic multipotency of Pax5-deficient precursor B-cell clones. *Blood*, **99**, 2760–2766.

Weng AP, Ferrando AA, Lee W *et al.* (2004) Activating mutations of NOTCH1 in human T cell acute lymphoblastic leukemia. *Science*, **306**, 269–271.

Yang MY, Liu TC, Chang JG, Lin PM, Lin SF. (2003) JunB gene expression is inactivated by methylation in chronic myeloid leukemia. *Blood*, **101**, 3205–3211.

## The CSC niche

Broxmeyer HE, Orschell CM, Clapp DW *et al.* (2005) Rapid mobilization of murine and human hematopoietic stem and progenitor cells with AMD3100, a CXCR4 antagonist. *Journal of Experimental Medicine*, **201**, 1307–1318.

Fleming HE, Janzen V, Lo Celso C *et al.* (2008) Wnt signaling in the niche enforces hematopoietic stem cell quiescence and is necessary to preserve self-renewal in vivo. *Cell Stem Cell*, **2**, 274–283.

Ishikawa F, Yoshida S, Saito Y *et al.* (2007) Chemotherapy-resistant human AML stem cells home to and engraft within the bone-marrow endosteal region. *Nature Biotechnology*, **25**, 1315–1321.

Iwamoto S, Mihara K, Downing JR, Pui CH, Campana D. (2007) Mesenchymal cells regulate the response of acute lymphoblastic leukemia cells to asparaginase. *Journal of Clinical Investigation*, **117**, 1049–1057.

Muller-Tidow C, Steffen B, Cauvet T *et al.* (2004) Translocation products in acute myeloid leukemia activate the Wnt signaling pathway in hematopoietic cells. *Molecular and Cellular Biology*, **24**, 2890–2904.

Nie Y, Han YC, Zou YR. (2008) CXCR4 is required for the quiescence of primitive hematopoietic cells. *Journal of Experimental Medicine*.

Qian H, Buza-Vidas N, Hyland CD *et al.* (2007) Critical role of thrombopoietin in maintaining adult quiescent hematopoietic stem cells. *Cell Stem Cell*, **1**, 671–684.

Spoo AC, Lubbert M, Wierda WG, Burger JA. (2007) CXCR4 is a prognostic marker in acute myelogenous leukemia. *Blood*, **109**, 786–791.

Tavor S, Petit I, Porozov S *et al.* (2004) CXCR4 regulates migration and development of human acute myelogenous leukemia stem cells in transplanted NOD/SCID mice. *Cancer Research*, **64**, 2817–2824.

Yoshihara H, Arai F, Hosokawa K *et al.* (2007) Thrombopoietin/MPL signaling regulates hematopoietic stem cell quiescence and interaction with the osteoblastic niche. *Cell Stem Cell*, **1**, 685–697.

## Targeting CSCs

Bhatia R, Holtz M, Niu N *et al.* (2003) Persistence of malignant hematopoietic progenitors in chronic myelogenous leukemia patients in complete cytogenetic remission following imatinib mesylate treatment. *Blood*, **101**, 4701–4707.

Billottet C, Grandage VL, Gale RE *et al.* (2006) A selective inhibitor of the p110delta isoform of PI3-kinase inhibits AML cell proliferation and survival and increases the cytotoxic effects of VP16. *Oncogene*, **25**, 6648–6659.

Chaudhary PM, Roninson IB. (1991) Expression and activity of P-glycoprotein, a multidrug efflux pump, in human hematopoietic stem cells. *Cell*, **66**, 85–94.

Copland M, Hamilton A, Elrick LJ *et al.* (2006) Dasatinib (BMS-354825) targets an earlier progenitor population than imatinib in primary CML but does not eliminate the quiescent fraction. *Blood*, **107**, 4532–4539.

Guzman ML, Rossi RM, Karnischky L *et al.* (2005) The sesquiterpene lactone parthenolide induces apoptosis of human acute myelogenous leukemia stem and progenitor cells. *Blood*, **105**, 4163–4169.

Jin L, Hope KJ, Zhai Q, Smadja-Joffe F, Dick JE. (2006) Targeting of CD44 eradicates human acute myeloid leukemic stem cells. *Nature Medicine*, **12**, 1167–1174.

Linenberger ML, Hong T, Flowers D *et al.* (2001) Multidrug-resistance phenotype and clinical responses to gemtuzumab ozogamicin. *Blood*, **98**, 988–994.

Nagai Y, Garrett KP, Ohta S *et al.* (2006) Toll-like receptors on hematopoietic progenitor cells stimulate innate immune system replenishment. *Immunity*, **24**, 801–812.

Okkenhaug K, Bilancio A, Farjot G *et al.* (2002) Impaired B and T cell antigen receptor signaling in p110delta PI3-kinase mutant mice. *Science*, **297**, 1031–1034.

Pearce DJ, Taussig D, Simpson C *et al.* (2005) Characterization of cells with a high aldehyde dehydrogenase activity from cord blood and acute myeloid leukemia samples. *Stem Cells*, **23**, 752–760.

Sievers EL, Larson RA, Stadtmauer EA *et al.* (2001) Efficacy and safety of gemtuzumab ozogamicin in patients with CD33-positive acute myeloid leukemia in first relapse. *Journal of Clinical Oncology*, **19**, 3244–3254.

Storms RW, Trujillo AP, Springer JB *et al.* (1999) Isolation of primitive human hematopoietic progenitors on the basis of aldehyde dehydrogenase activity. *Proceedings of the National Academy of Sciences of the United States of America*, **96**, 9118–9123.

Tamburini J, Elie C, Bardet V *et al.* (2007) Constitutive phosphoinositide 3kinase/AKT activation represents a favourable prognostic factor in de novo AML patients. *Blood*.

Taussig DC, Pearce DJ, Simpson C *et al.* (2005) Hematopoietic stem cells express multiple myeloid markers: implications for the origin and targeted therapy of acute myeloid leukemia. *Blood*, **106**, 4086–4092.

Yalcintepe L, Frankel AE, Hogge DE. (2006) Expression of interleukin-3 receptor subunits on defined subpopulations of acute myeloid leukemia blasts predicts the cytotoxicity of diphtheria toxin interleukin-3 fusion protein against malignant progenitors that engraft in immunodeficient mice. *Blood*, **108**, 3530–3537.

# Chapter 30 Molecular basis of transplantation

## Francesco Dazzi

*Stem Cell Biology, Department of Haematology, Imperial College London, UK*

## Introduction

Transplantation is a successful therapeutic modality for a variety of diseases of different etiology and pathogenesis. Liver, heart, and kidney failure are common indications that would be even more widely pursued should donor availability not be so limited. Although the basic general principle underlying transplantation is replacement of a malfunctioning tissue with a healthy one, in the case of hematopoietic stem cell transplantation (HSCT) the procedure is associated with a number of other beneficial effects that can be exploited not only to restore hematopoietic failure itself but also to treat cancer and autoimmune diseases.

## Principles and clinical indications of HSCT

Hematopoietic stem cells (HSCs) have the capacity to self-renew and give rise to all formed elements in the blood. Because of this property, they can be used to rescue the hematopoietic system from the intensification of anticancer cytotoxic therapies. HSCT can be autologous when donor and recipient are the same individual or allogeneic if another individual is selected as HSC donor. In autologous HSCT, patients are subjected to lethal doses of chemoradiotherapy to eradicate the tumor and then receive their own HSCs harvested beforehand to restore the otherwise permanently ablated hematopoietic system. Although autologous HSCT is useful in some solid tumors, its efficacy in the treatment of hematopoietic malignancies is limited by contamination of the harvested stem cells by the original tumor and/or by

insufficient activity of the chemotherapy in eliminating the tumor itself. However, such an approach maintains some efficacy, because normal HSCs have a temporary growth advantage in repopulating the recipient compared with neoplastic stem cells.

A more recent application of autologous HSCT has been the treatment of severe autoimmune diseases, whereby repopulation of the immune system with primitive HSCs is believed to re-educate the disordered immune system. Phase I/II trials have reported high response rates in systemic lupus erythematosus, systemic sclerosis, rheumatoid arthritis, and multiple sclerosis. Randomized studies are ongoing to compare these achievements with conventional immunosuppressive therapies.

When a compatible donor is available, the use of allogeneic HSCT has profoundly modified the outcome of several hematological malignancies. The conditioning regimens contribute to eradication of the abnormal cells and ensure sustained engraftment of the healthy allogeneic stem cells. However, the efficacy of this approach cannot simply be ascribed to the chemoradiotherapy and to the administration of healthy HSCs, but is greatly dependent on immune recognition of the tumor by the lymphocytes contained in the donor stem cell preparation.

From these preliminary considerations it is clear how several mechanisms contribute to the outcome of HSCT and these involve HSC engraftment, expansion, and differentiation as well as, in the case of allogeneic HSCT, the interplay between donor and recipient immune responses.

## Non-immunological factors regulating HSCT

HSCs normally face four different outcomes: self-renewal, differentiation, mobilization, or programmed cell death. All

*Molecular Hematology*, 3rd edition. Edited by Drew Provan and John Gribben.
© 2010 Blackwell Publishing.

these process are tightly regulated and play a fundamental role during transplantation. Since HSCs are the source of every blood cell, their self-renewal and lifespan must be securely controlled. For this reason, a proportion of HSCs remains quiescent but available to contribute to blood homeostatic renewal. These HSCs reside in specialized areas in the bone marrow where they receive signals required for their homeostatic quiescent and stationary state. These HSC niches are constituted by endosteal bone-lining osteoblasts and other stromal cells that are responsible for generating the signals. The niche saves stem cells from depletion, while protecting the host from unnecessary stem cell proliferation (Plate 30.1).

## The hematopoietic stem cell

Probably the best definition of an HSC is functional and refers to a cell capable to provide lifelong reconstitution of all blood cell lineages after serial transplantation into lethally irradiated recipients (see Chapter 3).

In mice, the phenotype of HSCs is characterized by the surface expression of stem cell antigen (Sca)-1, c-Kit (receptor for stem cell factor) with associated low levels of Thy-1 (CD90) expression and the absence of other lineage-specific markers: $Lin^-Thy1.1^{+lo}c\text{-}Kit^+Sca1^+$. The biological activity of the candidate mouse HSC population has been enumerated by in vitro assays and in vivo competitive repopulation assays. These functional assays have shown that extensive self-renewal potential and proliferation ability are gradually lost during commitment and have defined a hierarchy in hematopoiesis. Long-term HSCs give rise to short-term HSCs that self-renew for 6–8 weeks only, then progress to multipotent progenitors with very limited self-renewal ability and inability to durably engraft in lethally irradiated mice.

In humans, HSC have been characterized by the expression of cell surface antigen CD34, c-Kit, Thy1 (CD90) and the absence of CD38 and other lineage-specific markers and are therefore styled as $Lin^-c\text{-}Kit^+Thy1^+CD38^-CD34^+$. The phenotype is the result of functional studies conducted not only in vitro but also using strains of immunodeficient mice suitable for human HSC engraftment.

Further studies have identified the heterogeneity of the HSC compartment and identified new markers, such as CD133, which is unique to a rare CD34⁻ subset with long-term HSC function in vivo and can similarly identify stem cells of other tissue origin. Very recently, a new classification of HSCs and early progenitors has been proposed based on the selective expression of SLAM (signaling lymphocyte activation molecule) family receptors. Highly enriched bone marrow HSC populations are marked by the expression of CD150 and the absence of CD224 and CD48, whereas multipotent progenitors and restricted B-cell progenitors selectively express only CD224 and CD48, respectively. A similar expression pattern of SLAM receptors has been described in fetal hematopoiesis.

The number of HSCs infused after the conditioning regimen remains a major prognostic factor for predicting the outcome of clinical HSCT. The larger the number of HSCs administered, the faster the recovery of recipient hematopoiesis and the lower the transplant-related mortality. Therefore, much effort is being invested in expanding the number of HSCs ex vivo with a variety of cytokine cocktails, although very limited success has been achieved thus far because expansion is almost invariably associated with differentiation.

## The hematopoietic niche

In the postnatal marrow, stromal cells form a three-dimensional network investing marrow sinusoids. Four main cell types of marrow stromal tissue are known to take part in supporting hematopoiesis: one is of hematopoietic origin (macrophages), whereas the others derive from mesenchymal progenitors (reticular cells, adipocytes, and osteoblasts). Among the various players it appears that a particular subset of osteoblasts (i.e., those expressing N-cadherin) is the most important component of the niche.

Osteoblast control of HSC proliferation within the niche is regulated by both cell contact mechanisms and soluble factors that mediate their effects via transcription factors, cell cycle regulators, adhesion molecules and chromosomal modifiers. These include a series of molecules that regulate the quiescent state of HSCs and their population size, including Notch1/Jagged1, the Wnt/β-catenin signaling pathways, Tie-2/Ang-1, osteopontin, and tenascin C. Animals deficient in these molecules have reduced number and function of HSCs. A wide variety of cytokines is produced by stromal cells, which maintain HSCs in quiescence or promote their self-renewal rather than differentiation. These include stem cell factor, leukemia inhibitory factor, the SDF-1/CXCL12 chemokine axis, bone morphogenetic protein (BMP)-4, the cytokine fms-like tyrosine kinase-3 (Flt-3), and transforming growth factor (TGF)-β. Stroma also produces a variety of interleukins and, under certain circumstances, cytokines which act on more mature hematopoietic progenitors, such as granulocyte macrophage colony-stimulating factor (GM-CSF) and granulocyte colony-stimulating factor (G-CSF). Lastly, adhesion molecules also play an important role in the control of HSC proliferation because engagement of β1 integrins prevents the progression of CD34⁺ cells from the $G_1$ to S phase of the cell cycle, thus inhibiting progenitor proliferation.

Although osteoblasts are ultimately the stromal cell making contact with and regulating the HSC compartment, bone is continuously subject to bone remodeling, a process generated by the cooperation of osteoblasts, the bone-forming cells, and osteoclasts, the bone-resorbing cells. As part of this tightly regulated process, osteoblasts regulate osteoclast maturation and proliferation and there is emerging evidence that the hematopoietic niche is the result of this process. In fact, pharmacological agents with the ability to modulate the number and/or functions of these cells have an impact on the number of HSCs and their ability to engraft in myeloablated recipients. Therefore, clinical trials are ongoing to test the effects of pretreating donors of HSC with drugs like parathormone on the transplantation outcome.

## Mobilization and homing of HSCs

The function of the niche is not confined to controlling the size of HSCs but also their mobilization. The ability to migrate is a fundamental property of HSCs throughout their development. During ontogeny, blood formation occurs in distinct extra-embryonic and embryonic sites that involve, in sequence, the yolk sac, aorta–gonad–mesonephros, placenta and fetal liver, before hematopoiesis finally takes place only in the bone marrow. Migrating from one site to another is critical, as demonstrated by the fact that mice made genetically deficient for CXCL12, a chemokine responsible for the homing of HSCs to the bone marrow, or its receptor CXCR4 have normal production of fetal liver HSCs but fail to transition to hematopoiesis in the marrow space.

The migratory nature of HSCs is maintained in adulthood, during which HSCs are found in the blood even under homeostatic conditions. Following the administration of cytokines, including G-CSF, GM-CSF and interleukin (IL)-8, the number of HSCs in the peripheral blood changes dramatically, with different kinetics depending on the mechanism involved. For example, G-CSF can modify niche cells by reducing the production of CXCL12 by osteoblasts, despite the absence of G-CSF receptors on these cells. Of particular interest is the observation that mice with altered sympathetic nervous system function lack the ability to mobilize stem cells from the bone marrow in response to G-CSF, indicating the possibility that stem cells might be able to "sense" changes such as those occurring distantly at the site of an injury.

Further developments in the area of HSC mobilization have recently identified the use of chemokine antagonists as an alternative and probably more effective strategy than G-CSF. AMD3100, a specific antagonist of the chemokine receptor CXCR4, is currently in clinical development and clinical trials have demonstrated its efficacy even in patients or donors refractory to G-CSF.

## The concept of bone marrow space and cell competition

A large number of studies in both animals and humans have shown that recipients of HSCs must receive some form of myeloablation for the HSCs to engraft, irrespective of whether there is an underlying malignancy to eradicate or an allogeneic immune system to suppress. This has introduced the notion that the quantitative reduction of host cellular components provides space for the incoming HSCs to expand and compete more favorably with recipient cells reduced in number by the conditioning regimen. Furthermore, there is also evidence that such homeostatic expansion might also affect some of the immunological mechanisms involved in transplantation tolerance that we discuss later.

However, "opening space" is not the only mechanism for engraftment. High levels of long-term marrow engraftment are obtained with infusion of high levels of marrow cells in untreated mice. This indicates that syngeneic engraftment is also determined by stem cell competition in the hematopoietic niche.

## Exploiting HSCT for resetting the immune system

Whilst the long-term efficacy of autologous HSCT in malignancies is confined to a minority of tumors, the fact that HSCs are also the precursors of immune cells has prompted investigators to test the ability of autologous HSCT to treat conditions characterized by abnormal immune responses. In support of this initiative is evidence that the maturation of new T cells in the thymus continues, albeit at a decreased rate, also in adult life.

Autologous HSCT is currently being explored with remarkable success in severe forms of autoimmune diseases, including multiple sclerosis, systemic lupus erythematosus, systemic sclerosis, rheumatoid arthritis and Crohn's disease. The main rationale for applying HSCT to autoimmune diseases has been the idea that intensive immune depletion could eliminate the pathogenic repertoire, and that reconstitution of a new immune system from hematopoietic precursors could restore immune tolerance, halting ongoing inflammatory activity and preventing relapses.

Recent studies have confirmed the notion that HSCT induces alterations in the immune system that are beyond the effects of a dose-escalating immunosuppressive approach. HSCT has been shown not only to affect the B-cell populations associated with the production of autoantibodies, but also to profoundly perturb the T-cell compartment, as illustrated by the normalization of the deregulated T-cell receptor (TCR) repertoire in multiple sclerosis. Furthermore, it appears that following myeloablation a subset of T cells (regulatory T cells) with the specific function of controlling immunity to self antigen selectively expands and could contribute to the control of the underlying autoimmune disease.

In contrast, the immune reconstitution following allogeneic HSCT remains incomplete for several months or years depending on the histocompatibility differences between donor and recipient. This is one of the several problems associated with the various immune responses generated in an allogeneic setting.

## Basic concepts in the immunology of allogeneic HSCT

Allogeneic HSCT triggers a network of immune responses that fundamentally affects the outcome of the procedure in terms of both complications and therapeutic success. Whereas recipient anti-donor immune responses (host-versus-graft) are important in solid organ transplantation, in allogeneic SCT they are profoundly inhibited by the conditioning regimen. The immunologically competent cells, present in the HSC preparation, play a more important role because they mediate a reaction against the host that targets recipient normal tissues (graft-versus-host), but also mediate the effect as the basis of the eradication of residual neoplastic cells (graft-versus-leukemia).

## The major histocompatibility complex

The major histocompatibility complex (MHC) defines a genetic region that includes genes encoding class I and class II membrane-bound cell surface glycoproteins. The function of MHC proteins is to present peptide antigens to T cells, a vital part of initiating an antigen-specific immune response. MHC proteins are also involved in the recognition of virally infected cells, or those cells in which genetic anomalies arise, by natural killer (NK) cells.

There are two major classes of genes within the MHC region, namely class I and class II genes. In addition to these, the MHC class III region encodes other proteins of the immune system, like certain complement and cytokine genes. In humans the MHC region is found on the short arm of chromosome 6 and encodes the human leukocyte antigens (HLA). Different loci are designated by a letter; thus the major class I loci are HLA-A, HLA-B and HLA-C. HLA class II genes are collectively designated HLA-D, and individual loci identified by a second letter, HLA-DR, HLA-DP, HLA-DQ. In addition to the classical class I and class II MHC genes, there exists a number of non-classical MHC genes,

such as HLA-E, HLA-F and HLA-G with functions that have not yet been fully elucidated.

The role of MHC molecules is to present peptide antigens to T cells. Class I molecules present endogenous peptides, virus- or tumor-encoded, that are generated in the cytosol, transported to the endoplasmic reticulum, and finally presented to the cell surface. HLA class II molecules are assembled in the endoplasmic reticulum, then transported through the Golgi to endosomal compartments where they load peptides that have entered the cell via endocytosis or receptor-mediated internalization. The selection of peptides by MHC molecules is dictated by the sequence of the MHC antigen-binding groove. Although MHC molecules have limited polymorphism compared with TCRs, they exhibit different avidity for different peptides, thus accounting for individual variability to respond to the same antigen and against different moieties.

## Mechanisms of allorecognition

Allorecognition is a particular form of antigen presentation that occurs only after transplantation of tissues between genetically disparate individuals of the same species (or after *in vitro* simulation of such). Host-versus-graft reactions refer to the immune response of the host to disparate antigens expressed on donor cells that result in graft rejection. Current understanding of host-versus-graft responses derives mainly from studies of solid organ transplantation in which the host does not receive any conditioning prior to the transplant and thus maintains the ability to reject it.

Two pathways of allorecognition have been described, namely direct and indirect allorecognition (Plate 30.2). The term "direct allorecognition" was initially used to describe the recognition by host T cells of intact donor MHC–peptide complex directly on the surface of donor antigen-presenting cells (APCs), but was also later extended to include the recognition of other donor-derived transplantation antigens (minor histocompatibility antigens) presented on donor APCs by an MHC molecule that is shared between donor and recipient. The frequencies of alloreactive T cells using this pathway has been estimated as 0.1–10% compared with approximately $10^{-5}$ for nominal peptide antigens. An explanation for such a high frequency is that direct allorecognition arises as a consequence of cross-reactivity of self-MHC-restricted T cells.

Indirect allorecognition is the recognition of donor-derived antigens that have been processed and which are presented on the cell surface of host APCs in the context of self-MHC. Therefore, the distinction between direct and indirect presentation is the source of the APCs on which alloantigens are presented. The mechanism of indirect allorecognition is indistinguishable from the physiological processing and presentation of pathogen-derived peptide antigens. Donor MHC molecules may be processed and peptide fragments presented to T cells by host APCs. Although only approximately 5–10% of alloreactive T cells are specific for indirectly presented donor antigens, they are still thought to play a major role in chronic allograft rejection, which occurs at a time when donor APCs are no longer thought to be present. The mechanisms by which indirectly primed T cells mediate graft rejection are unclear. Following organ transplantation, the donor endothelial layer is repopulated with recipient cells. One theory is that donor antigen is presented to direct pathway T cells by recipient MHC class I by the recipient endothelium. An alternative hypothesis is that graft destruction is the result of bystander killing following re-encounter of antigen on the surface of graft-infiltrating APCs.

## Transplantation tolerance

The establishment of tolerance to antigens expressed by donor tissues is a major goal of allogeneic transplantation. There are three main mechanisms that contribute to transplantation tolerance: clonal deletion, anergy and regulation (Plate 30.3).

During T-cell ontogeny, intrathymic clonal deletion of self-reactive T cells is the primary process for the selection of the mature T-cell repertoire. The transplantation of donor HSCs into sublethally or lethally myeloablated recipients gives rise to an immune system that is immunologically tolerant to donor antigens. The chimerism is established not only at the level of the bone marrow but also in the thymus, where recipient T cells learn to recognize the donor as self. Since mainly based on clonal deletion, such tolerance is long term and does not require immunosuppression but for the first months from the transplant. There is now plenty of anecdotal evidence that patients undergoing allogeneic HSCT can subsequently receive an organ from the original HSCT donor without the need for immunosuppression. Clonal deletion can also occur in extrathymic sites and can account for the removal of mature alloreactive T cells, thus leading to the establishment and maintenance of donor-specific tolerance in experimental models of mixed chimerism induction following MHC-mismatched HSCT. T cells are deleted in the periphery by either activation-induced cell death or passive cell death, both leading to apoptosis.

T-cell anergy describes a persistent state of unresponsiveness of T cells to their cognate antigen. This functional inactivation occurs as a consequence of TCR engagement in absence of full costimulatory signals. T cells receive costimulatory signals via ligation of surface CD28 with B7 molecules expressed on APCs. Other costimulatory pathways include CD40/CD40 ligand (CD154). Furthermore, signaling

through CTLA-4 (CD152) has also been implicated in the generation of hyporesponsive T cells. Anergic T cells fail to produce sufficient IL-2 and to proliferate in response to antigen, but the unresponsive state can be overcome by the exogenous addition of IL-2 or if anergic T cells are cultured in the absence of their cognate antigen. The blockade of costimulatory pathways has been widely exploited as a mechanism to induce tolerance in solid organ transplantation and HSCT. In the context of experimental models of allogeneic HSCT, the administration of anti-CD154 monoclonal antibody has been shown to induce mixed lymphohematopoietic chimerism and subsequent permanent skin graft acceptance if used as a single agent, in combination with reduced-intensity HSCT, or in combination with the antagonists of CTLA-4. However, there is little evidence in support of a role for anergy in the induction of transplantation tolerance.

Since the demonstration that tolerance to allogeneic graft can be transferred to naive recipients by T cells derived from a tolerant hosts, induction and maintenance of transplantation tolerance has largely been ascribed to immunoregulation. The initial problems in the identification of a suppressor T cell in the 1970s has been partially overcome more recently with the discovery of a distinct CD4$^+$ T-cell subset constitutively expressing CD25. Besides CD25, regulatory T cells (Treg) are characterized by the expression of CTLA-4, glucocorticoid-induced tumor necrosis factor receptor, the transcription factor Foxp3 and, most recently, folate receptor (FR)-4. CD4$^+$CD25$^+$ naturally occurring Treg cells are thymic-derived and have been shown to be important for maintaining self-tolerance, regulating the homeostasis of the peripheral T-cell pool, and contributing to tolerance induction in various models of solid organ transplantation as well as in allogeneic HSCT. *In vivo* depletion of Treg cells in animal models increases the incidence of autoimmune diseases and immune responses to tumors. It has also been observed that in myeloablation there is a selective advantage in the homeostatic expansion of Treg cells as compared with effector T cells. The presence of donor antigens during this phase skews the Treg repertoire toward the preferential expansion of Treg cells recognizing the donor antigens, thus accounting for the induction of transplantation tolerance. However, although a proportion of Treg cells specifically recognize allogeneic antigens, their overall suppressive activity is not limited to cells expressing their cognate antigens, thus enhancing their ability to prevent graft rejection but also implicating the possibility of undesirable effects of virus- or tumor-specific immunity.

The precise mechanism(s) of Treg activity remains to be elucidated. Direct cell-to-cell contact with the suppressed cells appears necessary, at least for the naturally occurring Treg cells, but other CD4$^+$CD25$^+$ regulatory cells with similar phenotype have been described that exert their suppressive activity via inhibitory cytokines such as TGF-β or IL-10. It is likely that a combination of naturally occurring and reactive regulatory cells are involved in transplantation tolerance.

## Graft-versus-host and graft-versus-leukemia

A unique and prominent feature of allogeneic HSCT, as compared with solid organ transplantation, is the presence in the graft of immunologically competent cells that have the ability to recognize normal and malignant recipient tissues. As a consequence, donor lymphocytes mediate a reaction against normal tissues, defined as graft-versus-host disease (GVHD), but also mediate the fundamental therapeutic effect by eradicating residual neoplastic cells, the graft-versus-leukemia (GVL) effect. It is not surprising therefore that the molecular targets of graft-versus-host (GVH) and GVL largely overlap.

### The immunological targets of GVHD and GVL

We have previously discussed how differences between donor and recipient at the MHC level produce vigorous immune responses. Since genetic differences are the major factors influencing the outcome of allogeneic HSCT, selection of the donor is of crucial importance and where possible it should be an MHC-identical sibling or an MHC-matched unrelated donor. However, MHC matching is not sufficient for long-term graft survival and/or to prevent GVH reactions without the use of potent immunosuppressive regimens. The existence of additional histocompatibility loci, first indicated in inbred mice, was then clearly demonstrated in humans in HSCT, where they were associated with severe GVH reactions. In this genetic situation, immune responses are directed against alloantigens encoded by histocompatibility (H) loci outside the MHC, the so-called minor H loci. Minor H antigens are polymorphic self-derived peptides expressed on the cell surface in association with MHC class I and II molecules. The fact that they are recognized, as are viruses, by MHC-restricted T cells with specificity for peptides brought to the cell surface during biosynthesis of MHC class I and II molecules makes their identification more difficult. Unlike in vitro T-cell responses to MHC antigens, which can be measured readily by proliferation in mixed lymphocyte reactions without previous exposure to antigen, responses against minor H antigens need prior in vivo immunization.

Although there are a large number of polymorphic proteins, not all give rise to peptides recognized as minor H antigens. Furthermore, there are several factors that appear in practice to severely limit the number of minor H antigens eliciting an in vivo response in a particular donor/recipient combination. In fact, it is clear that there is a hierarchy of responsiveness. In a genetic situation where there are many minor H disparities, one or a few are immunodominant, with clones of CD8+ T cells responding to such an antigen expanding selectively whereas T cells against others appear transiently early in the response or not at all. In most models, immunodominance results from competition for APC resources among responding CD8+ T cells, because it disappears when competing epitopes are presented on different APCs or when APCs are present in large excess. There is strong statistical and genetic evidence that this also occurs in human immune responses to multiple minor H antigens, thus in principle making it possible to predict, measure and manipulate the immune response following allografting.

### Graft-versus-leukemia

Clinical studies and experimental animal models have shown that the efficacy of allogeneic HSCT in hematological malignancies is related not only to intensive chemoradiotherapy but also to an immunological antitumor effect exerted by the graft itself. This effect, referred to as GVL, has been initially recognized because patients who received T-cell-depleted HSC preparations with the intention of reducing GVHD had a much higher incidence of leukemia recurrence after the transplant. Further lines of evidence support this concept. For example, the risk of relapse is higher if donor and recipient are identical twins and some reports have indicated that remission can be re-established by the withdrawal of post-transplant immunosuppressive treatment and/or by the recurrence of GVHD. The proof of principle of the GVL effect came from evidence that the infusion of lymphocytes from the original stem cell donor could restore complete remission in patients with chronic myeloid leukemia (CML) relapsed after allogeneic HSCT. These data support the requirement of two main components for GVL to occur: the presence of T cells in the donor preparation and the existence of antigenic differences between donor and recipient.

Although the GVL effect of donor lymphocyte infusion (DLI) is extremely successful in CML (the response rate is more than 90%), the experience in other malignancies is not as good and in some cases rather disappointing. However, the introduction of reduced-intensity conditioning has extended the indications for allogeneic HSCT, and thus promoted the use of DLI in several diseases. The rate of response after reduced-intensity-conditioning allografts in patients with high-risk acute myeloid leukemia (AML) and myelodysplastic syndrome (MDS) has been reported to be comparable with the results obtained using myeloablative regimens. However, a GVL effect was demonstrated after DLI only in patients with low tumor burdens. Durable responses that exceed the response durations seen both after conventional transplantation and following previous chemotherapy cycles have been reported in a small cohort of patients with Hodgkin lymphoma and in low-grade non-Hodgkin lymphoma. Initial enthusiasm with multiple myeloma has been subsequently disappointing, since it has become apparent that responses can be achieved only in association with severe GVHD. It is possible that higher doses of donor lymphocytes are necessary but then they would be incompatible with the side effects.

Exploitation of the beneficial effect of allogeneic immune responses in non-hematological malignancies has established the susceptibility of renal cell carcinoma to a graft-mediated effect. There are only anecdotal reports of such an effect following non-myeloablative HSCT in patients with metastatic breast carcinoma, colon carcinoma, pancreatic carcinoma, and osteosarcoma.

The reason for the different sensitivity to DLI among various diseases remains unclear. A possible explanation for the low susceptibility to DLI of acute lymphoid leukemia has been attributed to the limited duration and magnitude of leukemia-specific T-cell response generated *in vivo*, which has been ascribed to clonal exhaustion. As suggested by studies on solid cancers, other mechanisms implicated in tumor evasion of immune surveillance might be involved in the resistance to graft-versus-tumor responses.

## Tumor-specific T cells generated after allografting: the case of chronic myeloid leukemia

There is evidence that the immune system can mount a response against a tumor by recognizing antigens that are either specific or associated with the tumor. Tumor-specific antigens include antigenic peptides generated by genetic mutations specific to an individual cancer. Tumor-associated antigens come from normal non-polymorphic proteins overexpressed or aberrantly expressed in the tumor.

Almost all patients with CML harbor a specific molecular abnormality, the reciprocal chromosome translocation t(9;22)(q34;q11), which juxtaposes *BCR* and *ABL* genes. The fusion gene encodes for a chimeric protein, namely p210$^{BCR-ABL}$. Peptides derived from p210$^{BCR-ABL}$ can be presented by both MHC class I and class II molecules on CML cells *in vitro*, and p210$^{BCR-ABL}$-specific CD8$^+$ T cells have been detected in the peripheral blood of CML patients. However, it is unclear whether these T cells have any purpose in the control of the leukemia. Early-phase clinical trials using

p210$^{BCR-ABL}$ vaccination have showed some encouraging results. In patients with CML receiving a peptide-based vaccination, the development of BCR-ABL peptide-specific immune responses was associated with clinical responses and/or further reduction of residual disease.

Other non-polymorphic proteins, such as proteinase (Pr)3 and Wilms tumor (WT)1 have also been investigated as targets for T cells in CML because of their high expression levels in this leukemia. The presence of Pr3- or WT1-specific T cells at very low frequency has been identified in patients in remission after allogeneic HSCT but the significance of these findings remains to be clarified.

## Graft-versus-host disease

GVHD is the main drawback of allogeneic HSCT and is largely responsible for transplant-related mortality. In relation to the time of onset, GVHD can be acute or chronic, depending on whether it develops within 100 days from the transplant. However, although there are clearly two types of diseases in terms of symptoms, organ involvement, and pathological changes, there is not necessarily a temporal correlation. The uncertainty in the clinical classification is the result of the poor understanding of the pathogenesis of the disease.

### Acute GVHD

Acute GVHD is a potentially severe disease that usually targets skin, liver and gastrointestinal tract. The typical pathological finding in the skin is epithelial apoptotic damage, with characteristic nuclear alterations and a small inflammatory infiltrate. In the liver, the first injury involves vascular endothelial cells and later the biliary epithelium is destroyed as a result of portal lymphocytic infiltration. In the gastrointestinal tract there is destruction of intestinal crypts, with acute or chronic inflammatory infiltrates and flattening of the villous architecture. The clinical score is graded at four levels, with grade 4 very often being lethal.

The cellular effectors of alloreactivity after HSCT are cytotoxic T cells and NK cells. Cytotoxic T cells are activated CD8$^+$ T cells that recognize their specific antigen bound to MHC class I molecules on the target cells. They exert their functions through two main contact-dependent cytolytic pathways: Fas/Fas-ligand (Fas–FasL, CD95–CD178)-mediated apoptosis and the release of cytotoxic granules containing perforin/granzyme. Studies performed in mice genetically deficient for these molecules showed that the perforin/granzyme pathway plays a significant, but not exclusive, role in GVHD-induced organ damage. In contrast, the same pathway appears to be critical for the GVL effect, suggesting that it may be possible to selectively impair the alternative pathways to inhibit GVHD without compromising GVL. In fact, during experimental and clinical GVHD, FasL expression on donor T cells is increased and elevated serum levels of soluble FasL and Fas are correlated with severity of GVHD. Inhibition of the Fas–FasL pathway markedly reduces GVHD of the liver in animal models.

NK cells mediate direct cytotoxicity using the same pathways of cytotoxic T lymphocytes (Fas/FasL or performing granzyme) but their activation is largely dependent on the lack of recognition of particular epitopes on self-MHC class I molecules (so-called "missing self" hypothesis). Experimental studies have shown that NK cells are neither necessary nor sufficient to induce GVHD, but in the setting where GVHD is already underway, NK cells contribute to the overall outcome. The effect of donor NK-mediated cytotoxicity *in vivo*, in the absence of alloreactive T cells, is shown to be confined to recipient lympho-hematopoietic cells. Although the mechanism responsible for such selectivity is unclear, it has been hypothesized that donor "alloreactive" NK cells could prevent GVHD manifestations by killing host dendritic cells, thus avoiding alloantigen presentation to donor T cells. Furthermore, the involvement of "alloreactive" NK cells in GVL, suggested in preclinical models, has been corroborated in clinical studies, where the transplantation of haploidentical NK-"alloreactive" donors in high-risk AML patients was shown to prevent disease relapse and improve survival as an independent factor.

## Chronic GVHD

Chronic GVHD is a syndrome characterized by multiorgan involvement and is clinically similar to an autoimmune disorder. It usually involves skin, liver, gastrointestinal tract and the respiratory mucosa, but several immunological functions are impaired. The incidence of chronic GVHD ranges from 6 to 80% mainly depending on the degree of disparity in the major histocompatibility antigen and the previous appearance of acute GVHD. Pathological findings are not typical and are characterized by epithelial atrophy, increased hyaline deposits, fibrosis and chronic inflammatory infiltrates. Historically, chronic GVHD was classified as limited or extensive on the basis of the results of a small retrospective study, but the classification has been shown to be neither reproducible nor predictive of the clinical outcome and a new scoring system is being proposed.

## Pathogenesis of GVHD

Donor T cells recognizing major and/or minor H antigen disparities on recipient tissues are certainly critical in the induction of acute GVHD. However, other factors need to be taken into account. In particular, the incidence of acute

GVHD has been reported to be much higher if allogeneic donor lymphocytes are administered concomitantly with the conditioning regimen than if they are infused a few months later in the form of DLI. The reason for this is that the injuries produced by the cytotoxic agents and the infections at the time of transplantation activate the innate immune system and induce proinflammatory changes in endothelial and epithelial cells. This process, described as the "cytokine storm," consists of three main phases.

*Acute GVHD and the cytokine storm* In the first phase, the destruction of natural barriers by the conditioning regimens and the release of inflammatory cytokines like tumor necrosis factor (TNF)-α and IL-1 allows bacterial products to permeate the tissues. T cells exposed to bacterial products like lipopolysaccharide exhibit enhanced migration and survival. In accord with this notion, the use of low intensity preparatory regimens substantially reduces the incidence of acute GVHD.

The second step in the cytokine storm involves the activation of dendritic cells and the presentation of alloantigens. The inflammatory changes promoted in recipient tissues by conditioning regimens can initiate dendritic cell maturation and license them to potently induce T-cell responses. While host APCs are necessary and sufficient for GVHD development, the role of donor APCs appears confined to the intensification of ongoing disease. The differential role of donor and recipient APCs can be accounted for by the fact that endogenously synthesized minor H antigen-derived peptides are presented to CD8+ T cells on host MHC class I (induction phase). Subsequently, the same antigens can be processed by donor APCs through the exogenous route of antigen processing and presented to T cells, thus accounting for the augmentation of the GVHD initiated by host APCs (maintenance phase). This two-step process is similar to that described for the rejection of solid organ transplants (direct and indirect alloresponses).

For its full development GVHD finally requires cellular effectors to be recruited. Although activated donor T and NK cells effect the killing of host cells by contact-dependent cytotoxicity, the release of inflammatory cytokines also play an important role. In accordance, target organ injury can be partially prevented by the neutralization of TNF-α and IL-1 in animal models and the blockade of TNF-α is of some efficacy in pilot clinical studies. The importance of multiple inflammatory effectors in GVHD suggests that inhibition of several pro-inflammatory cytokines simultaneously is required for reducing systemic GVHD.

*Acute GVHD and T-cell trafficking* Although essentially all tissues express transplantation antigens, the clinical manifestations of acute GVHD display remarkable tissue tropism, involving primarily gut, liver and skin. Recent studies have suggested that the skewed organ involvement is related to the homing properties of activated allogeneic T cells and the presence of local tissue inflammation.

Naive T cells injected in lethally irradiated allogeneic recipients are initially retained within secondary lymphoid tissues where, activated by recipient-derived APCs, they undergo a rapid burst of proliferation, enter the peripheral circulation, and subsequently accumulate in the gut, liver and skin. However, local inflammation also appears crucial in permitting the entry of activated T cells to target tissues, because the infusion of alloreactive T cells produces GVHD in irradiated recipients but not in recipients in which mixed hematopoietic chimerism has already been established, despite similar levels of alloreactive T cells in the periphery. To confirm the role of local inflammation, GVHD can also be induced in mixed chimeric mice if inflammatory stimuli are administered together with the donor T-cell transfer.

*Chronic GVHD*  The pathogenesis of chronic GVHD largely remains to be elucidated. Mature donor alloreactive T cells infused with the graft are also supposed to play a key role in chronic GVHD. Similarly, APCs have been shown to be important, although in contrast to acute GVHD the development of the chronic form is dependent on the APCs of donor rather than recipient origin, thus justifying the possibility of a broader repertoire of antigens and more widespread organ involvement.

However, one of the most remarkable features of chronic GVHD is the clinical and pathological similarities with systemic autoimmune disease. Elevated levels of serum autoantibodies (i.e., antinuclear, anti-dsDNA, anti-smooth muscle antibodies) in up to 70% of chronic GVHD patients support the hypothesis that functionally relevant autoreactive T and B cells can be generated during chronic GVHD. It has been suggested that antibodies to ubiquitously expressed minor H antigens may be analogous to pathogenic autoantibodies in systemic autoimmune diseases, thus justifying the similarities of tissue pathology. The importance of B-cell responses in chronic GVHD was documented by clinical improvement following B-cell depletion with anti-CD20 monoclonal antibody.

Studies in animal models have been carried out with the aim of investigating the autoimmune manifestations of chronic GVHD. Using an HSCT model in which donor and recipient differed for multiple minor H antigens, it was possible to isolate from mice developing chronic GVHD autoreactive CD4$^+$ T cells with specificity for an MHC class II-encoded determinant common to donor and recipient. Moreover, donor CD4$^+$ T cells isolated from recipients with chronic GVHD cause autoimmune disease if transferred to new syngeneic recipients. The development of donor T cells that recognize antigens shared by donor and host has also been attributed to impaired mechanisms of deletion or regulation during chronic GVHD. It has been hypothesized that autoreactive T cells may be the consequence of a damaged recipient thymus, unable to select the new T-cell repertoire following pretransplant therapy or acute GVHD. However, it seems also that thymectomized animals can develop GVHD.

Not dissimilarly from the acute disease, cytokine dysregulation has a causative role in chronic GVHD. High levels of IL-1β, IL-6, interferon (IFN)-γ, TNF-α, and low levels of the inhibitory cytokine IL-10 are associated with more severe forms. Multiple cytokines produced by activated T cells, such as IFN-γ and TGF-β, have been shown to promote increased collagen deposition in preclinical models. Other soluble mediators, such as the CCL2 and CCL3 chemokines, seem to modulate collagen turnover and deposition by sending signals to fibroblasts via macrophages or indirectly through stimulation of TGF-β.

## Can GVHD and GVL be dissected?

Currently, the major aim in allogeneic HSCT is to identify a way to the separate the beneficial GVL from GVHD (summarized in Plate 30.4). Several attempts have been made during the last 15 years, either by selectively controlling GVHD or selectively inducing GVL.

### Control of GVHD

The simplest and most pragmatic approach is to escalate the dose of donor lymphocytes until a clinical response is achieved. This reduces the incidence of GVHD to less than 20% of cases and has proved more useful than depleting T-cell subsets like CD8$^+$. Alternatively, the route of selectively depleting *in vitro* recipient-reactive donor T cells before their infusion is valuable and its application has been successfully tested in haploidentical transplantation.

Active immune regulation of donor/recipient-reactive cells is emerging as a key mechanism for inducing and maintaining tolerance to alloantigens. Treg cells are probably the main player in this process and a few studies in animal models have documented that their adoptive transfer can also prevent and partially treat GVHD. There are also suggestions that Treg cells may preserve GVL activity, but data obtained in patients after HSCT have failed to show a significant correlation with GVHD and found that leukemia relapses were associated with an increment in the number of Treg cells in the peripheral blood of patients. Similarly, the amount of Treg infiltration seems to correlate with bad prognosis in ovarian cancer.

The possibility of interfering with the non-specific effects of the cytokine storm with neutralizing monoclonal antibodies is currently under scrutiny and the topic has been discussed before.

A more recent approach to diminish GVHD has been based on the exploitation of mesenchymal stromal cells (MSCs) of bone marrow origin. These cells exhibit a potent immunosuppressive activity *in vitro* and *in vivo* that targets virtually any cells of the immune system. Their effect is not cognate dependent, thus not requiring MHC identity between MSCs and immune cells. Third-party MSCs have been infused into patients with steroid-resistant acute GVHD with extremely encouraging results. This is even more interesting in the light of the observation that MSCs are precursors of the hematopoietic niche and that indeed they favor the engraftment of hematopoietic cells in the bone marrow. Therefore, their use at various stages of the transplantation procedure could ultimately improve the outcome of HSCT.

### Induction of selective GVL

It is generally true that minor H antigens are the targets of both GVHD and GVL, in principle making separation of the two processes impossible. However, there are two strategies for pursuing selectivity. One is based on the fact that not all minor H antigens are equally expressed on the various tissues and some of them are preferentially, if not exclusively, expressed on hematopoietic tissues. In the case of leukemia, for example, the generation of T cells with specificity against hematopoietic polymorphisms may limit the collateral damage by confining the GVH activity to that tissue and sparing the others. Further selectivity could be achieved by concentrating on lineage-specific polymorphisms as demonstrated for B-cell malignancies (Plate 30.5).

The alternative is to exploit the phenomenon of immunodominance, previously described. T cells directed against a broadly expressed minor H antigen but specific for the immunodominant epitope appear able to exert a powerful GVL effect selectively without GVHD. The mechanisms for this tumor-specific effect largely remain unknown.

Ultimately, the best solution would be to identify tumor-specific antigens. Unfortunately, most tumor antigens are self-antigens against which the T cells of a tumor-bearing host are immunologically tolerant. However, the recent progress in gene therapy has made it possible to transduce T lymphocytes with a gene encoding an antigen receptor against these weak antigens and early studies in melanoma patients have suggested this as a promising, though elaborate and expensive strategy.

## Further reading

### Indications for HSCT

Barrett AJ, Savani BN. (2008) Allogeneic stem cell transplantation for myelodysplastic syndrome. *Seminars in Hematology*, **45**, 49–59.

Dazzi F, van Laar JM, Cope A, Tyndall A. (2007) Cell therapy for autoimmune diseases. *Arthritis Research and Therapy*, **9**, 206.

Demirer T, Barkholt L, Blaise D et al. (2008) Transplantation of allogeneic hematopoietic stem cells: an emerging treatment modality for solid tumors. *Nature Clinical Practice. Oncology*, **5**, 256–267.

Koca E, Champlin RE. (2008) Peripheral blood progenitor cell or bone marrow transplantation: controversy remains. *Current Opinion in Oncology*, **20**, 220–226.

### The hematopoietic niche

Kollet O, Dar A, Lapidot T. (2007) The multiple roles of osteoclasts in host defense: bone remodeling and hematopoietic stem cell mobilization. *Annual Review of Immunology*, **25**, 51–69.

Morrison SJ, Spradling AC. (2008) Stem cells and niches: mechanisms that promote stem cell maintenance throughout life. *Cell*, **132**, 598–611.

Scadden DT. (2007) The stem cell niche in health and leukemic disease. *Best Practice and Research. Clinical Haematology*, **20**, 19–27.

### Transplantation tolerance

Fehr T, Sykes M. (2004) Tolerance induction in clinical transplantation. *Transplantation Immunology*, **13**, 117–130.

Sakaguchi S. (2005) Naturally arising Foxp3-expressing CD25+CD4+ regulatory T cells in immunological tolerance to self and non-self. *Nature Immunology*, **6**, 345–352.

Waldmann H, Chen TC, Graca L et al. (2006) Regulatory T cells in transplantation. *Seminars in Immunology*, **18**, 111–119.

### GVHD and GVL

Dazzi F, Horwood NJ. (2007) Potential of mesenchymal stem cell therapy. *Current Opinion in Oncology*, **19**, 650–655.

Shlomchik WD. (2007) Graft-versus-host disease. *Nature Reviews. Immunology*, **7**, 340–352.

van den Brink MR, Burakoff SJ. (2002) Cytolytic pathways in hematopoietic stem-cell transplantation. *Nature Reviews. Immunology*, **2**, 273–281.

# Appendix 1 Glossary

**Adenine (A)** Nitrogenous (purine) base. One member of the base pair A–T (adenine–thymine).

**Allele** Alternative forms of a gene occupying the same locus on homologous chromosomes; segregate at meiosis.

**Allogeneic BMT** *Allogeneic bone marrow transplantation.* Marrow from an HLA-matched donor (related or unrelated) is administered to the patient following "conditioning" (usually chemotherapy with radiotherapy). Cf. autologous BMT.

**Alu sequences** DNA sequences recognized by the restriction enzyme *Alu* I; Alu sequences are represented about 300 000 times in the human genome.

**Anergy** Immunological unresponsiveness to specific antigenic rechallenge.

**APC** *Antigen-presenting cell.* Cells capable of triggering naive T-cell response to antigen, leading to clonal T-cell expansion. APCs include dendritic cells, activated B cells and macrophages.

**Apoptosis** Programed cell death involving nuclear DNA fragmentation.

**ARMS** *Amplification refractory mutation system*: a PCR method that allows amplification of a single specific allele due to specific primers used, i.e., the primers bind only to the mutant allele.

**Autologous BMT** Patient's own bone marrow is collected following treatment (presumed disease-free) and reinfused in order to reconstitute the hematopoietic system.

**Autoradiography** Detection of radioactively labeled molecules on radiographic film. For analysis of nucleic acids, single-stranded DNA is immobilized onto a membrane before adding radiolabeled probe. Allows analysis of length and number of DNA fragments after separation by gel electrophoresis.

**Autosome** Non-sex chromosome.

**BAC** Bacterial artificial chromosome; allows propagation of large DNA molecules (up to 300 kb).

**Base pair (bp)** A pair of complementary nucleotide bases in a duplex DNA or RNA molecule.

**bcl-2** Protein that inhibits apoptosis; overexpressed in, for example, follicular non-Hodgkin lymphoma carrying t(14;18).

**Cap** Structure at the 5′ end of mRNAs containing a methylated guanine residue.

**CDR** *Complementarity-determining region.* Those components of immunoglobulin and T-cell receptor (TCR) molecules that make contact with specific ligand; determine specificity. The CDR regions are the most variable portions of the immunoglobulin and TCR molecules.

**Centromere** Chromosome region to which spindle fibers attach during cell division.

**Chromosome painting** Labeling of whole chromosome using fluorescence *in situ* hybridization. Involves mixture of different sequences from single chromosome.

**Clonality** Determination of clonal origin of cells.

**Clone** Population of cells or DNA molecules arising from a single progenitor.

**Cloning** The process of asexually producing a group of cells (clones), all genetically identical, from a single ancestor. In recombinant DNA technology, the use of DNA manipulation procedures to produce multiple copies of a single gene or segment of DNA is referred to as cloning DNA.

**Cloning vector** DNA molecule from a virus, a plasmid, or the cell of a higher organism into which another DNA fragment of appropriate size can be integrated without loss of the vector's capacity for self-replication; vectors introduce foreign DNA into host cells, where it can be reproduced in large quantities.

**Codon** DNA or corresponding RNA sequence of three base pairs that codes for a particular amino acid or termination signal.

**Complementary DNA (cDNA)** DNA copy of a messenger RNA generated by reverse transcriptase.

**Consensus sequence** DNA or amino acid sequence that specifies the most commonly found DNA base or amino acid at each position in a sequence of similar DNA or amino acid sequences.

**Conserved sequence** DNA or protein sequence that has remained essentially unchanged throughout evolution.

**Contigs** Groups of clones representing overlapping genomic regions.

**Cosmid** Plasmid DNA containing Cos sites to enable it to be packaged into phage particles. For example, cosmids can be packaged in λ phage particles for infection into *E. coli.* May harbor inserts of about 40 kb.

**Cyclins** Family of proteins that are positive regulators of cell cycle.

**Cytosine (C)** Pyrimidine base of RNA and DNA; one of cytosine–guanine (C–G) pair.

**Diploid** Cell or organism containing two complete sets of homologous chromosomes (cf. haploid).

**DNA polymerase** Enzyme that adds nucleotides to a growing chain of DNA in a 5′ to 3′ direction during DNA replication using a DNA strand as a template to copy from.

**Domain** In a protein this refers to a discrete region of the protein which has a specific function associated with it.

**Electrophoresis** Method for separating large molecules (nucleic acids or proteins) from a mixture of similar molecules using an electric current. Molecules travel through agarose or polyacrylamide gel at varying rates depending on their electrical charge and size.

**Endonuclease** Enzyme that cleaves nucleic acid at internal sites in the nucleotide sequence.

**Epitope** That part of an antigen that binds to the antigen-binding region of an antibody.

**EST** Expressed sequence tag.

**Exon** Segment of a gene that is present in the fully mature RNA after transcription, i.e., contains coding sequences (cf. introns).

**FACS** *Fluorescence activated cell sorting*. Technique used to separate cells from a population on the basis of their expression of specific antigens.

**FISH** *Fluorescence in situ hybridization*. A technique used to visualize locations on chromosomes that hybridize to specific nucleotide probes. Biotin, digoxigenin or fluorescent dyes are incorporated into cDNA probes using nick-translation. Probes are then hybridized to metaphases or interphase nuclei thus defining gene number and location.

**Flow cytometry** Analysis of biological material by detection of the light-absorbing or fluorescing properties of cells or subcellular fractions (i.e., chromosomes) passing in a narrow stream through a laser beam. An absorbance or fluorescence profile of the sample is produced. Automated sorting devices, used to fractionate samples, sort successive droplets of the analyzed stream into different fractions depending on the fluorescence emitted by each droplet.

**Flow karyotyping** Use of flow cytometry to analyze and/or separate chromosomes on the basis of their DNA content.

**Frameshift** Mutation that shifts the reading frame of triplet codons in a gene during translation of mRNA.

**Gardos channel** Red cell transport system accounting for selective loss of potassium in response to increase in intracellular ionized $Ca^{2+}$.

**G banding** Technique used to visualize the band patterns of chromosomes on staining with Giemsa.

**Gene** Unit of heredity that specifies an RNA or mRNA. A gene will also contain intronic regions and regions that control transcription.

**Gene expression** Process by which a gene's coded information is converted into the structures present and operating in the cell. Expressed genes include those that are transcribed into mRNA and then translated into protein, and those that are transcribed into RNA but not translated into protein (e.g., transfer and ribosomal RNAs).

**Gene mapping** Construction of a map of different genetic loci based on their physical position with respect to each other.

**Gene therapy** Insertion of normal DNA directly into cells to correct a genetic defect.

**Genetic code** The sequence of nucleotides, coded in triplets (codons) along the mRNA, that determines the sequence of amino acids in protein synthesis. The DNA sequence of a gene can be used to predict the mRNA sequence, and the genetic code can, in turn, be used to predict the amino acid sequence.

**Genomic library** Collection of clones made from a set of randomly generated overlapping DNA fragments representing the entire genome of an organism.

**Genotype** The genetic composition of a cell or organism responsible for its appearance.

**Grb-2** *Growth factor receptor-bound protein 2*. Participates in downstream signaling after activation of a variety of cellular receptors. Binds to EDGF and PDGF.

**Guanine (G)** Purine base of RNA or DNA. One member of the base pair G–C (guanine and cytosine).

**Haploid** A single set of chromosomes (half the full set of genetic material), present in the egg and sperm cells of animals, and in the egg and pollen cells of plants (cf. diploid).

**Haplotype** Combination of closely linked genes. Usually inherited together as a "block" arising from one chromosome.

**Hemizygote** Diploid cell or organism that contains only one allele of a gene due to loss of one chromosome of a homologous chromosome pair.

**Heterodimer** A complex of two non-identical moieties, e.g., proteins such as the T-cell receptor.

**Heterozygote** Diploid cell or organism that contains different alleles of a gene at one locus on homologous chromosomes.

**Homeobox** A short stretch of nucleotides whose base sequence is virtually identical in all the genes that contain it. It has been found in many organisms from fruit flies to humans. In the fruit fly, a homeobox appears to determine when particular groups of genes are expressed during development.

**Homodimer** Complex of two identical moieties.

**Homotetramer** Tetramer comprising four identical subunits.

**Hybridization** The ability of complementary single-stranded DNA or RNA molecules to form a duplex.

***In situ* hybridization** Use of DNA or RNA probe to detect the presence of the complementary DNA sequence in cloned bacterial or cultured eukaryotic cells.

**Interphase** Period of the mitotic cell cycle between one mitosis and the next.

**Intron** Intervening sequence. Segments within the coding region of a gene that are not present in the fully mature RNA after transcription due to removal by splicing.

***In vitro*** Taking place outside a living organism (literally "in glass"; cf. *in vivo*).

***In vivo*** Taking place within a living organism ("in life").

**Karyotype** Photomicrograph of an individual's chromosomes arranged in a standard format showing the number, size and shape of each chromosome type.

**Kilobase (kb)** 1000 nucleotides.

**Kinase** An enzyme that phosphorylates a substrate.

**Knockout** The ability to remove a specific gene in a cell or organism by molecular techniques.

**Leucine zipper** Leucine-rich domain of a protein that allows protein–protein interaction.

**Library** An unordered collection of cloned DNA whose relationship to each other can be established by physical mapping.

**Linkage** The tendency for two genes in close proximity on a chromosome to be inherited together.

**Locus** The position of a gene on a chromosome.

**LOH** *Loss of heterozygosity.* Deletions believed to occur during tumor development. Identified as loss of an allele at a specific locus.

**Lyonization** X-chromosome inactivation in mammals. One X chromosome is randomly inactivated in each cell.

**Maternal inheritance** Preferential carriage of a gene by the maternal parent.

**Megabase (Mb)** $10^6$ nucleotides.

**Messenger RNA (mRNA)** The mature transcript from a gene transcribed by RNA polymerase which specifies the order of amino acids during mRNA translation to protein.

**Metaphase** Stage in mitosis when the parental and newly synthesized chromosomes are maximally condensed but prior to their segregation to opposite spindle poles.

**MHC** *Major histocompatibility complex.* A polymorphic family of genes involved in mediating T-cell immune responses; present peptides to T-cell receptor.

**Minimal residual disease** Low-level disease present following therapy; generally not detected using standard techniques such as light microscopy, but requires molecular techniques such as PCR for detection.

**Missense mutation** Single-base substitution causing incorporation of inappropriate amino acid into a protein.

**Monosomy** Condition in which one member of a chromosome pair is missing.

**Multidrug resistance (MDR)** Cell mechanism conferring drug resistance to a wide variety of chemotherapeutic agents.

**Mutation** A transmissible change in nucleotide sequence which leads to a change or loss of normal function encoded by that nucleotide sequence.

**Nonsense mutation** Mutation resulting in premature termination during protein synthesis.

**Northern blot** Technique that transfers RNA molecules after size fractionation on gels to filter papers for hybridization to specific probes.

**Nucleotide** A subunit of DNA or RNA consisting of a nitrogenous base (adenine, guanine, thymine or cytosine in DNA; adenine, guanine, uracil or cytosine in RNA), a phosphate molecule and a sugar molecule (deoxyribose in DNA and ribose in RNA).

**Oncogene** Mutated gene that is normally involved in the correct control of cell division such that disruption of the normal gene function leads to cell immortalization and transformation.

**Open reading frame** Series of triplet codons in the coding region of a gene that lie between the signals to start and stop translation.

**PBSC** *Peripheral blood stem cell.* Following administration of chemotherapy with or without growth factor (e.g., G-CSF), stem cells enter the peripheral circulation and are collected by leukopheresis.

**PCR** *Polymerase chain reaction.* Technique to amplify a target DNA sequence by multiple rounds of DNA synthesis. Involves a heat-stable DNA polymerase (e.g. *Taq*, isolated from the hot spring bacterium *Thermus aquaticus*) and two oligonucleotide primers (generally about 20 bases), one complementary to the (+) strand at one end of the sequence to be amplified and the other complementary to the (−) strand at the other end. Newly synthesized DNA can subsequently serve as additional templates for the same primer sequences, allowing a million-fold increase in DNA sequence after 30 cycles of primer annealing, strand elongation, and DNA melting.

**PFGE** *Pulsed field gel electrophoresis.* An electrophoretic technique to separate very large molecules of DNA by periodically altering the direction of the electric field through which the samples are migrating.

**Phenotype** The observable characteristics of a cell or organism resulting from the expression of the cell's genotype.

**Plasmid** A circular, autonomously replicating, extrachromosomal DNA molecule. Some plasmids are capable of integrating into the host genome.

**Pleckstrin homology domain** First noted in platelet protein pleckstrin, 100 residues, function unknown.

**Polymorphism** DNA sequence variation among individuals. May be used as linkage marker.

**Positional cloning** Method for identifying the gene responsible for a genetic disease in the absence of a transcript or protein product; relies on the use of markers tightly linked to the target gene.

**Primer** Short oligonucleotide sequence that provides the starting point for polymerases to copy a nucleotide sequence and make a double strand.

**Probe** DNA or RNA molecules (single stranded) of specific base sequence; may be labeled radioactively (e.g., $^{32}$P) or non-radioactively (e.g., digoxigenin) to detect complementary sequence on Southern blot, etc.

**Promoter** DNA sequence that targets RNA polymerase to a gene for transcription.

**Proto-oncogene** Refers to a normal gene involved in controlling cell division which, when mutated, becomes an oncogene.

**Pseudogene** A duplicated gene that has become non-functional.

**Purine base** Organic base containing two heterocyclic rings that occurs in nucleic acids (adenine and guanine in DNA and RNA).

**Pyrimidine base** Organic base containing one heterocyclic ring that occurs in nucleic acids. Cytosine (C) and thymine (T) in DNA; cytosine (C) and uracil (U) in RNA.

**Q banding** Banding technique to visualize the banding patterns of chromosomes using quinacrine stain.

**Recombination** The process by which progeny derive a combination of genes different from that of either parent. In higher organisms, this can occur by crossing over. Also occurs in non-germline cells, e.g., B cells and T cells during production of immunoglobulin and T-cell receptor genes, respectively.

**Reporter gene** A gene encoding a product thta can be easily measured when introduced into cell, e.g., by transfection.

**Restriction enzyme** An endonuclease (usually bacterial) that recognizes specific short nucleotide sequences and cuts DNA at those sites.

**Restriction enzyme cutting site** Specific nucleotide sequence of DNA at which a particular restriction enzyme cuts the DNA. Some sites occur frequently in DNA (e.g., every several hundred base pairs), others much less frequently (rare-cutter, e.g., every 10 000 base pairs).

**Retrovirus** RNA virus that replicates by first converting its RNA genome to a double-stranded DNA copy using the enzyme reverse transcriptase.

**Reverse transcriptase** Enzyme used to make a DNA copy of RNA. Found in retroviruses allowing conversion of their RNA genome into double-stranded DNA which may then integrate into the host genome.

**RFLP** *Restriction fragment length polymorphism.* Heritable differences in the length of DNA fragments from a specific region of DNA generated by restriction enzymes due to DNA sequence differences.

**Ribozyme** An RNA molecule with properties of RNAse; cleaves single-stranded RNA.

**RNA polymerase** Enzyme that makes an RNA copy of a DNA template.

**RNA splicing** Removal of introns from transcribed RNA to generate a mature mRNA.

**RT-PCR** *Reverse transcriptase polymerase chain reaction.* Amplification of RNA by PCR after copying of the RNA→cDNA by reverse transcription.

**Sequencing** Determination of the order of nucleotides (base sequences) in a DNA or RNA molecule or the order of amino acids in a protein.

**Somatic mutation** Mutation arising in a somatic cell.

**Southern blot** Technique that transfers DNA molecules after size fractionation on gels to filter papers for hybridization to specific probes.

**Src homology 3 (SH3) domain** Protein domain on oncoprotein Src; binds to proline-rich domains on other proteins.

**Syngeneic** Genetically identical (e.g., identical twins).

**Taq polymerase** Heat-stable DNA polymerase used for DNA amplification (*see* PCR). More recent heat-stable polymerases include VENT and Tth.

**TATA box** Also called Hogness Box; DNA sequence found in many eukaryotic promoters that binds the TATA-binding protein in order to recruit RNA polymerase for transcription. Consensus sequence TATAAAA; specifies position where transcription is initiated.

**T-cell receptor** Membrane protein complexes expressed on T lymphocytes and which recognize specific antigens when associated with MHC molecules.

**Telomere** Specialized structures at the ends of chromosomes involved in the replication and stability of linear DNA molecules.

**Thymine (T)** Nitrogenous base. One member of the base pair A–T (adenine–thymine).

**Tolerance** Reduced ability to mount an immune response to specific antigens *in vivo*.

**Transcription** Process by which a DNA template (a gene) is copied to RNA by RNA polymerase.

**Transcription factor** Proteins, other than RNA polymerase, that are required for transcription of all genes.

**Transfection** The introduction of DNA into cells in culture.

**Translation** The mechanism by which mRNA is used as a template to synthesize protein on the ribosome.

**Tumor-suppressor gene** A gene that negatively regulates cell division such that mutation in these genes results in uncontrolled cell division and tumor progression, e.g., Rb, p53 genes.

**Tyrosine kinase** Enzymatic activity catalyzing the attachment of phosphate group to tyrosine residue within a protein molecule.

**Uracil (U)** Pyrimidine base that replaces the DNA base thymine in RNA molecules; forms base pair with adenine (A–U).

**Vector** DNA molecule in which DNA sequences can be cloned; agent used to deliver genes for gene transfer.

**VNTR** *Variable number of tandem repeats.* Variations in numbers of tandem repeat DNA sequences found at specific loci in different populations. May be used as genetic markers.

**Western blot** A technique that transfers protein molecules after size fractionation on gels to filter papers for analysis with antibodies.

**X inactivation** Inactivation of one of the X chromosomes in female somatic cells.

**YAC** *Yeast artificial chromosome.* Plasmid DNA which contains DNA sequences that allow plasmid maintenance in yeast cells permitting cloning of very large regions of DNA.

# Appendix 2  Cytogenetic glossary

**add**  Addition of chromosomal material of unknown origin to another chromosome

**del**  Deletion of chromosomal material

**der**  Derivative of a chromosomal rearrangement

**dup**  Duplication of chromosomal material; extra copy of part of a chromosome

**cen**  Centromere

**Hypo/hyperdiploid**  Human karyotype with <46 or >46 chromosomes, respectively

**i**  Isochromosome; chromosome whose arms are mirror images of each other

**ins**  Insertion of chromosomal material

**inv**  Rotation of chromosome segment by 180°

**mar**  Marker chromosome. Signifies any structurally rearranged chromosome

**p**  Short (petit) arm of chromosome

**q**  Long arm of chromosome

**p+/q+**  Addition of DNA to short/long arms, respectively

**p–/q–**  Deletion of DNA from short/long arms, respectively

**t**  Translocation; chromosome segment moves from one chromosome to another. May or may not be reciprocal

**ter**  Terminus (end); e.g., pter, qter indicates short arm and long arm ends, respectively

**+/–**  Gain/loss of chromosomal material, respectively

# Appendix 3 Cluster designation (CD) antigens used in this book

| CD | Expression | Comments |
|---|---|---|
| CD1a,b,c | Thymocytes, dendritic cells | Ligand for some $\gamma\delta$ T cells |
| CD3 | T cells | Complex of molecules that transduce signals from T-cell receptor |
| CD4 | T cells, monocytes, tissue macrophages, microglial cells, EBV-transformed B cells | Binds HLA class II Receptor for HIV env gp120 |
| CD5 | Thymocytes and T cells, most T-cell malignancies, B-CLL | Binds to CD72 |
| CD8 | T-cell subset | Binds MHC class I |
| CD10 | T- and B-cell precursors, BM stromal cells, pre-B ALL | Zinc metalloproteinase, marker for pre-B cell ALL (also termed common ALL antigen, CALLA) |
| CD15 | Neutrophils, eosinophils, monocytes | Also called Lewis-x (Le$^x$) |
| CD19 | B cells, B-cell malignancies | Function unknown |
| CD20 | B cells, B-cell malignancies | Function unknown |
| CD21 | Mature B cells, follicular dendritic cells | Complement control protein. Receptor for complement C3d, EBV |
| CD23 | Mature B cells, activated macrophages, eosinophils, follicular dendritic cells, CLL | Low-affinity receptor for IgE |
| CD28 | T-cell subsets, activated B cells | Receptor for costimulatory signal, binds CD80 (B7-1) and CD86 (B7-2) |
| CD34 | Hematopoietic precursors, capillary endothelium | Ligand for CD62L (L-selectin) |
| CD38 | Early B and T cells, activated T cells, germinal center B cells, plasma cells | Function unknown |
| CD43 | Leukocytes (except resting B cells) | Binds CD54 (ICAM-1) |
| CD55 | Hematopoietic and non-hematopoietic cells | Decay-accelerating factor (DAF). Binds C3b |
| CD56 | NK cells | Isoform of neural cell adhesion molecule (N-CAM) |
| CD59 | Hematopoietic and non-hematopoietic cells | Binds complement C8 and C9 |
| CD79a,b | B cells | Component of B-cell antigen (analogous to CD3) |
| CD80 | Antigen-presenting cells | Costimulation. Ligand for CD28 and CTLA-4 |
| CD86 | Antigen-presenting cells | Costimulation. Ligand for CD28 and CTLA-4 |

Abbreviations: see list on p. xiii

# Index

Note: page numbers in *italics* refer to figures, those in **bold** refer to tables

refractory anemia with ringed sideroblasts
(RARS) 146–7
refractory anemia with ringed sideroblasts
(RARS) with thrombosis 101
*JAK2* V617F gene mutation 108
regulatory RNAs 2
restriction enzymes 365–6, 392
restriction fragment length polymorphisms
(RFLPs) 393
hemophilia carrier testing 226
reticulocyte binding proteins 201–2
reticulocytopenia 205
retinoblastoma (RB) gene product 123
multiple myeloma 131, 136
retinoic acid receptor 43
retroviruses 320, *322*
Rh genes 266, 267, 268
Rh system 266–7
RhD immunogenicity 266–7
rheumatoid arthritis, treatment 303
rhoptry proteins 201–2
ribosomal RNA 363
ribosomes 363
ribozymes 331, 393
ring surface protein (RSP)-2 205
rituximab
ITP 301–2
multiple myeloma 131
RNA 363
blotting 366–7
extraction 365
RNA interference (RNAi) 331
RNA polymerase II 364, 393
RNases 365
romiplostim 312
*RPS14* gene 99
*RPS19* gene mutations 156
*RUNX1* gene 43, 89
mutations 47, 89, 253
RUNX1–RUNX1T1 fusion protein 43

Sanger, Fred *361*, 368
Scott syndrome 253
selectins 35–6
sequence-based typing (SBT) 260, 262
serial analysis of gene expression (SAGE) 355
severe combined immunodeficiency (SCID)
ADA deficiency 327
X-linked 327
severe congenital neutropenia 316
sickle cell anemia 17, 181–91, 198
age-dependency of complications *183*
anemia 183–4, 187
blood transfusion 187
clinical features 183–7
complications *183*, 184, Plate 15.1
genetics 181–2
painful crisis 184, 188

pathophysiology 185–7
red cell dehydration 186–7
severity 183, 184–5
α thalassemia co-inheritance 184
treatment 187–9
sickle gene 17
frequency 182
Indo-European mutation 182
spread 182
sickle red cells, adhesion to endothelium
185–6
sickle/β thalassemia 189
sickling disorders 17
sideroblastic anemias 144–8
ALAS2 deficiency 144–6
bone marrow failure-associated
conditions 148–56
classification **145**
Pearson marrow–pancreas syndrome
147–8, Plate 12.1
pyridoxine-responsive 146
X-linked with ataxia 146–7
siderosis 172
African **175**, 177–8
autosomal dominant **175**, 177
signal transducer and activator of
transcription (STAT) proteins 309
*see also individual named STATs*
signaling lymphocyte activation molecule
(SLAM) 381
single nucleotide polymorphisms (SNPs) 2,
364
array analysis 21–2
cytokines 294
genotype array 19
*JAK2* 109
lymphoma genetics 119–20
myelodysplastic syndromes 101
pharmacogenomics 337–8, 345
whole genome analysis 119–20
sirolimus 49
small molecule inhibitors, acute myeloid
leukemia 49
small nuclear RNAs 364
small nucleolar RNAs 364
small-cell lymphoma, molecular/cytological
pathogenesis *122*
smoldering myeloma 127, **128**
SOCS3 106
somatic mosaicism 226
Southam, Chester 370
Southern blotting 1, 366–7, 393
hemophilia 222–3, 224
lymphoma genetics 117, 118
minimal residual disease *58*, 59–60
spectral karyotyping (SKY) 20
splice site consensus sequences 8
splicing 363

Stahl, Franklin 363
STAT3 activation, multiple myeloma 134,
136
STAT5 78, *79*, 80
JAK2 signaling 105, 106
Steel factor (SF) 30, **33**
stem cell(s) 26–41
definitions 26
distinctions 26
plasticity 29
sources 26, *27*
transdifferentiation 29
types 26, *27*
*see also* hematopoietic stem cells
stem cell transplantation, CML treatment
80–1
storage pool disease 251–2
Stormorken syndrome 253
stromal derived factor (SDF)1 374, 375
structural hemoglobin variants 2, 16–18
abnormal oxygen transport 17
congenital cyanosis 17–18
genotype–phenotype relationships 17–18
molecular pathology 16
unstable 17
suicide gene therapy 332, *333*
super-Hb S 190–1
systemic lupus erythematosus (SLE) 295

T lymphocytes 28, 287, 290
activation 291
anergy 331, 384
antigen receptors 288–9
antigen recognition 291
autoreactive 291–2
tolerance 290–1
t(2;5)(p23;q35) translocation 68–9
t(4;14) translocation 130
t(8;13) translocation 111
t(8;14) translocation 121, 122
t(8;21) translocation 71–2
t(9;14) translocation 124
t(11;14) translocation 123
t(11;14)(q13;q32) translocation 68, 70
t(11;18)(q21;q21) translocation 124
t(12;21) translocation 71
t(14;18) translocation 68, 69, 70, 122
follicular lymphoma 123, *124*, Plate 10.2
t(14;18)(q32;q21) translocation Plate 10.2
t(15;17) translocation 71
TaqMan real-time PCR 66, 270
TATA box 364, 393
T-cell receptors (TCR) 65–6, 288–9, 291, 393
combinatorial association 65
genetic immunotherapy 330–1
signaling 291
tumor-associated antigens 330
*see also* TCR genes

MONKLANDS HOSPITAL
LIBRARY
MONKSCOURT AVENUE
AIRDRIE ML60JS
☎01236712005